HANDBOOK OF MIGRATION AND HEALTH

Handbook of Migration and Health

Edited by

Felicity Thomas

University of Exeter, UK

Edward Elgar PUBLISHING

Cheltenham, UK • Northampton, MA, USA

Published by
Edward Elgar Publishing Limited
The Lypiatts
15 Lansdown Road
Cheltenham
Glos GL50 2JA
UK

Edward Elgar Publishing, Inc.
William Pratt House
9 Dewey Court
Northampton
Massachusetts 01060
USA

A catalogue record for this book
is available from the British Library

Library of Congress Control Number: 2016944287

This book is available electronically in the **Elgar**online
Social and Political Science subject collection
DOI 10.4337/9781784714789

MIX
Paper from responsible sources
FSC® C013056

ISBN 978 1 78471 477 2 (cased)
ISBN 978 1 78471 478 9 (eBook)

Typeset by Servis Filmsetting Ltd, Stockport, Cheshire

Printed and bound in Great Britain by TJ International Ltd, Padstow, Cornwall

Contents

PART IV VULNERABILITY AND PRECARITY

PART V SPECIFIC HEALTHCARE NEEDS AND PRIORITIES

PART VI HEALTHCARE PROVISION

PART VII TRANSNATIONAL AND DIASPORIC NETWORKS

Figures

Boxes

Contributors

Sabrina Bacci is an expert in vaccine preventable disease at the European Centre for Disease Prevention and Control.

Loretta Baldassar is discipline chair of anthropology and sociology at the University of Western Australia and Adjunct Research Fellow at Monash University. Loretta has published extensively on transnational migration, caregiving and settlement. Her most recent books include, *Chinese Migration to Europe* (with Johanson, McAuliffe and Bressan, Palgrave, 2015); *Transnational Families, Migration and the Circulation of Care: Understanding Mobility and Absence in Family Life* (with Merla, Routledge, 2014); *Conflicting Identities: Refugee Protection and the Role of Law* (with Kneebone and Stevens, Routledge, 2014). Loretta is a board member of the ISA Migration Research Committee and a regional editor for the journal Global Networks.

Cyril Bennouna is a senior research associate at the CPC Learning Network and also at the Center on Child Protection (PUSKAPA) at the University of Indonesia. He has a Masters of Public Health from Columbia with a focus on humanitarian assistance, and currently lives in Jakarta, Indonesia.

Jessica R. Botfield is a senior research officer at Family Planning NSW, focusing on sexual and reproductive health programmes and qualitative research in Australia and the Indo-Pacific region. Prior to this she worked as a research associate with the Health, Rights and Development team (@HEARDatUNSW) at the School of Social Sciences, UNSW Australia, with a focus on global health and development research. She is also a registered nurse with experience in sexual and reproductive healthcare.

Elaine Chase is a senior lecturer in education, health promotion and international development at University College London Institute of Education. Her research broadly focuses on the sociological dimensions of wellbeing and rights of individuals and communities, particularly those most likely to experience disadvantage and marginalization.

Jennifer Cook is a cultural anthropologist engaged in applied and scholarly work focusing on US–Mexico migration, transnational migrant communities, il/legality, and agricultural labour. She is the founder and coordinator of a volunteer-based program which provides English language education to Spanish-speaking farmworkers in the state of Connecticut. Jennifer has a Master of Arts in International Studics, and is currently enrolled as a PhD student in the Department of Anthropology at the University of Connecticut.

Erika Duffell is an expert in viral hepatitis at the European Centre for Disease Prevention and Control.

Dr Ruth Evans is an associate professor in human geography, University of Reading. Her research focuses on caring relations in families affected by HIV and bereavement, and gendered and generational inequalities in access to land and other resources. Her publications include a co-authored book with Saul Becker, *Children Caring for Parents with HIV/AIDS: Global Issues and Policy Responses* (Policy Press, 2009) and articles on young caregiving, HIV and mobilities in African migrant families (*Population, Space and Place*, 2011), caring relations in families affected by HIV in East Africa (with Felicity Thomas, *Emotions, Space and Society*, 2009; *Area*, 2011; *Geoforum*, 2012) and an ethics of care in supporting disabled forced migrants (with Gudbjorg Ottosdottir, first author, *British Journal of Social Work*, 2014).

Jasmine Gideon is a senior lecturer in development studies at Birkbeck, University of London. She is the author of *Gender, Globalization and Health in a Latin American Context* (Palgrave Macmillan, 2014) and the editor of *The International Handbook on Gender and Health* (Edward Elgar, 2016). Her current research explores wellbeing among the Latin American community in the UK and the links between health, trans-national justice and exile.

Dr Kelly Hall is a lecturer in social policy at the University of Birmingham. Her broad research interests include migration, ageing, health/social care and the third sector. Her research into international retirement migration focuses on the migration and return of vulnerable, older British people within the EU. This includes her PhD (in collaboration with Age UK and Age Concern España), which explored the lived experiences of older British people in Spain and their access to informal and formal care and support.

Dr Anne-Cécile Hoyez has been a research fellow with the CNRS (Centre National de la Recherche Scientifique/National Center for Scientific Research) since 2008. A geographer specializing in health, she mainly works on the health practices of immigrant populations in France. She is the author or co-author in French and English of many works on these issues. She hosts an international network of social science and public health researchers and has initiated several research projects on migration in France.

David Ingleby is Emeritus Professor of intercultural psychology at Utrecht University and a researcher in the Centre for Social Science and Global Health, University of Amsterdam.

Hiranthi Jayaweera was a senior researcher, Centre on Migration, Policy and Society (COMPAS) in the University of Oxford from 2005 to 2015, and is currently a research associate at the School of Anthropology in the University of Oxford. She has a particular research interest in issues around global migration and health, and the integration of migrants, particularly in the UK, and has undertaken quantitative and qualitative research in both areas. Hiranthi has a DPhil in sociology and has researched, taught and written about issues related to social divisions, particularly gender and ethnic divisions in the UK. Before working at COMPAS she was a researcher at the National Perinatal Epidemiology Unit (NPEU) in the University of Oxford.

Marry-Anne Karlsen is a senior researcher at Uni Research Rokkan Centre and affiliated with the International Migration and Ethnic Relations (IMER) research unit at the University of Bergen. With a background in social anthropology and geography, her research focuses on the intersection between migration control and welfare policy and the encounter between migrants and service providers.

Majella Kilkey is reader in social policy, University of Sheffield, where she is co-director of the Migration Research Group. She researches at the intersection of migration and family studies. Recent publications include *Family Life in an Age of Migration and Mobility: Global Perspectives through the Life Course* (edited with Palenga-Mollenbeck, Palgrave) and *Gender, Migration and Domestic Work: Masculinities, Male Labour and Fathering in the UK and USA* (with Diane Perrons, Ania Plomien, Pierrette Hondagneu-Sotelo and Hernan Ramirez, Palgrave). She is editor of the journal *Social Policy and Society* (Cambridge University Press).

Ronald Labonté, PhD, holds a Tier 1 Canada Research Chair in globalization and health equity and is professor in the Faculty of Medicine, University of Ottawa. His earlier work focused on health promotion, community development, community empowerment and social determinants of health, building on his 15 years' experience with provincial, municipal and federal public health departments. For the past 25 years he has led research and scholarship on the health equity impacts of contemporary globalization. Present research interests include health equity impacts of health worker migration; medical tourism; comprehensive primary healthcare reforms; global health diplomacy; globalization, trade and tobacco control; austerity and health; and trade and food security. He has published more than 230 scientific papers and several hundred popular articles, books and book chapters.

Yao Lu is associate professor of sociology at Columbia University. Her research focuses on the causes and consequences of migration and immigration for different segments of population in sending and receiving societies. She has conducted studies based on data from diverse settings, including China, Indonesia, Mexico, South Africa, Canada and the United States.

Lenore Manderson is concurrently professor of public health and medical anthropology, School of Public Health, University of the Witwatersrand, Johannesburg, South Africa, and professor of anthropology at the Institute at Brown for Environment and Society, Brown University, Providence, RI, USA. Her research interests include both infectious and chronic diseases, gender and sexuality, the health of Indigenous and immigrant women, and inequality and access to care. Her research interests include both infectious and chronic diseases, gender and sexuality, the health of Indigenous and immigrant women, and inequality and access to care, and she has published extensively on these topics. Her most recent work includes, with Elizabeth Cartwright and Anita Hardon, *The Routledge Handbook of Medical Anthropology* (2016). She has been editor of the international journal *Medical Anthropology* since 2010.

Stephanie Mayell is a doctoral student in the Anthropology Department at the University of Toronto in Canada. Her research explores the mental health experiences of Jamaican migrant agricultural workers and their family members. Stephanie has also been active as a volunteer facilitating migrant workers' access to healthcare and other services.

Martin McKee is professor of European public health at the London School of Hygiene and Tropical Medicine and the European Observatory on Health Systems and Policies.

Janet McLaughlin is an assistant professor of health studies and a research associate with the International Migration Research Centre, at Wilfrid Laurier University in Ontario, Canada. For more than a decade, her research has focused on health issues among migrant agricultural workers in Canada. She is also co-founder of the Migrant Worker Health Project (www.migrantworkerhealth.ca), which aims to improve healthcare access for migrant workers.

Dr Celia McMichael is a lecturer in health geography at the University of Melbourne, Australia. She conducted her doctoral research in the area of refugee resettlement and psychosocial wellbeing. Her current research focuses on medical anthropology, forced migration, international health and climate change-related population displacement. She has conducted both fieldwork and applied development work in Peru, Angola, Indigenous Australia, Sri Lanka, Nepal and Fiji.

Laura Merla is professor of sociology at the Catholic University of Louvain (Belgium), where she is director of the Interdisciplinary Research Center on Families and Sexualities (CIRFASE). She is also Honorary Research Fellow at the University of Western Australia. Her main research areas are the sociology of the family, migration and social policies. Her research has been funded by two Marie Curie fellowships. She recently won an ERC Starting Grant. In 2014 Laura Merla published two edited volumes: *Transnational Families, Migration and the Circulation of Care: Understanding Mobility and Absence in Family Life*, published by Routledge (in collaboration with Loretta Baldassar); and *Distances et Liens*, published by Academia-L'Harmattan (in collaboration with Aurore François).

Sarah Meyer is an assistant professor of clinical population and family health at Columbia University's Mailman School of Public Health. She has led qualitative and quantitative research methods training and data collection in Cambodia, Rwanda, Uganda and Thailand, focusing on migration, child protection and mental health in humanitarian and low-income settings. She is currently the co-investigator on a joint study between the CPC Learning Network and UNHCR on measuring child protection in refugee settings. She has also published a review of the UNHCR's mental health and psychosocial support [MHPSS] activities, and led a review of the IASC MHPSS Guidelines.

Philipa Mladovsky is assistant professor in international development at LSE.

Christy E. Newman is an associate professor at the Centre for Social Research in Health, in UNSW Australia Arts and Social Sciences. With a background in health sociology and cultural studies, Christy has broad interests in expert and lived accounts, as well as social representations, of medicine 'at the margins'. Her research explores five distinctive but interesting domains: appreciating lived experiences of infectious disease; strengthening health workforce capacity to care for disadvantaged communities; enhancing wellbeing in the context of sexual diversity; understanding the place of sexual health in young adults' lives; and analysing representations of health, illness and medicine.

Louise Newman is the director of the Centre for Women's Mental Health at the Royal Women's Hospital and Professor of Psychiatry, University of Melbourne. She is a practising infant psychiatrist. Her research interests include the areas of infant mental health, attachment disorders trauma and prevention of child abuse and the impact of immigration detention on child asylum seekers. She is the convenor of the Alliance of Health Professions for Asylum Seekers and vice-president of Doctors for Refugees. She has been a government advisor on asylum seeker and refugee mental health and contributed to the development of policy for mental health screening and response to torture survivors.

Teymur Noori is an expert in HIV at the European Centre for Disease Prevention and Control.

Lorena Núñez Carrasco is a medical anthropologist and obtained her PhD from Leiden University in 2008. She is an associate professor in health sociology at the Department of Sociology, University of the Witwatersrand. Lorena has researched on the linkages between migration, livelihoods and HIV/AIDS and, more recently, on experiences of faith healing among African Independent and Pentecostal churches. In her work she explores urban diversity through the lens of religious practices. She also researches and writes on the topics of death, funeral, burials and end-of-life care among cross-border migrants.

Anna Odone is a medical doctor and PhD candidate in the Department of Clinical and Experimental Medicine, University of Parma.

Dina Oksen is an epidemiologist and project manager at the French National Institute for Health and Medical Research (INSERM).

Dr Siân Oram is lecturer in Women's Mental Health at the Institute of Psychiatry, Psychology & Neuroscience, King's College London. She holds a PhD from the London School of Hygiene and Tropical Medicine for research exploring the public policy response to the health needs of trafficked people. Her recent research concerns the health outcomes associated with human trafficking and other forms of violence, and related health services and policy responses.

Meghann Ormond is assistant professor in cultural geography at Wageningen University in the Netherlands. A human geographer, her research is mainly focused on the intersections of transnational mobility, health and care. She is the author of *Neoliberal Governance and International Medical Travel in Malaysia* (Routledge, 2013) and numerous journal articles and book chapters on 'medical tourism', migrant health, cross-border and intra-regional healthcare developments, personalized medicine and international retirement migration. Her work has appeared in such journals as *Social Science and Medicine*, *Health and Place*, *Globalization and Health*, *Maturitas* and *Mobilities*.

Gudbjorg Ottosdottir is an assistant professor, Faculty of Social Work, School of Social Sciences, University of Iceland where she has worked since 2013. Previously, Gudbjorg was a social worker in Iceland, working with migrants and refugees. She completed her PhD in human geography in 2015 at the University of Reading. Her research focused on the experiences of asylum seekers and refugees with disabilities and those caring for them in the south-east of England. Her main research interests lies in the area of migration, disability, care and social work. Her publications include 'Ethics of care in supporting disabled forced migrants: interactions with professionals and ethical dilemmas in health and social care in the south-east of England' (with Ruth Evans, *British Journal of Social Work*, 2014) and 'Disabled asylum seekers and refugees and access to social care in South-East England' (*Icelandic Journal of Social Work*, 2016).

Corinne Packer holds a PhD in international law from Utrecht University, the Netherlands. She is a senior research associate at the University of Ottawa in Canada. She has collaborated on a number of scholarly compilations, journals and conferences on health worker migration and medical tourism. She is co-editor of a book on globalization and health, and an upcoming volume on case studies of comprehensive primary healthcare.

Anastasia Pharris is an expert in HIV at the European Centre for Disease Prevention and Control.

Oliver Razum, Dr med, MSc epidemiology, is full professor and dean of the School of Public Health, Bielefeld University, Germany; he also heads the Department of Epidemiology & International Public Health. His main research field is social epidemiology, with a particular focus on the health of immigrants and on the role of contextual factors in the production of health inequalities. Before moving into epidemiology, Oliver worked as district medical officer in Zimbabwe.

Bernd Rechel is a researcher at the European Observatory on Health Systems and Policies and honorary senior lecturer at the London School of Hygiene and Tropical Medicine.

Anna Reeske is a health scientist with a PhD in public health. Her scientific interest lies within the field of migration and health with a particular focus on health inequalities during pregnancy and early life. She is currently employed at the Federal Institute for Occupational Safety and Health (BAuA), working on mental health and immigrants' psychosocial work conditions.

Alison Reid is an associate professor at the School of Public Health, Curtin University, Western Australia. She has a background in anthropology and demography and is an occupational epidemiologist with a specific interest in the occupational causes of disease and risks among subgroups of the population. Specifically she is interested in the working conditions and hazard risks of migrant workers. She has examined whether the incidence of fatal and non-fatal work-related accidents and injuries differed among foreign and Australian-born workers, and whether exposure to workplace carcinogens differs by ethnicity, country of birth or language spoken. Her other area of interest is low-dose asbestos exposure and asbestos-related diseases and she has studied these among women and children exposed to blue asbestos at Wittenoom, Western Australia.

Vivien Runnels, PhD, is a researcher with the Globalization and Health Equity Research Unit, Faculty of Medicine at the University of Ottawa in Canada. Her work includes studies on global health diplomacy, medical tourism, health worker migration from the perspectives of source and destination countries and, more recently, research on the international privatization of healthcare. She is also involved in research and programme evaluation of social and health interventions with marginalized populations.

Andreas Sandgren was employed as an expert in tuberculosis at the European Centre for Disease Prevention and Control at the time of this work. Currently he is an independent consultant.

Rebecca Shadwick was employed as a research associate at LSE Health at the time of this research and is now a global inequality campaign coordinator at Oxfam International.

Daniela Sime is reader in education and social policy, University of Strathclyde. Her research interests are in the areas of social justice and inequalities, with a focus on migration, education, poverty and marginalized groups, as well as children and young people's participation in society. She is currently principal investigator on an ESRC-funded study entitled *Here to Stay? Identity, Belonging and Citizenship among Eastern European Settled Migrant Children (A Decade After the EU Enlargement).*

Jacob Spallek, Dr PH, MSc epidemiology, epidemiologist and public health researcher, is full professor at the Department of Public Health at the Brandenburg University of Technology Cottbus-Senftenberg, Germany. Jacob has expertise in both social epidemiology and migrant health. He is also principal investigator of the migrant birth cohort BaBi-Study in Bielefeld, Germany.

Dr Denise L. Spitzer is a medical anthropologist and professor with the Institute of Feminist and Gender Studies at the University of Ottawa (Canada) where from 2005 to 2015, she was the Canada Research Chair in Gender, Migration, and Health and a principal scientist affiliated with the Institute of Population Health. Professor Spitzer examines how global processes – intersecting with gender, racialization, migration status and other social identifiers – are implicated in health and wellbeing and has published in journals such as *Sociology*, *Gender & Society*, *Medical Anthropology Quarterly* and *the Canadian Journal of Public Health*, among others. Her edited collection, *Engendering Migrant Health: Canadian Perspectives*, was published by the University of Toronto Press in 2011 and was recognized by the Women's and Gender Studies Association in 2013 with a WGSRF Outstanding Scholarship citation.

Lindsay Stark is an associate professor in the Program on Forced Migration and Health at Columbia University's Mailman School of Public Health. She has more than a decade of experience leading applied research on protection of women and children in humanitarian settings, and is the author of multiple publications on the rehabilitation and resiliency of former child soldiers and survivors of sexual violence. Lindsay serves as the executive director of the Child Protection in Crisis (CPC) Learning Network, a consortium of agencies and academic institutions that work together on global learning associated with children in disaster and war settings.

Jonathan E. Suk is an expert in emerging threats and preparedness at the ECDC and holds an honorary lectureship with the Global Public Health Unit, University of Edinburgh.

Dr Felicity Thomas is a senior research fellow at the University of Exeter. With a background in medical anthropology and geography, her work focuses on health inequalities, particularly in relation to migrants and to low-income communities. Other research interests include the medicalization of mental distress, sexual health and HIV, environmental injustice and the promotion of healthy schools.

Alice Tianbo Zhang is a PhD candidate in Sustainable Development at Columbia University. Her doctoral research seeks to improve the understanding of how large-scale natural and social processes affect human welfare. Her current research projects include studies on the environmental justice impacts of the Superfund programme, forced migration and labour market outcomes, and causes and consequences of education inequality. She is also collaborating with an interdisciplinary team of researchers on a global assessment of climate change impacts.

Taavi Tillmann is a medical doctor and PhD candidate in the Faculty of Population Health Sciences, University College London.

Dr Katherine Vasey is a medical anthropologist currently affiliated with the University of Melbourne, Australian Catholic University, Monash University and Brown University. She was formally a research fellow in the School of Social Sciences, Faculty of Arts, Monash University, where she conducted research into refugee wellbeing and resettlement, immigrant and parenting with Iraqi families and the emotional experiences of early parenthood with diverse migrant groups. Her research interests include the health and wellbeing of Indigenous and immigrant women, and inequality and access to care, especially borderless healthcare. She is also interested in new technologies and human-centred design.

Jo Vearey holds a PhD in public health and is an associate professor with the African Centre for Migration & Society, University of the Witwatersrand and holds a Senior Fellowship with the Center for Peace, Democracy and Development, McCormack Graduate School of Policy and Global Studies, University of Massachusetts, Boston. Jo's research focuses on migration and health in southern Africa; she has published widely and is involved in a range of international partnerships including with the VU University, Amsterdam; University of Edinburgh; and the London School of Hygiene and Tropical Medicine.

Raelene Wilding is a sociologist at La Trobe University, where she is deputy director of the Transforming Human Societies Research Focus Area and leads the Mobilities and Migration (Ancient and Current) Research Cluster. Her research examines the transnational relationships of migrants and refugees in Australia, with a particular focus on the role of communication technologies in exchanging care and support. Her recently completed Australian Research Council (ARC)-funded project examined the role of communication technologies in the transnational settlement experiences of refugee youth. She is now commencing a new ARC-funded project on the transnational care and support experiences of older Australians. Her work is published in a range of journals, including *Journal of Refugee Studies*, *Global Networks*, *Continuum*, *Journal of Ethnic and Migration Studies* and *Journal of Family Studies*.

Sarah S. Willen, PhD, MPH is assistant professor of anthropology at the University of Connecticut, where she is also director of the Research Program on Global Health and Human Rights at the university's Human Rights Institute. A medical and sociocultural anthropologist, she has authored more than 25 articles and book chapters and edited or co-edited seven volumes, including the books *Transnational Migration to Israel in Global Comparative Context* (Lexington, 2007), *Shattering Culture: American Medicine Responds to Cultural Diversity* (Russell Sage, 2011), and *A Reader in Medical Anthropology: Theoretical Trajectories, Emergent Realities* (Wiley-Blackwell, 2010), as well as special issues of *Culture, Medicine, and Psychiatry* (2013), *Social Science & Medicine* (2012), *Ethos* (2012), and *International Migration* (2007). Her monograph *Indignity and Indignation: Migrants' Lives on Israel's Margins*, is forthcoming from the University of Pennsylvania Press.

Gemma A. Williams is a PhD candidate in health economics at the Department of Social Policy, LSE, and a global health researcher within LSE Health.

Hajo Zeeb is an epidemiologist at the University of Bremen (Germany) and the Leibniz Institute for Prevention Research and Epidemiology-BIPS where he heads the Department of Prevention and Evaluation. Studies on migrant health in the broader context of diversity and its association with health is one of his main research areas.

Anthony B. Zwi is professor of global health and development at UNSW Australia. He is particularly interested in global health and development policy and their interface with equity, social justice and human rights. He seeks to promote mechanisms to facilitate evidence-informed health and development policy. Anthony and colleagues have worked on the ethics of research in conflict-affected settings, and the role of service providers and community members, including young people, in shaping and influencing responses to conflict and disasters. Anthony convenes a research and advocacy group focused on Health, Rights and Development (@HEARDatUNSW).

Acknowledgements

Thanks are due to Victoria Chow, and to Malcolm Baylis, Alex O'Connell and Sarah Brown of Edward Elgar Publishing for their support in the production of the book. Thanks are also due to the authors and publishers who gave permission to reprint various figures in some of the chapters in this book:

- Figure 3.2, Jacob Spallek, Hajo Zeeb and Oliver Razum, 'Life course epidemiology: a conceptual model for the study of migration and health', in *Migration and Health: A Research Methods Handbook* by Marc B. Schenker, Xochitl Castaneda and Alfonso Rodriguez-Lainz © 2014 by the Regents of the University of California. Published by the University of California Press.
- Figures 13.1 and 13.2 from *Population Facts: The Number of International Migrants Worldwide Reaches 232 Million*, by the Department of Economic and Social Affairs, © 2013 United Nations. Reprinted with the permission of the United Nations.
- Figure 20.1 is reprinted with the permission of the Inter-Agency Standing Committee (IASC), UN.

PART I

INTRODUCTION

1 Migration and health: an introduction

Felicity Thomas

Migration is now firmly embedded as a leading global policy issue of the twenty-first century. In 2015, an estimated 244 million people were international migrants, an increase of 71 million since the year 2000 (UNDESA 2015). A further 740 million are estimated to migrate within their own country (IOM 2015). Many millions more people, while not themselves moving, are directly affected by migration, both as social networks extend within and across national borders, and as labour markets and service provision become increasingly entangled within the wider global political economy.

Migration therefore plays an integral role within the lives of a sizeable portion of today's global population. While not a new phenomenon, it has altered significantly in recent decades, with changing demographics, geopolitics, conflict, climate change and patterns of global development shaping new types of migration. Such movement involves an increasingly diverse group of people, as well as shifting countries of origin, transit and destination in what is often a complex, multi-staged and, at times, lengthy process.

Alongside such changes, migration is increasingly recognised as an important social determinant of health and wellbeing (Davies et al. 2010; Castañeda et al. 2015). Most governments recognise health as an essential human right, and many have signed up to a range of rights-based conventions and legal instruments to help ensure that certain groups of migrants have comparable rights to citizens. Yet despite such developments, the global policy arena on migrant health remains largely uncoordinated and inconsistent, with major inconsistencies between migration and health-related policy and practical need. Where polices do exist, they often operate in isolation at national level and cover only partial, disjointed and often overly simplistic snapshots of people's lives, experiences and priorities (Zimmerman et al. 2011).

At the same time, there is an ongoing tendency for migration to be considered and responded to as a 'new' phenomenon, rather than as an embedded characteristic of many communities and countries. Indeed, in a context in which population movement is increasingly politicised and security-focused, and as the current era of global economic austerity plays out, there is an amplified tendency for policymakers and sectors of the popular media to view and react to many types of migrants as both a public health and a security 'threat' to be monitored, controlled and contained. Perhaps nowhere has this been more blatant in recent times than in the context of the current European migrant crisis, where political rhetoric, increasingly protectionist policies and (in)action have combined with very real and all too often adverse consequences for the health and lives of those involved.

Largely in response to concerns regarding migrant welfare, recent decades have seen a considerable literature emerging across a range of academic disciplines, including public health, development studies, anthropology, geography and law, which stress the importance of understanding how best to conceptualise and respond practically to ensure the health-related rights and entitlements of migrants (Thomas and Gideon 2013; Ingleby et al. 2012). Such work recognises that while migration itself is not necessarily risk-laden, weak and uncoordinated policy and hostile receptivity can leave many migrants facing vulnerabilities, such as poor living and working conditions, social and cultural isolation, and discrimination. It also highlights the importance of considering the subjective perceptions and experiences, and the health and wellbeing-related priorities of migrants themselves, and using this information to deliver culturally competent forms of healthcare (MacFarlane et al. 2014). Such approaches not only draw attention to the agency of migrants, but also recognise the need for academic debate and practical and policy responses that more clearly differentiate between forms of migration and the diverse social groups involved within this. Importantly, there is also growing recognition of the need for attention to be placed on the more positive benefits that migration and migrants themselves can bring, not only for the individuals concerned, but for their social networks and the wider societies in which they are located (Aggleton et al. 2014).

It is against this evolving, yet politically charged backdrop that this *Handbook* has been developed, to offer in one location an authoritative overview of key debates that underpin and progress understandings of migration and health in a contemporary global context. Bringing together the contributions of 58 leading researchers, the *Handbook* is intended as a scholarly, yet accessible reference tool for researchers, students and practitioners. In addition to providing insightful knowledge, theoretical reflection and empirical evidence relating to a diversity of carefully selected topics, the chapters offer a wealth of disciplinary perspectives, presenting critical insights into a diversity of approaches to understanding migration and health across a wide variety of geographical settings and sociocultural contexts.

The book is organised into six further sections: theories and models of migration; rights and deservingness; vulnerability and precarity; specific healthcare needs and priorities; healthcare provision; and transnational and diasporic networks. Each of these sections is underpinned by three common themes. The first theme is concerned with the intersectional nature of migration and health. Such a stance recognises that experiences of migration and health cannot be viewed separately from other intersecting axes of identity such as gender, age, religion, class and country of origin, because people experience the world holistically, with their various social identities interacting on multiple and often simultaneous levels. Importantly, and as a number of the chapters in this volume make clear, recognition of the intersectional nature of migrant experience and the ways this plays out across the life-course enables more critical insight into the processes that create and reinforce indicators of social stratification, and the ways that health-related opportunities as well as injustices and inequalities are enacted on a multidimensional basis.

The second theme is concerned with the broad neoliberal context within which many experiences of migration and health now take place and, in particular, how the 'functional ignorance' (Mladovsky et al. 2012) of those with power to enact positive change can impact directly on lived experience and health and wellbeing outcomes. A number of the chapters in this book demonstrate how, in an era in which border controls are being increasingly tightened for all but those deemed either 'deserving', 'necessary' or 'useful' to help meet wider economic ends, accountability for meeting basic human rights becomes elusive and avoidable. Indeed, as is evidenced in this volume, many immigration-related policies demonstrably contradict individual and public health needs and entitlements, which are in many instances now having to be addressed through more informal, and often less secure routes.

The final cross-cutting theme reiterates the importance of looking beyond host country responses and biomedical frameworks of understanding to consider how diverse sociocultural influences can shape the health and wellbeing-related experiences of migrants and those within wider transnational and diasporic networks. Central within this is a need to move beyond the kind of 'one-size fits all' approach to health and healthcare that problematises cultural difference to recognise how subjective perspectives, priorities and responses feed in to ideas about, and experiences of, health, treatment-seeking and care. The analysis provided within a number of the chapters in this volume demonstrates that while such influences can enhance experiences of health, and provide an important channel of social support, they can also be a source of tension, particularly in situations in which unequal power hierarchies are reinforced.

THEORIES AND MODELS OF MIGRATION

The chapters in Part II of this book examine and seek to extend some of the main theoretical and conceptual paradigms in which migration and health have been examined. A clear theme that emerges from these chapters is the complex ways in which migration and health are linked, and the empirical challenges faced in both quantitative and qualitative analyses as it relates to causal identification of these interconnections.

In Chapter 2, Yao Lu and Alice Tianbo Zhang draw on evidence from across the globe to examine three major mechanisms that underlie the relationship between migration and health. This involves examination of the ways that different individuals are selected into migration by health conditions, and the ways that health influences decisions to return; the ways that socioeconomic and psychosocial factors influence migrant experiences of health; and the ways in which migration is linked to the health of people left behind in origin communities. While the evidence presented generally supports the 'healthy migrant hypothesis', the authors call for more rigorous data collection that enables the causal link between migration and health to be more definitively unpacked.

Commonly used explanatory models of migration and health are examined in Chapter 3. Here, Jacob Spallek, Anna Reeske, Hajo Zeeb and Oliver Razum critique the healthy migrant hypothesis and the model of migration as health transition that have commonly been used within the migration field. Instead, they argue for the benefits of a life-course approach that incorporates the temporal dimension of health. Using examples from Germany, they demonstrate how a life-course approach enables consideration of health-related exposures in critical periods of the life-course as well as risk accumulation over time. Such an approach, they argue, permits much-needed understanding that moves beyond snapshot assessments of migrant health while also enabling consideration of migrant heterogeneity and the social determinants and processes that combine to influence the outcomes of health inequalities.

This complex interplay is examined further in Chapter 4 in relation to health behaviour. In this discussion, Hiranthi Jayaweera explores how the health outcomes of migrants relate to 'risky' health behaviours. Viewing morbidity, mortality and birth outcome patterns of migrants within a framework that encompasses both sending and receiving country contexts and other social determinants, the chapter identifies some of the weaknesses of the widely used 'acculturation' approaches that often dominate research and commentary on migrant health behaviour. Jayaweera presents a convincing case for moving beyond a simplistic linear focus relating to health behaviour change to formulate interventions that relate more closely to the dynamic contexts and influences shaping the health behaviours and outcomes of migrants.

In common with the other chapters in this section, Chapter 5 challenges overly simplistic generalisations that homogenise the health experiences of all migrants. In this chapter, Denise Spitzer considers how the application of an intersectional lens enables richer understanding of the dynamic interactions between gender, race, socioeconomic class, ethnicity and country of origin. Drawing on examples from across the globe, she demonstrates how gendered and racialised ideologies and discourse can interact to influence the health experiences and outcomes of migrants in the context of neoliberal globalisation and labour force demands.

RIGHTS AND DESERVINGNESS

The chapters in Part III of the book are concerned with examining the ways that rights and entitlements to health are predicated both on wider scale processes of governance and accountability, and on deeply embedded ideas regarding morals, ethics and 'deservingness'. Sarah S. Willen and Jennifer Cook examine the notion of health-related deservingness in considerable depth in Chapter 6, providing valuable insight into the competing array of moral stances that influence whose health, and whose lives matter – and whose do not. Drawing on examples from the US, Europe and the Middle East, the authors outline an analytical framework for examining the roles played by the array of *stakeholders* involved in deciding deservingness (e.g., policymakers, media, advocacy groups, citizens, migrants), the *contexts* in which such debates take place and the *evaluative criteria* employed. Underpinning these themes is a call for greater understanding of the ways that vernacular and often implicit ways of reckoning deservingness influence discourse, policy and practice, with very real impacts on the bodies, lives and life chances of migrants and the communities in which they live.

Notions of governance and accountability underpin Chapter 7, where Vivien Runnels, Corinne Packer and Ronald Labonté explore the complex and competing web of rights, duties and responsibilities incumbent on health workers, states and the international community to protect the health and wellbeing of citizens. The migration of healthcare workers, they argue, becomes both an ethical and a humans rights issue when skilled personnel move away from countries where healthcare is in short supply, yet is complicated by the coexisting rights of populations in wealthier countries, and the rights of migrant workers who wish to pursue opportunities for themselves and their families by relocating overseas. The authors place particular focus on the feminisation of healthcare labour, and the deskilling that often accompanies this when female migrants move abroad. They end by emphasising the growing trend in many countries towards healthcare privatisation. As they state, it is vital that more attention is given to understanding the implications of such changes – not only for the supply of global healthcare, but also in terms of global ethics and healthcare equity.

In Chapter 8, Marry-Anne Karlsen demonstrates the tensions and ambiguities that exist between a state's obligations to universal rights conventions, and the way that migration and healthcare policy is translated into daily, situated practice on the ground. As she states, children are generally positioned in Western discourse as particularly needing, and deserving of protection. Yet, 'irregular' migrant children are increasingly negatively impacted by the attempts of many countries to manage and control unwanted migration by restricting access to basic welfare. Drawing on research undertaken in Norway, she demonstrates how the state's commitment to protecting migrant children has been undermined by a restrictive immigration policy that obscures responsibility and downplays the controversial nature of official policy. Integral to this is the delegation of often life-changing healthcare decisions to healthcare providers who, Karlsen argues, become reconfigured not only as border guards, but as 'petty sovereigns' who face major ethical and practical dilemmas in their use of the discretionary powers that have been placed upon them.

In the final chapter in this section (Chapter 9), Anne-Cécile Hoyez demonstrates the practical and socio-spatial challenges facing many migrants as they seek to access basic resources in their day-to-day lives, and the additional burdens faced when migrants are undocumented or have longer-term healthcare needs. Drawing on work undertaken in France, she examines how the principles of universalism enshrined within state policy and national rhetoric are simultaneously undermined by government policy while being positively renegotiated by committed and compassionate individuals at the frontline of healthcare provision. At the centre of this is the provision of outreach work to ensure vulnerable migrants are brought into the healthcare system. Whilst the chapter demonstrates the vital role played by dedicated individuals and informal networks, it raises important questions regarding health-related accountability as well as concerns over the sustainability of relying on acts of benevolence to deliver healthcare.

VULNERABILITY AND PRECARITY

It is important to recognise that people migrate for many different reasons, and that not all of those who move are especially vulnerable. However, many groups of migrants face specific inequalities in their everyday lives and in accessing formal healthcare services. The chapters in the fourth section of the book are concerned with understanding more about the groups of migrants that are especially vulnerable to impaired health and wellbeing outcomes, and the kinds of circumstances that result in experiences of precarity. In Chapter 10, Katherine Vasey, Lenore Manderson and Louise Newman provide a wide-ranging overview of the concept of 'survival migration' to highlight the diverse array of challenges facing those forced into migration through persecution, conflict, violence or human rights violations. In this, they emphasise the very real dilemmas and consequences that are created for survival migrants through the imposition of predefined, immigration-related administrative categories, and the securitisation of asylum seeking. The authors provide insight into the health and wellbeing risks and instabilities facing survival migrants across different stages of the migration 'process', including those confronted in transit, in refugee camps, in detention centres and during resettlement. Attention is also given to ways that such experiences are compounded by gender, and the implications this can have for children and young people. This theme is examined in greater depth in Chapter 11, where Elaine Chase outlines the multiplicity of interacting factors that influence young people's wellbeing and vulnerability to adversity as they make the complex shift in status from being an 'unaccompanied minor' to being considered an 'adult' within immigration and social care systems. In so doing, she draws important distinctions between vulnerability, precariousness and precarity for the young people and the ways these issues are played out at different institutional, spatial and temporal scales. While the chapter clearly demonstrates the politically induced nature of precariousness and the extreme circumstances in which physical and psychological loss and harm manifest, it also emphasises how precarity can be a rallying point for resistance among young people caught up in a complex web of immigration-related policy and practice.

In Chapter 12, Siân Oram provides an overview of the health risks faced by trafficked people, and the consequences of this for their physical, sexual, reproductive and psychological wellbeing. As she argues, evidence here is focused mainly around research with women forced into sex work, who have been found to suffer high levels of depression and post-traumatic stress disorder. Oram identifies a number of gaps in knowledge relating to the health needs of women trafficked for other forms of exploitation, as well as the needs of trafficked men and children. While calling for greater attention to be given to research that focuses on improving trafficked people's physical and psychological recovery, Oram urges policymakers, practitioners and academics to also consider what can be learned from best practice relating to survivors of torture and domestic violence.

The next two chapters in this section focus on the health and wellbeing experiences of labour migrants. Labour migrants play a central role in the contemporary global economy, and a number of international instruments have been put in place to recognise and protect their rights. Yet, as these chapters demonstrate, their health considerations remain largely neglected in both policy and practice, and questions relating to responsibility and accountability for migrant health remain vague. In Chapter 13, Stephanie Mayell and Janet McLaughlin provide an insightful overview of contemporary transnational labour migration, and the health vulnerabilities faced by migrants at each stage of the migratory process. Drawing on extensive primary research with migrants from Mexico and the Caribbean who labour in the Canadian agricultural sector, the authors illustrate the structural vulnerabilities and poor health outcomes that accrue from cumulative exposure to risk. This theme is explored further in Chapter 14, where Alison Reid compares the occupational health and safety of migrant workers to those of native-born populations. In this, she examines the different scales at which work-related risk is played out, from national policy through to workplace practice and the attributes of individual workers themselves. Focusing on the tendency of young, unskilled migrants to undertake precarious and often poorly regulated work involving high rates of exposure to a range of occupational hazards, workplace injustices and work-related accidents and injuries, Reid provides a compelling case for strengthening and enforcing legislation to protect migrant workers.

In the final chapter in this section (Chapter 15) Celia McMichael examines the complex role of climate change in shaping human migration, and discusses the implications of this for human health and wellbeing. As she demonstrates, climate-related migration presents both opportunities and threats for migrant health, as well as for host and home communities. Drawing on case studies from the Northwest Arctic region, Morocco, Sri Lanka and the South Pacific, McMichael provides informative insight into climate-related risks, vulnerabilities and opportunities at different stages of the migration process. She concludes by calling for nuanced and improved policymaking that builds resilience to climate change in home communities, more effective governance and management that protects the rights and wellbeing of migrants, expanded development assistance and funding mechanisms, and institutional change that effectively responds to the health needs of affected communities.

SPECIFIC HEALTHCARE NEEDS AND PRIORITIES

The chapters in the fifth section of the book provide insight into the experiences, needs and priorities of migrants living with particular healthcare requirements, and the conceptual debates that underpin policy and programmatic responses to this. In Chapter 16, Gudbjorg Ottosdottir and Ruth Evans discuss a neglected area within the migration literature, namely the healthcare situation facing migrants with disabilities and/or chronic illness. Here, they provide insight into key conceptual understandings of disabilities and chronic illness, and critique the policy context within which this is framed in relation to migration. Demonstrating the value of social, rather than purely medical approaches to understanding health and wellbeing, the authors provide in-depth insight into the complex linkages between migration, disability, chronic illness and care support. Using empirical data from the UK, they reveal the major barriers to accessing appropriate health, social care and welfare experienced by asylum seekers and the impact of this on the wellbeing of informal family carers such as children and young people.

Another relatively neglected issue within the field of migration relates to the mental health experiences and needs of migrants. What work has been done has tended to apply Western biomedical models of post-traumatic stress disorder and depression to quantify and categorise migrant experience, with little discussion around subjective conceptualisations and the way these may be mediated by temporal health needs, and factors such as gender, age, race, class and sexuality. These issues are examined in depth in Chapter 17, where Jasmine Gideon discusses the mental health experiences, needs and coping strategies of long-term Chilean exiles in the UK. Placing particular focus on the gendered nature of migrant experience, she argues for greater attention to be given to understanding the complex causes of health complaints and the ongoing sociocultural, economic and political context in which mental health issues are experienced.

In Chapter 18, Jo Vearey draws on research from southern Africa to examine the complex and contested relationship between HIV and migration. As she argues, most programmatic and policy responses to HIV continue to exceptionalise migration, even within contexts where mobility within or across borders is a prevalent norm – and to consider migrants as a problematic, high-risk population. Such responses not only fail to engage with the complexity and heterogeneity of diverse population movements, they also pay little consideration to the broader contextual factors that are likely to be affecting aspects of the management of HIV associated with mobility, including treatment continuity and combination prevention approaches. Vearey concludes by proposing recommendations for action through migration-aware programming to assist in strengthening approaches to HIV.

The final chapter in this section (Chapter 19) explores the burden of infectious diseases in migrant populations in the European Union and the European Economic Area (EU/EEA). As Gemma A. Williams and colleagues argue, understanding the changing epidemiology of infectious diseases in Europe is important, not only given the large-scale population movement currently taking place, but also in terms of the effective planning and delivery of health services. Williams et al. point to available evidence that indicates that migrants in the EU/EEA have a higher burden of some infectious diseases than the native-born population, and a comparatively lower burden of others. Examining HIV, TB, hepatitis B, measles, rubella and Chagas disease, they demonstrate the extent to which different migrant populations are affected by infectious diseases, and how this depends on the disease in question, the country or region of origin, and the country of destination. The chapter concludes with recommendations on how future policy and public health responses in the EU/EEA can be improved to reduce the infectious disease burden in vulnerable migrant groups.

HEALTHCARE PROVISION

Although many migrants struggle to access formal healthcare, particularly when they have crossed an international border, it is important to recognise that many are able to, and do, make use of a range of healthcare services. Part VI of this volume therefore examines the provision of healthcare interventions for different groups of migrants. Particular attention is given to the logistical and resource-based issues this can entail for both migrants and health providers, and the perceived relevance of existing service provision for diverse migrant groups. The first chapter in this section (Chapter 20) examines some of the main health issues faced when refugee camps intended as temporary protection for refugees awaiting more 'durable' solutions become long-term, often multigenerational settlements that require sustained health service provision. Sarah Meyer, Cyril Bennouna and Lindsay Stark explore the realities of trying to implement interventions aimed at meeting healthcare needs in what are often poorly resourced, low-income settings. Discussing a range of health issues including those relating to communicable disease, maternal and reproductive health, child health, nutrition, mental health, HIV and violence and abuse, the authors outline the key risk factors for adverse health outcomes in refugee camps, as well as the effective interventions that have been developed and implemented in such settings.

While many migrants are young, healthy and have limited contact with the health systems of the countries they move to, the situation can be quite different for older people who have frequent and often coexisting health requirements. In Chapter 21, Kelly Hall considers the health and wellbeing issues facing retired people who spend at least some of their time each year living abroad. In this chapter, Hall examines the health and care issues faced by elderly and frail British retirees in Spain. Central within this discussion are the unanticipated differences in healthcare rights and provision across areas of the European region, and the ways that tensions between expectations and reality are underpinned by different cultural understandings of care.

In Chapter 22, Daniela Sime argues the case for incorporating migrant children and young people's participation and 'voice' into healthcare provision. Using research with newly arrived Eastern European migrants in the UK, she demonstrates the key role played by many children and young people in facilitating access to healthcare for family members and the importance of listening to the views and experiences of children and young people as a matter of social justice. The experiences of young people also form a central tenet of Chapter 23, where Jessica Botfield, Anthony Zwi and Christy Newman examine the sexual and reproductive health needs of migrants, refugees and international students in Australia. While the migration backgrounds of these groups differ substantially, all are at potentially heightened risk of poor sexual and reproductive health, and tend to underutilise available health services in these areas. The authors assess the complexities of designing and implementing effective sexual healthcare that engages with and is culturally relevant to the needs of migrant groups. This theme is extended further in the final chapter in this section (Chapter 24), where Felicity Thomas examines the concept of culturally competent healthcare for migrant groups, and assesses what this means in the context of large-scale migration such as that currently witnessed across the European region. Particular attention is given to the need for health practitioners to move beyond biomedical models of understanding, to consider subjective experiences of health and wellbeing and the potential role that cultural mediation can play within this.

TRANSNATIONAL AND DIASPORIC NETWORKS

The final section of this volume focuses on the complex – and to some extent, reciprocal – relationships that influence the health of both migrants and those in their transnational and diasporic networks. Inherent within these chapters is recognition that migrant health and wellbeing is shaped not only by local care and policy regimes, but by the wider, transnational social, cultural and economic systems in which they are situated. In Chapter 25, Loretta Baldassar, Majella Kilkey, Laura Merla and Raelene Wilding explore the notion of transnational families, and examine how feelings of collective welfare and unity impact on wellbeing. In particular, the chapter focuses on the ability of family members to practice caregiving as a key feature of migrant wellbeing, and identifies a range of factors that facilitate or impede this. This includes the role of new communication technologies, the ways that policy mediates families' capabilities to care across distance, the way that the care burden is unevenly distributed within families subject to cultural norms, and the way that policy intersects with the care regimes of the countries and communities within which families and migrants reside. A central theme underlying this chapter is the need for social protection systems to be better adapted to the realities of transnational lives.

In Chapter 26, Meghann Ormond reviews the concept of 'medical tourism' as it relates to migrant health, and examines the role of migrant health workers in the development of medical tourism industries in the Global South. Particular emphasis is placed on understanding the ways that the knowledge accumulated by migrants can feed into local healthcare delivery in countries of origin and, at the same time, respond effectively to the needs and interests of other mobile populations seeking to become involved in these emerging medical tourism industries.

As this volume attests, contemporary literature on migration and health has overwhelmingly, and for good reason, been concerned with enabling and maintaining health and wellbeing. The final chapter in this volume, however (Chapter 27), addresses a vital, but generally overlooked issue – that of end-of-life care and the death of migrants. As Lorena Núñez Carrasco explains, most of what literature does exist in this area is concerned with ensuring formal palliative care and repatriation is conducted with culturally sensitivity. Yet in many parts of the world, and for many migrants, relying on such formal services is not an option, and needs to be understood alongside wider circumstances of inequality and poverty. Using her research with migrants facing death in South Africa, Núñez Carrasco explores the strategies they use to mobilise symbolic, emotional and material resources to try to ensure a 'good' death. Particular attention is given to the role of informal actors such as hospices, churches and bus drivers in providing crucial forms of support to migrants as they seek to avoid a death or burial 'out of place', by returning – or being returned – to their home community. In advocating the need for more compassionate end-of-life care and support for migrants, the author calls for more attention to be given to understanding how responsibility and accountability for migrant health can be more effectively addressed.

In conclusion, the chapters presented in this *Handbook* identify some of the most important concepts and themes that underpin contemporary understandings of migration and health. The detailed case studies and examples used in this volume point clearly to the ways in which these issues are intrinsically caught up with wider political, economic and social processes and how this, in turn, can result in critical inconsistencies between migration and health-related policy, practice and experience on the ground. It is hoped that in bringing together the contributions that make up this *Handbook*, the volume offers a scholarly, yet accessible overview and a timely source of reference for understanding the diverse and evolving field of migration and health.

REFERENCES

Aggleton, P., S.A. Bell, A. Kelly-Hanku (2014), 'Mobile men with money': HIV prevention and the erasure of difference, *Global Public Health*, **9**, 257–270.

Castañeda, H., S. M. Holmes, D. S. Madrigal, M-E. De Trinidad Young, N. Beyeler and J. Quesada (2015), Immigration as a social determinant of health, *Annual Review of Public Health*, **36**, 375–392.

Davies, A. A., A. Basten and C. Frattini (2010), Migration: a social determinant of migrants' health, *Eurohealth*, **16**(1), 10–12.

Ingleby, D., A. Chiaenza and W. Deville (2012), *Inequalities in Health Care for Migrants and Ethnic Minorities*, vol. 2, COST Series on Health and Diversity, Garant: Antwerpen-Apeldoom.

IOM (2015), *World Migration Report 2015, Migrants and Cities: New Partnerships to Manage Mobility*, Geneva: IOM.

MacFarlane, A., M. O'Reilly-de Brun, R. de Brun, C. Dowrick, C. O'Donnell, F. Mair, W. Spiegel, M. van den Muijsenbergh, E. van Weel Baumgarten, C. Lionis, C. Clissmann and the RESTORE consortium (2014), Healthcare for migrants, participatory health research and implementation science – better health policy and practice through inclusion. The RESTORE project, *European Journal of General Practice*, **20**, 148–152.

Mladovsky, P., D. Ingleby and B. Rechel (2012), Good practices in migrant health: the European experience, *Clinical Medicine*, **12**(3), 248–252.

Thomas, F. and J. Gideon (eds.) (2013) *Migration, Health and Inequality*, London: Zed Books.

UNDESA (2015) *Trends in International Migrant Stock: The 2015 Revision*, available online at www.un.org/en/development/desa/population/migration/data/estimates2/estimates15.shtml.

Zimmerman, C., L. Kiss and M. Hossain (2011), Migration and health: a framework for 21st century policy-making, *PLoS Medicine*, **8**(5), e1001034.

PART II

THEORIES AND MODELS OF MIGRATION

2 The link between migration and health

Yao Lu and Alice Tianbo Zhang

INTRODUCTION

The objective of this chapter is to delineate the myriad mechanisms through which two important population processes, migration and health, are interconnected. Fueled by the larger processes of urbanization and globalization, migration, both moving within and across national boundaries, has become an unprecedented phenomenon in the modern world and an integral aspect of life in many countries (Lucas 1997; Massey et al. 1999). Between 2000 and 2010, the world has witnessed an annual increase of 4.6 million international migrants, more than doubling the average 2 million annual increase during the period 1990–2000 (United Nations 2013). Facilitated by the advances in information and technology, individuals and households are able to achieve greater geographical mobility by moving within a country or by emigrating to more developed countries. Internal migration, especially rural-to-urban labor migration, happens at a larger scale than international migration. An estimated 763 million people are internal migrants compared to the 232 million international migrants in 2013; together, one in seven people in the world is a migrant (United Nations, 2013). As some of the world's most populous regions, such as Asia and Africa, undergo rapid urbanization, rural-to-urban migration has become a dominant feature of population movement and resulted in wide-ranging socioeconomic and cultural repercussions.

Three Explanatory Mechanisms

Against this backdrop, the link between migration and health is an important component of the puzzle in understanding the determinants and consequences of such large-scale social phenomenon. We focus on three main underlying mechanisms of this relationship. As depicted in Figure 2.1, individuals may be differentially selected into migration in terms of pre-migration health conditions due to the physical and psychological strains resulting from undertaking the move and settlement. People who successfully migrate and are able to settle at their destination may have superior health prior to migration compared to non-migrants at the origin (1a: healthy migrant bias). Alternatively, migrants may return to the origin in

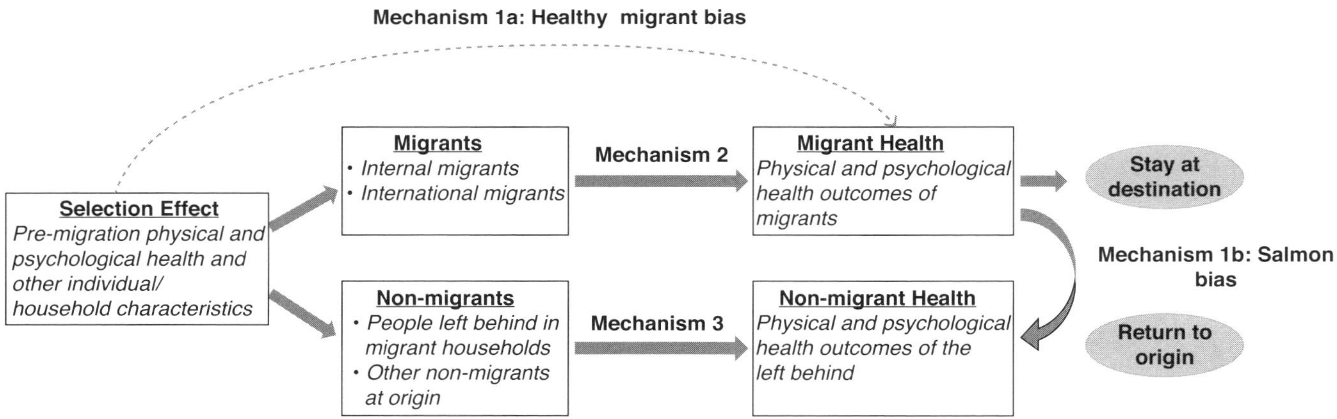

Source: Adapted from Lu (2010a) and Nauman et al. (2015).

Figure 2.1 Interconnections between migration and health through three mechanisms

consideration of health deterioration (1b: salmon bias). The next section of this chapter elaborates on these two selection processes and discusses empirical findings that support or refute these propositions. The main effect of migration on health is portrayed in mechanism 2. The process of migration may affect health directly through changes in the physical environment or indirectly through socioeconomic, psychosocial or behavioral pathways. The third section of this chapter details the possible mediating factors for the health effect of migration and highlights the multifaceted role of migration for different dimensions of health and through different underlying mechanisms. While moving to more developed areas often entails improvements in socioeconomic status and better sanitation, migrants may not experience significant physical or psychological health improvements due to the loss of social support, pressures from work, lack of health utilization and literacy or increased exposure to risk behaviors that may compromise health.

The economic and social benefits and costs associated with the process of migration not only affect the health and economic outcomes of those who move, but they may also have important implications for the physical and psychosocial health of those family members left behind by migrants. Mechanism 3 demonstrates the effect of migration on the left-behind. On the one hand, migrant remittances provide additional sources of income and increase the standard of living of people in left-behind households. On the other hand, as left-behind households face reduced labor supply and a loss of social support resulting from family separation, migration may bring about stress and a deterioration of emotional health for those who stayed behind. The final section of this chapter illustrates these competing factors through which migration can contribute to better or worse health outcomes for the left behind.

HEALTH SELECTION OF MIGRATION AND RETURN MIGRATION

Understanding the health selection effect among migrants offers crucial insights into the underlying mechanisms that give rise to migratory behavior. A primary question of interest is whether people are differentially selected into migration by health conditions and how health facilitates or constrains people's decision to move. This question has intrigued social scientists and epidemiologists alike, leading to claims of an "epidemiological paradox." First coined by Markides and Coreil (1986), the epidemiological paradox refers to the finding that despite having lower education and socioeconomic status, Hispanic immigrants in the United States are generally healthier than the native population, as manifested in longer life expectancy, lower infant mortality rate, fewer chronic conditions and better mental health (Halliday and Kimmitt 2008; Hayward and Heron 1999; Markides and Eschbach 2011; Riosmena and Dennis 2012; Rubalcava et al. 2008; Villa et al. 2012; Farley et al. 2005).

Healthy Migrant Hypothesis

Among the many explanations for this paradox, the most prominent one is the "healthy migrant hypothesis." This hypothesis posits that health selection among the migrant-sending population results in a process of "migration of the fittest," such that only the healthiest and most competent individuals can endure the strenuous emotional, physical, and institutional challenges incurred in the migratory journey and in the subsequent adaptation to the new environment. For example, Kuo and Tsai (1986) suggested that those who chose to migrate not only tended to have better physical and mental health, but were also more capable of enduring the stress of relocation and overcoming the barriers of cultural and social assimilation. Formal health screening in the context of international migration, especially with respect to communicable diseases and risk, may further contribute to the health selection among potential migrants (Chiswick et al. 2008). As a result, migrants tend to be positively selected on the basis of health (Chiswick et al. 2008; Palloni and Morenoff 2001). This positive health selection holds even for migrants from underdeveloped origins with generally high rates of mortality and morbidity (Abraído-Lanza et al. 1999; Markides and Eschbach 2011).

Bilsborrow et al. (1984) and Jasso et al. (2004) nicely summarized the empirical challenges in studying the selection process of migration. The difficulty lies not only in conceptualizing the appropriate comparison group, but also in disentangling the selection effect from possible reverse causality. Most studies on the epidemiological paradox have compared the health status of migrants with that of the native population at destination (Anson 2004; Feranil 2005; Marmot et al. 1983, 1984; Palloni and Morenoff 2001). While these studies serve to inform public health professionals about the health of immigrants in relative terms compared with native-born populations, they often lack credible strategies for identifying the selection effect. This commonly adopted identification strategy essentially confounds two processes: the health selection of migration and the effect of migration on health for migrants.

A more plausible research design for testing the health selection process needs to take into account the health conditions prior to migration and compare people who migrated with those who stayed from the same communities. Timing also plays an important role in the extent to which one can interpret the results as indicating a selection or migration effect. These considerations highlight the shortcomings of previous studies on immigrant health that rely heavily on cross-sectional data with only post-migration health outcomes.

Assisted by the availability of longitudinal data with pre-migration health characteristics, a growing (although still limited) body of research has empirically and directly tested the healthy migrant hypothesis. In theory, one would expect the health selection effect to be larger among international migrants compared to internal migrants, because the former experience greater barriers to migration, more disruption in social networks and are more likely to be subjected to pre-arrival health screening. However, studies do not necessarily support such a hypothesis. Rubalcava et al. (2008), for example, studied the health selection among Mexican immigrants to the US using nationally representative longitudinal data from a sample of the Mexican population over time, some of whom moved to the US between waves of the survey. They generally found weak evidence for the health selection of migrants, and the selection applied only to females and rural males.

Studies based on internal migration have found stronger support for the healthy migrant hypothesis, and reveal that the process is more complex than originally conjectured. Lu (2008) is one of the first such attempts. The paper draws on longitudinal data in the context of internal migration in Indonesia. To investigate whether migrants are healthier than those who stay behind (direct test for the "healthy migrant hypothesis"), the author used logistic regressions of migration status between 1997 and 2000 based on health status and other factors associated with migration status that were measured in 1997 before migration took place. The study examined a wide range of health indicators and separated age groups (prime age adults versus older respondents).

The results highlight important heterogeneity in terms of how health affects the likelihood of migration. The first dimension of heterogeneity lies in the choice of health indicators. While more severe health conditions (i.e., problems with activities of daily living, ADL) significantly affected the likelihood and type of migration, health conditions that were less salient and progress more gradually, such as anemia and hypertension, did not seem to affect migration. Moreover, the direction of health selection varied by the age of migrants. Younger migrants and labor migrants tended to be positively selected on health. In contrast, older adults tended to be negatively selected on health, presumably because they migrated mostly in search of better medical care or relatives who could be caregivers. While migration was often an economic strategy for young people, therefore, it was more likely to reflect a response to health deterioration for older people.

Tong and Piotrowski (2012) adopted a similar strategy and examined the healthy migrant hypothesis in China, using longitudinal data over a decade and contrasting migrants and non-migrants at the origin. They showed that migrants were positively selected on health, especially self-reported health. However, they found that the level of health selection of migration declined over time as migrants became acculturated into the host population.

Salmon Bias Hypothesis

A second explanation for the epidemiological paradox is the "salmon bias hypothesis" or selective return migration. This hypothesis suggests that migrants return to the origin selective on health, in such a way that unhealthy migrants or those who suffer from deteriorating health conditions have a greater tendency to return or move closer to their origin communities than their healthier counterparts (Abraído-Lanza et al. 1999). Migrants facing health problems are less capable of achieving high productivity in destination labor markets, which could lead to reduced earnings and a lower standard of living. These factors, along with constraints in affording and effectively utilizing healthcare services, lack of a supportive network, and various sources of work-related stress in the destination, may in turn render return a more attractive option to migrants (Lu and Qin, 2014).

Direct empirical testing of this hypothesis, however, is even scarcer than that for the healthy migrant hypothesis. This is largely due to the lack of data tracking migrants who returned and those who stayed. Ullmann et al. (2011) compared returned migrants and non-migrants in Mexico while controlling for their early-life health profiles. Their study showed worse health for return migrants than non-migrants in terms of obesity, smoking, and psychological health. Turra and Elo (2008), meanwhile, presented one of the first direct assessments of salmon bias in Hispanic migration to the US, and found very modest evidence for the hypothesis. Their study also called for the use of longitudinal surveys that follow individuals in and out of migrant destinations for a better evaluation of selective return processes. However, the salmon bias hypothesis is not always supported. For example, Sander (2007) examined return migration from Germany to Turkey and suggested that for male migrants, those with poorer health were less likely to return than those with better health.

Lu and Qin (2014) examined the presence and magnitude of both the healthy migrant and salmon bias hypotheses in the context of internal migration in China. The study used a nationally representative longitudinal survey and health measures prior to migration or prior to return. When testing the salmon bias hypothesis, the authors compared the health (at a previous wave) of migrants who remained at destinations with those who by the next wave returned or moved closer to their home villages. They included both a dichotomous measure of migration status and a measure indicating the distance of migration. The results provided clear evidence for a negative health selection of return migration, such that less healthy migrants were more likely to return or move closer to home than healthier migrants. The health selectivity (both in migration and in return) among migrants in China appeared to be stronger than that in other developing countries, or even than international migration, which the authors attributed to specific institutional arrangements in the country that imposed structural and social barriers for migrants to thrive and settle down in cities.

EFFECT OF MIGRATION ON HEALTH OF MIGRANTS

The impact of migration on the health of migrants is multifaceted and can be mediated through various underlying mechanisms, whether via change in socioeconomic conditions and physical environment or via social and emotional support and stressors. A growing body of research has focused on international migration and examined mechanisms that contribute to differential health outcomes between immigrants and the native-born population (Hayward and Heron 1999; Marmot et al. 1984; Singh and Siahpush 2001). Such studies usually find that, despite their socioeconomic disadvantages, immigrants appear healthier than the native population as indicated by various dimensions of health and health behaviors (Marmot et al. 1984; Williams and Collins, 1995). Immigrants' health advantage, however, tends to diminish over the course of acculturation into the host societies (Landale et al. 2000; Abraído-Lanza et al. 2005). Although not all immigrants undergo the same process, this pattern of declining advantage largely results from various socioeconomic and psychosocial processes accompanying migration, including the loss of social support, added work stressors, various legal and social barriers and the detrimental effect of acculturation stress (Bhugra 2004; Takeuchi et al. 2007). The mechanisms through which immigrants initially exhibit a health advantage followed by a health deterioration may also be applicable to internal migration.

Most existing studies on the health outcomes of migration rely on cross-sectional data and are plagued by inadequate research design that does not warrant causal inference. As illustrated in the previous section, one major challenge for identifying the causal effect of migration on health lies in the possible "healthy migrant hypothesis" and the unavailability of health status prior to migration that would allow researchers to take into account baseline health of migrants and their change over time (before and after migration) (Lu 2008; Rubalcava et al. 2008). For instance, if migrants are favorably selected on health, one may conclude that migration has a positive effect on health even when migrants' health conditions remain stable or slightly deteriorate after migration. Additionally, identification hinges on convincingly establishing the appropriate counterfactual and control group. Since the native-born population is likely different from migrants in important unmeasured ways, they are not the proper group for comparison. Rather, the appropriate research design should compare changes in the health of people who migrated with that of people who stayed in the sending communities that share similar background but then undergo different migratory experiences.

Physical Health: Effect and Mechanisms

Investigating physical health and psychological health separately sheds light on the complex mechanisms through which migration affects health. Unfortunately, data limitations mean that there are very few existing studies based on an appropriate research design. Most existing work focuses on the context of internal migration, where it is easier to follow migrants over time. One exception however, is Lu's (2010a) study, which demonstrates that the impact of migration on health is multifaceted and can be mediated through socioeconomic, psychological and behavioral pathways. In terms of the socioeconomic impacts, the study found that moving from rural to urban areas might improve the standard of living of migrants. Urban areas were also found to have higher-quality medical facilities and be equipped with more modern infrastructure, such as electrification, indoor plumbing, and refrigeration (Lu, 2010a). However, improvements in economic status and sanitation may be offset by the inability of migrants to navigate or utilize the complex health system in cities due to limited health literacy (Newbold 2005) or legal residency restrictions (Wong et al. 2007). For example, rural migrant workers in China have limited access to healthcare services and other welfare programs due to restrictions imposed by the *Hukou* system (Wong et al. 2007). Additionally, migrant workers are often involved in informal labor contracts that put them in precarious working conditions and long hours that are detrimental to health (Walsh and Walsh 1987).

Rural migrants may also be more susceptible to infectious and communicable diseases, as their immune systems may not be well adapted to the local natural or built environments and the related pathogens (Apostolopoulos and Sönmez 2007). Rural-to-urban migration also has implications for the sexual behavior of migrants, especially among young adults who are susceptible to the prevailing social and cultural norms at the destination. Research in Thailand and Nigeria, for example, has found that this has resulted in an earlier age of sexual debut (Anglewicz et al. 2014; Mberu and White 2011). In the absence of effective community and parental oversight, young migrants with inadequate knowledge of reproductive health may become especially vulnerable to contracting STIs (Chamratrithirong et al. 2007). A growing body of literature, for example, has highlighted the vulnerabilities of internal migrants to infectious diseases such as HIV (Lurie et al. 2003; Yang and Xia 2006).

Overall, the effect of migration on physical health depends in large part on the competing effects discussed above and summarized in Figure 2.2.

Recent longitudinal studies employing data on pre-migration health and socioeconomic conditions of migrants generally attribute the physical health advantages enjoyed by migrants to the "healthy migration effect" rather than the process of migration itself (Lu 2010a; Nauman et al. 2015). Two prominent studies in this area have been conducted in the context of rural-urban migration in Indonesia and Thailand. Lu (2010a), for example, examined the effect of rural–urban migration in Indonesia on physical and psychological health and explored the various socioeconomic, psychosocial, and behavioral pathways mediating the effect. The study found little effect of migration on short- and medium-term physical health, after taking into account the superior health of migrants before migration. Similarly, Nauman et al. (2015) demonstrated better health of rural migrants in Kanchanaburi, Thailand, which was largely explained by their health advantage before moving to urban areas compared to rural non-migrants from the same region.

Lu (2010a) further probes into the underlying mechanism that may have attributed to the lack of effect on physical health. The results suggest that there are complex and competing mechanisms that may have attenuated the net effect of migration on physical health. While labor migrants earned about 1.3 times as much as rural non-migrants, they also worked 15 hours more per week. This suggests that the improvement in earnings may not translate into better health outcomes due to work-related stressors. In addition, even though migrants were more likely to have insurance coverage, they often failed to adequately utilize preventative healthcare services, largely owing to their low health literacy and unfamiliarity with local health facilities. These work-related stressors coupled with limited

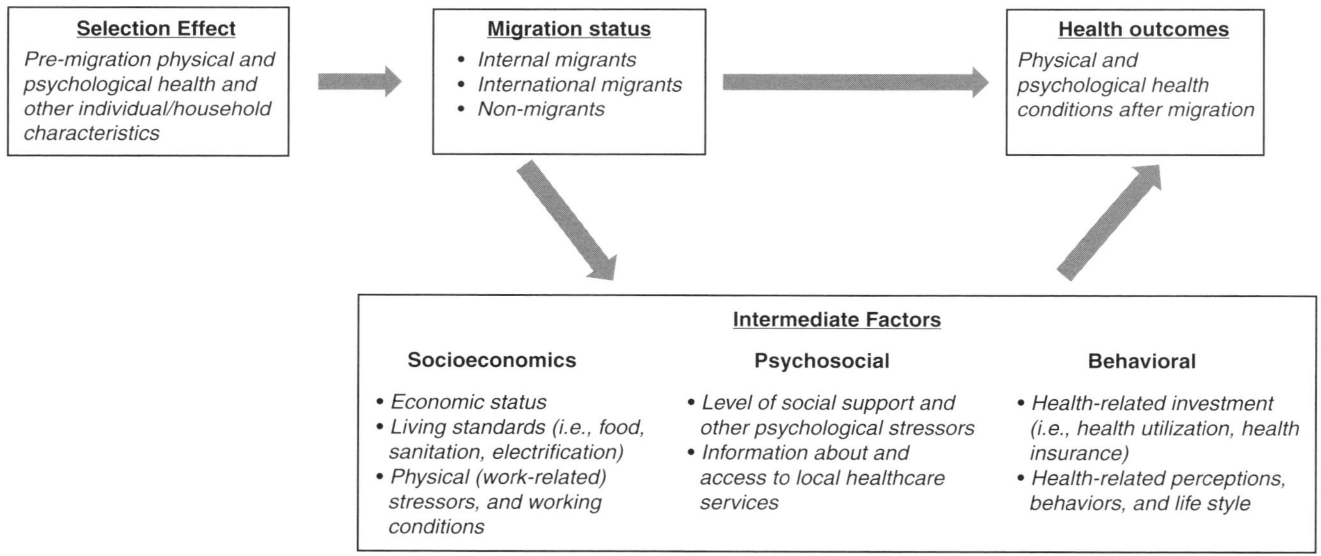

Source: Adapted from Lu (2010a).

Figure 2.2 Post-migration health of migrants as a function of pre-migration health, migration status, and intermediating factors

healthcare utilization were found to undermine the beneficial effect of higher earnings and sanitation on overall physical health status.

An empirically challenging question is the effect of migration on longer-term health. Previous studies using longitudinal data are limited by the short duration between consecutive waves of surveys. While the short time window between surveys reduces sample attrition, it poses several major limitations: it confines the sample size of individuals or households who could possibly migrate within that time frame, restricts the external validity and statistical power of the analysis, and overlooks health effects that take longer to manifest (Nauman et al. 2015). Very little research has attempted to link migration to long-term health outcomes, with one notable exception. Black et al. (2011) examined the extent to which the Great Migration—the relocation of millions of African-Americans from the South to the North, Midwest and West in the United States in the early twentieth century—affected mortality risks later in life. Despite positive selection into migration, they found that migration lowered longevity, although it was not clear what the underlying mechanisms were.

Mental Health and Risk Behaviors: Effect and Mechanisms

Another important dimension of health potentially related to migration is mental health and health-related risk behaviors. While the previous discussion underlines the detrimental impact of migration on psychological health, it is not immediately clear what the underlying stressors and mechanisms are and whether they manifest differently between males and females or across time. Limited work has been done on the mental health consequences of internal migration and the findings are often mixed (Almeida-Filho et al. 1995; Wong et al. 2008). Migration could lead to wide-ranging sources of physical, social, cultural and institutional stressors that may affect the emotional wellbeing of migrants. Despite the potential gains in income, a dire reality facing migrants is the loss of social support as they are uprooted from origin communities and embark on an often solitary journey to the destination. The separation between labor-migrants and their families may cause considerable anxiety. The initial difficulty in establishing a supportive social network may further contribute to the feelings of loss, inadequacy or loneliness and may exacerbate work-related stress (Bhugra 2004). The elevated stress from work coupled with the pressure to assimilate to the host population culturally and socially put migrants at a higher risk of emotional strain. As migrants become detached from their close social circles and other accountability systems in their places of origin, they may engage in riskier behavior and become more prone to external influences that are adverse to health (Shuval 2001).

Unfavorable institutional arrangements and unfamiliar social orders pose formidable challenges for migrants to quickly assimilate to the local population. Although the destinations are likely equipped with overall better sanitation and infrastructure, migrants may not be able to take advantage of the local services due to cost, discrimination, or legal barriers. Finch et al. (2000) showed that discrimination could lead to low self-esteem and negatively affect health. Discrimination could also manifest in residential segregation, wage differentials, or limited access to health services, which together contributed to the emotional toll on migrants.

In addition to understanding the underlying mechanisms through which migration affects psychological health, an equally important question is whether the impact differs between demographic groups. Unlike voluntary migration, forced migration arising from political instability or natural disasters tends to be more traumatic and unpredictable. As such, refugees likely suffer from worse health consequences than other types of migrants (Watters 2001). Furthermore, several studies have shown that gender plays an important role in terms of how stress affects health. Gove and Tudor (1973) and Needham and Hill (2010) demonstrate the ramifications of gender roles for mental health and attribute the higher levels of emotional vulnerability observed among women to their gendered socialization experiences. Their work found that different social norms regarding acceptable emotional expression meant that men tended to distract themselves from psychological distress or externalize it through unhealthy lifestyles such as substance abuse and cigarette smoking. On the other hand, women may be more likely to internalize their emotions and show more depressive symptoms (Needham and Hill, 2010).

Lu's (2010a, 2010b) studies on the effect of rural–urban labor migration on mental health and risk behaviors in Indonesia demonstrate that rural–urban labor migrants are significantly more likely to report depressive symptoms than rural non-migrants. The detrimental effect of migration on mental health is strongly associated with family separation and reduced social support. Due to the psychological distress, migrants are also more likely to exhibit risky behaviors as measured by levels of smoking. Although there was no clear impact of migration on the uptake of smoking, migrants, mostly men, were found to smoke significantly more cigarettes per day compared to their smoking intensity before migration. Combined with the observation that migrants tended to be younger and were more often men and single, this result highlighted the fact that men were more likely to express psychological distress through externalized unhealthy behaviors such as smoking.

In contrast, Nauman et al. (2015) found that rural-to-urban migration from Kanchanaburi province, western Thailand significantly improved the mental health of young adults. While rural young adults scored lower in their mental health status prior to migration than the non-migrant comparison group, moving to urban areas was strongly associated with an improvement in their psychological wellbeing. The authors speculated that young adults were dissatisfied with life back in their rural homes and chose to move to urban areas to enjoy greater social, cultural, and financial autonomy. These mixed findings underscore the existing gap in the literature and the limited extent to which one can generalize findings across regions and across diverse groups of migrants.

Migration-related stress manifests differently among women and men. Lu (2010b) found that while female migrants were more likely to report depressive symptoms, male migrants tended to become heavier smokers. There is suggestive evidence that for both men and women, the loss of social support as indicated by moving without family members aggravate the detrimental impact of migration on mental health among women and on smoking intensity among men. The negative impact of migration is the most acute for recent migrants and becomes attenuated for those who have stayed longer (Lu 2010b). This points to the beneficial effects of cultural assimilation on the mental health of migrants as they begin to adapt to the local environment and establish new social networks.

EFFECT OF MIGRATION ON HEALTH OF PEOPLE LEFT BEHIND

Improved income and family disruption that commonly arise in the context of labor out-migration not only affect the health of those who moved, but also have important and mixed implications for the health of those left behind. Figure 2.3 illustrates the socioeconomic, psychosocial, and behavioral intermediating factors through which migration may affect the health of family members left behind. On the one hand, remittances sent back from migrant members of the family provide additional sources of income and increase the standard of living of those who remained. On the other hand, the impact of out-migration may not extend beyond the short-term improvements in consumption, as rural households face reduced labor supply in agricultural activities and a loss of emotional and social support from family separation. Such changes in the family structure may lead to stress and a deterioration of psychological health for those who stayed behind.

Despite being a key component in the migration–health nexus, only recently have researchers begun to examine the health implications of migration for people left behind. Most existing studies here focus on

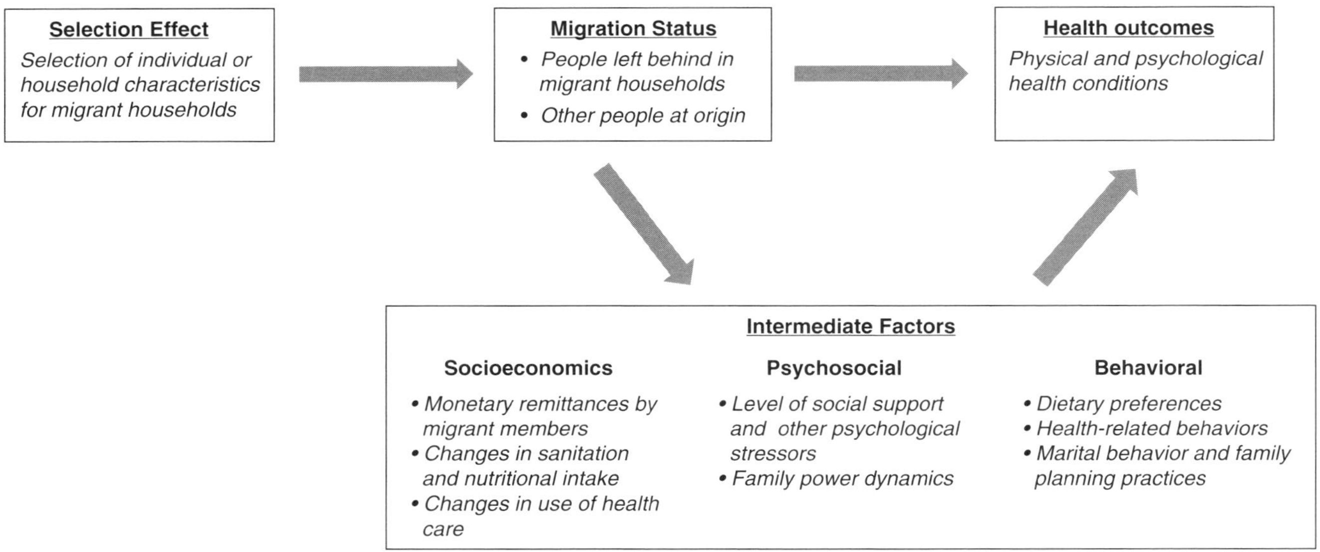

Figure 2.3 Post-migration health of people left behind in migrant households and intermediating factors

children's health. Kanaiaupuni and Donato (1999), for example, reported higher rates of infant mortality in Mexican communities with higher levels of migration by any household member—including the head, spouse, and resident children—to the US, although this negative effect diminished with the level of remittances. By contrast, other studies on Mexico (Frank and Hummer 2002; Hildebrandt and McKenzie 2005) found that children in households with emigrants had lower risks of low birth weight and child mortality. The limitation of these studies is that they do not distinguish different relationships between the migrants and children. For example, there is reason to believe that the out-migration of parents, especially mothers, is more detrimental than that of other relatives, who are often not the main caregivers for children.

There is growing but limited evidence on the adult population. Kuhn's study in Bangladesh (2005) for example, showed a strong positive effect of adult children's migration on their parents' physical functioning and survival. However, Roy and Nangia's study in rural Bihar, India (2005) found that wives left behind reported a higher prevalence of reproductive morbidity, which was considered to result from husbands' risky sexual behaviors at migratory destinations and wives' poor health-seeking behavior at home. These conflicting results suggest that the effect of migration on health may be highly heterogeneous depending on whether the migrants are parents, spouses, or adult children of those left behind.

Remittance and Health

There is a rich literature on the economic gains of emigration for those who stayed through monetary remittance. According to the New Economics of Labor Migration (NELM), migration decisions are made collectively by members of the households to maximize economic benefits and diversify risk, especially in less developed countries with inadequate credit systems and little institutionalized provision for insurance against crop failure or loss of productivity in old age (Stark and Bloom 1985). As a result, while some of the family members work in the field, others go out to work in wage labor and send a large proportion of their income home through remittances (Azam and Gubert 2006). For instance, in the late 1990s, 25 percent of rural households in Indonesia relied on labor migration and remittances (Hugo 2002). Remittances can play a crucial role in reducing the level of poverty and offer a strong potential for regional economic development (Adams 2006). The accompanied social transfers of knowledge, attitudes, and practices may further improve awareness of the benefits of nutrition, sanitation, and healthcare (Levitt 1998), thus affecting health practices and moderating the impact of monetary remittances.

A growing literature focusing on children and women left behind in Mexico has linked household migration with children's birthweight and mortality, women's reproductive health, and health utilization (Frank and Hummer 2002; Hirsch et al. 2002; Hildebrandt and McKenzie 2005; Amuedo-Dorantes et al. 2007) demonstrating that remittances improve the material standard of living of spouses, children, or older parents staying at home and increase household consumption, while generating savings that could be directed toward preventative healthcare and improved health utilization. However, internal migration or emigration can also have detrimental morbidity and mortality implications. For example, higher calorie intake among the wealthy—those in left-behind households benefiting from improved economic resources—could contribute to changes in dietary preferences toward more processed, sugary, and high-fat food or a more sedentary lifestyle (Popkin 1998).

Lu (2013) examines the link between household out-migration and left-behind adults' nutritional status in the context of internal migration in Indonesia. Results suggested a beneficial role of migration on the nutritional health of left-behind household members, as adults in migrant households were 40 percent less likely to suffer from malnutrition than those in non-migrant households. The effect was driven mostly by labor-migrant households and increased with the number of migrants within a household, suggesting that remittance might have contributed to the improved living standards and increased calorie intake. It is important to note that there is a time lag in the relationship between migration and nutritional benefits, as the effect is only marginally significant within the first two years of out-migration and becomes more significant over time. Interestingly, there was no evidence of a lifestyle change associated with migration that might increase the risk of being overweight, possibly suggesting that dietary preferences were stable over the short run. This study also revealed the moderating role of gender, with women more likely to secure nutritional benefits from the out-migration of other household members than men. This is presumably a result of women's greater propensity to invest in health, especially when they are left behind and thus empowered to manage resource allocation.

Psychosocial Processes

Although remittances sent by migrants to their family members can increase the standard of living of those left behind, such as improving their nutrition status, the extent to which monetary transfers can contribute positively to health may be limited by other competing psychosocial factors. The psychosocial consequences of out-migration on those left behind are likely to be multifaceted with competing channels of influence. One the one hand, out-migration not only changes the social structure within households by diminishing the social support between family members, but also reduces labor supply in agricultural activities that further aggravate the physical and emotional burden from separation (Taylor et al. 1996). Prolonged separation between family members and the subsequent loss of social and emotional support creates anxiety and stressors that are detrimental to physical and psychological wellbeing. On the other hand, those who are left behind may experience beneficial effects on emotional health through restructuring of the power dynamics within the family (Parreñas 2005). For example, as men go out to urban areas in search of work, women who remain in the countryside may enjoy more autonomy and gain more decision-making power.

The discussion so far has masked the specific repercussions of migration for the elderly, women, and children. The literature has offered mixed evidence regarding the consequences of adult children's migration on the health of their parents. As adult children move away from home, elderly parents who are left behind may enjoy socioeconomic benefits from the remittances and a higher standard of living. However, the absence of their children as caregivers may be draining on the elderly parents, who depend on them to provide physical and emotional support. Kuhn et al. (2011) found a positive association between children's internal migration and old-age health of parents who were left behind in rural areas in Indonesia. Antman (2010), however, suggested a statistically significant relationship between children's migration to the US and poor self-reported physical and mental health and greater risks of suffering from a heart attack and stroke for parents left behind in Mexico. Antman (2015) attempted to provide a causal interpretation of this negative relationship by addressing the possible endogeneity problem between children's decision to move and parental health. The evidence supported the earlier finding that having a child migrate to the US raised the likelihood of experiencing loneliness and depressive symptoms for elderly parents left behind.

However, existing studies haven't established the process through which children's migration affect the level of caregiving and emotional support received by the elderly parents left behind. A closer look at the different channels that may have contributed to the health effect, such as changes in the level of remittances, financial and time commitments provided by siblings who remain at home (Antman, 2015), the distance between home and destination for migrant children and the extent to which they could go back home and visit, would help reconcile the conflicting empirical evidence mentioned earlier. Lu et al. (2012), for example, showed that the detrimental effect of migration on psychosocial health of those left behind, as manifested in higher levels of depressive symptoms, was larger for households that did not receive remittances. Heterogeneity in the underlying causes of migration between internal and international migrants, as well as the different family structures and social norms for old-age support may also have contributed to the disagreements.

Family separation due to temporary and seasonal labor migration may have unintended consequences on marital relationships, family structure, and reproductive behaviors, some of which persist even after the migrant's return. Agadjanian et al. (2011), for example, found that married women in southern Mozambique had lower birth rate during the absence of their husbands, and the reduction in lifetime fertility rates was larger for wives whose husbands spent longer accumulated times away from home. But the decline was partially compensated for by an increase in birth rate once the period of migration ended. This result, they suggest, represents a normative trade-off between the socioeconomic gains made through remittances and the disruption in family life, which is well expected by communities with longstanding traditions of labor migration.

Migratory success may also affect family power dynamics. It is suggested, for example, that wives of highly successfully male migrants become increasingly dependent on remittances and lose decision-making power (Menjívar and Agadjanian 2007). Because the economic success of migrants can magnify gender inequality, women may become less capable of negotiating sexual practices and become more vulnerable in contracting STIs from their husbands, who may engage in risky extramarital sexual behaviors while away from home (Sevoyan and Agadjanian 2010). In contrast, for men who are less successful in migration, their wives tend to show greater autonomy that increases with their cumulative migration duration, which may persist even after their return (Yabiku et al. 2010). On the other hand, women's migration success may help them achieve greater economic autonomy that may positively impact on gender equality. For example, Parrado and Flippen (2005) found that Mexican immigrant women in the United States experience more egalitarian gender relations by having more employment opportunities. However, female migrants may become more rather than less dependent on their partners, as they often work in low-wage and low-skill service jobs and are marginalized in the US labor market. This calls for more empirical work to document the determinants and evolution of gender relations and family dynamics throughout the course of migration.

The absence of male labor migrants can also have unintended consequences for child outcomes. In the context of Mozambique for example, Yabiku et al. (2012) found that while monetary support sent to the families left behind might help a child's survival, the effect on child health differed by men's migratory success. When discounting the degree of success in migration, children of male labor migrants showed no discernable difference in mortality patterns compared to children of non-migrants. When the wives' perceptions of their husbands' migration success were considered, children of successful migrants exhibited the lowest mortality rate, followed by children of non-migrant men, while children of unsuccessful migrants had the highest mortality rate. Combined with results from Yabiku et al. (2010), these studies highlight the contingent effect of parental migration on child health. Children whose fathers are less successful at channeling economic resources back home fare poorly in health, as their mothers are more likely to be working outside home to make ends meet, while they bear the consequences of limited parental attention and support.

Studies have identified important moderating factors. As Lu (2012) has suggested, kinship linkages, usually reflected in co-residence of extended family members, may influence an individual's adaptation to migration. Emigration may have a weaker effect on psychosocial health when extended families are able to fill the roles normally assigned to the absent migrants by offering emotional and instrumental support. The effect of depressive symptoms is reduced by half for individuals in extended family arrangements. This suggests that emotional and social support from extended family members provide a buffer against the stress created by separation from spouses or adult-children who migrated (Lu 2012). Over time, as family members become more accustomed to the absence of the emigrant, they will likely develop better coping mechanisms that alleviate the health impacts of migration. As such, we may observe an inverted U-shaped curve, in which the psychosocial impact of out-migration initially increases during the early phases of migration and then slowly diminishes over the long run. However, this has not yet been supported by empirical evidence. Lu (2012) found that the detrimental effect of migration on health for people who were left behind tended to accumulate over time, such that the initial impact was relatively small and increased with prolonged separation (1–3 years). However, there is insufficient evidence for the long-term health impact of migration, as any coping mechanism of those left behind to become more emotionally resilient would be confounded by diminishing physiological functioning as people age.

The role of out-migration for health hinges on the specific family relations under scrutiny and varies by gender. Lu (2012) found that people left behind in Indonesian migrant households tended to experience a 3 percent and 5 percent increase, respectively, in the probability of developing hypertension and depression. When a primary household laborer and caregiver migrated for work, parents left behind were especially vulnerable to developing hypertension and depressive symptoms, compared to spouses left behind, whose health costs existed largely with respect to depressive symptoms. Moreover, there is suggestive evidence that gender roles manifest in different levels of health costs between men and women in Indonesia (Lu 2012). While women tended to have a higher risk of experiencing depressive symptoms, men were more vulnerable to hypertension that resulted from greater work obligations and longer hours while experiencing household labor shortages. Women were also found to be more effective at mobilizing social support from kin and co-villagers than men.

CONCLUSIONS AND FUTURE DIRECTIONS

As migration becomes an unprecedented phenomenon in the modern world and an integral aspect of life in many societies, a comprehensive understanding of the complex processes and consequences linking migration and health is crucial. To this end, this chapter has highlighted three possible linkages between the processes of migration and health: the health selection of migration, the effect of migration on health for migrants, and the effect of migration on health for people left behind. Empirical studies using longitudinal data to compare the pre-migration health of migrants and non-migrants generally support the "healthy migrant hypothesis" that healthier individuals are more likely to move than their peers who are less healthy. The process of migration in turn affects migrants' health directly through changes in the physical environment or indirectly through socioeconomic, psychosocial, or behavioral pathways. While moving to more-developed areas can entail improvements in socioeconomic status and better sanitation, migrants may not experience significant physical or psychological health improvements due to the loss of social support, pressures from work, lack of health utilization and literacy, or susceptibility to infectious diseases. In addition, economic improvement and family disruption in the context of labor out-migration affect the psychosocial wellbeing of people left behind through complex pathways. Although remittances sent back by migrants provide additional sources of income and increase the standard of living of those who remained, such improvement in the quality of life may only be limited to short-term gains in material consumption. Studies have documented a deterioration of psychological and physical health outcomes due to the loss of emotional and social support from family separation.

Despite a growing number of studies examining this link, important gaps remain in the following areas. First, we need to use more suitable data (longitudinal data with information on health prior to migration and on the appropriate groups of comparison) to be able to more definitively pin down the causal link between migration and health. Second, going beyond assessing the net effect of migration, to identifying potential mediating and moderating mechanisms is particularly important in fully unpacking the black box linking migration with health. Third, studying internal and international migration in a unified rather than separate framework will allow a more in-depth understanding of the similarities and differences in the implications of these two migratory processes for health. Lastly, considerable insights can be gained by cross-country comparisons. Most existing studies mentioned in this review consider internal migration in a specific country. While labor migration streams are likely driven by similar underlying economic forces in other countries, cross-country comparative studies will be useful not only in establishing the external validity of the identified relationships between migration and different dimensions of physical and psychosocial health, but also in achieving a contextualized understanding of the migration–health nexus. Institutional variation across different socioeconomic contexts may impose a different set of constraints for internal migrants in different countries. For instance, while internal rural-to-urban migrants in Indonesia face no systematic barrier and enjoy a relatively 'open' environment, restrictive migration policies and the associated legal and social barriers pose considerable challenges to within or cross-country mobility. Notable examples include the *Hukou* system and internal migration in China, the population influx control in South Africa during apartheid, and the stringent immigration policies applied within developed countries in Europe and North America. Future work should address the extent to which internal and international migrants share similar experience in terms of health and how the impacts manifest differently across the diverse socioeconomic and legal spectrum across countries.

REFERENCES

Abraído-Lanza, A. F., B. P. Dohrenwend, D. S. Ng-Mak and J. B. Turner (1999), The Latino mortality paradox: a test of the "salmon bias" and healthy migrant hypotheses, *American Journal of Public Health*, **89**(10), 1543–1548.

Abraído-Lanza, A. F., M. T. Chao and K. R. Flórez, (2005), Do healthy behaviors decline with greater acculturation? Implications for the Latino mortality paradox, *Social Science & Medicine*, **61**(6), 1243–1255.

Adams Jr, R. H. (2006). *Migration, Remittances and Development: The Critical Nexus in the Middle East and North Africa*, United Nations Expert Group Meeting on International Migraton and Development in the Arab Region, UN Secretariat, Beirut, 15–17 May 2006.

Agadjanian, V., S. T Yabiku and B. Cau (2011), Men's migration and women's fertility in rural Mozambique, *Demography*, **48**(3), 1029–1048.

Almeida-Filho, N., J. J. Mari and E. Coutinho (1995), Rural–urban migration and

mental health in Latin America: the debate continues, in T. Harpham and I. Blue (eds.), *Urbanization and Mental Health in Developing Countries*, Avebury: Brookfield, pp. 41–60.
Amuedo-Dorantes, C., T. Sainz and S. Pozo (2007), *Remittances and Healthcare Expenditure Patterns of Populations in Origin Communities: Evidence from Mexico*, Working Paper Documento de Trabajo ITD.
Anglewicz, P., M. VanLandingham and D. Phuengsamran (2014), Rural-to-urban migration and sexual debut in Thailand, *Demography*, **51**(5), 1955–1976.
Anson, J. (2004), The migrant mortality advantage: a 70-month follow-up of the Brussels population, *European Journal of Population/Revue Europenne de Demographie*, **20**(3), 191–218.
Antman, F. M. (2010), Adult child migration and the health of elderly parents left behind in Mexico, *American Economic Review*, **100**(2), 205–208.
Antman, F. M. (2015), *How Does International Migration Affect the Health of Elderly Parents Left Behind? Evidence from Mexico*, available online at http://spot.colorado.edu/~antmanf/Antman_Migration&ElderlyHealthMar2013.pdf.
Apostolopoulos, Y. and S. Sönmez (2007), *Population Mobility and Infectious Disease*, Boston, MA: Springer US.
Azam, J.-P. and F. Gubert (2006), Migrants' remittances and the household in Africa: a review of evidence, *Journal of African Economies*, **15**(S2), 426–462.
Bhugra, D. (2004), Migration and mental health, *Acta Psychiatrica Scandinavica*, **109**(4), 243–258.
Bilsborrow, R. E., A. S. Oberai and G. Standing (1984), *Migration Surveys in Low-Income Countries: Guidelines for Survey and Questionnaire Design*, Beckenham: Croom Helm.
Black, D., S. Sanders and E. Taylor (2011), The impact of the Great Migration on mortality of African Americans: evidence from the Deep South, *American Economic Review*, **105**(2), 477–503.
Chamratrithirong, A. (2007), Research on internal migration in Thailand: the state of knowledge, *Journal of Population and Social Studies*, **16**(1), 1–20.
Chiswick, B. R., Y. L. Lee and P. W. Millar (2008), Immigrant selection systems and immigrant health, *Contemporary Economic Policy*, **26**(4), 555–578.
Farley, T., A. Galves, L. M. Dickinson and M. de Jesus Diaz Perez (2005), Stress, coping, and health: a comparison of Mexican immigrants, Mexican-Americans, and non-Hispanic Whites, *Journal of Immigrant Health*, **7**(3), 213–220.
Feranil, A. B. (2005). Anaemia among migrant and non-migrant mothers in disadvantaged areas in the Visayas, the Philippines, in S. Jatrana, M. Toyota and B. S. A. Yeoh (eds.), *Migration and Health in Asia*, London: Routledge, pp. 100–115.
Finch, B. K., B. Kolody and W. A. Vega (2000), Perceived discrimination and depression among Mexican-origin adults in California, *Journal of Health and Social Behavior*, **41**(3), 295–313.
Frank, R. and R. A. Hummer (2002), The other side of the paradox: the risk of low birth weight among infants of migrant and nonmigrant households within Mexico, *International Migration Review*, **36**(3), 746–765.
Gove, W. R. and J. F. Tudor (1973), Adult sex roles and mental illness, *American Journal of Sociology*, **78**(4), 812–835.
Halliday, T. J. and M. C. Kimmitt (2008), Selective migration and health in the USA, 1984–93, *Population Studies*, **62**(3), 321–334.
Hayward, M. D. and M. Heron (1999), Racial inequality in active life among adult Americans, *Demography*, **36**(1), 77.
Hildebrandt, N. and D. J. McKenzie (2005), The effects of migration on child health in Mexico, *Economía*, **6**(1), 257–289.
Hirsch, J. S., J. Higgins, M. E. Bentley and C. A. Nathanson (2002), The social constructions of sexuality: marital infidelity and sexually transmitted disease – HIV risk in a Mexican Migrant community, *American Journal of Public Health*, **92**(8), 1227–1237.
Hugo, G. (2002), Effects of international migration on the family of Indonesia, *Asian and Pacific Migration Journal*, **11**(1), 13–46.

Jasso, G., D. S. Massey, M. R. Rosenzweig and J. P. Smith (2004), Immigrant health: selectivity and acculturation, in N. B. Anderson, R. A. Bulatao and B. Cohen (eds.), *Critical Perspectives on Racial and Ethnic Differences in Health in Late Life*, Washington, DC: National Academies Press, pp. 227–266.
Kanaiaupuni, S. M. and K. M. Donato (1999), Migradollars and mortality: the effects of migration on infant survival in Mexico, *Demography*, **36**(3), 339–353.
Kuhn, R. S. (2005). A longitudinal analysis of health and mortality in a migrant-sending region of Bangladesh, in S. Jatrana, M. Toyota and B. S. A. Yeoh (eds.), *Migration and Health in Asia*, London: Routledge.
Kuhn, R., B. Everett and R. Silvey (2011), The effects of children's migration on elderly kin's health: a counterfactual approach, *Demography*, **48**(1), 183–209.
Kuo, W. H. and Y. M. Tsai (1986), Social networking, hardiness and immigrant's mental health, *Journal of Health and Social Behavior*, **27**(2), 133–149.
Landale, N. S., R. S. Oropesa and B. K. Gorman (2000), Migration and infant death: assimilation or selective migration among Puerto Ricans? *American Sociological Review*. http://doi.org/10.2307/2657518.
Levitt, P. (1998), Social remittances: migration driven local-level forms of cultural diffusion, *International Migration Review*, **32**(4), 926.
Lu, Y. (2008), Test of the "healthy migrant hypothesis": a longitudinal analysis of health selectivity of internal migration in Indonesia, *Social Science and Medicine*, **67**(8), 1331–1339.
Lu, Y. (2010a), Rural–urban migration and health: evidence from longitudinal data in Indonesia, *Social Science and Medicine*, **70**(3), 412–419.
Lu, Y. (2010b), Mental health and risk behaviours of rural-urban migrants: longitudinal evidence from Indonesia, *Population Studies*, **64**(2), 147–163.
Lu, Y. (2012), Household migration, social support, and psychosocial health: the perspective from migrant-sending areas, *Social Science and Medicine*, **74**(2), 135–142.
Lu, Y. (2013), Household migration, remittances and their impact on health in Indonesia, *International Migration*, **51**(S1), e202–e215.
Lu, Y. and L. Qin (2014), Healthy migrant and salmon bias hypotheses: a study of health and internal migration in China, *Social Science and Medicine*, **102**, 41–48.
Lu, Y., P. Hu and D. J. Treiman (2012), Migration and depressive symptoms in migrant-sending areas: findings from the survey of internal migration and health in China, *International Journal of Public Health*, **57**(4), 691–698.
Lucas, R. E. (1997), Internal migration in developing countries, *Handbook of Population and Family Economics*, **1**, 721–798.
Lurie, M. N., B. G.Williams, K. Zuma, D. Mkaya-Mwamburi, G. Garnett, A. W. Sturm and S. S. Abdool Karim (2003), The impact of migration on HIV-1 transmission in South Africa: a study of migrant and nonmigrant men and their partners, *Sexually Transmitted Diseases*, **30**(2), 149–156.
Markides, K. S. and J. Coreil (1986), The health of Hispanics in the southwestern United States: an epidemiologic paradox, *Public Health Reports*, **101**(3), 253–265.
Markides, K. S. and K. Eschbach (2011), Hispanic paradox in adult mortality in the United States, in R. G. Rogers and E. M. Crimmins (eds.), *International Handbook of Adult Mortality*, Dordrecht: Springer Netherlands, pp. 227–240.
Marmot, M. G., M. A. Adelstein and L. Bulusu (1983), Immigrant mortality in England and Wales 1970–78, *Population Trends*, **33**, 14–17.
Marmot, M. G., A. M. Adelstein and L. Bulusu (1984), Lessons from the study of immigrant mortality, *The Lancet*, **323**(8392), 1455–1457.
Massey, D., J. Arango and G. Hugo (1999), *Worlds in Motion : Understanding International Migration at the End of the Millennium*. Oxford: Clarendon Press.
Mberu, B. U. and M. J. White (2011), Internal migration and health: premarital sexual initiation in Nigeria, *Social Science & Medicine*, **72**(8), 1284–1293.
Menjívar, C. and V. Agadjanian (2007), Men's migration and women's lives: views from rural Armenia and Guatemala, *Social Science Quarterly*, **88**(5), 1243–1262.

Nauman, E., M. VanLandingham, P. Anglewicz, U. Patthavanit and S. Punpuing (2015), Rural-to-urban migration and changes in health among young adults in Thailand, *Demography*, **52**(1), 233–257.
Needham, B. and T. D. Hill (2010), Do gender differences in mental health contribute to gender differences in physical health? *Social Science & Medicine*, **71**(8), 1472–1479.
Newbold, B. (2005), Health status and health care of immigrants in Canada: a longitudinal analysis, *Journal of Health Services Research & Policy*, **10**(2), 77–83.
Palloni, A. and J. D. Morenoff (2001), Interpreting the paradoxical in the Hispanic paradox, *Annals of the New York Academy of Sciences*, **954**(1), 140–174.
Parrado, E. A. and C. A. Flippen (2005), Migration and gender among Mexican women, *American Sociological Review*, **70**(4), 606–632.
Parreñas, R. S. (2005), The gender paradox in the transnational families of Filipino migrant women, *Asian and Pacific Migration Journal*, **14**(3), 243–268.
Popkin, B. M. (1998), The nutrition transition and its health implications in lower-income countries, *Public Health Nutrition*, **1**(1), 5–21.
Riosmena, F. and J. A. Dennis (2012), A tale of three paradoxes: the weak socioeconomic gradients in health among Hispanic immigrants and their relation to the Hispanic health paradox and negative acculturation, in J. L. Angel, F. Torres-Gil and K. Markides (eds.), *Aging, Health, and Longevity in the Mexican-Origin Population*, Boston, MA: Springer US, pp. 95–110.
Roy, A. K. and P. Nangia (2005), Reproductive health status of wives left behind by male out-migrants: a study of rural Bihar, India, in S. Jatrana, M. Toyota and B. S. A. Yeoh (eds.), *Migration and Health in Asia*, Routledge, London.
Rubalcava, L. N., G. M. Teruel, D. Thomas and N. Goldman (2008), The healthy migrant effect: new findings from the Mexican Family Life Survey, *American Journal of Public Health*, **98**(1), 78–84.
Sander, M. (2007), Return migration and the "healthy immigrant effect," *SOE Papers on Multidisciplinary Panel Data Research*.
Sevoyan, A. and V. Agadjanian (2010), Male migration, women left behind, and sexually transmitted diseases in Armenia, *International Migration Review*, **44**(2), 354–375.
Shuval, J. T. (2001), Migration, health and stress, in *The Blackwell Companion to Medical Sociology*, Oxford: Wiley-Blackwell, pp. 126–145.
Singh, G. K. and M. Siahpush (2001), All-cause and cause-specific mortality of immigrants and native born in the United States, *American Journal of Public Health*, **91**(3), 392–399.
Stark, O. and D. E. Bloom (1985), The new economics of labor migration, *The American Economic Review*, **75**(2), 173–178.
Takeuchi, D. T., M. Alegría, J. S. Jackson and D. R. Williams (2007), Immigration and mental health: diverse findings in Asian, black, and Latino populations, *American Journal of Public Health*, **97**(1), 11–12.
Taylor, J. E., J. Arango, G. Hugo, A. Kouaouci, D. S. Massey and A. Pellegrino (1996), International migration and community development, *Population Index*, **62**(3), 397–418.
Tong, Y. and M. Piotrowski (2012), Migration and health selectivity in the context of internal migration in China, 1997–2009, *Population Research and Policy Review*, **31**(4), 497–543.
Turra, C. M. and I. T. Elo (2008), The impact of salmon bias on the Hispanic mortality advantage: new evidence from social security data, *Population Research and Policy Review*, **27**(5), 515–530.
Ullmann, S. H., N. Goldman and D. S. Massey (2011), Healthier before they migrate, less healthy when they return? The health of returned migrants in Mexico, *Social Science & Medicine*, **73**(3), 421–428.
United Nations (2013), *International Migration Report 2013*, Geneva: United Nations.
United Nations (2014), *World Urbanization Prospects: The 2014 Revision*, available online at http://esa.un.org/unpd/wup/Highlights/WUP2014-Highlights.pdf.
Villa, V. M., S. P. Wallace, S. Bagdasaryan and M. P. Aranda (2012), Hispanic baby boomers: health inequities likely to persist in old age, *The Gerontologist*, **52**(2), 166–176.

Walsh, A. and P. A. Walsh (1987), Social support, assimilation, and biological effective blood pressure levels, *International Migration Review*, **21**(3), 577–591.
Watters, C. (2001), Emerging paradigms in the mental health care of refugees, *Social Science and Medicine*, **52**(11), 1709–1718.
Williams, D. R. and C. Collins (1995), US socioeconomic and racial differences in health: patterns and explanations, *Annual Review of Sociology*, **21**, 349–386.
Wong, D. F. K., C. Y. Li and H. X. Song, (2007), Rural migrant workers in urban China: living a marginalised life, *International Journal of Social Welfare*, **16**(1), 32–40.
Wong, D. F. K., X. He, G. Leung, Y. Lau and Y. Chang (2008), Mental health of migrant workers in China: prevalence and correlates, *Social Psychiatry and Psychiatric Epidemiology*, **43**(6), 483–489.
Yabiku, S. T., V. Agadjanian and A. Sevoyan (2010), Husbands' labour migration and wives' autonomy, Mozambique 2000–2006, *Population Studies*, **64**(3), 293–306.
Yabiku, S. T., V. Agadjanian and B. Cau (2012), Labor migration and child mortality in Mozambique, *Social Science and Medicine*, **75**(12), 2530–2538.
Yang, X. and G. Xia (2006), Gender, migration, risky sex, and HIV infection in China, *Studies in Family Planning*, **37**(4), 241–250.

3 Models of migration and health

Jacob Spallek, Anna Reeske, Hajo Zeeb and Oliver Razum

INTRODUCTION

Being a migrant or member of an ethnic minority group can impact on an individuals' health and has been strongly associated with health inequalities (Razum and Samkange-Zeeb 2014; Rechel et al. 2013; WHO 2011). International migration is generally understood as the temporary or permanent change of residence across state borders. Migration can be voluntary and planned; for example, to improve an individual or household's economic outlook or to follow family members or spouses. Migration can also be forced and involuntary, due to political persecution, war, hunger, environmental catastrophes, or other circumstances. The global number of migrants has continuously grown since the 1960s. Today there are about 200 million migrants worldwide, corresponding to 3.5 percent of the world population (UN 2013). More than half of all migrants are female (IOM 2005).

The population of Europe is becoming more diverse, largely due to increasing migration movements. In 2011, about 10.1 percent of the EU population were either foreign born or a citizen of another country (Eurostat 2012). In Western European countries, a considerable part of the population has a migration history or is part of an ethnic minority group. In Germany, for example, one in five residents has a so-called 'migrant background' (Statistisches Bundesamt 2014), and this proportion is even higher among newborns (Razum et al. 2008). 'Migration background' not only comprises persons who have migrated themselves, but also their offspring and, depending on the definition, even grandchildren, i.e., the "third generation." However, attempts to harmonize these definitions across Europe have not been successful, and there is still debate about their proper use (Bhopal 2004; Urquia and Gagnon 2011; EMN 2014).

People who migrated, even if this was decades ago, or whose parents had migrated, may still be influenced by the culture of their country of origin. This influence can be passed on from generation to generation ("cultural inheritance"). However, a process of acculturation may also take place, whereby migrants adapt to the culture of their new home country—generalizations relating to migrant experience are therefore neither possible nor useful.

In this chapter we discuss the ways in which the health situation of individuals with a migrant background differs from that of the autochthonous, non-migrated population. We focus on current explanatory models, using the healthy migrant effect and the model of migration as health transition as our examples. Furthermore, we present selected empirical evidence and describe further factors, notably socioeconomic status and gender, as well as methodological aspects that are important for a valid description, analysis, and interpretation of the health of migrants. Importantly, we argue for a life-course model of migrant health that incorporates these aspects, moving well beyond snapshot assessments of health status of migrants.

HEALTH RISKS AMONG MIGRANTS: MODELS AND EMPIRICAL EVIDENCE

It is important to note that migrants are a heterogeneous group, along categories such as country of origin, rationale for migration, time of migration and duration since arrival, age, gender, social status, etc. Consequently, their health situation is also bound to differ, even within groups.

In order to capture the complex association between migration and health and to describe mechanisms that influence the health of migrants, various models have been developed in recent decades, among them the concept of the "healthy migrant," the model of health transition and the life-course model of migration and health (Razum and Twardella 2002; Spallek et al. 2011).

Healthy Migrant Effect

The concept of the healthy migrant and the "healthy migrant effect" postulate that it is predominantly healthy and active persons who migrate (Wallace and Kulu 2014; Lu and Qin 2014). Thus it can be expected that migrants will have better health when compared to non-migrants (and to the general population in their country of origin), at least close to the time of arrival. However, this model has several weaknesses. In particular, it does not take into account that classical migration and health research compares their health to the overall population in the target country (and not in the country of origin, as the selection hypothesis would require). Additionally, migrants can become "statistically immortal" if they leave a country without their departure being registered. They thus remain in the population registry, and if they die outside the country they have moved to (e.g., return migration to their country of origin), this death potentially escapes notification. This can lead to spuriously low mortality estimates in the migrant population (Ringbäck Weitoft et al. 1999) and may in part help account for the claims made regarding the "healthy migrant" effect. However, the phenomenon of comparatively lower mortality among migrants has also been observed in studies where this statistical artifact can be excluded (Abraído-Lanza et al. 1999; Razum 2009; Singh and Hiatt 2006). Thus, data errors are likely to play only a limited role for the explanation of migrant health advantages such as mortality. However, it is worth emphasizing that in all models of understanding, high-quality health and social data are of utmost importance for valid and useful migrant health assessments.

Migration as Health Transition

Some of the limitations of the healthy migrant concept are addressed in the model of migration as health transition (Razum and Twardella 2002). This conceptualizes migration from a less-affluent to a more-affluent country (following, for example, the classical pattern of work-related migration) as a rapid health transition. The incidence of, and mortality from, infectious diseases as well as from complications of pregnancy and childbirth declines quickly in the migrant population as compared to the situation in their country of origin, because hygiene and healthcare in the target country are of a higher standard (Razum and Twardella 2002). Morbidity and mortality from chronic diseases such as breast and bowel cancer or myocardial infarction, however, remain on the (often lower) level of the country of origin for an extended lag period, probably due to nutritional or other factors constituting a more "healthy" lifestyle. Together with the long latency periods between exposures to a "unhealthy" lifestyle in many target countries and disease onset, this may lead to relatively lower rates of chronic disease among migrants over extended periods of time after migration relative to the host population, even if they are socioeconomically disadvantaged—an apparent paradox (Razum 2009; Razum and Twardella 2002). It should be noted that these considerations predominantly apply to South to North migration, and the current developments with massive South–South migration are not adequately mirrored. Thus, new theories and models tested against empirical evidence are required.

Life-course Models

The life-course model of migration and health derives from the health transition model and extends earlier models by introducing a life-course perspective (Spallek et al. 2011). The earlier models had not included the temporal dimension of effects influencing the health of migrants. By explicitly addressing this temporal component, the life-course model aims to describe how exposures in critical periods of the life-course as well as risk accumulation over the entire lifespan affect health outcomes. The objective of life-course epidemiology is to identify and explore biological as well as environmental, behavioral, and psychosocial factors and processes and to explain how these factors act over the lifetime or even over generations to influence morbidity and mortality (Lynch and Davey Smith 2005). This approach has generated new insights into the explanation of health inequity (e.g., Davey Smith 2008). For instance, the social environment may act upon the course of pregnancy (stress, complications) and influence the risk of adverse outcomes. This in turn may act upon chronic disease risk in later life. For example, Barker (1998) showed an association between low birthweight and the occurrence of adiposity in adult age.

Applying this to the health situation of migrants means that the respective individual and social situation leads to a clustering of negative and positive factors over time and on different levels. The timing of exposures (generally understood as processes with health relevance) and their importance for the development of diseases depends on the type of health problem and the relevant critical periods for its occurrence over the life-course.

In consequence, the development of health inequalities can be explained by an interaction of risk accumulation and the actual imprinting occurring during critical periods for disease development. From this viewpoint, biological factors influencing health can also be perceived as part of the social processes leading to health inequalities, since biological and social elements are regarded as "reciprocally constitutive" under the life-course framework (Davey Smith 2008).

Migrants thus often have life-course exposures that differ from those of the non-migrant population. A cross-sectional "snapshot" at a single time-point after migration is not sufficient (Lynch and Davey Smith 2005; Spallek and Razum 2008; Spallek et al. 2011). For some illnesses, such as specific cancers, the risk for an incident disease in later life is already determined through exposures in early childhood; for example, by infectious exposures or nutritional programming (Spallek et al. 2011). This makes an investigation of the whole life-course of migrants indispensable if one aims to understand their health situation (e.g., the pattern of cancers among a migrant group).

From an epidemiological perspective, the life-course of migrants may be split in three phases: phase (1) prior to, (2) during, and (3) after migration (see Figure 3.1). In all three phases, exposures act upon their health

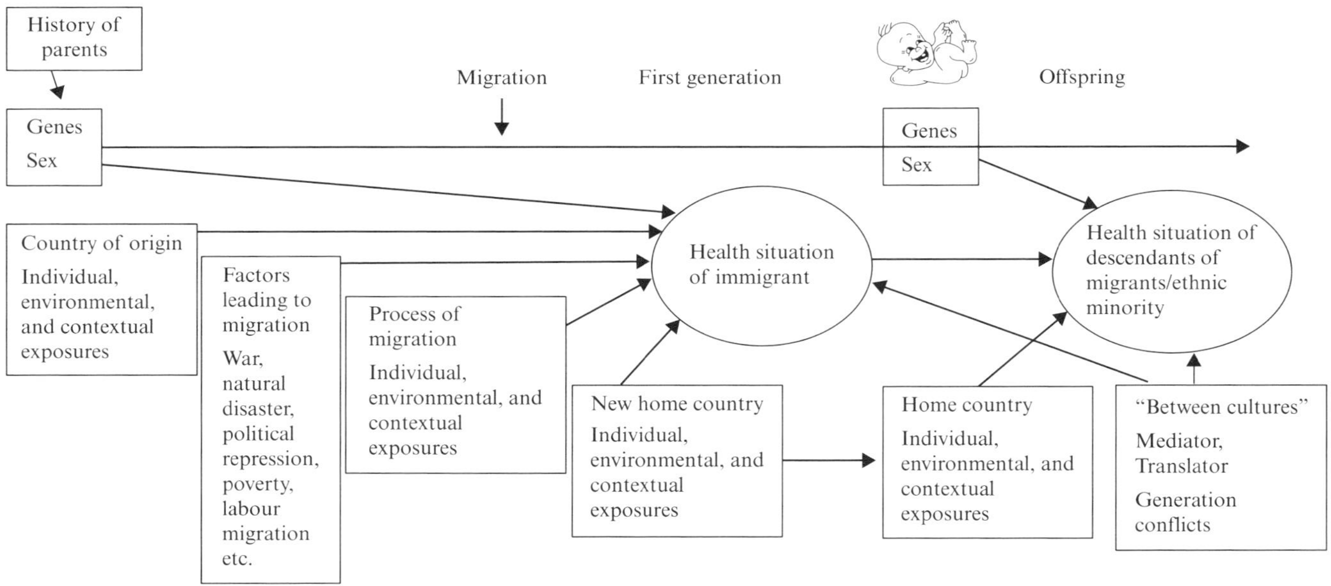

Source: Spallek et al. 2014.

Figure 3.1 Different exposures act on health during the life-course of migrants

and can have acute or long-term influences on health. A typical example for an extended latency between exposure and disease onset is the influence of early life programming of metabolism on the occurrence of adult metabolic syndrome (Barker 1998). A further example is the influence of various infectious agents including hepatitis B virus, papillomavirus, and Helicobacter pylori on cancer risk; for example, for liver, cervical and stomach cancer. As the exposure situation of migrants to such agents may differ in all three phases (1)–(3) due to different environmental situation and living conditions, hygiene, or prevalence of infections as compared to non-migrants, different health outcomes may be the result (Spallek et al. 2011). Thus it is important to consider the different phases when assessing health of migrants, even though empirical data over the whole life-course may frequently be lacking.

Elevated or decreased disease or mortality risks among migrants can converge towards the average risks among the majority population over time, as risks are often determined both by early and later life influences. This has been demonstrated for breast and lung cancer—for example, among Turkish migrants in Hamburg, Germany (Spallek et al. 2009)—as well as cancer risk among offspring of migrants in the Netherlands (Stirbu et al. 2006) or in British Columbia, Canada (Au et al. 2004). In the Hamburg study, first-generation female Turkish migrants had a significantly lower breast cancer risk when compared to the general female population. This advantage was lost in the subsequent generations. As a possible reason is the change in reproductive behavior, with a decreased number of children and later first pregnancy, as in the non-migrant population discussed (Spallek et al. 2009). Lung cancer risks follow the changes in smoking prevalence. At the time of the first migration wave in Germany in the 1960s, Turkey had high smoking prevalence among men, while smoking was rare among women. This led to low lung cancer rates among Turkish migrant women when compared to German women. Over time, smoking among Turkish migrant women has increased (e.g., Reeske et al. 2009), and so too have lung cancer rates. Among Turkish migrant men, no major changes in smoking prevalence and lung cancer rates were found (Reeske et al. 2009).

HEALTH RISKS AMONG SECOND AND THIRD GENERATIONS

Offspring of migrants, sometimes called the second or third generation, may also experience particular health risks due to biological or "cultural" inheritance of relevant traits or factors. Genetically determined characteristics such as skin color may lead to low disease risks for skin cancer, for example, but may also influence the health and wellbeing situation if this leads to forms of discrimination. Subsequent generations are also influenced by parental, often culturally determined behaviors and characteristics that may include attitudes and norms regarding nutrition, smoking, and alcohol consumption as well as sexual behaviors or attitudes towards physical activity (Hosper et al. 2007; Afable-Munsuz et al. 2010). Specific traditions may be maintained over decades and thus continue to differ from the non-migrant population.

Similarly, the socioeconomic situation of the parent generation has been long been found to strongly influence the social, health, educational, and environmental circumstances of subsequent generations (Bourdieu and Passeron 1977; Osler et al. 2005). However, acculturation or segregation of migrants from other community members as well as the lack of specific health-relevant exposures that affected the parent generation prior to migration may also lead to a quite different overall health situation in the offspring.

Members of the second or third generation may find themselves in a situation "between cultures," i.e., between the culture of their parent's country of origin and of their own country of birth. This may lead to various adaptation processes, located on a continuum from strongly leaning towards the parental culture to strong identification with the culture of the host country. Thus, from a public health perspective, this group may also have health needs that require particular attention. For example, children who identify more with the host culture than their parents might experience a degree of role reversal whereby parents depend on them for navigating in the new culture and society. This in turn may have negative influences on the children's health, as parental control is diminished.

Members of the second generation, however, are not only influenced by biology and other characteristics of the preceding generations, but in turn also play a role in shaping the health of their parents. For example, children can act as mediators, as translators of language and of culture when issues of access to societal institutions including access to healthcare arise for first-generation migrants.

OBESITY AMONG IMMIGRANT CHILDREN: APPLYING THE LIFE-COURSE MODEL

The usefulness and limitations of the life-course model in migrant research can best be shown using a concrete example. We here focus on the issue of overweight and obesity among children with a migrant background.

An interaction of genetic factors, fetal programming during abnormal metabolic environment *in utero* and social factors such as restrictive infant feeding practices and risk factors related to diet and physical activity in early life are currently thought to explain the high obesity prevalence in some migrant groups, such as black and Hispanic children in the USA or children from Turkish parents in Germany (Taveras et al. 2010; Robert Koch-Institut 2008).

Results from various studies support the hypothesis that migrant background is an independent risk factor for (infant) weight gain among the offspring of migrants. In Germany, for example, migrant children show a notably higher prevalence of overweight and obesity (19.5 percent) than non-migrants (14.1 percent), with highest prevalence rates among girls and boys originating from Turkey (Robert Koch-Institut 2008). The important question is how cultural and lifestyle-related factors in pregnancy and early life may act upon the development of overweight and obesity in migrants. As previously described, critical periods, which may place migrants at particular risk, lie in pregnancy and early infancy (Dietz 1994; Gillman 2004). However, timing of mother's migration and migrant generation may also affect their children's vulnerability (Robert Koch-Institut 2008).

The health of pregnant women with migration experience can still be affected by exposures and access to healthcare prior to migration. For example, pregnant migrant women may carry the burden of the high prevalence of (pre-pregnancy) overweight and high gestational weight gain during pregnancy from their country of origin, with both being strong risk factors for overweight in the offspring (Taveras et al. 2010). In the Dutch multiethnic ABCD study, for example, maternal pre-pregnancy body mass index (BMI) was a strong predictor for overweight at the age of two and also explained higher rates of overweight in children of Turkish and Moroccan origin (de Hoog et al. 2011).

Second-generation women of childbearing age might still be affected by the culture and habits of their parents' country of origin. Hence, the observed ethnic differences in childhood obesity may also be explained by differences in cultural beliefs and practices related to food and physical activity (Kumanyika 2008). These practices have an effect on the offspring, especially when it comes to early feeding practices and role models. For example, during the critical infancy period, rapid weight gain in combination with potentially detrimental infant feeding practices (e.g., short duration of exclusive breastfeeding, early supplementary feeding and early introduction of solid food) comprises a risk factor for later childhood obesity. We found differences in weight at birth and after six months (weight measured as mean weight standard deviations scores) when comparing infants from migrant families to infants with parents born in Germany (Reeske et al. 2013). Among children from parents originating from Turkey or Eastern European countries, weight was largely similar to that of non-migrants, but was markedly increased six months later (Reeske et al. 2013). Several studies support this notion, demonstrating an earlier introduction of solid food and sweet beverages among Turkish mothers compared to the non-migrant population (Bulk-Bunschoten et al. 2008; de Hoog et al. 2011). However, infant feeding patterns in immigrant families are apparently similar to those among highly educated mothers in Turkey who also breastfeed at a lower prevalence or for shorter time periods than women with low education (Bulk-Bunschoten et al. 2008; Alikaşifoğlu et al. 2001). Among Turkish migrants, such patterns seem to be associated with the culturally related belief that a chubby child represents health, wealth, and good motherhood (de Hoog et al. 2011; Bulk-Bunschoten et al. 2002). However, reasons for discontinued breastfeeding could also be due to the child's health or the mother's occupational situation.

The example shows that health and lifestyle of the offspring of migrants is partly determined by genetically and culturally induced characteristics and (health) behaviors of the parent generation, starting with exposures prior to the migration of the mothers, which still may have an influence in future generations. Exposures in early life may have long-term effects on the health of the second and third generation, and thus explain health differences when compared to the non-migrant population. The onset of health differences in early life emphasizes the need to study migrant health from a life-course perspective.

SOCIAL DETERMINANTS

The models discussed indicate the complexity of factors shaping the health of migrants. Migration adds substantially to societal diversity and heterogeneity, and migrants have both health advantages and disadvantages when compared to the non-migrant majority population.

Social determinants of health affect all population groups, at least to some degree. With regard to the association of migration and health, social status may act as a mediator or as a confounder. Figure 3.2 shows how various factors interact. It becomes clear that without socioeconomic status information that includes occupation, education, but also gender and endowment with social capital, a differentiated analysis of the migration and health link is hardly possible. Social status influences this association strongly and through several pathways, and even the initial step of deciding to migrate is clearly linked to social factors in most instances.

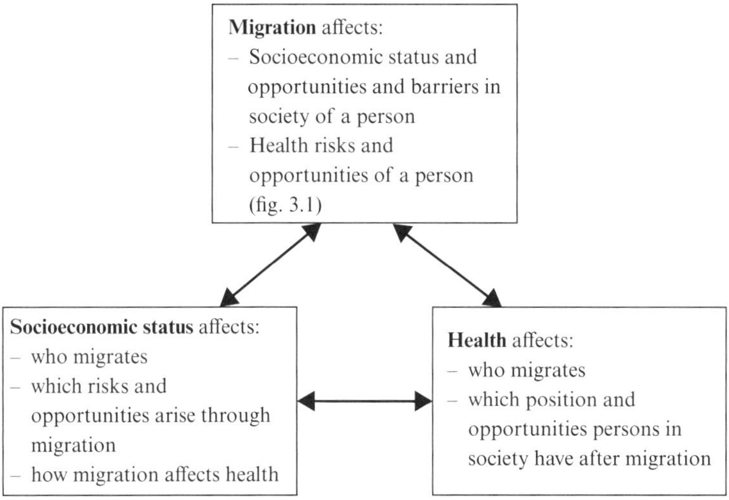

Figure 3.2 Interaction of migration, socioeconomic status, and health

Frequently, health-related differences between migrants and non-migrants are considered to be solely due to socioeconomic differentials. Migrants more frequently (but obviously by no means always) belong to lower socioeconomic strata, and this is known to be associated with less favorable health outcomes as compared to high socioeconomic status. There is clear and persuasive evidence that socioeconomic inequalities have a profound influence on health (Siegrist and Marmot 2006; CSDH WH 2008; Marmot and Allen 2014). People with lower socioeconomic status die earlier and are more often affected by adverse health than individuals with higher socioeconomic positions (Marmot and Wilkinson 2006; Mackenbach et al. 2008; Bleich 2012).

On average, migrants often have less advanced education and poorer access to material resources than the majority population (Spallek et al. 2010). A higher unemployment rate and less well paid and more dangerous or strenuous jobs exemplify this point in developed countries (Razum and Samkange-Zeeb 2014). Migrants are often young and healthy on arrival, but over time as they live and work under worse conditions than the majority population, their health may become jeopardized due to this chronic burden. However, this similarly applies to non-migrants under the same conditions, and reiterates the role of socioeconomic conditions in influencing health outcomes. The same applies to the housing conditions and average size of homes or flats, often smaller than in the majority population overall, but not when compared to people of similar social status (Razum et al. 2008). However, an additional burden limiting further the spending power of migrant households in their new home country may be due to transnational resource flows (money remittances) back to the country of origin (Faist et al. 2013).

Biological Sex and Gender

Factors of high explanatory relevance, but with strong potential to be neglected when considering the health of migrants, are sex and gender. More than half of all migrants worldwide are women (De Leon Siantz 2013). However, with some important exceptions, relatively few studies specifically differentiate migrant health issues by gender (Binder-Fritz and Rieder 2014). Sex and gender also determine who migrates, and why. Depending on the country, the legal, social, and financial circumstances relevant for migration may vary markedly between men and women. Under a life-course perspective, there may be long-lasting effects of conditions prevalent in the country of origin, one of the most dramatic being female genital mutilation, which is still performed in several African countries (Sauer and Neubauer 2013). Women are also faced with particular risks during migration; for example, through sexual violence and related crimes. In the host country, the social and income situation and issues of autonomy may change for both women and men, and in particular the role of women in the family and society may be subject to substantial challenges and changes (Spallek and Razum 2016). Migration may mean more freedom, independence, and empowerment for women, but at the same time their experiences may involve risks, including exploitation, isolation, discrimination, and stigmatization, with serious repercussions for health (Jolly and Reeves 2005). Of note, gender aspects of health and migration also include potential status and autonomy loss and their implication for health, issues that may be particularly relevant for male migrants.

Social Cohesion

Persons of similar origin or ethnicity often provide strong mutual support in the diaspora. These forms of reciprocal support have been described in detail, for example, among Turkish migrants in Germany (White 1997). Strong social cohesion can result in health advantages (Wilkinson and Marmot 2003), and this enhanced cohesion may be characteristic for migrant groups and thus confer health gains. However, there is little medical evidence on this issue so far, and further work is needed to examine the longer-term impact this may have across the life-course.

CONCLUSIONS

Having a migrant background is an important social determinant of health that is needed to describe and analyze health inequalities. The health situation of migrants and their offspring often differs from that of the non-migrant population. The multidimensional relationship between migration and health can only be understood when the many underlying mechanisms and processes are adequately integrated into explanatory frameworks that also take the dimension of time into account. Migrants may have been exposed in ways that differ from those of the non-migrant population over their whole life-course, including the period before migration, the migration process, and the period after migration. A cross-sectional snapshot of their health situation at one or several time-points after migration is thus often not sufficient (Lynch and Davey Smith 2005; Spallek et al. 2011). Detailed data both for the migrant population of interest as well as for comparison populations are required for a comprehensive, theory-based assessment of the changing health of migrants (Spallek et al. 2011).

REFERENCES

Abraído-Lanza, A. F., B. P. Dohrenwend, D. S. Ng-Mak and J. B. Turner (1999), The Latino mortality paradox: a test of the "salmon bias" and healthy migrant hypotheses, *American Journal of Public Health*, **89**, 1543–1548.

Afable-Munsuz, A., N. A. Ponce, M. Rodriguez and E. J. Perez-Stable (2010), Immigrant generation and physical activity among Mexican, Chinese and Filipino adults in the US, *Social Science and Medicine*, **70**, 1997–2005.

Alikaşifoğlu, M., E. Erginoz, E. T. Gur, Z. Baltas, B. Beker and A. Arvas (2001), Factors influencing the duration of exclusive breastfeeding in a group of Turkish women, *Journal of Human Lactation*, **17**, 220–226.

Au, W. Y., R. D. Gascoyne, R. E. Gallagher, N. Le, R. D. Klasa, R. H. S. Liang, C. Choy, W. Foo and J. M. Connors (2004), Hodgkin's lymphoma in Chinese migrants to British Columbia: a 25-year survey, *Annals of Oncology*, **15**, 626–630.

Barker, D. J. P. (1998), *Mothers, Babies and Health in Later Life*, Edinburgh: Churchill Livingstone.

Bhopal, R. (2004), Glossary of terms relating to ethnicity and race: for reflection and debate, *Journal of Epidemiology and Community Health*, **58**, 441–445.

Binder-Fritz, C. and A. Rieder (2014), *Zur Verflechtung von Geschlecht, sozioökonomischen Status und Ethnizität im Kontext von Gesundheit und Migration*. Bundesgesundheitsbl 57: 1031–1037.

Bleich, S. N., M. P. Jarlenski, C. N. Bell and T. A. LaVeist (2012), Health inequalities: trends, progress, and policy, *Annual Review of Public Health*, **33**, 7–40.

Bourdieu, P. and J. C. Passeron (1977), *Reproduction in Education, Society and Culture*, London and Beverly Hills: Sage Publications.

Bulk-Bunschoten, A. M., S. van Bodegom, J. D. Reerink, P.C. de Jong and C. J. de Groot (2002), Weight and weight gain at 4 months (The Netherlands 1998): influences of nutritional practices, socioeconomic and ethnic factors, *Paediatric and Perinatal Epidemiology*, **16**, 361–369.

Bulk-Bunschoten, A. M., P. C. Pasker-de Jong, J. P. van Wouwe and C. J. de Groot (2008), Ethnic variation in infant-feeding practices in the Netherlands and weight gain at 4 months, *Journal of Human Lactation*, **24**, 42–49.
CSDH WH (2008), *Closing the Gap in a Generation: Health Equity through Action on the Social Determinants of Health*, Final Report of the Commission on Social Determinants of Health, Geneva: WHO.
Davey Smith, G. (2008), Die Bedeutung einer Lebenslaufperspektive für die Erklärung gesundheitlicher Ungleichheit, in U. Bauer, U. Bittlingmayer and M. Richter (eds.) *Health Inequalities*. Wiesbaden: VS Verlag für Sozialwissenschaften.
de Hoog, M. L., M. van Eijsden, K. Stronks, R. J. Gemke and T. G. Vrijkotte (2011), Overweight at age two years in a multi-ethnic cohort (ABCD study): the role of prenatal factors, birth outcomes and postnatal factors, *BMC Public Health*, **11**, 611.
De Leon Siantz, M. L. (2013), Feminization of migration: a global health challenge, *Global Advances in Health and Medicine*, **2**, 12–14.
Dietz, W. H. (1994), Critical periods in childhood for the development of obesity, *American Journal of Clinical Nutrition*, **59**, 955–959.
EMN (2014), *Asylum and Migration Glossary 3.0 – a Tool for Better Comparability*, available online at http://ec.europa.eu/dgs/home-affairs/what-we-do/networks/european_migration_network/index_en.htm.
Eurostat (2012), *Non-National Population by Group of Citizenship and Foreign-Born Population by Country of Birth*, 1 January 2012, available online at http://epp.eurostat.ec.europa.eu/statistics_explained/index.php?title=File:Non-national_population_by_group_of_citizenship_and_foreign-born_population_by_country_of_birth,_1_January_2012_YB14.png&filetimestamp=20131204140111.
Faist, T., M. Fauser and E. Reisenauer (2013), *Transnational Migration*, Oxford and New York: Polity Press.
Gillman, M. W. (2004), A life course approach to obesity, in D. Kuh and Y. Ben-Shlomo (eds.), *A Life Course Approach to Chronic Disease Epidemiology*, New York: Oxford University Press, pp. 189–217.
Hosper, K., V. Nierkens, M. Nicolaou and K. Stronks (2007), Behavioural risk factors in two generations of non-Western migrants: do trends converge towards the host population? *European Journal of Epidemiology*, **22**, 163–172.
IOM (2005), *World Migration 2005: Costs and Benefits of International Migration*, available online at www.iom.int/cms/en/sites/iom/home.html.
Jolly, S. and H. Reeves (2005), *Gender and Migration*, BRIDGE Overview Report, Brighton: Institute of Development Studies.
Kumanyika, S. K. (2008), Environmental influences on childhood obesity: ethnic and cultural influences in context, *Physiology & Behaviour*, **94**, 61–70.
Lu, Y. and L. Qin (2014), Healthy migrant and salmon bias hypotheses: a study of health and internal migration in China, *Social Science and Medicine*, **102**, 41–48.
Lynch J. and G. Davey Smith (2005), A life course approach to chronic disease epidmiology, *Annual Review of Public Health*, **26**, 1–35.
Mackenbach, J. P., I. Stirbu, A. R. Roskam, M. M. Schaap, G. Menvielle, M. Leinsalu and A. E. Kunst (2008), Socioeconomic inequalities in health in 22 European countries, *New England Journal of Medicine*, **358**, 2468–2481.
Marmot, M. and J. J. Allen (2014), Social determinants of health equity, *American Journal of Public Health*, **104**(S4), S517–S519.
Marmot, M. and R. G. Wilkinson (2006), *Social Determinants of Health*, Oxford. Oxford University Press.
Osler, M., A. M. Andersen, G. D. Batty and B. Holstein (2005), Relation between early life socioeconomic position and all cause mortality in two generations: a longitudinal study of Danish men born in 1953 and their parents, *Journal of Epidemiology & Community Health*, **59**, 38–41.
Rechel, B., P. Mladovsky, D. Ingleby, J. P. Mackenbach and M. McKee (2013), Migration and health in an increasingly diverse Europe, *Lancet*, **381**, 1235–1245.

Razum, O. (2009), Migration, Mortalität und der Healthy-migrant-Effekt, in M. Richter and K. Hurrelmann (eds.), *Gesundheitliche Ungleichheit. Grundlagen, Probleme, Perspektiven*, Wiesbaden: VS Verlag für Sozialwissenschaften.
Razum, O. and F. Samkange-Zeeb (2014), *Populations at Special Health Risk: Migrants*, Reference Module in Biomedical Sciences, London: Elsevier.
Razum, O. and D. Twardella (2002), Time travel with Oliver Twist—towards an explanation for a paradoxically low mortality among recent immigrants, *Tropical Medicine and International Health*, **7**, 4–10.
Razum, O., H. Zeeb, U. Meesmann, L. Schenk, M. Bredehorst, P. Brzoska, T. Dercks, S. Glodny, B. Menkhaus, R. Salman, A-C. Saß and R. Ulrich (2008), *Migration und Gesundheit. Schwerpunktbericht der Gesundheitsberichterstattung des Bundes*, Berlin: Robert Koch-Institut.
Reeske, A., S. Spallek and O. Razum (2009), Changes in smoking prevalence among first- and second-generation Turkish migrants in Germany – an analysis of the 2005 Microcensus, *International Journal for Equity in Health*, **8**, 26.
Reeske, A., J. Spallek, K. Bammann, G. Eiben, S. De Henauw, Y. Kourides, P. Nagy and W. Ahrens (2013), Migrant background and weight gain in early infancy: results from the German study sample of the IDEFICS study, *PLoS ONE*, **8**(4), e60648.
Ringbäck Weitoft, G., A. Gullberg, A. Hjern and M. Rosén, M. (1999), Mortality statistics in immigrant research: method for adjusting underestimation of mortality, *International Journal of Epidemiology*, **28**, 756–763.
Robert Koch-Institut (2008) *KiGGS 2003–2006: Kinder und Jugendliche mit Migrationshintergrund in Deutschland*, Berlin: Robert Koch-Institut.
Sauer, P. J. and D. Neubauer (2013), Female genital mutilation: a hidden epidemic (statement from the European Academy of Paediatrics), *European Journal of Pediatrics*, **173**, 237–238.
Siegrist, J. and M. G. Marmot (2006), *Social Inequalities in Health: New Evidence and Policy Implications*, Oxford: Oxford University Press.
Singh, G. K. and R. A. Hiatt (2006), Trends and disparities in socioeconomic and behavioural characteristics, life expectancy, and cause-specific mortality of native-born and foreign-born populations in the United States, 1979–2003, *International Journal of Epidemiology*, **35**, 903–919.
Spallek, J. and O. Razum (2008), Gleich und gerecht? Erklärungsmodelle für die gesundheitliche Situation von Migrantinnen und Migranten, in U. Bauer, U. H. Bittlingmayer and M. Richter (eds.), *Health Inequalities. Determinanten und Mechanismen gesundheitlicher Ungleichheit*, Wiesbaden: VS Verlag für Sozialwissenschaften.
Spallek, J. and O. Razum (2016), Migration und Gesundheit aus Geschlechterperspektive, in P. Kolip and K. Hurrelmann (eds.), *Handbuch Geschlecht und Gesundheit – Männer und Frauen im Vergleich*, Bern: Hans Huber.
Spallek, J., M. Arnold, S. Hentschel and O. Razum (2009), Cancer incidence rate ratios of Turkish immigrants in Hamburg, Germany: a registry based study, *Cancer Epidemiology*, **33**, 413–418.
Spallek, J., H. Zeeb and O. Razum (2010), Prevention among immigrants: the example of Germany, *BMC Public Health*, **10**, 92.
Spallek, J., H. Zeeb and O. Razum (2011), What do we have to know from migrants' past exposures to understand their health status? A life course approach, *Emerging Themes in Epidemiology*, **8**, 6.
Spallek, J., H. Zeeb and O. Razum (2014), Life course epidemiology: a conceptual model for the study of migration and health, in M. B. Schenker, X. Castaneda and A. Rodriguez-Lainz (eds.), *Migration and Health: A Research Methods Handbook*, Berkeley, CA: University of California Press.
Statistisches Bundesamt (2014), Pressemitteilung Nr. 402/14.
Stirbu, I., A. E. Kunst, F. A. Vlems, O. Visser, V. Bos, W. Deville, H. G. Nijhuis and J. W. Coebergh (2006), Cancer mortality among 1st and 2nd generation migrants in the Netherlands: convergence towards the rates of the native Dutch population, *International Journal of Cancer*, **119**, 2665–2672.

Taveras, E. M., M. W. Gillman, K. Kleinman, J. W. Rich-Edwards and S. L. Rifas-Shiman (2010), Racial/ethnic differences in early-life risk factors for childhood obesity, *Pediatrics*, **125**, 686–695.
UN (2013), *Department of Economic and Social Affairs, Population Division: Trends in International Migration Stock, the 2013 Revision*, available online at http://esa.un.org/unmigration/TIMSA2013/migrantstocks2013.htm.
Urquia, M. L. and A. J. Gagnon (2011), Glossary: migration and health, *Journal of Epidemiology and Community Health*, **65**, 467–472.
Wallace, M. and H. Kulu (2014), Low immigrant mortality in England and Wales: a data artefact? *Social Science and Medicine*, **120**, 100–109.
White, J. B. (1997), Turks in the New Germany, *American Anthropologist*, **99**, 754–769.
WHO (2011), *Migration and Health in the European Union*, New York: Open University Press.
Wilkinson, R. G. and M. Marmot (2003), *Social Determinants of Health: The Solid Facts*, Copenhagen: WHO.

4 Migration and health behaviour

Hiranthi Jayaweera

INTRODUCTION: WHAT IS HEALTH BEHAVIOUR?

Most current research and writing on health-related behaviour refer to lifestyle-associated modifiable individual or group actions such as dietary preferences, physical exercise, smoking, alcohol consumption, recreational drug use and sexual behaviour. Such behaviours could either be health-enhancing or health-impairing, the latter implicated as 'risk factors' for morbidity and mortality with respect to a range of diseases (Conner 2002). Public health approaches – for instance, National Institute for Health and Clinical Excellence (NICE) guidance – characterise health behaviour as not entirely attributable to individual responsibility and free choice but as needing to be viewed in relation to the structures and contexts in which it occurs (NICE 2007). However, academic and health policy accounts of health behaviour vary according to the emphasis placed on individualistic lifestyle approaches versus a broader perspective connecting the individual to his or her physical and social environment with an emphasis on structural constraints as well as choices (Duncan et al. 1996).

MIGRATION AND HEALTH BEHAVIOUR

Around 1 billion people are at present mobile globally, and about a quarter of these are international migrants (IOM 2014). There is considerable research and policy interest in the relationship between migration and health behaviour, much of it revolving around the impact of health behaviour on health outcomes when people move from one place to another (Jayaweera 2014). Both internal and international migration have been studied, particularly in relation to the role of health behaviour in the occurrence of disease and in causes of mortality of migrants (McKay et al. 2003). Research and policy concern is directed towards two empirically somewhat separate areas of health behaviour, both of which are seen to have serious public health implications including on the provision and cost of health services. One strand is the way health behaviour of migrants is implicated in the transmission of infectious diseases such as TB and HIV, and more recently the spread of virus-borne diseases such as pandemic flu and Ebola. The focus here may for instance be on 'risky' communication associated with mobility and/or on healthcare-seeking attitudes and behaviour once migrants are in receiving contexts. The second strand relates to the increasing 'global burden' of non-communicable (chronic) diseases (NCDs) such as cardiovascular illnesses and cancers (Lim et al. 2012), and its link to migration. However, maternal health behaviour that impacts on birth and infant outcomes could also be included. The emphasis in this strand is on health behaviour of recent migrants and possible behavioural changes among migrants over time in destination countries – for example in diet and physical activity, smoking and alcohol consumption – that constitute a significant positive or negative effect on NCD morbidity and mortality and/or on maternal health and birth outcomes. That is, health behaviour is seen as an explanation of risk in these outcomes.

The aim of this chapter is to provide a broad overview of theoretical approaches and empirical evidence on the second research and policy-related strand, the relationship between migration and migrants' health behaviour with regard to NCD mortality, prevalence and risk, and to an extent with regard to maternal health and birth outcomes, as similar types of health behaviour are implicated in both areas. The chapter will be limited to international migration in keeping with the largest proportion of studies in this area (McKay et al. 2003). Crossing national borders has specific implications for the health of migrants that require separate consideration from health issues that are linked with internal migration. While taking a 'receiving country' perspective, with emphasis on migrants in high-income countries in the Global North, the chapter reflects on the importance of countries of origin of migrants for gaining a better understanding of their health behaviour and its contribution to health outcomes.

Migrant Mortality and Morbidity

Reviews of international studies on migrant mortality and morbidity patterns show that to a greater or lesser extent the health of migrants is likely to differ, initially at least, from that of non-migrants both in the country they migrate to and in the country they migrate from (McKay et al. 2003; Agyemang et al. 2013). As McKay et al. (2003) point out, both sending and receiving contexts and the migration process itself are key influences on migrant health status. There is no evidence of a definitive pattern in the direction of change as to whether migrants' health is better or worse than that of non-migrants in countries of origin or destination country-born populations, and many factors affect outcomes at individual, group, local area and country levels. The evidence is complicated by the way data is collected and analysed in different countries (Rafnsson and Bhopal 2009).

For instance, in the UK, while death registration is according to country of birth, hospital data and cancer and cardiovascular disease (CVD) registers record ethnicity but not country of birth, which makes it difficult to understand NCD patterns among migrants. Better data linkage as in the case of Scandinavian countries (Bo et al. 2015; Hedlund et al. 2007) is, however, increasingly making a significant difference to knowledge (Bhopal et al. 2010; Harding 2004). Further, many epidemiological studies group people according to regional categories such as 'South Asian' and 'African', partly because of small numbers in some groups. This practice tends to mask heterogeneity in country of birth, ethnicity and religion, which have been shown to be associated with differences in health outcomes and risk factors (Zaman and Bhopal 2013). Variable quality in numerator (disease incidence) and denominator (population) data in countries migrants come from also makes comparison difficult (Agyemang et al. 2013; McLennan and Jayaweera 2014).

Patterns of disease incidence and cause-specific mortality among migrants in receiving countries vary by country of birth of the migrants and by the disease examined. This can be seen very clearly in the case of outcomes that have been linked with health behaviour. For example, in the early 2000s in England and Wales, the highest death rates from coronary heart disease (CHD) were among migrants from the Indian subcontinent while the highest stroke mortality rates were among migrants of Caribbean and African origin. At the same time, Caribbean migrants had around half the coronary mortality rate of people born in England and Wales (Harding et al. 2008). Similar high rates of coronary disease incidence among South Asian-origin men and women compared to other population groups have been reported in Scotland, although more recent analyses suggest that longer-term survival rates among South Asians are no worse than for other groups despite higher prevalence of diabetes (Zaman and Bhopal 2013). Hypertension and diabetes are closely linked with CVD outcomes and there is evidence of higher rates of hypertension among West African migrants in Europe compared to white populations, which clearly contribute to higher stroke risk among the former (Agyemang et al. 2013). The highest age-adjusted diabetes mortality rates were recorded among South Asian migrants, especially Pakistanis, in Denmark and in England and Wales (Vandenheede et al. 2012).

Associations have been found between differences in CVD outcomes in migrant groups and different patterns of health behaviour, although the evidence specifically for migrants is limited. For example, a more favourable cholesterol profile among African-descent populations in Europe has been considered to contribute towards their lower coronary mortality and morbidity risk compared to other populations, and there is evidence that older African-Caribbeans, who are more likely to have migrated to the UK, have a higher intake of a more traditional Caribbean diet of fruits and vegetables than their younger, UK-born counterparts, thus contributing to a protective effect on heart disease (Agyemang et al. 2009). However, other risk factors such as genetic predisposition and physiological differences, such as metabolism and adiposity, in interaction with behavioural factors such as physical activity and calorie intake have also been discussed; for example, with references to the greater susceptibility of South Asian groups compared to some other migrant and receiving country populations to Type 2 diabetes and heart disease (Bhopal 2012; Zaman and Bhopal 2013).

Mortality from all cancers combined appears highest among people born in Scotland and Ireland who have migrated to England and Wales, and relatively low among migrants from most other countries, compared to people born in England and Wales (Wild et al. 2006). There are sex and country of birth differences in relation to individual cancers, and changes across generations. For example, higher mortality ratios were reported for breast cancer among West African born women than for women born in England and Wales and those born in the Indian subcontinent (Wild et al. 2006). In Scotland, while lung cancer incidence rates were lower for most ethnic minority groups compared to white Scottish, rates for women were lower than for men and Scottish-born people in most ethnic minority groups had higher rates than those born abroad (Bhopal et al. 2012). There is evidence that in general, age-standardised mortality rates among migrants rise with increasing length of residence in receiving countries and that declines in death rates over time are smaller for many migrant groups compared to the receiving country-born population, at least in England and Wales (Harding 2003a, 2004; Harding et al. 2008). As discussed later in the chapter, while changes in health behaviour may play an important part in migrants' vulnerability to ill health over time in the receiving country, other – non-biological, non-genetic – risk factors such as access to healthcare, poverty, uncertain legal status, stress and racism have been identified in studies (McLennan and Jayaweera 2014). For example, Harding found that downward social mobility was associated with reported limiting long-term illness more among South Asian and Caribbean migrants in England and Wales than among all others in the study (Harding 2003b).

Less attention has been given to how migrant health outcomes in receiving societies compare with those among populations 'left behind' in countries of origin. The 'healthy migrant thesis' posits that generally it is the healthiest and most able-bodied among local populations who migrate in search of better opportunities than can be found in countries of origin. Lower mortality and morbidity rates among some migrant groups relative to receiving country populations have also been cited as evidence to support this thesis (Abraído-Lanza et al. 2005; Razum et al. 1998; Norredam et al. 2012). However, as shown earlier, there is no uniform evidence that migrants are healthier than people in countries they move to; there are too many variables to be accounted for including socioeconomic factors before and after migration (McLennan and Jayaweera 2014). Similarly, it is clear that there are many reasons for migration, including the need to flee political persecution or environmental disasters, or for family unification (Blinder 2014), and health may not be a primary determining factor. While country-of-origin health evidence for migrants from lower-income to higher-income countries is limited and variable, there is evidence that NCD prevalence and mortality is increasing in lower- and middle-income countries in the Global South, especially in urban areas. Globally, almost three-quarters of NCD-related deaths and 82 per cent of NCD deaths below age 70 occur in low- and middle-income countries (WHO 2015). For instance, a population-based survey in Sri Lanka showed both high national rates of hypertension, diabetes and obesity as key risk factors for CVD and regional and sex differences in the prevalence of these conditions (Wijewardene et al. 2005). A study comparing Sri Lankans in Kandy, Sri Lanka and Oslo, Norway showed unfavourable if different CVD risk factors among participants in both locations: migrant Sri Lankans in Oslo had higher rates of obesity while the local sample in Kandy had higher cholesterol levels (Tennakoon et al. 2010). A comparative study of overweight and obesity among Ghanaians living in both rural and urban areas in Ghana and among Ghanaian migrants in the Netherlands found that there was an increasing gradient in overweight and obesity among migrants from rural areas to urban areas in Ghana (and to Amsterdam), even when adjusted for age and education (Agyemang et al. 2008).

The lack of a uniform pattern of NCD mortality and morbidity among migrants compared to populations in receiving countries and in countries of origin highlighted in the above section shows that it is important to consider many possible factors that have been identified that may be associated with health outcomes for migrants in receiving countries. Following a brief consideration of birth outcomes for migrant mothers in the next section, this chapter turns to explanations that have been put forward for migrant health outcomes, and the role of health behaviour in such explanations.

Migrant Mothers and Birth Outcomes

The number of births to migrant mothers in high income countries in Europe and North America is increasing. In the UK in 2014, more than a quarter of births (27 per cent) were to mothers born outside the UK, and somewhat similar percentages are found in other countries (Office for National Statistics 2015; Zeitlin et al. 2013; Urquia et al. 2010a). In some London boroughs, the percentage of births to non-UK born mothers is more than half of total births (Office for National Statistics 2015), thus highlighting the public health importance of attention to maternal and infant health outcomes of migrants. Studies have investigated birth outcomes such as birthweight, gestational age at birth of infants and perinatal mortality of infants born to migrant mothers but fewer studies have investigated the perinatal health of migrant mothers themselves (Urquia et al. 2010a, 2010b; Leon and Moser 2012; Gagnon et al. 2011). In this chapter we are concerned with research that has examined a possible link between maternal health behaviour and birth outcomes and/or maternal health among migrants, rather than the much broader topic of birth outcomes in themselves. As in the case of adult migrant mortality, some studies highlight an 'epidemiological paradox' in better birth outcomes relating to foetal growth (for example birthweight, gestational age) among migrant mothers than can be expected given the socioeconomic disadvantages of many migrant groups compared with receiving country populations; this phenomenon has especially been noted with reference to Hispanic migrant mothers in the United States who have more favourable birth outcomes than either US-born non-Hispanic white women or US-born Hispanic women (Flores et al. 2012). The reasons for both such seemingly paradoxical birth outcomes and their erosion in subsequent generations in the receiving country have been the subject of debate, as shown later in this chapter. However, international reviews of migrant mothers have documented mixed patterns depending on the country or region of birth of the mother, and receiving country. Notably, black or Hispanic migrant mothers in the United States were less likely to have low birthweight or preterm babies than black or Hispanic mothers born in the US but there was little difference for Asian mothers, suggesting convergence to prevailing differential patterns of ethnic and socioeconomic inequality in birth outcomes in the US rather than a uniform loss of a protective effect of migration in subsequent generations (Urquia et al. 2010a).

Other studies document poorer outcomes for babies of migrant mothers, such as infant mortality and low birthweight. For instance, infant mortality rates in the UK are highest among Caribbean-born and Pakistan-born mothers, although there is some evidence of lower infant mortality among babies of non-UK born mothers compared to babies born to UK-born women in the same broad ethnic groups of white, Asian and black (Gray et al. 2009; Oakley et al. 2009). Risk factors for infant death include socioeconomic, genetic and maternal behavioural factors, which also vary according to ethnicity and country of birth of babies' parents and are difficult to disentangle from each other (Gray et al. 2009). These risk factors may also be implicated in patterns of low birth. For instance Leon and Moser's secondary analysis of national linked routine data showed that mean birthweight among Bangladeshi, Indian and Pakistani mothers in England and Wales is lower than among white British mothers irrespective of whether the former is a migrant or not (although babies of the migrants were slightly heavier than babies of UK-born counterparts), suggesting the possible importance of genetic effects that may not change much across generations, over any significant health advantages of being a migrant (Leon and Moser 2012). On the other hand, a study in urban Ontario, Canada showed a linear increasing risk of preterm birth in migrant mothers from lower to higher than that of non-migrants (rather than convergence) according to length of residence of migrants from most world regions (Urquia et al. 2010b), suggesting that time in the receiving country rather than generational change may be useful for examining other, non-biological factors such as health behaviour.

Explanations of Migrant Health Outcomes

Within a broader framework, the key determinants of morbidity and mortality at a population level in any country are seen in the literature to include genetic, physiological, behavioural/lifestyle and psychosocial factors and access to and quality of healthcare (WHO 2015). Among these, change in health behaviour is viewed in many accounts as one of the most prominent risk factors for both NCD and birth outcomes among migrants but it is important to consider the contribution of behaviour to health outcomes in relation to other possible contributors.

The risk factors for health outcomes set out in Box 4.1 apply to both migrants and non-migrants anywhere in the world. Note that biological factors such as hypertension, diabetes and obesity are health outcomes in themselves, affected by behavioural, socioeconomic and service access risks, and are on the pathway to NCDs such as heart disease/stroke or poorer birth outcomes. In the case of migrants, risks for health outcomes operate within a framework of legal migration status that may have significant impact on socioeconomic circumstances, health behaviour and access to healthcare, such as in the case of irregular migrants (Davies et al. 2011). The focus of the remaining part of this chapter is on health behaviour as

BOX 4.1 RISK FACTORS FOR HEALTH OUTCOMES

- **Genetic/intra-uterine**: includes sex, age, and 'race' as well as individual/family genetic make-up
- **Biological**: high blood pressure (hypertension), high blood sugar (diabetes), lipid levels, obesity
- **Behavioural**: insufficient uptake of healthy foods especially vegetables and fruit; tobacco, alcohol, physical inactivity, stress
- **Socioeconomic**: economic activity, occupation, income, living conditions, area of residence (includes availability of green spaces, prevalence of junk food eating places)
- **Access to and uptake of health services**
- **Ethnic density and social support**

a risk factor for health outcomes. It considers health behaviour in relation to other risk factors set out in Box 4.1 and the extent to which some of the other risk factors are in themselves determinants of health behaviour.

As shown earlier in the chapter, associations have been made in studies, between health outcomes of migrant groups and patterns of health behaviour as risk factors for these outcomes. However, making associations and correlations in quantitative terms is different from exploring such associations in more depth and attempting to view these within conceptual frameworks. It is to such an approach that the following section turns.

MIGRANT HEALTH BEHAVIOUR AND ACCULTURATION

Many studies reviewed incorporate the premise that as people migrate to a new society they become vulnerable to unhealthy lifestyles such as smoking, alcohol consumption and nutritionally deficient diet (Davies et al. 2011; Hawkins et al. 2008). However, it is important to examine the validity of this claim more closely with reference to research evidence *and* to the way evidence is framed and explained in studies. A commonly employed theoretical framework surrounding changes in health behaviour of migrants as risk factors for health outcomes is that of 'acculturation'. Deriving from broader twentieth-century anthropological and sociological approaches on migrants' loss of original culture and the adoption of values, beliefs and behaviour prevalent in receiving societies (Hunt et al. 2004), it has largely been applied in health research as an attempt to explain the decline – over time or by other indicators – of initially positive health behaviour and risk factor profiles of Latin American migrants in the US (Abraído-Lanza et al. 2005). However, the concept is also present in the literature on the health of other migrant groups in the US, and migrants in other countries (Davies et al. 2011; Delavari et al. 2013), and often used loosely as 'a given' term with reference to changes in migrants' health after migration, even in studies that do not necessarily engage with it more theoretically. The aim of this part of the chapter is to subject this widely used concept of acculturation in its application to migrant health behaviour to critical scrutiny predominantly with regard to types of health behaviour that have been highlighted in the literature as being important for NCD and birth outcomes as discussed above, particularly smoking, alcohol consumption and diet.

First, there may not be a strong indication of a singular pattern of migrant health behaviour in receiving countries that is prior to, or the result of, perceived 'acculturation'. There is evidence that smoking and alcohol consumption patterns vary according to ethnicity, country of origin (including exposure prior to migration), and general population demographic determinants of such behaviour including sex and age (Bhopal et al. 2012; Agyemang et al. 2009, 2013). While migrant-specific data on health behaviour is limited in high-income countries in Europe, heterogeneity in smoking prevalence has been found among both African and South Asian-descent populations. A unique analysis of intergenerational patterns of health behaviour in the Health Survey for England (HSE) 1999 and 2004, for example, reported percentages of non-smokers that varied widely across ethnic groups (black Caribbean, Indian, Pakistani, Bangladeshi, Chinese, Irish, white) and between migrants and the UK-born within the different ethnic minority groups. The age and sex-adjusted odds of smoking for the second generation versus the first generation also varied considerably, the highest odds being among black Caribbeans and the lowest among Chinese (Smith et al. 2009). Smoking rates among African-Caribbean men and women in the HSE 2004 were similar to those in the general population but there were lower rates among sub-Saharan men, and especially women (Agyemang et al. 2009). Similarly, in the same survey, Bangladeshi men had far higher smoking rates than whites, Pakistanis and Indians, but Bangladeshi women – in common with other South Asian women – had very low rates (Zaman and Bhopal 2013).

Alcohol consumption has been found to vary by religion, with Muslims among ethnic minority groups reporting lower consumption compared to other religious groups (Mckeigue and Karmi 1993). Research in countries of origin of South Asian migrants, such as the global case-control Interheart study of coronary risk factors, showed very similar patterns to those among migrant counterparts in receiving countries: for instance, high rates of current and former smoking among Bangladeshi men, lower levels of smoking and alcohol consumption among women in all South Asian countries, and low alcohol consumption in predominantly Muslim countries of Pakistan and Bangladesh (Joshi et al. 2007). These patterns suggest that changes in health behaviour after migration, and according to ethnicity in the UK, may not be as clear-cut or uniform as set out in the acculturation thesis. A multivariate analysis of migrant mothers of infants in a UK national population survey in 2001/2002 showed that while lower rates of smoking and alcohol consumption remained among many minority ethnic groups compared to white British mothers even after adjusting for length of residence and sociodemographic circumstances, a linear trend of increasing smoking and alcohol consumption according to length of residence in the UK disappears after adjusting for ethnicity and sociodemographic variables (Jayaweera and Quigley 2010). A recent review of pregnancy diets of women in low-income countries also examined whether women change their dietary practices in pregnancy when they migrated to high-income countries. This showed a mixed response, with varying influences of transnational connections, networks of co-ethnics in receiving countries and advice of health professionals (D'Souza et al. 2015).

Second, alongside the premise that the adoption of unhealthy behaviour by migrants is inevitable when they move to affluent Western societies, there is an idea inherent in some acculturation accounts of essentially one mainstream receiving country behavioural pattern that migrants are adopting. This assumption has been heavily criticised by commentators. In a systematic review of articles on Hispanic health and acculturation in the US, for example, Hunt et al. point out that none of the articles attempted a definition of 'mainstream' culture, instead relying on 'pervasive references to an unexamined, presumably homogenous dominant society . . . to which the ethnic group members are thought to be adapting' (Hunt et al. 2004: 977). Given that in any society there are demographic and socioeconomic differences or gradients in population health outcomes and health behaviour, as, for example, in the socioeconomic gradients in smoking, obesity, lack of physical exercise and unhealthy diet in England (Marmot et al. 2010), it is far more likely that migrants, for whatever reason, manifest health behaviours that are common to specific groups, whether these are, for example, economic, ethnic or locality based. 'Segmented assimilation' approaches may provide a more useful framework to understand these behavioural processes, emphasising the existence of different reference groups and varied patterns of interaction (Abraído-Lanza 2006). More ethnographic research in local areas is needed to understand specific patterns of, and influences on, health behaviour among different migrant populations.

Third, most studies of acculturation and health behaviour use proxy indicators to measure acculturation. Commonly these are length of residence in the receiving country, proficiency in the language of the receiving country or generational status, although some studies build these and other indicators such as participation in receiving country networks, into standardised acculturation scales (Delavari et al. 2013; Reiss et al. 2015). It is reported that some health behaviours of migrants, such as smoking, may change the longer they live in the receiving country or by receiving country language proficiency or educational level (Reiss et al. 2015), although the evidence on migrant mothers in the UK cited above shows that it is not possible to generalise to all migrants. It is however, difficult to see a logical progression from a tangible, empirically tested, association – say between time in the country and smoking behaviour – to a more nebulous conclusion that the migrants are 'more acculturated' or 'less acculturated' in terms of adopting the 'culture' of the receiving society presumed as different from the 'culture' of a migrant's country of origin (Hunt et al. 2004). There may be more valid and empirically testable reasons why changes in behaviour take place, including the role of structural opportunities or constraints. Obesogenic environmental factors such as the proliferation of cheap neighbourhood fast food outlets catering to religious preferences have, for example, been shown to be associated with dietary practices among adolescent children of migrant Bangladeshi parents in a deprived East London area (Lofink 2010). This research study brings out the complex way in which *home* (parental food practices) interacting with *school* (limited food choice and lack of policies on sweet and fatty food consumption) and *street* (country of origin food availability in the local area as well as the easy availability of local fast food) environments contribute to increasing likelihood of overweight and obesity among young people. Rather than operating within a reductive 'acculturation' approach, this and other studies of changes in food behaviour of migrants in receiving countries suggest the importance of explanations that bring together physical, economic, cultural and political factors; for instance, the possible impact of time poverty in sourcing and preparing healthy food resulting from employment patterns such as shift work and long working hours or the complex interaction between food, transnational identity, and social life in the new environment (Jayaweera 2014; Basnayake and Chenhall 2013). Other research has focused on the positive effect of the availability of social support, mainly from family and relatives, on some health behaviours such as diet quality among pregnant Mexican-American women who are long-stay migrants in the US (Harley and Eskenazi 2006) or the protective effect of living in an area where large numbers of co-ethnics live (ethnic density) on the decreased likelihood of alcohol consumption across ethnic groups in England (Becares et al. 2009). Such findings challenge simplistic linear acculturation arguments and show the importance of considering complex ways in which multiple factors affect health behaviour and outcomes.

ACCESS TO HEALTHCARE

As set out in Box 4.1, health behaviour is only one, if key, factor affecting NCD and birth outcomes of migrants. It is beyond the scope of this chapter to unravel the complexities around the relative contribution of medical (genetic, physiological), social, cultural, economic and political influences on health outcomes. However, one risk factor that is useful to mention here is access to and uptake of healthcare as it also interacts with health behaviour; for instance, in seeking treatment for health conditions. Stratification of rights to healthcare for migrants in many high-income receiving countries leads to a situation where undocumented migrants or those with uncertain legal status lack access to essential health services on the same basis as citizens or permanent residents, thereby negatively affecting their healthcare-seeking behaviour, with implications for poorer health outcomes (Kelly et al. 2005; Doctors of the World 2010). While there is limited evidence according to migration variables – country of birth, length of residence, legal status in the receiving country – ethnic inequalities in uptake of cancer screening and antenatal care have been documented in the UK (Webb et al. 2004; Jayaweera and Quigley 2010). Attendance at appointments is affected by lack of information, limited provision of interpreting services, travel constraints because of poverty, as well as stereotyping and discrimination by healthcare providers, rather than simple behavioural choice (Thomas et al. 2005). Counterbalancing migrants' own health with life stressors and transnational obligations may also be a factor affecting access to healthcare, thus highlighting contextual influences related to migration. For example, a qualitative study of migrant women's participation in mammography screening in Denmark showed that beyond direct destination country influences such as language and travel barriers and lack of translation/interpreting support, other factors such as time, finances and attention focused on important family commitments in countries of origin had impact on lower participation in screening compared to Danish-born women (Kessing et al. 2013).

CONCLUSION

This chapter has attempted to relate particular health outcomes of migrants in receiving countries, namely chronic diseases such as CVD and cancers as well as birth outcomes of migrant mothers, to health behaviours that have been demonstrated in research to constitute a risk to these outcomes, alongside other risk factors. By viewing morbidity and mortality patterns of migrants and birth outcomes within a framework that encompasses both sending and receiving country contexts and complex, varied determinants, this chapter has tried to point out some of the weaknesses of the widely used 'acculturation' approaches that to a greater or lesser extent dominate research studies and commentaries with regard to migrant health behaviour. This chapter has also reiterated the importance of moving beyond associations between health behaviour and health outcomes among migrants to exploring multifaceted explanations of change in health behaviour and health outcomes. This account suggests the importance for health policy of going beyond a simple linear focus on change in health behaviour of migrants in receiving countries, for example from 'low' to 'high' smoking levels or 'healthy' to 'unhealthy' diets, and on individual responsibility and choice in change, to formulate interventions that relate more to the contexts and influences that shape health behaviour and health outcomes of migrants.

REFERENCES

Abraído-Lanza, A. F., M. T. Chao and K. R. Florez (2005), Do healthy behaviours decline with greater acculturation? Implications for the Latino mortality paradox, *Social Science and Medicine*, **61**(2005), 1243–1255.

Abraído-Lanza, A. F., A. N. Armbrister, K. R. Flórez and A. N. Aquirre (2006), Toward a theory-driven model of acculturation in public health research, *American Journal of Public Health*, **96**(8), 1342–1346.

Agyemang, C., E. Owusu-Dabo, A. de Jonge, D. Martins, G. Ogedegbe and K. Stronks (2008), Overweight and obesity among Ghanaian residents in the Netherland: how do they weigh against their urban and rural counterparts in Ghana? *Public Health Nutrition*, **12**(7), 909–916.

Agyemang, C., J. Addo, R. Bhopal, G. Aikins Ade and K. Stronks (2009), Cardiovascular disease, diabetes and established risk factors among populations of sub-Saharan African descent in Europe: a literature review, *Globalization and Health*, **5**, 7.

Agyemang, C., A. de-Graft Aikins and R. Bhopal (2013), Ethnicity and cardiovascular health research: pushing the boundaries by including comparison populations in countries of origin, *Ethnicity and Health*, **17**(6), 579–596.

Basnayake, P. and R. Chenhall (2013), Social, cultural and emotive functions of food patterns among a group of South Asians with diabetes, in *Evolving Humanity, Emerging Worlds (IUAES2013): Interdisciplinary perspectives on identity, food and wellbeing of migrants (MMM11)*, 5–10 August, Manchester.

Becares, L., J. Nazroo and M. Stafford (2009), The ethnic density effect on alcohol use

among ethnic minority people in the UK, *Journal of Epidemiology and Community Health*, **65**, 20–25.
Bhopal, R. (2012), A four-stage model explaining the higher risk of Type 2 diabetes mellitus in South Asians compared with European populations, *Diabetic Medicine*, **30**, 35–42.
Bhopal, R., C. Fischbacher, C. Povey, J. Chalmers, G. Mueller, M. Steiner, H. Brown, D. H. Brewster and N. Bansal (2010), Cohort profile: Scottish Health and Ethnicity Linkage Study of 4.65 million people exploring ethnic variation in disease in Scotland, *International Journal of Epidemiology*, **40**, 1168–1175.
Bhopal, R, N. Bansal, M. Steiner and D. H. Brewster (2012), Does the 'Scottish effect' apply to all ethnic groups? All-cancer, lung, colorectal, breast and prostate cancer in the Scottish Health and Ethnicity Linkage Cohort Study, *BMJ Open*, **2**(5), e001957.
Blinder, S. (2014), *Immigration by Category: Workers, Students, Family Members, Asylum Applicants*, Oxford: Migration Observatory at the University of Oxford.
Bo, A., L. Zinckernagel, A. Krasnik, J. H. Petersen and M. Norredam (2015), Coronary heart disease incidence among non-Western immigrants compared to Danish-born people: effect of country of birth, migrant status and income, *European Journal of Preventive Cardiology*, **22**(10), 1281–1289.
Conner, M. (2002), Health behaviors, available onlune at http://userpage.fu-berlin.de/~schuez/folien/conner2002.pdf.
Davies, A. A., C. Blake and P. Dhavan (2011), Social determinants and risk factors for non-communicable diseases (NCDs) in South Asian migrant populations in Europe, *Asia Europe Journal* (2011), **8**, 461–473.
D'Souza, L., H. Jayaweera and K. E. Pickett (2015), Pregnancy diets, migration and birth outcomes, *Health Care for Women International*, in press.
Delavari, M., A. L. Sonderlund, B. Swinburn, D. Mellor and A. Renzaho (2013), Acculturation and obesity among migrant populations in high income countries – a systematic review, *BMC Public Health*, **13**(458).
Doctors of the World (2010), *Impact Report: 2009–2010*, London: Doctors of the World UK.
Duncan, C., K. Jones and G. Moon (1996), Health-related behaviour in context: a multi-level modelling approach, *Social Science and Medicine*, **42** (6), 817–830.
Flores, M.E.S., S. Simonsen, T. A. Manuck, J. M. Dyer and D. K. Turok (2012), The 'Latina epidemiologic paradox': contrasting patterns of adverse birth outcomes in US-born and foreign-born Latinas, *Women's Health Issues*, **22**(5), e501–e507.
Gagnon, A., S. McDermott, J. Rigol-Chachamovich, M. Bandyopadhyay, B. Stray-Pedersen and D. Stewart (2011), International migration and gestational diabetes mellitus: a systematic review of the literature and meta-analysis, *Paediatric and Perinatal Epidemiology*, **25**(6), 575–592.
Gray, R., J. Headley, L. Oakley, J. J. Kurinczuk, P. Brocklehurst and J. Hollowell (2009), *Towards an Understanding of Variations in Infant Mortality Rates between Different Ethnic Groups in England and Wales*, Inequalities in Infant Morality Project Briefing Paper 3, Oxford: National Perinatal Epidemiology Unit.
Harding, S. (2003a), Mortality of migrants from the Indian subcontinent to England and Wales: effect of duration of residence, *Epidemiology*, **14**, 287–292.
Harding, S. (2003b), Social mobility and self-reported limiting long-term illness among West Indian and South Asian migrants living in England and Wales, *Social Science and Medicine*, **56**, 355–361.
Harding, S. (2004), Mortality of migrants from the Caribbean to England and Wales: effect of duration of residence, *International Journal of Epidemiology*, **33**, 382–386.
Harding, S., M. Rosato and A. Teyhan (2008), Trends for coronary heart disease and stroke mortality among migrants in England and Wales, 1979–2003: slow declines notable for some groups, *Heart*, **94**, 463–470.
Harley, K. and B. Eskenazi (2006), Time in the United States, social support and health behaviours during pregnancy among women of Mexican descent, *Social Science and Medicine*, **62**, 3048–3061.
Hawkins, S. S., K. Lamb, T. J. Cole and C. Law (2008), Influence of moving to the UK on

maternal health behaviours: prospective cohort study, *British Medical Journal*, **336**(7652), 1052–1055.

Hedlund, E., A. Lange and N. Hammar (2007), Acute myocardial infarction incidence in immigrants to Sweden: country of birth, time since immigration and time trends over 20 years, *European Journal of Epidemiology*, **22**, 293–503.

Hunt, L.M., S. Schneider and B. Comer (2004), Should 'acculturation' be a variable in health research? A critical review of research on US Hispanics, *Social Science and Medicine*, **59**, 973–986.

IOM (2014), *Global Migration Trends: An Overview*, Geneva: International Organization for Migration Migration Research Division.

Jayaweera, H. (2014), *Health of Migrants in the UK: What Do We Know*, Oxford: Migration Observatory at the University of Oxford.

Jayaweera, H. and M. A. Quigley (2010), Health status, health behaviour and healthcare use among migrants in the UK: evidence from mothers in the Millennium Cohort Study, *Social Science and Medicine*, **71**, 1002–1010.

Joshi, P., S. Islam, P. Pais, S. Reddy, P. Dorairaj, K. Kazmi, M. R. Pandey, S. Hague, S. Mendis, S. Rangarajan and S. Yusuf (2007), Risk factors for early myocardial infarction in south asians compared with individuals in other countries, *JAMA*, **297**(3), 286–294.

Kelly, R., G. Morrell and D. Sriskandarajah (2005), *Migration and Health in the UK*, London: Institute for Public Policy Research.

Kessing, L. L, M. Norredam, A-B. Kvernrod, A. Mygind and M. Kristiansen (2013), Contextualising migrants' health behaviour – a qualitative study of transnational ties and their implications for participation in mammography screening, *BMC Public Health*, **13**, 431.

Leon, D. A. and K. A. Moser (2012), Low birth weight persists in South Asian babies born in England and Wales regardless of maternal country of birth. Slow pace of acculturation, physiological constraint or both: analysis of routine data, *Journal of Epidemiology and Community Health*, **66**(6), 544–551.

Lim, S. S. et al. (2012), A comparative risk assessment of burden of disease and injury attributable to 67 risk factors and risk factor clusters in 21 regions, 1990–2010: a systematic analysis for the Global Burden of Disease Study 2010, *Lancet*, **380**(9859), 2224–2260.

Lofink, H. E. (2010), 'The worst of the Bangladeshi and the worst of the British': exploring eating patterns and practices among British Bangladeshi adolescents in East London, *Ethnicity & Health*, **17**(4), 385–401.

Marmot, M., J. Allen, P. Goldblatt, T. Boyce, D. McNeish, M. Grady and I. Geddes (2010), *Fair Society, Healthy Lives*, London: The Marmot Review.

McKay, L., S. Macintyre and A. Ellaway (2003), *Migration and Health: A Review of the International Literature*, Glasgow: MRC Social and Public Health Sciences Unit.

Mckeigue, P. M. and G. Karmi (1993), Alcohol consumption and alcohol-related problems in Afro-Caribbeans and South Asians in the United Kingdom, *Alcohol & Alcoholism*, **28**(1), 1–10.

McLennan, A. K. and H. Jayaweera (2014), *Non-Communicable Diseases and Risk Factors in Migrants from South Asian Countries*, Oxford: Centre on Migration, Policy and Society.

NICE (2007), *Behaviour Change: General approaches*, Manchester: National Institute for Health and Clinical Excellence.

Norredam, M., M. Olsbjerg, J. Petersen, K. Juel and A. Krasnik (2012), Inequalities in mortality among refugees and immigrants compared to native Danes – a historical prospective cohort study, *BMC Public Health*, **12**, 757.

Oakley, L., N. Maconochie, P. Doyle, N. Dattani and K. Moser (2009), Multivariate analysis of infant death in England and Wales in 2005–06, with focus on socio-economic status and deprivation, *Health Statistics Quarterly*, **42**, 22–39.

Office for National Statistics (2015), *Births in England and Wales by Parents' Country of Birth, 2014*, Statistical Bulletin, Titchfield, Hampshire: Office for National Statistics.

Rafnsson, S. B. and R. Bhopal (2009), Large-scale epidemiological data on cardiovascular diseases and diabetes in migrant and ethnic minority groups in Europe, *European Journal of Public Health*, **19**(5), 484–491.

Razum, O., H. Zeeb, H.S. Akgün and S. Yilmaz (1998), Low overall mortality of Turkish residents in Germany persists and extends into a second generation: merely a healthy migrant effect? *Tropical Medicine and International Health*, **3**(4), 297–303.

Reiss, K., J. Lehnhardt and O. Razum (2015), Factors associated with smoking in immigrants from non-western to western countries – what role does acculturation play? A systematic review, *Tobacco Induced Diseases*, **13**, 11.

Smith, N. R., Y. J. Kelly and J. Y. Nazroo (2009), Intergenerational continuities of ethnic inequalities in general health in England, *Journal of Epidemiology and Community Health*, **63**, 253–258.

Tennakoon, S. U. B., B. N. Kumar, D. B. Nugegoda and H. E. Meyer (2010), Comparison of cardiovascular risk factors between Sri Lankans living in Kandy and Oslo, *BMC Public Health*, **10**, 654.

Thomas, V. N., T. Saleem, and R. Abraham (2005), Barriers to effective uptake of cancer screening among black and minority ethnic groups, *International Journal of Palliative Nursing*, **11**(11), 562–571.

Urquia, M. L., R. H. Glazie, B. Blondel, J. Zeitlin, M. Gissler, A. Macfarlane, E. Ng, M. Heaman, B. Stray-Pedersen and A. J. Gagnon (2010a), International migration and adverse birth outcomes: role of ethnicity, region of origin and destination, *Journal of Epidemiology and Community Health*, **64**, 243–251.

Urquia, M. L., J. W. Frank, R. Moineddin and R. H. Glazier (2010b), Immigrants' duration of residence and adverse birth outcomes: a population-based study, *BJOG*, **117**, 591–601.

Vandenheede, H., P. Deboosere, I. Stirbu, C. O. Agyemang, S. Harding, K. Juel, S. B. Rafnsson, E. Regidor, G. Rey, M. Rosato, J. P. Mackenbach and A. E. Kunst (2012), Migrant mortality from diabetes mellitus across Europe: the importance of socio-economic change, *European Journal of Epidemiology*, **27**(2), 109–117.

Webb, R., J. Richardson, A. Esmail and A. Pickles (2004), Uptake for cervical screening by ethnicity and place of birth: a population-based cross-sectional study, *Journal of Public Health*, **26**(3), 293–296.

Wijewardene K., M. R. Mohideen, S. Mendis, D. S. Fernando, T. Kulathilaka, D. Weerasekara and P. Uluwitta (2005), Prevalence of hypertension, diabetes and obesity: baseline findings of a population based survey in four provinces in Sri Lanka, *Ceylon Medical Journal*, **50**(2), 62–70.

Wild, S. H, C. M. Fischbacher, A. Brock, C. Griffiths and R. Bhopal (2006), Mortality from all cancers and lung, colorectal, breast and prostate cancer by country of birth in England and Wales, 2001–2003, *British Journal of Cancer*, **94**, 1079–1085.

WHO (2015), *The Determinants of Health*, Health Impact Assessment, World Health Organization, available online at www.who.int/hia/evidence/doh/en.

Zaman, M. J. and R. Bhopal (2013), New answers to three questions on the epidemic of coronary mortality in south Asians: incidence or case fatality? Biology or environment? Will the next generation be affected? *Heart*, **99**, 154–158.

Zeitlin, J., A. Mohangoo and M. Delnord (2013), *European Perinatal Health Report: Health and Care of Pregnant Women and Babies in Europe in 2010*, Paris: Euro-Peristat Project.

5 Migration and health through an intersectional lens

Denise L. Spitzer

INTRODUCTION

As one of every 33 people on this planet is a migrant (Levitt and Lamba-Nieves 2013), mobility has become a dominant feature of contemporary societies across the globe. The movements of peoples, households and communities, however, are not uniform, nor are their experiences of wellbeing or their subsequent health outcomes. In this chapter, I unpack some of the prominent characteristics of gender as it intersects with other elements of social stratification that are implicated in the relationship between migration and health status. I begin by situating migration within the current context of neoliberal globalisation and considering its gendered implications. Next I introduce intersectionality and demonstrate how it is implicated in the dynamics of migration and health. Having established the context and explicated key concepts, I move on to an examination of the interactions between intersectionality, migration and health, and argue that an embodied intersectional perspective is vital to understanding responses – and resistance – to the impacts of migration on health and wellbeing.

SETTING THE CONTEXT: MIGRATION AND NEOLIBERAL GLOBALISATION

While migration has been a feature of human history, it has expanded dramatically in recent decades concomitant with both the multitude of political and environmental upheavals that have spurred the departure of populations from their homelands, and the rise of neoliberal globalisation (Cymbal and Bujnowski 2010; Van Hear 2010). Neoliberal globalisation is characterised by intensified, multi-sited, and uneven flows of people, materials and ideas across boundaries and borders, and the demand for an increasingly flexible and migratory labour force to serve attenuated global commodity chains that are strewn across the world's low-income landscapes (Spitzer and Piper 2014). Since the 1970s, the neoliberal agenda that underpins contemporary globalisation has encouraged the withdrawal of state investment in public services in favour of privatisation and global production along with the reduction of state intervention in social protection and in economic trade (Glick Schiller 2009). The multiple impacts of these shifts in the terrain of capital accumulation, production, and decision-making – in essence rapid changes in the sites of political and economic power and who wields it – suggests that 'there are multiple gendered globalisations which have context-specific ramifications [that] are socially constructed, and are locked into an intimate and hierarchical relationship with one another' (Eschle 2004: 116). These globalisations engender restructuring both of sites of production and reproduction, and of trans- and intra-national relations as people traverse borders following movements of capital, production and employment (Dejardin 2008).

A critical examination of neoliberal globalisation including how it operates and how it impacts the peoples and places it encounters requires the deployment – most basically – of a gender lens. As Piper (2011 in Spitzer and Piper 2014) asserts, three major trends of feminisation coalesce under neoliberal globalisation: the feminisation of poverty, work and migration. Notably, women are situated in the most low-waged and precarious positions in global production chains where they are less apt to secure employment benefits and are more vulnerable to lay-offs during economic downturns (Dejardin 2008). Moreover, as migrant workers, women are often recruited into the legions of foreign domestic labourers who serve as the avatars of more prosperous (sometimes only *minimally* more prosperous) women who relinquish their gendered household roles to their foreign-born employees (Özyegin and Hondagneu-Sotelo 2008; Williams and Gavanas 2008).

In countries such as the Philippines and Indonesia, female migrant workers are regarded as economic heroes for contributing to the coffers of national economies and to the budgets of local households who contend with high unemployment and underemployment, increasing costs of living, and low wages in nation-states whose health and social programmes have been degraded in allegiance to neoliberal ideology (Spitzer and Piper 2014). However, counter-discourses are also promulgated wherein overseas women workers are suspected of shirking their gendered responsibilities as mothers, wives and daughters at home; therefore, forwarding remittances to their families helps to mitigate these negative images through the performance of the widely entrenched gender role of the dutiful woman dedicated to family and kin (Spitzer 2014a).

While neoliberal globalisation has indeed led to the increased exploitation of predominantly female labour and furthered the impoverishment of women most notably from the Global South (Hu-Dehart 2003), Davids and Van Driel (2009) caution that the dominant circulating image of the poor 'Third World' woman crushed by global forces effaces complex global-local interactions and possibilities for agency, resistance, and multiple – even contradictory – subjectivities. Furthermore, attention to gender in the context of migration has most generally focused on women and on low-waged women in domestic service in particular, which, although constituting a significant portion of the migrant workforce, does not illuminate the diversity of gendered circumstances and policies under which women and men move, and the variety of jobs they occupy – the range of which deserve our attention (Kofman 2004). The complexity, fluidity and diversity of migratory experiences and the nexus of relations that they generate in which these experiences are situated, as well as the implications for the shifting pastiche of collectivities that are affected by these phenomena, are best understood in the context of intersectionality.

INTERSECTIONALITY AND MIGRATION: AN OVERVIEW

Intersectionality highlights how social indicators or axes of power and domination, such as socioeconomic class, racialisation, ethnicity, gender, sexualities, ability, geographic location, indigenous and immigrant status are composed within broader historical and current systems of colonialism, neo-colonialism and globalisation, and operate as interactive, mutually constituted identity markers that situate individuals and groups within social hierarchy and produce social location (CRIAW 2006b; Varcoe et al. 2007; Webber and Parra-Medina 2003; Yuval-Davis 2007). Possessing both explanatory power and operating as an analytical lens, intersectionality emerged from critical race theory that demonstrates how racism operates subtly and structurally, and advocates that we trouble issues of race and racism rather than mask inequalities by insisting that institutions are 'colour blind' (Warner 2006). Intersectionality is also an outgrowth of gender-based analysis that most often highlights gender as a determinant of life experiences and outcomes, even though in its basic conceptualisation gender-based analysis was also meant to consider factors such as racialisation,[1] socioeconomic class and sexuality (Hankivsky et al. 2010; Spitzer 2006). Further informed by feminist postcolonial thought, intersectional analysis recalls the ways in which colonialism has helped shape the contemporary social landscape, and attends to the shifting power arrangements in neo- and postcolonial contexts that lead to different forms of oppression (Brown et al. 2007).

Simply stated, intersectional analysis is grounded in the notion that different dimensions of social life cannot be segregated as individuals experience the world holistically, as the totality of subject positions. It demands consideration of space, time and historical and localised specificities to understand how persons experience their location in the social landscape (Hankivsky et al. 2010). As Warner (2006) asserts, axes of power and hegemony are interconnected; therefore, we cannot privilege one particular identity without referencing others as is evidenced by the discernibly disparate ways against which individuals and groups are discriminated. An intersectional lens also focuses on the processes that create and reinforce markers of social stratification and illuminates their linkages to individual and communal identities, behaviours and health statuses (Webber and Parra-Medina 2003).

With regards to our topic, intersectionality disrupts the 'god's eye view' of globalisation by insisting on attention to both the multiplicity of standpoints and to the processes as to how these positions were constructed at different scalar levels (Davids and Van Driel 2009; Eschle 2004; Mahler and Pessar 2001). Moreover, given the gendered and racialised stereotypes that inform recruitment of disposable migrant workers from the 'nimble-fingered' Latin American and Asian women who are deemed suited to monotonous factory work (Hu-Dehart 2003) to the childlike and obedient domestic workers from the Philippines (Pratt 1997), intersectional analysis enables us to unpack the interactive nature of these social markers and how they are deployed in the service of neoliberal globalisation. The complexity and dynamics of migration and globalisation cannot be readily explained by dichotomous pairings such as global–local, macro–micro, etc. that permeate migration studies but that are best regarded, as Van Hear (2010) advocates, by examining the complex interplay among these phenomena.

THE INTERSECTIONAL DYNAMICS OF MIGRATION AND WORK

The dynamic interactions of gender, racialised status, socioeconomic class, ethnicity and/or country of origin, underpin the hierarchy that generally constitutes the global migrant labour force. In addition to those who labour in rural areas where they are subject to dispossession of land, women from the Global South engaged in casual and informal labour, the service sector or industries such as textile and clothing that are vulnerable to upheavals in the world market are most apt to pursue work opportunities abroad, although some may migrate for personal and social reasons as well (Lestari 2012; Piper 2004; Spitzer and Piper 2014).

Often the precariousness of their work situations in their homelands is replaced by precarious employment in a new setting where as migrant labourers they earn low wages, are seldom granted employment benefits and have little control over their work environments. In countries such as Canada, more than 40 per cent of all women's jobs can be regarded as precarious, representing a more than 30 per cent increase since the 1980s (Menéndez et al. 2007). Compounding these conditions, migrant workers contend with the added burden of precarious migration status, which often precludes their ability to claim workplace rights and seek redress for workplace abuses through formal channels, to change employers, to be joined by family or to resettle permanently, among other issues. Taken together, these issues act as chronic stressors that, given their diminished access to social resources such as social support, can have profound negative effects on their health and wellbeing, as will be described in further detail in the next section.

In contrast to the predominant relegation of women from the Global South to low-skilled, low-waged migrant labour (and not to deny the experiences of men who are engaged in fields such as construction, agriculture and fisheries, etc.), migrants, primarily men who embody neoliberal values and possess technological skills are increasingly enticed across borders (Jones 2004; Ong 2005). Ong (2005, 2006) deploys the term 'flexible citizenship' to identify the ways in which citizenship has become imbued with notions of entrepreneurship, self-reliance and individualism, which opens doors for desirable individuals to cross borders with ease and entitlements.

Re(productive) Labour

Following Van Hear (2010), I concur that we cannot disaggregate gendered productive and reproductive (both biological and social) roles and encourage us to remain cognizant of how these issues are interactive and mutually constituted. As Wee and Sim (2004: 168) write about these interrelations, 'a labour vacuum emerges which is filled by the insertion of migrant women workers, whose work thereby fits into the prevailing gender division of labour, as well as the existing dichotomisation of state and family responsibilities, respectively for formal economic production and informal social reproduction'.

In addition to their role in productive labour, women are also assigned the responsibility for the work of both social and biological reproduction. Increasingly women in middle- and upper-class households in Europe, the Americas and the Middle East, expanding to working-class households in countries such as Malaysia, delegate social reproductive duties to migrant workers. In the Philippines and Indonesia, the two major migrant-sending countries in Asia, women comprise 60–80 per cent of migrant workers as they are primarily destined to labour in private households as domestic workers regardless of their educational status or occupational background (Rahman and Fee 2009). Foreign domestic workers are particularly vulnerable to economic, social, sexual and physical abuse, as they are sequestered in the homes of their employers, which are generally regarded as private spaces rather than workplaces (Piper 2004; Spitzer and Torres 2008). The duties of domestic workers are closely associated with female gender roles and are presumed to have little monetary value as carrying out these tasks is construed as a labour of love. Moreover, the gendered nature of this work is reflected in policies; for example, countries such as Malaysia prohibit men from entering the country as foreign domestic workers (Immigration Department of Malaysia 2015; Piper 2004).

Even as women workers assume productive roles in the public sphere or in the private homes away from their families, they are still compelled to enact the roles of social reproduction, including transnational parenting, organising care labour and transmitting values and traditions (Kusakabe and Pearson 2010; Parreñas 2005). In the households of migrant women, it is often daughters or other female relatives who take on household responsibilities even when adult men are present. While some men will become more active parents, others – preferring to rely on their wives' remittances – leave their jobs, find other intimate partners and/or move to another location (Carling et al. 2012; Parreñas 2005; Petrozziello and Robert 2010; Spitzer 2014b).

With regards to biological reproduction, some authors suggest that migration provides women with greater opportunities to negotiate sexual boundaries and assert greater control over sexuality and reproduction as they take on new economic and social roles (Espin 1999). Others, however, assert that women are compelled to act as gatekeepers of collective (family, ethnic, religious) boundaries, a role that places them under even greater surveillance from the local community and potentially influences reproductive decision-making (Alvadj 2007). For migrant workers in particular, this surveillance can be more than metaphoric. In Singapore, for instance, foreign domestic workers are subject to biannual pregnancy screenings and are deported should they test positive (Ministry of Manpower 2015; Sobritchea and de Guzman 2006). Moreover, Saudi Arabia in 2003 forbade hospitals from admitting women preparing to give birth without being accompanied by a male who acknowledged paternity – a policy that community activists regarded as targeting migrant women (CARAM Asia 2006). The realities of circular migration also impact workers' reproductive choices as returning to their homelands to carry out a pregnancy may not be an option for them, particularly if family members pressure them to remain abroad to ensure an incoming flow of remittances (Spitzer 2014a). That said, migration may also allow some to circumvent either social and/or familial pressure to bear children or to conform to compulsory heterosexuality and hetero-normative performance. However, both temporary and permanent migrants are still subject to surveillance by members of local ethno-cultural communities, which may further influence expressions of sexuality and reproductive outcomes (Alvadj 2007; O'Neill and Sproule 2011).

THE IMPACTS OF INTERSECTIONALITY AND MIGRATION ON HEALTH

Social Stratification and Migrant Health

Given the stamina required to migrate temporarily or permanently, and the medical screening that is generally required, data from immigrant receiving countries in the Global North at least, demonstrate that migrants are generally in better health than the native-born population (Ng 2011; Ng et al. 2005). Notably, over time this health advantage can decline, with racialised women reporting the most precipitous deterioration in health status (Spitzer 2011; Vissandjée, et al. 2004). This trend can best be explained by the way in which gender, racialisation and migration status interact to populate the dominant hierarchy that informs the global gendered division of labour, and that is reflected in gradations of material and social disadvantage – that is to say, poverty – that underpins health inequities most significantly (Menéndez et al. 2007; Raphael et al. 2005).

Migrants are commonly relegated to jobs that the local population is unwilling to perform, often in poorly regulated work environments where they are subject to noxious occupational hazards – both biological and social (Calderon et al. 2012; Krieger et al. 2006; Rosenstock et al. 2005). Most often, women are thrust into precarious informal labour that can best be described as 'peripheral, insecure, hazardous, and low-paying' (International Labour Organization 2003 in Menéndez et al. 2007: 778). Racialised migrants to Canada, women in particular, are most likely to report a substantial gap between their current employment and their prior education and work experience contributing to a prolonged process of deskilling (Haan 2008; Spitzer and Torres 2008). Importantly, immigrant women in Canada are better-educated than their native-born counterparts; however, both their human and social capital is found lacking by potential employers (Bauder 2003; Chen et al. 2011). While foreign credentials of both women and men are denigrated in comparison to local national standards, women may face additional challenges if the presentation of their social bodies (accents, mode of dress, etc.) is judged as unsuitable for the workplace (VanderPlaat 2007). Job mismatch – where one's employment and education skills are greater than required in one's position – is linked to poor mental health, with each degree of over-qualification enhancing the risk, even when migrants' expectations are already lowered (Chen et al. 2011). In addition, migrant workers frequently experience downward social and economic mobility that in itself has health consequences contributing to conditions such as depression, hypertension and Type 2 diabetes (Krieger et al. 2001; Özyegin and Hondagneu-Sotelo 2008).

The social organisation of labour also has a significant impact on health. For example, control over one's work, the precarity of one's employment status and access to complaint mechanisms that offer remedy to improve working conditions have implications for health and wellbeing contributing to injuries, poor mental health and increased rates of musculoskeletal conditions (Lewchuk et al. 2003; Menéndez et al. 2007; Siviö et al. 2012). Additionally, the global, predominantly female, foreign domestic workforce faces particular challenges as they labour in private households that are generally not recognised as workplaces and are vulnerable to the demands of their employers who may control their workers' rest hours and sleeping arrangements, the quantity and quality of their food, access to health services and to social support including contact with family and friends and rendering myriad forms of abuse (Spitzer and Torres 2008).

Manifestations of racism and sexism further complicate and exacerbate many of the health outcomes that result from the intersections of gender, racialised status, migration and low-income. Racism not only influences the attitudes of healthcare providers and subsequently the care and treatments patients are offered, but it can contribute to a heightened and prolonged stress response that can depress immune function thereby enhancing risk to myriad diseases (Hyman 2009). These stressors, exacerbated by material deprivation, are likely to lead to gendered coping strategies that may result in disparate trends in morbidity and mortality as men are apt to resort to negative health behaviours such as immoderate alcohol and tobacco consumption, while women tend to suppress their emotions and are more likely to succumb to stress-related disorders such as heart disease (Benach et al. 2001).

Social Relationships, Health and Wellbeing

The presence of loved ones and the availability of social support is a powerful determinant of health and wellbeing, particularly for foreign-born members of a society (Dunn and Dyck 2000; Stewart et al. 2008). Familial separation, a common feature of life for migrant workers, can lead to poor mental health and risk-taking behaviours (Calderon et al. 2012; McGuire and Martin 2007). For asylum-seekers and claimants, these sentiments may be particularly acute as they may feel guilt about their relative safety and concomitantly concerned about the whereabouts and wellbeing of family members and friends who may be languishing in refugee camps or whose whereabouts are unknown (Spitzer 2006). 'Worry work' is generally relegated to women who are most often charged with family caregiving responsibilities such as attending to the welfare of their children, parents, siblings or extended family; therefore, women migrants are particularly vulnerable to feelings of guilt and anxiety. Even as women migrant workers from disparate contexts both individually and collectively provide remittances more often and in greater amounts than their male counterparts (Petrozziello and Robert 2010; Rahman and Fee 2009), their physical absence is held responsible for intra-familial tensions and at times the dissolution of spousal relationships (Bernhard et al. 2005; Torres et al. 2012).

Migrants who are reunited with family members on foreign soil may find the joys of reunification tempered by the strains of resettlement that their loved ones confront. As the resident household expert, the (former) sojourner is often burdened with serving as the main source of support for family members as they navigate their new society. Gender ideologies further influence roles and expectations. Female migrants may be expected to tend more closely to family needs and to assume household responsibilities, often while still engaged in precarious work and continuing to forward remittances to those still at home. As Menéndez et al. (2007: 779) state: 'A gender-segregated distribution of non-standard arrangements may be an important determinant of the social patterning of exposures and health outcomes such as mortality, self-perceived health status, mental health, dissatisfaction, or other indicators of quality of life and well-being.' Moreover, in some instances, male partners may resent the need to rely on their wives to orient them to their new setting. The erosion of men's sense of masculinity may contribute to greater marital disharmony, while intergenerational tensions may develop as children negotiate their identities that may differ from those of their parents (Pratt 2006; Spitzer 2014b). Notably, similar disorientation and adjustment can occur when migrants return to their families and home communities (Calderon et al. 2012).

Access to Health Services

Chee and Wong (2009) describe how access to healthcare is informed by the interactions of the characteristics of the community seeking care, the organisation of the healthcare system, and the attitudes and behaviours of health professionals, which are situated within the macro-social context that includes government policies, economic development and gender ideologies. In addition, migrants' access to healthcare services are generally structured by both formal issues (i.e., immigration status, health policy, cost of services) and informal matters (i.e., availability, stigma, racism) that work to constrain or facilitate service uptake. Whereas dominant discourses suggest that migrants are bearers of disease who burden public health systems, the reverse is a more accurate reflection of reality in that migrants tend to underutilise rather than overutilise health services (Calderon et al. 2012; VanderPlaat 2007). Moreover, where migrants' access to healthcare services may be nebulous, underscoring their liminal legal status, health service personnel and healthcare providers can act as either gatekeepers or facilitators negotiating their entry into the system (Villegas 2013).

In addition to migrant status, gender, language, working conditions, socioeconomic status, the organisation of the healthcare system and the coherence between the patients' and the practitioners' conceptualisations of health and medicine, all influence health- and help-seeking behaviours. As female gender often overlaps with low-income and as women are enculturated to place the needs of others ahead of themselves, they are apt to forgo medical assistance in favour of expenditures on other household members (Chee and Wong 2009). Cost and availability of services in terms both of geographic location and hours of operation may inhibit healthcare service uptake, particularly as migrant workers are often engaged in labour over which they have neither control nor health benefits, making it difficult to attend appointments or wait in long queues at public facilities during work hours (Webber et al. 2012). While individuals may make use of self-care or medication available from pharmacists or paraprofessionals, these remedies too may be costly.

Stress: the Embodiment of Inequality

In the context of Western biomedicine, stress generally serves as the black box – the label applied to a host of embodied responses to the world that underscore the connection between mind and body. Exposure to gendered and structural racism, engagement with precarious labour, policies that restrict access to both social support and health services, situated in poverty that influences nutrition, health expenditures and heightens worries, are all informed by gender ideologies. Responses to these issues coalesce with the frequent disappointments faced by individuals who struggle for a better life, but whose efforts are so often unrewarded, generating chronic stress that can have significant negative health effects (Spitzer 2012). As Scheder (1988: 269) concludes in her examination of migrant farmworkers, 'frequent adjustment to stressful life events and life change, compounded by social inequality and psychosocial stress inherent in the migrant lifestyle, act via a series of physiological responses to culminate in hyperglycemia'. Notably, the interactive social and physical assaults on the body have effects that may or may not result in a set of symptoms that are classified as a disease such as Type 2 diabetes or hypertension, but are instead experienced as amorphous pains that like the migrants themselves, travel throughout the body (Coker 2004).

Freund (2006) suggests that the body's response to the social environment is mediated by the neuro-hormonal interactions. Persistently high levels of stress hormones, for example, are linked to reduced immunity and coronary diseases among other conditions, while the ability to cope with the onslaught of stressors is also socially organised and distributed. Various aspects of employment conditions such as high demand–low control situations or effort–reward imbalance engender physiological effects while the disparity between what one has worked for and one's current situation, (i.e., job mismatch as experienced by numerous migrant workers) leads to heightened arousal of the sympathetic nervous system. For racialised, migrant women, and other marginalised individuals and communities such as indigenous peoples and others, the body's response to ongoing social and material disadvantage and injustice can result in symptoms and/or conditions that can best be regarded as the embodiment of inequality (Spitzer 2011).

INTERSECTIONAL AND EMBODIED MIGRANT HEALTH

Health and wellbeing are determined not by the presence or absence of pathogens, symptoms or diagnostic labels, but by perceptions of illness and wellness and the psychosocial, biogenetic and physiological coping mechanisms that can be harnessed in response to the body's expression of its relationship with the world. Situated at once in physical, social, historical, political-economic and individual context, the body is located in global and local social hierarchies upheld by gender ideologies and ethno-racialist constructions. Neoliberal globalisation both structures and profits from maintaining these hierarchies, shaping and reshaping the organisation of productive and reproductive work and allocating and reallocating workers to this labour depending upon their location in the global socioeconomic hierarchy. As noted, racialised migrant women are most likely to be relegated to the lowest echelons of this economic order where poverty, gender and migration coalesce and where they are most vulnerable to precarious employment and migration status.

These processes are facilitated and these structures maintained through discourses imbued by gender, racialist and neoliberal ideologies that promote migration as the key to economic prosperity and women as the financial saviours of family and nation (Spitzer 2014a). It follows that migrant women – many carrying out reproductive labour as productive waged labour in private households – are neither able to relinquish nor fully control their own roles in biological and social reproduction as they remain tasked with earning for their families and embedded in transnational care-work. While there may be genuine satisfaction and pleasure in both providing material and emotional support for loved ones and in fulfilling one's gendered and cultural expectations, these sentiments may yet coincide with disappointments, dissatisfaction and anger as one's efforts and expectations for a better life are frequently met with frustration.

Importantly, the trends portrayed here are brushed in broad strokes and represent in essence a shorthand description that highlights only gender and racialised status. However we must recall how other elements that contribute to social stratification such as migration status, age, socioeconomic class, education, geographic location, ethnic origins, linguistic ability, sexual identity, dis/ability, religion, literacy, among others, result in varied experiences that are best understood through the lens of intersectionality rather than through gender alone. Simply illustrated, a university-educated Filipino lesbian woman from Manila working as a caregiver in a small town in Canada may have a different set of responses to her experiences characterised by deskilling, downward mobility and isolation than a rural born Indonesian woman with elementary education and four children who works as a domestic labourer in Hong Kong who may be overwhelmed by the urban atmosphere and by the relative wealth of her employers, but who may have access to a larger community of support than someone working in small-town Canada. Assuredly, their shared gender and migration status does not allow us to ascribe commonality of experience or outcomes. Furthermore, in either situation, disaggregating each element that composes their current social location is unhelpful as they are mutually constitutive, mutable and are experienced as a whole.

Back to the Body

Returning to the body, the locus of human experience within and from which we inhabit, take up and respond to the world and the context in which we live, is essential. Claimed by the body politic, projecting one's status and identities through – and being responded to because of – our social markers, the individual body inhabits and responds to the multiple and multilayered contexts in which it is situated. That context is determined by the intersections of social stratifiers that influence not only position within the social landscape, but also the availability of personal, social, political, economic and cultural resources from which one can draw – ranging from food, friends and personal fortitude to a strong belief system, 'good' genes and sense of identity. Termed 'resistance resources' by Dressler (1991), these assets can be mobilised to mitigate stress, whether resulting in a constellation of signs and symptoms that can be organised under a nosological category for which one may obtain remediation or as expressed in the inchoate manner that defies such categorisation that I term the embodiment of inequality. In summary, the stress of migration and the subsequent health outcomes that result there from, is wrought – and contextualised – by neoliberal globalisation and informed by gendered, racialist and neoliberal ideologies and discourses. The social distribution of these effects suggests that an intersectional lens is essential in order to comprehend the complexity of the interactions among gender, health and migration in our current context. While the resources through which individuals can moderate these effects are similarly unequally distributed, they are by no means fixed. Social support and social solidarity are critical elements that can be deployed to counter the stressful effects of migration and neoliberal globalisation.

NOTE

1. Racialisation refers to the political and ideological processes of Othering individuals and groups of individuals through relegation to (presumably) immutable racial categories that are, in reality, sociopolitical identities based on biocultural distinctions such as phenotype, ethnic background accent, culture or religion that are linked to particular characteristics and that are assigned a particular social value (CRIAW 2006b; Li 2001; Spitzer 2004). I employ the term, 'racialisation' and 'racialised' to highlight this process and to reinforce the notion 'that race is not an objective biological fact, but rather a social and cultural construct that potentially exposes individuals to racism' (Hyman 2009: 5).

REFERENCES

Alvadj, T. (2007), Immigrant women and fertility: gender under re-construction, in P. Liamputtong (ed.), *Reproduction, Childbearing and Motherhood A Cross-Cultural Perspective*, New York: Nova Science Publisher, pp. 35–46.

Bauder, H. (2003), 'Brain abuse', or the devaluation of immigrant labour in Canada, *Antipode*, **35**(4), 699–717.

Benach, J., Y. Yasui, C. Correll, M. Sáez, and M. Pasarin (2001), Material deprivation and leading causes of death by gender: evidence from a nationwide small area study, *Journal of Epidemiology and Community Health*, **55**, 239–245.

Bernhard, J., P. Landolt and L. Goldring (2005), *Transnational, Multi-Local Motherhood: Experiences of Separation and Reunification Among Latin American Families in Canada*, CERIS Working Paper, Toronto: Joint Centre of Excellence for Research in Immigration and Settlement.

Brown, A., V. Smye and C. Varcoe (2007), Postcolonial-feminist theoretical perspectives and women's health, in M. Morrow, O. Hankivsky and C. Varcoe (eds.), *Women's Health in Canada: Critical Perspectives on Theory and Policy*, Toronto: University of Toronto Press, pp. 124–142.

Calderon, J., B. Rijks and D. Rannveig Aguinas (2012), *Asian Labour Migrants and Health: Exploring Policy Routes*, Bangkok: IOM and MPI.

CARAM Asia (2006), *State of Health of Migrants: Access to Health*, Kuala Lumpur: CARAM Asia Berhad.

Carling, J., C. Menjivar and L. Schmalzbauer (2012), Central themes in the study of transnational parenthood, *Journal of Ethnic and Migration Studies*, **38**(2), 191–217.

Chee, H. L. and Y. L. Wong (2009), Women's access to health care services in Malaysia, in H. L. Chee and S. Barraclough (eds.), *Health Care in Malaysia: The Dynamics of Provision, Financing and Access*, London: Routledge, pp. 137–153.

Chen, C., P. Smith, and C. Mustard (2011), The prevalence of over-qualification and its association with health status among occupationally active new immigrants to Canada, *Ethnicity & Health*, **6**, 601–619.

Coker, E. (2004), 'Traveling pains': embodied metaphors of suffering among southern Sudanese refugees in Cairo, *Culture, Medicine, and Psychiatry*, **28**, 15–39.

CRIAW (2006a), *Fact Sheet*, available online at http://criaw-icref.ca/WomenAndPoverty.

CRIAW (2006b), *Intersectional Feminist Frameworks: An Emerging Vision*, Ottawa: CRIAW.

Cymbal, W. and S. Bujnowski (2010), Migration patterns and trends: a quantitative snapshot, *Health Policy Research Bulletin*, **17**, 7–11.

Davids, T. and F. Van Driel (2009), The unhappy marriage between gender and globalization, *Third World Quarterly*, **30**(5), 905–920.

Dejardin, A. (2008), *Gender Dimensions of Globalization*, Geneva: International Labour Organization.

Dressler, W. (1991), *Stress and Adaptation in the Context of Culture: Depression in a Southern Black Community*, Albany, NY: State University of New York Press.

Dunn, J. and I. Dyck (2000), Social determinants of health in Canada's immigrant population: results from the National Population Health Survey, *Social Science & Medicine*, **51**, 1573–1593.

Eschle, C. (2004), Feminist studies of globalisation: beyond gender, beyond economism? *Global Society*, **18**(2), 97–125.

Espin, O. (1999), *Women Crossing Boundaries: A Psychology of Immigration and Transformations of Sexuality*, London: Routledge Press.

Freund, P. (2006), Socially constructed embodiment: neurohormonal connections as resources for theorizing about health inequalities, *Social Theory & Health*, **4**, 85–108.

Glick Schiller, N. (2009), A global perspective on migration and development, *Social Analysis*, **53**(3), 14–37.

Haan, M. (2008), The place of place: location and immigrant economic well-being in Canada, *Population Research and Policy Review*, **27**, 751–771.

Hankivsky, O., C. Reid, R. Cormier, C. Varcoe, N. Clark, C. Benoit and S. Brotman (2010), Exploring the promises of intersectionality for advancing women's health research, *International Journal for Equity in Health*, **9**(5), 1–15.
Hu-Dehart, E. (2003), Globalization and its discontents: exposing the underside, *Frontiers* **24**(2/3), 244–260.
Hyman, I. (2009), *Racism as a Determinant of Immigrant Health*, Ottawa: Public Health Agency of Canada and Metropolis.
Immigration Department of Malaysia (2015), Foreign domestic helper, available online at www.imi.gov.my/index.php/en/main-services/foreign-domestic-helper.
Jones, S. (2004), Canada and the globalized immigrant, *American Behavioral Scientist*, **47**(10), 1263–1277.
Kofman, E. (2004), Gendered global migrations: diversity and stratification, *International Feminist Journal of Politics*, 6(4), 643–665.
Krieger, N., J. Chen and J. Selby (2001), Class inequalities in women's health: combined impact of childhood and adult social class – a study of 630 US women, *Public Health*, **115**, 175–185.
Krieger, N., P. Waterman, C. Hartman, L. Bates, A. Stoddard, M. Quinn, G. Sorenson, and E. Barbeau (2006), Social hazards on the job: workplace abuse, sexual harassment, and racial discrimination – a study of black, Latino, and white low-income women and men workers in the United States, *International Journal of Health Services*, **36**(1), 51–85.
Kusakabe, K. and R. Pearson (2010), Transborder migration, social reproduction and economic development: a case study of Burmese women workers in Thailand, *International Migration*, **48**(6), 13–43.
Lestari, E. (2012), Impacts of the economic crisis on women migrants, in *Women Resisting Crisis and War*, Quezon City: Asia Pacific Research Network, pp. 65–70.
Levitt, P. and D. Lamba-Nieves (2013), Rethinking social remittances and the migration-development nexus from the perspective of time, *Migration Letters*, **10**(1), 11–22.
Lewchuk, W., A. de Wolff, A. King, and M. Polyani (2003), From job strain to employment strain: health effects of precarious employment, *Just Labour*, **3**, 23–35.
Li, P. (2001), The racial subtext in Canada's immigration discourse, *Journal of International Migration and Integration*, **2**(1), 77–97.
Mahler, S. and D. Pessar (2001), Gendered geographies of power: analyzing gender across transnational spaces, *Identities*, **7**(4), 441–459.
McGuire, S. and K. Martin (2007), Fractured migrant families: paradoxes of hope and devastation, *Family and Community Health*, **30**(3), 178–188.
Menéndez, M., J. Benach, C. Muntaner, M. Amable and P. O'Campo (2007), Is precarious employment more damaging to women's health than men's? *Social Science & Medicine*, **64**, 776–781.
Ministry of Manpower, Singapore Government (2015), Sixth-monthly medical exam for FDWs, available online at www.mom.gov.sg/passes-and-permits/work-permit-for-foreign-domestic-worker/eligibility-and-requirements/six-monthly-medical-examination.
Ng, E. (2011), The healthy immigrant effect and mortality rates, *Health Reports*, **22**(4), 1–5.
Ng, E., R. Wilkins, F. Gendron, and J-M. Berthelot (2005), *Dynamics of Immigrants' Health in Canada: Evidence from the National Population Health Survey*, Ottawa: Statistics Canada.
O'Neill, B. and K. Sproule (2011), Enhancing social inclusion: settlement services in relation to lesbian, gay and bisexual newcomers, in D. L. Spitzer (ed.), *Engendering Migrant Health: Canadian Perspectives*, Toronto: University of Toronto Press, pp. 62–77.
Ong, A. (2005), Ecologies of expertise: assembling flow, managing citizenship, in A. Ong and S. Collier (eds.), *Global Assemblages: Technology, Politics and Ethics as Anthropological Problems*, Malden, MA: Blackwell Publishing, pp. 337–353.
Ong, A. (2006), Mutations in citizenship, *Theory, Culture & Society*, **23**(2–3), 499–505.
Özyegin, G. and P. Hondagneu-Sotelo (2008), Conclusion: domestic work, migration and

the new gender order in contemporary Europe, in H. Lutz (ed.), *Migration and Domestic Work: A European Perspective*, Aldershot: Ashgate Publishing, pp. 195–208.
Parreñas, R. S. (2005), *Children of Globalization: Transnational Families and Gendered Woes*, Berkeley: University of California Press.
Petrozziello, A. and E. Robert (2010), *Migration, Remittances and Gender-Responsive Local Development: Case Studies: Albania, the Dominican Republic, Lesotho, Morocco, the Philippines, and Senegal*, Santo Domingo: UN-INSTRAW and UNDP.
Piper, N. (2004), Gender and migration policies in Southeast and East Asia: legal protection and sociocultural empowerment of unskilled migrant women, *Singapore Journal of Tropical Geography*, **25**(2), 216–231.
Pratt, G. (1997), Stereotypes and ambivalence: the construction of domestic workers in Vancouver, British Columbia, *Gender, Place and Culture*, **4**(2), 159–178.
Pratt, G. (2006), Separation and reunification among Filipino families in Vancouver, *Canadian Issues*, Spring, 46–49.
Rahman, M. M. and L. K. Fee (2009), Gender and the remittance process; Indonesian domestic workers in Hong Kong, Singapore and Malaysia, *Asian Population Studies*, **5**(2), 103–123.
Raphael, D., J. Macdonald, R. Colman, R. Labonté, K. Hayward and R. Torgerson (2005), Researching income and income distribution as determinants of health in Canada: gaps between theoretical knowledge, research practice, and policy implementation, *Health Policy*, **72**, 217–232.
Rosenstock, L., M. Cullen and M. Fingerhut (2005), Advancing worker health and safety in the developing world, *Journal of Occupational and Environmental Medicine*, **47**, 132–136.
Scheder, J. (1988), A sickly-sweet harvest: farmworker diabetes and social equality, *Medical Anthropology Quarterly*, **2**(3), 251–277.
Siviö, A., E. Ek, J. Jokelainen, M. Koiranen, T. Järvikoski and A. Taanila (2012), Precariousness and discontinuous work history in association with health, *Scandinavian Journal of Public Health*, **40**, 360–367.
Sobritchea, C. and O. de Guzman (2006), *Life and Death on the Move: The Sexual and Reproductive Health Status and Needs of Filipino Women Migrant Domestic Workers*, Quezon City, Philippines: Action for Health Initiative.
Spitzer, D. L. (2004), In visible bodies: minority women, nurses, time and the new economy of care, *Medical Anthropology Quarterly*, **18**(4), 490–508.
Spitzer, D. L. (2006), The impact of policy on Somali refugee women in Canada, *Refuge*, **23**(2), 42–49.
Spitzer, D. L. (2011), Work, worries and weariness: towards an embodied and engendered migrant health, in D. L. Spitzer (ed.), *Engendering Migrant Health: Canadian Perspectives*, Toronto: University of Toronto Press, pp. 23–39.
Spitzer, D. L. (2012), Oppression and im/migrant health in Canada, in E. McGibbon (ed.), *Oppression: A Social Determinant of Health*, Halifax: Fernwood Publishing, pp. 113–122.
Spitzer, D. L. (2014a), *No (Wo)man's Land: Migration, Gender, and the Making of the Entrepreneurial Subject in the Philippines and Indonesia*, paper presented to CIRCEM, 21 January, Ottawa, Canada.
Spitzer, D. L. (2014b), *Familiar Strangers: Migrant Family Reunification in Canada*, report presented to the United Nations North American Experts' Group Meeting, Mexico City, Mexico.
Spitzer, D. L. and N. Piper (2014), Retrenched and returned: Filipino migrant workers during times of crisis, *Sociology*, **48**(5), 1007–1023.
Spitzer, D. L. and S. Torres (2008), *Gendered Barriers to Settlement and Integration for Live-in Caregivers: A Review of the Literature. CERIS Working Paper No. 71*, Toronto: CERIS.
Stewart, M, J. Anderson, E. Mwakarimba, A. Neufeld, L. Simich and D. L. Spitzer (2008), Multicultural meanings of social support among immigrants and refugees, *International Migration*, **46**(3), 123–159.
Torres, S., D. L. Spitzer, K. Hughes, J. Oxman-Martinez and J. Hanley (2012), From

temporary worker to resident: the LCP and its impact through an intersectional lens, in P. Lenard and C. Straehle (eds.), *Legislated Inequality: Temporary Foreign Migrants in Canada*, Ottawa: McGIll-Queen's University Press, pp. 227–244.

VanderPlaat, M. (2007), *Integration Outcomes for Immigrant Women in Canada: A Review of the Literature 2000–2007, AMC Working Paper*, Halifax: Atlantic Metropolis Centre.

Van Hear, N. (2010), Theories of migration and social change, *Journal of Ethnic and Migration Studies*, **36**(10), 1531–1536.

Varcoe, C., O. Hankivsky and M. Morrow (2007), 'Introduction: beyond gender matters', in M. Morrow, O. Hankivsky and C. Varcoe (eds.), *Women's Health in Canada: Critical Perspectives on Theory and Policy*, Toronto: University of Toronto Press, pp. 3–30.

Villegas, P. (2013), Negotiating the boundaries of membership: health care providers, access to social good, and immigration status, in L. Goldring and P. Landholt (eds.), *Producing and Negotiating Citizenship: Precarious Legal Status in Canada*, Toronto: University of Toronto Press, pp. 221–237.

Vissandjée, B., M. Desmeules, Z. Cao, S. Abdool and A. Kazanjian (2004), Integrating Ethnicity and Immigration as Determinants of Canadian Women's Health, *Women's Health Surveillance Report: Supplementary Chapters*, Ottawa: Canadian Institutes for Health Research, pp. 5–7.

Warner, R. (2006). *Theoretical Framework for the Racism, Violence and Health Project: a Working Paper*, available online at http://rvh.socialwork.dal.ca/resources.html.

Webber, L. and D. Parra-Medina (2003), Intersectionality and women's health: charting a path to eliminating health disparities, *Advances in Gender Research*, **7**, 181–230.

Webber, G., D. L. Spitzer, R. Somrongthong, T. Dat and S. Kounnavongsa (2012), Facilitators and barriers to accessing reproductive health care for beer promoters in Cambodia, Laos, Thailand and Vietnam: a mixed methods study, *Globalization and Health*, **8**(21).

Wee, V. and A. Sim (2004), Transnational networks in female labour migration, in A. Ananta and E. Arifin (eds.), *International Migration in Southeast Asia*, Singapore: Institute of Southeast Asian Studies Publications, pp. 166–198.

Williams, F. and A. Gavanas (2008), The intersection of childcare regimes and migration regimes: a three-country study, in H. Lutz (ed.), *Migration and Domestic Work: A European Perspective on a Global Theme*, Aldershot: Ashgate Publishing, pp. 15–28.

Yuval-Davis, N. (2007), Intersectionality, citizenship and contemporary politics of belonging, *Critical Review of International Social and Political Philosophy*, **10**(4), 561–574.

PART III

RIGHTS AND DESERVINGNESS

6 Health-related deservingness

Sarah S. Willen and Jennifer Cook

INTRODUCTION

In 2003, 17-year-old Jesica Santillan underwent a heart and lung transplant at Duke University Medical Center in Durham, North Carolina. Just after the surgery, routine post-operative blood tests revealed a terrible mistake; Santillan had received organs of an incompatible blood type. In a frantic effort to correct the error, her doctors procured another set of organs and performed a second transplant. Yet the damage was too great for her already weakened system, and she died several days later.

The story of the "bungled transplant" (Wailoo et al. 2006) made local and national headlines. How could such a mistake occur in one of the nation's premier medical institutions, the American public wanted to know. Who was to blame? As the media dug deeper into the details of the case, the tone of the conversation shifted, and spectators began asking a decidedly more contentious question: did Santillan even deserve a transplant in the first place?

From a clinical standpoint, physicians establish eligibility for organ transplantation using sophisticated biomedical algorithms. In Santillan's case, post-mortem eligibility debates revolved not around biology, but around biography—especially the fact that Santillan and her mother had entered the United States without legal authorization when she was 13. Commentators labeled Santillan an "illegal immigrant" and debated whether or not she deserved the medical care she had received. Some contended that only citizens should have access to "citizen organs" (Chavez 2006: 292) and declared Santillan and other "illegals" inherently undeserving. Others pointed to Santillan's youthful innocence and life-threatening illness as evidence of her deservingness. The tragedy of Jesica Santillan's death and ensuing controversy highlight an important but under-examined issue: the impact of vernacular deservingness assessments on broader debates about migration and health.

Conceptions of "health-related deservingness" (Willen 2012a, 2012b) always emerge in specific social, historical, and ideological contexts. Debates about health-related deservingness involve divergent and often competing moral stances about whose health—whose bodies, lives, and life chances—matters. The focus of such debates can range from questions of individual access to a particular form of clinical treatment, as in the Santillan case, to questions of system-wide access for entire populations. The *absence* of public debate itself speaks volumes—for instance, when policymakers ignore occupational health risks that predominantly affect migrants (like prolonged pesticide exposure among agricultural workers), or developmental health risks common among migrants' children (like long-term "warehousing" in unregulated daycare settings that endanger health and human development).

In this chapter, we propose that any meaningful effort to influence the tone, tenor, or outcome of debates about migrants' health will depend on the ability to identify, uncover, and analyze the often-hidden values and presumptions they entail. To this end, we aim to operationalize the concept of health-related deservingness and illuminate its significance in debates about migration[1] and health in diverse settings and at multiple levels of analysis. We begin by considering how the notion of deservingness has been conceptualized in recent social science scholarship, where migrants comprise but one among many groups whose deservingness regularly comes into question. We then offer a framework for analyzing deservingness debates, with a particular focus on debates involving migrants' health. The framework involves three core elements: the *stakeholders* involved, the *contexts* in which such debates take place, and the *evaluative criteria* employed. In the final section, we put this framework into action by analyzing health-related deservingness debates in three migration settings: one in North America, one in Western Europe, and a third in the Middle East.

Overall, we aim to provide strong scaffolding for broad-ranging, interdisciplinary inquiry into both how health-related deservingness is reckoned and how local deservingness assessments can affect the health of individuals and the communities in which they live.

CONCEPTUALIZING DESERVINGNESS

In an important sense, deservingness can be understood as the flip-side of rights. Whereas rights claims are expressed in a formal *juridical* discourse that presumes fundamental equality before the law, deservingness claims are articulated in a vernacular *moral* register that is situationally specific and context-dependent. Put differently, deservingness debates often have less to do with empirical evidence than with competing everyday responses to normative questions. These vernacular responses generally mix subjective attitudes and presumptions with taken-for-granted truths regarded as collective "common sense." For instance, a debate might revolve around the question of "Who should have access to this particular healthcare service?" or "Should this person receive financial support in accessing this service?" In many instances, the vernacular reasoning deployed in such debates is but loosely tethered to empirical realities. Often it carries a powerful emotional charge.

How do rights claims and deservingness assessments differ? Both are social constructions (Schneider and Ingram 2005), but they diverge in key respects. First, unlike rights discourses, which presume blindness to individual particularities, deservingness assessments typically are *relational*. One assesses others' relative deservingness on the basis of two key factors: an implicit sense of one's own deservingness, and a sense of (actual or presumed) social connection to those whose deservingness is in question.

Second, deservingness assessments are often *conditional* on presumed or actual features of those whose deservingness is in question—intrinsic or extrinsic, mutable or immutable—regardless of their salience. In short, rights are presumed to have universal significance, even when they are not universally enjoyed in practice, whereas deservingness is always reckoned in conditional terms.

Third, conceptions of deservingness never emerge in a vacuum. Rather, they are always grounded in a particular social and political *context*. Fourth, deservingness assessments are *syncretic*; they are simultaneously grounded in multiple sources of moral insight and experience. For instance, they may reflect an amalgamation of professional expertise, "common sense," and personal beliefs and experiences. Fifth they are *infused with affect*, or emotion. Finally, they are *mutable*; they are liable to shift and change in response to new knowledge and evolving circumstances.

In short, vernacular ways of reckoning deservingness in general, and health-related deservingness in particular, involve complex forms of moral reasoning. The impact of such assessments is neither arcane nor trivial. At the local and national levels, questions of "who deserves what" are pivotal, if implicit, throughout the political process. They shape the discourse and practice of legislators and policymakers (Chock 1991; Guetzkow 2010; Heyman 1998), healthcare institutions (Horton 2004; Wailoo et al. 2006), clinicians (Holmes 2012; Marrow 2011; Vanthuyne et al. 2013; Huschke 2014), the media (Yoo 2002, 2008), and ordinary citizens (Gilens 1999; Katz 1989; Will 1993). At an international level, such questions challenge us to confront the profound health implications of contemporary patterns of global inequality.

DESERVINGNESS AND WELFARE

The most robust body of research on deservingness to date takes welfare as its focus. Some social scientists have sought to operationalize deservingness in terms of measurable variables or normative criteria (Appelbaum 2001; Appelbaum et al. 2003; de Swaan 1988; Feather 1999; van Oorschot 2000, 2006). Others have explored the impact of recipient characteristics like racial or ethnic background (Gilens 1999; Guetzkow 2010; Horton 2004; Morgen and Maskovsky 2003; Yoo 2008); the social positioning, demographic characteristics, or emotional state of deservingness "evaluators" (Olsen et al. 2003; Verkuyten 2004); level of responsibility for, or degree of control over, the circumstances producing a need for support (Appelbaum 2001; Appelbaum et al. 2003; de Swaan 1988; van Oorschot 2000; Will 1993; Scott 2008); and real or presumed associations with criminality (Morgen and Maskovsky 2003; Olsen et al. 2003) on deservingness assessments. Other scholars have examined the impact of context, including economic factors such as unemployment levels (Blekesaune and Quadagno 2003) as well as national and personal ideological frameworks (van Oorschot 2000). Additional avenues of inquiry include the impact of neoliberal influences on welfare and healthcare policy and practice (Bambra and Smith 2010; Guetzkow 2010; Horton 2004; Rylko-Bauer and Farmer 2002) and the impact of the media on public perception (Gollust et al. 2010). Still other influential studies examine how constructions of "undeservingness" ignore structural inequalities and reproduce negative, often racialized stereotypes (Gilens 1999; Katz 1989; Yoo 2008). In general, deservingness assessments seem to vary based on perceptions of social proximity between the subjects of debate and those rendering their evaluations (Grove and Zwi 2006; Newton 2005).

HEALTH-RELATED DESERVINGNESS

In contrast to this robust welfare literature, relatively little is known about how deservingness is reckoned in the health domain (cf. Gollust and Lynch, 2010; Gollust et al. 2010; Lynch and Gollust 2010; Scott 2008). This is a complex matter of great significance, especially in an era of neoliberal pressures toward healthcare privatization and commoditization, soaring healthcare costs, growing health disparities both within countries and between rich and poor regions, and massive waves of unregulated migration over land and sea. In countries with historically strong commitments to universal healthcare and social service protections, existing rights and entitlements are increasingly imperiled (Larchanché 2012).

Important research questions abound: how do divergent stakeholders—the privileged and the disadvantaged, policymakers and voters, clinicians and patients—reckon health-related deservingness? What criteria influence deservingness assessments, and what role does ideology play? Who is responsible for providing healthcare, and how should costs be covered? How do moral questions of deservingness intersect with juridical questions of rights? How do they relate to questions of "fairness" (Daniels 2008; Lynch and Gollust 2010)? Are inclusive deservingness assessments purely aspirational, or are they grounded in precedent, policy, or law?

In pursuing these questions, it is important to remember that health involves far more than just the presence or absence of disease or injury—and, moreover, more than just access to curative care. Equally important, if not more so, are the *social determinants of good health*: the upstream factors and structural conditions that predispose certain individuals and communities to be healthy in the first place (WHO Commission on Social Determinants of Health 2008). For example, given the "structural vulnerability" (Quesada et al. 2011) many migrants endure, their access to social determinants may be as limited as their access to curative care (Castañeda et al. 2015). Furthermore, structural vulnerability renders many migrants less capable of addressing their health needs than their citizen counterparts. Failure to recognize these interlocking forms of disadvantage can perpetuate the tacit politics of blame that lead many stakeholders to deem migrants undeserving.

Not surprisingly, migrant health has become a central theme in the emerging literature on health-related deservingness. Scholars have asked, for instance: how do local and national policies, especially in the domains of immigration and health, affect local conceptions of deservingness (Marrow 2011; Marrow and Joseph 2015; Haas 2012; Oliverio-Lauderdale 2014)? How do healthcare professionals' often unspoken moral assumptions about their migrant patients influence clinical interactions (Holmes 2012; Larchanché 2012; Marrow 2011; Vanthuyne et al. 2013)? How do migrant health advocates deploy notions of human rights, humanitarianism, and other "idioms of social justice mobilization" (Willen 2011) in claiming migrants' deservingness, and with what effect (Gottlieb et al. 2012; Tiedje and Plevak 2014)? How is migrants' deservingness framed, and contested, in scholarly public health literature (Viladrich 2012)? And what about migrants' perspectives? Do different migrant groups regard *themselves* as deserving of access to healthcare, or to the social determinants of good health? How are they affected by others' negative assessments (Chavez 2012; Larchanché 2012)? These are all crucial questions that demand further inquiry.

HEALTH-RELATED DESERVINGNESS: A FRAMEWORK FOR ANALYSIS

Deservingness debates involve conversations, either in public or behind closed doors, in which divergent stakeholders express or enact competing views about whether a particular person or social group deserves a certain kind of attention, investment, or care. Although professional considerations and empirical evidence may play a role, such debates frequently hinge on vernacular assumptions that rely less on empirical evidence than "common-sense" knowledge and subjective moral commitments. Despite the pivotal role such assumptions play and their tangible effects, they tend to remain unspoken and implicit.

Elsewhere we have proposed that these vernacular forms of moral reasoning urgently require investigation—from multiple stakeholder and disciplinary perspectives, in different contexts and professional settings, and using a range of research methods (Willen 2012a). We develop this argument below. Our project is framed not by normative *philosophical* questions—for instance, about health and distributive justice—but rather by empirical *social scientific* questions: how are moral assessments and ethical decisions made in everyday social contexts? How do they find expression in particular forms of discourse and social practice? What sort of consequences do they effect?

Below we offer a model for investigating how different forms of vernacular moral reasoning inform local conversations about the kinds of health-related attention, investment, and care migrants do or do not deserve, and on what grounds. To parse the assumptions implicated in such debates, three key considerations demand attention: the range of relevant *stakeholders*, the multiple layers of *context* in which debates unfold, and the *evaluative criteria* stakeholders employ.

STAKEHOLDERS

The array of *stakeholders* engaged in local deservingness debates varies depending on the migrant group involved, the health resource in question, the domain in which a point of tension or contention arises, and the personal stakes for individual stakeholders. These may include *policymakers* (elected and appointed), *politicians*, the *media* (journalists, pundits, etc.), *advocacy groups*, and members of the broader public in their capacities as *citizens*, *voters*, and *media consumers*. In the health domain, other key stakeholders include not just *healthcare providers* (physicians, nurses, allied health professionals, etc.), but also *public health professionals*, *clinical office staff*, *insurance administrators*, and other "*street level bureaucrats*" (Lipsky 1980) who serve important gatekeeping functions. *Ethicists*, including bioethicists and public health ethicists, may be stakeholders as well. *Migrants* are, of course, key stakeholders in all such debates—and the fact that their voices so often are muted demands careful scrutiny.

Although professional considerations influence many stakeholders' views, subjective commitments play a crucial role as well. Politicians, for instance, are elected to represent their constituents, but their own moral values—and concern for their political futures—also play a role. Public health workers hold core professional commitments (e.g., to make wise use of public resources, to follow scientific best practices), but also face political considerations and personal interests, some moral and some tactical (e.g., to protect one's professional credibility—or job security). In healthcare settings, administrative staff must juggle professional expectations, institutional mandates, and personal views. For example, a hospital's chief financial officer may insist that the billing office require up-front payment from undocumented patients as a way to offset daily operating costs. Administrators processing health insurance applications may thus take it upon themselves to scrutinize the paperwork of patients they suspect to be undocumented.

Clinicians, like administrators, also are beholden to professional, personal, and political commitments, but they are bound by ethical codes that impose additional obligations as well (e.g., the Hippocratic Oath). Advocates, activists, and private citizens are also important stakeholders in deservingness debates. They may be more open and explicit about their political and moral commitments than those acting in a professional role.

To date, scholarship on deservingness has tended to focus primarily on relatively advantaged stakeholders—those with power, influence or, at the very least, public voice. This, we contend, is insufficient. Instead, future research will need to investigate how deservingness is reckoned both *in relation to* and, furthermore, *from the perspectives of* those most directly affected: individuals and groups commonly represented as undeserving. Research on migrants' perspectives may reveal appreciable differences between their own ethical calculus and modes of moral reasoning, on one hand, and those of other, non-migrant stakeholders, on the other. Moreover, their views of their own and others' relative deservingness are likely to influence their care-seeking behavior as well as their overall health and wellbeing (see, for example, Larchanché 2012).

CONTEXT

Context is another key element in deservingness debates. Four contextual domains are especially significant when migrants' health-related deservingness is at stake: history, law, politics, and economics. Below we highlight a few considerations that arise in each, recognizing that these domains themselves overlap and entwine.

From an *historical* perspective, one might ask: how have past experiences—either negative (e.g., drought, famine, political turmoil, war) or positive (e.g., France's legacy as home of the *Droits de l'homme*)—influenced current views of migrants and migration? Does a particular locale have its own history as a "receiving" community, a "sending" community—or perhaps both at different times? Has it historically been welcoming or restrictive toward migrants? How do views of current migrant populations compare with attitudes toward earlier arrivals, and why is this so?

The *legal* realm is extraordinarily complex in its own right. At the international level, to what relevant international treaties and conventions is a given country signatory, and how do those international commitments influence policymaking, advocacy efforts, and public opinion? At the national level, who is and is not permitted either to enter the country or to immigrate, and under what conditions? How does national migration law influence public opinion regarding newcomers' opportunities, or lack of opportunities, for membership and social inclusion?

The impact of political and economic context on local deservingness debates cannot be underestimated. In the *political* realm, to what degree is migration a local concern, and in what respects? What role do political ideologies and other value systems (e.g., religion) play in framing local debate? How do such commitments inform the views of influential political parties? Vocal minorities? The courts? Advocacy and activist groups? Do migrants themselves play an active role in local political conversation?

In *economic* terms, how is the local economy performing, and what economic role do migrants play? Are they regarded as a boon or a threat to the local economy? As a valued source of labor, or unwelcome competitors for citizen-workers? The economic health of the local public health and clinical care systems also demands consideration. What health services can migrants access, and who foots the bill? Are these systems overburdened, or perceived to be, and if so, how are migrants' health needs conceptualized and discussed?

EVALUATIVE CRITERIA

Finally, what *evaluative criteria* inform local debates about migrants' health-related deservingness? In reckoning migrants' relative deservingness, stakeholders often rely on *presumptions* about migrants' lives and life circumstances that draw on a mixture of collective "common sense," personal attitudes, and politicized forms of emotion. The connections between such presumptions and empirical realities may be tenuous at best. Below we highlight five areas of presumption that figure frequently in local debates about who migrants are and what they do, or do not, deserve: *migration motive*, *legal status*, *moral character*, *vulnerability*, and *social proximity* to members of the broader society. Although these characteristics figure in general assessments of migrants' deservingness, they are especially salient in reckoning their deservingness of health-related attention, investment, or care.

Migration Motives

Migrants' presumed motives feature prominently in local deservingness debates. An especially bright line is assumed to distinguish "economic migrants" (who ostensibly left their country primarily to pursue economic opportunity) from "forced migrants" (presumed to have fled violent conflict, political persecution, or natural disaster). Although this distinction is typically presented as clear-cut and self-evident, realities are considerably more complex (see, for example, Yarris and Castañeda, 2015). For instance, asylum-seekers who have faced violence or oppression but fail to translate their experiences into bureaucratically legible categories will likely find their claims denied. Other migrants leave home fleeing poverty, including impoverishment resulting from climate change, only to find that their migration circumstances are not deemed worthy of recognition or status in their new countries of residence.

People identified as either "economic" or "forced" migrants tend to be viewed and treated in very different ways. "Forced" migrants generally are represented as unfortunate, faultless victims of circumstance who deserve society's attention and material support. This logic is often invoked to mobilize humanitarian and human rights commitments at the national and international levels. "Economic" migrants, in contrast, are often assumed to have chosen freely to migrate and, on these grounds, are deemed responsible for their own fates.

This pattern of moral valuation can vary; for instance, when national policies themselves influence how particular groups' deservingness is reckoned. Policies that prohibit asylum-seekers from working while their petitions are pending, for example, force them to rely on interim government support. As a result, migrants who would otherwise be regarded as faultless and hence deserving victims may be reimagined as a burden to society (Sales 2002; Watters 2007).

Legal Status

Presumptions about migrants' legal status also figure centrally in local deservingness debates. Although the very notion of legal status would seem to hinge on a straightforward distinction, such matters often are far from clear-cut. Deservingness debates rarely account for this complex fluidity.

There is, of course, nothing natural or self-evident about legal statuses; they are human creations designed to meet political demands. They are also varied, amenable to change, and differentially enforced. A wide range of possible statuses exists both across migration settings and even within a single country. For instance, some residence visas permit study but forbid work, and some time-delimited work permits forbid permanent residence or family reunification. Migrants seeking asylum or refugee status may hold a temporary status valid only while their petitions are pending. And in countries that grant citizenship on the basis of *jus soli* (birthright citizenship), statuses may vary within a single household or family. Often, violating the terms of one's authorization can automatically trigger a loss of legal status and consequent slip into "illegality."

Yet legal status is more than just a juridical category. It is also morally charged, and different forms of status are imbued with different moral valences. Unauthorized border-crossing, for instance, may be seen as evidence of immorality—or, worse still, of criminality. In either case, presumptions about legal status powerfully influence stakeholder assessments.

Moral Character

Debates about health-related deservingness hinge on impressionistic judgments about multiple aspects of migrants' moral character. For instance, stakeholders may make presumptions about a migrant's or migrant community's *economic productivity*, *personal responsibility*, *fulfillment of family obligations*, and *associations with criminality*. Are migrants presumed to contribute to the economy, or to society, through their labor, whether skilled or unskilled? To pay taxes? To depend on welfare, social support, or government programs? Are they seen as willing to integrate into the broader society? On all of these counts, vernacular presumptions influence deservingness debates, even when they are contradicted by empirical evidence (Chauvin et al. 2013; Chauvin and Garcés-Mascareñas 2014).

The same holds true for family status. How are migrants' family configurations imagined in comparison to idealized notions of a "normal" family? Are parents viewed as more morally upstanding, and hence more deserving, than single adults? Mothers more deserving than fathers? Parents who live with their children more deserving than those who have entrusted their children to the care of extended family members?

The element of *criminality* is a complicated one, especially given the recent convergence of immigration enforcement efforts and criminal justice in what has been described as "crimmigration law" (Stumpf 2006). When migrants with precarious legal status engage in informal or illicit activities as a survival strategy (e.g., working or selling goods without a permit, using other people's identification documents, etc.), their actions may be interpreted as signs of immorality and hence undeservingness. Associations between migrants and criminality, even when spurious, often are bandied about with the explicit goal of inflaming xenophobic sentiment.

Vulnerability

Presumptions of vulnerability also figure prominently in deservingness debates. Migrants considered especially vulnerable may be more likely to draw sympathy and, as a result, may be regarded as more deserving than those viewed as less vulnerable.

Various criteria are used to gauge migrants' vulnerability including gender, sexual orientation, or sexual identity; physical or mental disability; past experiences of victimization (i.e., status as a survivor of violent crime, domestic violence, or sex trafficking); life stage; and health status. Certain individuals—for instance, women, children, the elderly, the severely ill, people with disabilities, and individuals with non-conforming gender or sexual identities—may be regarded as more vulnerable than other migrants and, on that basis, more deserving. Depending on local context and relevant stakeholders' views, however, certain migrants' claims of vulnerability may be deemed suspect—for instance, because they fail to conform to social norms, are perceived as attempts to "cheat the system," or bear some form of social stigma. Migrants living with HIV/AIDS, for example, may not be seen as deserving despite the severity of their disease due to irrational fears of disease transmission. Alternatively, stakeholders may question the morality of those afflicted by HIV/AIDS because of stereotypical associations, for instance with homosexuality or promiscuity. The example of HIV reveals how evaluations of migrant morality and discussions of vulnerability can intersect in ways that affect deservingness assessments more broadly.

The relative visibility of one's source of vulnerability or affliction can also play a role in how deservingness is assessed. Sometimes a visible ailment (e.g., a missing limb from a landmine accident) is more likely to garner a sympathetic evaluation than a condition that is less visible (e.g., mental illness).

Social Proximity

Perceived social proximity between migrant populations and citizens is another key criterion in local deservingness debates. Proximity may be reckoned in terms of ostensibly intrinsic features (e.g., race/ethnicity, language, or religion) or extrinsic features (e.g., willingness to learn the local language, follow local gender norms, or otherwise endeavor to integrate into the broader society). Presumptions of social proximity generally lead migrants regarded as more "like us" to be deemed more deserving than others. On the other hand, in some contexts, stakeholders may invoke societal values like diversity or multiculturalism in an attempt to advocate for inclusiveness.

Assessments of social proximity are deeply influenced by local context. In relatively homogenous societies, for instance, racial, ethnic, religious, or cultural difference may be regarded as a threat to the collective. In countries with a long history of immigration, new migrants may be discursively aligned with older migrant groups with whom they share, or are presumed to share, key features. Aspects of local ideological, political, and historical context can influence perceptions of social proximity and heighten concern about particular groups (e.g., about migrants of color in majority white societies, or about Muslim migrants in societies that are predominantly Christian).

HEALTH-RELATED DESERVINGNESS: THREE DEBATES

How do these forms of vernacular moral reasoning figure in localized debates about migrants' health-related deservingness? To address this question, we turn now to three cases: one from North America, one from Western Europe, and one from the Middle East. In discussing each case, we engage all three elements of the framework introduced above (stakeholders, context, and evaluative criteria) while foregrounding one of the three. Each case provides a vivid illustration of how vernacular conceptions of health-related deservingness can be implicated in the domains of migrant health research, policy, or practice.

Organs for the Undocumented? A "Bungled Transplant" in the United States

The tragic case of Jesica Santillan, the 17-year-old immigrant from Mexico who died in the United States in 2003 after a "bungled" transplant, spurred high-profile debate among an impassioned array of stakeholders. Should she have received a heart and lung transplant in the first place? After the botched transplant that led those organs to fail, should she have received a second? Pundits and the general public seized on Santillan's story as an opportunity to debate a broader set of questions. Should undocumented immigrants receive healthcare in the United States at all? If so, what kind of care ought they to receive, under what conditions, and with what limitations, if any? Finally, who should pay?

In Santillan's case, as in any deservingness debate, context matters. Despite the country's "melting pot" origin myth, the history of restrictive immigration policy and anti-immigrant sentiment in the US runs deep (Ngai 2004). Especially in times of economic vulnerability, US public opinion has tended to portray migrants and immigrants, and unauthorized migrants in particular, as a drain on resources and a threat to national sovereignty (Chavez 2012; Portes et al. 2012). When Santillan and her family moved to the largely agricultural southern state of North Carolina in 2003, a new wave of Latino migrants seeking agricultural work had just begun to arrive (Kochhar et al. 2005). Although US citizens generally have been loath to take up jobs in the agricultural sector, fears of economic competition and cultural and demographic change have at times fueled xenophobic sentiment, especially in places like North Carolina, where Latino immigrants are a relatively new population (Marrow 2011).

A wide range of stakeholders participated in the stormy debates that erupted around Santillan's treatment and subsequent death, among them the two medical institutions involved in her care, the media, right-wing political pundits, and a white, middle-aged, local businessman named Mack Mahoney who first learned of Santillan's illness from the local newspaper. Compelled by her plight, Mahoney founded a charity to support her medical care and became the family's informal, if self-appointed, spokesman. In his public statements, Mahoney cited Santillan's youthful innocence as well as her frail, deteriorating body as evidence that she was a deserving candidate for transplant surgery. At times, he even infantilized her by describing her as a dying "baby" even though at 17 she was nearly a legal adult (Wailoo et al. 2006: 304).

Following her death, a heated media debate focused on Santillan's unauthorized migration status. Conservative commentators leveraged her story to intervene politically in national conversations about immigration. Right-wing pundit Michelle Malkin, for instance, contended that Santillan symbolized a larger problem in the US where "[t]he costs of illegal alien healthcare are crippling hospitals across the country" (Malkin 2003). In Malkin's narrative, Santillan was one of millions of "illegal aliens" flooding the country seeking access to already scarce resources.

Yet Malkin's account ignored several key facts. First, unlike most unauthorized migrants in the US, Santillan's mother was covered by an employment-based private health insurance policy. Given the US's employment-based insurance system, Santillan therefore was covered as her dependent. Additional costs were covered by private donations generated through Mahoney's charity.

Another conservative columnist, Joe Kovacs, compared Santillan to a different young woman awaiting a lung transplant, Lauren Averitt. According to Kovacs, Averitt—a desperately ill, law-abiding citizen—clearly was more deserving than Santillan. "[Il]legal aliens like Santillan," he wrote, "are able to leapfrog ahead of the many thousands of U.S. citizens patiently waiting and praying for their own personal miracle" (Kovacs 2003). From his standpoint, citizenship is more than a legal status; it is imbued with moral meaning—with life-or-death implications. Santillan's unauthorized border-crossing is portrayed as both criminal and immoral, as is her supposed desire and ability to jump ahead of US citizens on the transplant waiting list. In this account, Santillan herself is assigned culpability despite her youth and vulnerability, and even though her mother (and not she herself) initiated their migration.

The institutional stakeholders, Duke Medical Center and the United Network for Organ Sharing (UNOS), took a markedly different tactic. In their official responses, neither addressed Santillan's legal status. Each issued a carefully worded public statement in a cool, professional tone that contrasted sharply with the heated media fervor. Duke's response was particularly measured, likely due to concerns about legal liability for Santillan's death.

Much can be learned from this case about how migrants' health-related deservingness is reckoned. Above all, the contentious conversation following Santillan's death reveals just how low the threshold can be for involvement as a stakeholder—and, moreover, how quickly a relatively distant set of stakeholders can turn a localized discussion about a particular individual's health needs into a lightning rod for much broader public debate.

Not Sick Enough: Illness, Vulnerability, and Deservingness in Western Europe

In 2008, a very different deservingness debate unfolded in the United Kingdom about Ama Sumani,[2] a 39-year-old woman of Ghanaian origin and mother of two who was forcibly removed from her hospital bed in Cardiff, Wales, where she was being treated for malignant myeloma, a form of cancer (Lawrance 2012). Five British Home Office agents moved her into a wheelchair, drove her to Heathrow Airport, and put her on a plane to Ghana against her will. Before her "removal"[3] from the UK, Sumani had appealed the decision and petitioned to remain on compassionate grounds due to the life-threatening nature of her illness and lack of accessible treatment in her home country. Her appeal was denied. Unable to access treatment in her country of origin, she died two months later.

Sumani's case highlights the critical impact of context on local deservingness debates and their outcomes. How did historical, political, and legal circumstances influence her treatment by the British authorities? How might her fate have been different had her case been adjudicated in France? We explore these questions below.

In the heated public debate about Sumani's case, some British physicians and other sympathetic observers argued that her forcible removal would constitute a gross human rights violation. A *Lancet* editorial labeled it an act of "atrocious barbarism" and rightly anticipated that her deportation would precipitate her death (*Lancet* 2008). Yet several Members of Parliament vocally supported the Home Office actions. Without denying the likelihood of her imminent death, they claimed her case failed to meet the necessary threshold of "very exceptional" suffering required to activate the country's humanitarian relief mechanism.

In the UK, healthcare provision to migrant populations historically has been uncontroversial, and until relatively recently access to care was virtually the same for all. After an increase in asylum applications in the 1970s and 1980s, however, anxieties about growing migrant populations spurred the passage of laws distinguishing between "ordinary residents" eligible for free healthcare through the National Health Service and "non-ordinary residents" who can access only certain health services, and only for a fee (*Lancet* 2008). Seriously ill migrants ordered to leave the UK may seek relief from removal through appeal under Article 3 of the European Convention on Human Rights, which prohibits any action that would constitute "inhuman treatment" (Council of Europe, 1950). Decisions regarding humanitarian relief are made by an immigration judge on a case-by-case basis. Sumani's case was deemed unexceptional, and her appeal was denied (Lawrance 2012).

How might Sumani's fate have been different in France? In both countries, unauthorized migrants often are regarded with suspicion. Yet French policies regarding sick migrants have tended to be more favorable than their British analogs. In 1998, following an intensive campaign by a coalition of advocacy organizations, an informal, discretionary practice of granting temporary residency permits to seriously ill migrants became institutionalized (Ticktin 2011; Fassin 2012). The resulting new arrangement, an "illness residency permit," was created precisely to prevent the deportation of people with serious illnesses who would lack access to appropriate care following repatriation—people like Ama Sumani.

On the surface, the contours of the French and UK policies are similar. Both revolve around the same questions: Does the migrant's illness meet the threshold of "life-threatening" severity? Would appropriate treatment be accessible in his or her home country? What differs is the deservingness threshold, which would appear to be lower in France. Importantly, medical experts play an integral role in the French context, whereas immigration officers are the primary adjudicators in the UK (Fassin 2011; Larchanché 2012; Ticktin 2011). In Ama Sumani's case, context made all the difference.

"Pirate" Daycares and Infant Deaths in Israel[4]

During a six-week period in early 2015, five infants died in Tel Aviv in what advocates and the Israeli media describe as "pirate" daycares, or "child warehouses," in the city's neglected southern neighborhoods. Among them were two four-month-old babies who died within a 48-hour period. The local media were quick to publicize the circumstances of their deaths (see, for example, David 2015; Kashti, 2015; Vilnai 2015a, 2015b, 2015c), both involving infants born in Israel to Eritrean parents who had arrived, without authorization, seeking asylum.

In the first of these cases, a baby girl was left alone in a crib with a bottle of formula (Vilnai 2015b), possibly tied to her head (David 2015), and choked to death. The next day, in an adjacent neighborhood, a baby boy died of suffocation; his death went unnoticed until his mother came to pick him up after work and found him lying on his stomach, unresponsive. Immediately after this pair of deaths, migrant advocacy organizations and human rights groups demanded swift government action, and the media reported on "marathon meetings" in the subsequent days "among the relevant government ministries, in collaboration with the municipality" (Vilnai 2015c). Had the deceased infants been born to Jewish-Israeli citizen parents rather than non-Jewish asylum seekers from Africa, how might their fates have been different?

For nearly two decades, "pirate" daycares like these have been the only viable option for most infants and toddlers (age 0–3) born in Israel to unauthorized migrant parents, including both migrants who arrived explicitly in search of work and those, like the Eritrean parents of these unfortunate children, who arrived seeking asylum. Although asylum-seekers in Israel are officially forbidden to work, they receive no benefits from the government and therefore must find employment in order to sustain themselves and their families. Their employment options are thus sharply limited, pay is low, work conditions are often harsh, and parents have little flexibility in determining their work schedules. As a result, some children are in daycare for 15 hours per day or more—or even overnight, in some cases for multiple nights in succession.

Significantly, no public daycare frameworks are provided for any children in this age bracket, including Israeli citizens' children. Yet the private daycares that serve Israeli parents face tighter scrutiny—not only from the authorities, but also from parents who, as citizens, risk little in voicing their concerns.

As of 2015, an estimated 70–80 "pirate" daycares were operating in the Tel Aviv area, serving approximately 2,500 children and charging as little as 500 Israeli shekels (approximately US$132) per month for care that often exceeds what counts as "full-time" by Israeli standards (Vilnai 2015b; Mesila staff, personal interview). For Israeli politicians, the media, and the broader public, this spate of deaths came as no surprise; in the preceding two years, at least ten others had been recorded in similar settings (Vilnai 2015c). Indeed, the risks and dangers of these unregulated daycares had been detailed, and roundly condemned, in the State Comptroller's 2013 annual report (Office of the State Comptroller, 2013).

Thousands of children do survive these settings, but the short- and long-term risks are legion—and well-known. In many such daycares, a single adult, usually a woman with a migrant background, is responsible for as many as 20 or even 30 children (Office of the State Comptroller, 2013) whereas the national average ratio in Israel is one to six (David 2015). As a result, children tend to spend as much as 12–15 hours each day isolated in a crib with no daily routine and with minimal attention, physical contact, or direct interaction with others, whether children or adults. Neither do they receive much stimulation (e.g., stories, toys, music, art activities, outdoor playtime), although televisions are sometimes present. Most facilities are located in crumbling residential buildings, often in private apartments where rents are cheap. Among other hazards, many lack fire escapes and adequate ventilation, and some have unauthorized electrical connections, unsecured doors or gates, and unsafe balconies.

From a health standpoint, the long-term impact of spending one's critical first years in a setting like these is almost universally devastating. According to Mesila, a municipally-run social welfare organization in South Tel Aviv that had been responding to these unregulated care settings and their effects for more than a decade: "By the time they enter formal educational settings, every one of these children suffers at least one if not more forms of developmental delay" (Mesila Aid and Information Center 2006). They continue: "we are convinced that the overwhelming majority of infants and young children in these frameworks meet the criteria for children at risk as a result of spending most hours of the day in an atmosphere of physical and emotional deprivation that severely delays their development" (Mesila Aid and Information Center 2006). These conclusions were echoed in the 2013 State Comptroller report.

What "common-sense" assumptions and moral commitments make it possible for key stakeholders in the political and policy realms to ignore these well-known risks for years, even decades? The infants who died certainly could not be suspected of poor *moral character*. In terms of *migration motive*, they were neither economic nor forced migrants; although their parents fled countries in tumult, they were born in Israel. Since Israel has no *jus soli* provision, however, they are not eligible for Israeli citizenship.

One might expect that their young age and associated *vulnerability* would garner concern for their health and development, and in some respects, this has been the case. Since the 2000s, children of migrant parents have been among the few members of migrant communities for whom national and municipal stakeholders have expressed concern. For example, a small network of supervised private daycares (Unitaf) was established under the supervision of Mesila in 2005, with major philanthropic (as opposed to government) support. Unitaf daycares are roughly comparable to those serving Jewish-Israeli children, but they are more expensive for parents than the informal arrangements described above—and they serve just 350 children in total, with a waiting list of many more.

Changes benefiting these children have been driven both by pressure from local migrant and child advocacy groups and, not insignificantly, by a cultural emphasis on children and reproduction that has long found expression in the country's robust and institutionalized tradition of (selective) pronatalism (Kahn 2000; Kanaaneh 2002). Yet the overriding factor shaping Israeli attitudes toward children of migrant parents is *social proximity*. The clearest illustration of how proximity is reckoned in Israel is the country's "Law of Return." Established to invert the genocidal logic of the Nazi regime, this legal provision offers full citizenship benefits to anyone with a bureaucratically legible tie to the Jewish people. For those who lack such a tie, however, citizenship, and even permanent resident status, are almost completely unattainable regardless of country of origin or current legal status.

On the basis of this ethnonational logic, virtually everyone residing in Israel falls into one of three groups: ratified citizens (Jewish-Israelis, including the native-born and immigrants arriving under the Law of Return); Palestinians (who are represented as the country's "real" Others); and "other" Others—global migrants who have arrived in Israel for a variety of economic and/or political reasons and cannot readily be slotted into either of the first two groups (Willen 2010). For the vast majority of politicians, policymakers, and citizens, societal attention, investment, and care ought to focus primarily—some would say exclusively—on the country's Jewish-Israeli citizens. Other groups are constructed not simply as undeserving, but as a threat to the country's economy, identity, and even in some instances its existential security.

Immediately after this wave of infant deaths, the Prime Minister's Office announced it would begin working with Mesila to scale-up the small network of Unitaf daycares (which would continue to rely heavily on support from private philanthropy) (Mesila Aid and Information Center 2015). It is impossible to know precisely how key stakeholders' responses might have differed had the deceased infants been born to Jewish-Israeli citizen parents rather than African asylum seekers. Given the contours of Israel's local moral economy (Willen 2015), however, it seems likely that state, local, and non-government actors, under pressure from citizens and the media, would have responded much sooner—and with considerably greater decisiveness.

CONCLUSION: OPERATIONALIZING HEALTH-RELATED DESERVINGNESS

In this chapter, we have outlined an analytical framework for inquiry into a crucial but under-examined issue: health-related deservingness, especially as it applies in migration settings. By highlighting the key role played by *stakeholders*, *contextual factors*, and *evaluative criteria* in debates about deservingness, we aim to set the stage for broader interdisciplinary investigation of the moral, ideological, and political assumptions that undergird local debates about the health status of migrants as well as other vulnerable groups.

Our preliminary efforts to apply this framework highlight several insights that merit further inquiry. First, conceptions of deservingness are fundamentally expressed in a *moral* register; they are *vernacular* expressions of value as opposed to juridical notions of right. As such, deservingness inevitably is reckoned in ways that are *relational*, *conditional*, *context-dependent*, *syncretic*, *affect-laden*, and *mutable*.

Second, because deservingness is reckoned in fundamentally moral and relational terms, stakeholders' presumptions can play at least as powerful a role as empirical data, if not more so. Indeed, given the ease, and speed, with which information—including misinformation—can be disseminated through digital media, the diminishing role of empirical evidence in public and political debate is a matter of grave concern.

Yet deservingness assessments are not purely subjective; for some stakeholders, professional expertise plays an influential role, and professional and personal commitments can become deeply entwined. As such, efforts to change the tone, tenor, or outcome of debates about migrants' health-related deservingness may well depend on researchers' ability to uncover these hidden values and assumptions and demonstrate their impact in multiple domains, including the domains of public discourse, social policy, program implementation, and clinical practice.

One final insight merits particular attention. At the moment, we know altogether too little about how different migrants and members of other vulnerable groups conceptualize their own health-related deservingness. What sort of social contracts do they perceive, or envision? How do they participate in, or respond to, the often contentious deservingness debates transpiring in their communities of residence? What barriers, if any, impede their participation? Migrants' role as stakeholders, their views of the contexts and communities in which they live, and *their* deservingness criteria—as well as their engagement with and reactions to criteria espoused by others—constitute critical areas for future research.

ACKNOWLEDGEMENTS

Portions of this chapter draw from two of the first author's earlier publications (Willen 2012a, 2012b).

NOTES

1. Although the terms "migrant" and "immigrant" often are used interchangeably, they are not synonymous. Often these terms are employed as ostensibly neutral, empirically grounded descriptors of particular individuals or groups, yet different terms convey different ideological messages about who is expected to keep moving and who deserves to stay. Since individuals on the move often do not—and perhaps cannot—know whether their residence in a given location is temporary or permanent, or what sort of status will ultimately be available to them, the open-ended terms "migrants" and "migration" hew

closest to the variability, as well as the uncertainty, associated with many contemporary patterns of human mobility.
2. Sumani arrived in the UK in 2003 on a tourist visa. She later obtained a student visa and enrolled in finance classes, but her poor English skills and insufficient educational preparation prevented her from completing her course of study. Her myeloma was diagnosed in 2006, and she was placed on dialysis after the cancer spread to her kidneys. The Home Office ordered her "removal" to Ghana, arguing that her employment violated the terms of her student visa (Lawrance 2012).
3. In the UK, the response to visa violations is "removal," which does not affect a migrant's opportunity to apply for future visas, rather than "deportation," which does. Migrants may be deported if they have committed crimes or entered illegally (Blinder 2015).
4. Data for this section draw on ethnographic research conducted by the first author in Tel Aviv in 2014, supplemented by official reports and media coverage. This research phase, part of a larger study initiated in 2000, included interviews with staff at Mesila; visits to three "pirate" daycares; and an interview with the head of a Unitaf daycare.

REFERENCES

Appelbaum, L. D. (2001), The influence of perceived deservingness on policy decisions regarding aid to the poor, *Political Psychology*, **22**(3), 419–442.

Appelbaum, L. D, M. C. Lennon and J. L. Aber, (2003), How belief in a just world influences views of public policy, *National Center for Children in Poverty, Columbia University*, available online at www.nccp.org/publications/pub_553.html.

Bambra, C. and K. E. Smith (2010), No longer deserving? Sickness benefit reform and the politics of (ill) health, *Critical Public Health*, **20**(1), 71–84.

Blekesaune, M. and J. Quadagno (2003), Public attitudes toward welfare state policies, *European Sociological Review*, **19**(5), 415–427.

Blinder, S. (2015), *Briefing: Deportations, Removals, and Voluntary Departures from the UK*, 3rd revision, Oxford, Migration Observatory at the University of Oxford, available online at www.migrationobservatory.ox.ac.uk/sites/files/migobs/Briefing-Deportations.pdf.

Castañeda, H., S. M. Holmes, D. S. Madrigal, M.-E. DeTrinidad Young, N. Beyeler and J. Quesada (2015), Immigration as a social determinant of health, *Annual Review of Public Health*, **36**, 375–392.

Chauvin, S. and B. Garcés-Mascareñas (2014), Becoming less illegal: deservingness frames and undocumented migrant incorporation, *Sociology Compass*, **8**(4), 422–432.

Chauvin, S., B. Garcés-Mascareñas and A. Kraler (2013), Employment and migrant deservingness, *International Migration*, **51**(6), 80–85.

Chavez, L. R. (2006), Imagining the nation, imagining donor recipients, in Keith Wailoo, J. Livingston and P. Guarnaccia (eds.), *A Death Retold*, Chapel Hill, NC: University of North Carolina Press.

Chavez, L. R. (2012), Undocumented immigrants and their use of medical services in Orange County, California, *Social Science & Medicine*, **74**(6), 887–893.

Chock, P. P. (1991), 'Illegal aliens' and 'opportunity': myth-making in congressional testimony, *American Ethnologist*, **18**(2), 279–294.

Council of Europe (1950), *European Convention for the Protection of Human Rights and Fundamental Freedoms, as amended by Protocols Nos. 11 and 14*, ETS 5, available online at www.refworld.org/docid/3ae6b3b04.html.

Daniels, N. (2008), *Just Health*, Cambridge: Cambridge University Press.

David, A. (2015) Who will save the refugee children of Tel Aviv? *Ha'aretz*, 5 April, available online at www.haaretz.com/news/israel/.premium-1.650425.

de Swaan, A. (1988), *In Care of the State*, New York: Oxford University Press.

Fassin, D. (2012), *Humanitarian Reason*, Berkeley, CA: University of California Press.

Feather, N.T. (1999), *Values, Achievement, and Justice*, New York: Kluwer Academic/Plenum.

Gilens, M. (1999), *Why Americans Hate Welfare*, Chicago, IL: University of Chicago Press.

Gollust, S. E. and J. Lynch, (2010), *Who Deserves Health Care?* Robert Wood Johnson Foundation Working Paper Series (WP-48).

Gollust, S. E., P. M. Lantz and P. A. Ubel, (2010), The polarizing effect of news media messages about the social determinants of health, *American Journal of Public Health*, **99**(12), 2160–2167.

Gottlieb, N., D. Filc and N. Davidovitch (2012), 'Medical humanitarianism, human rights, and political advocacy,' *Social Science & Medicine*, **74**(6), 839–845.

Grove, N. J. and A. B. Zwi (2006), Our health and theirs: forced migration, othering, and public health, *Social Science & Medicine*, **62**, 1931–1942.

Guetzkow, J. (2010), Beyond deservingness: congressional discourse on poverty, 1964–1996, *Annals of the American Academy of Political and Social Science*, **629**, 173–197.

Haas, B. M. (2012), *Suffering and the Struggle for Recognition: Lived Experiences of the US Political Asylum Process*, PhD thesis in Anthropology, University of California, San Diego.

Heyman, J. (1998), *Finding a Moral Heart for US Immigration Policy*, Washington, DC: American Anthropological Association.

Holmes, S. M. (2012), The clinical gaze in the practice of migrant health, *Social Science & Medicine*, **74**(6), 873–881.

Horton, S. (2004), Different subjects, *Medical Anthropology Quarterly*, **18**, 472–489.

Huschke, S. (2014), Performing deservingness: humanitarian health care provision for migrants in Germany, *Social Science & Medicine*, **120**, 352–359.

Kahn, S. (2000), *Reproducing Jews*, Durham, NC: Duke University Press.

Kanaaneh, R. A. (2002), *Birthing the Nation*, Berkeley, CA: University of California Press.

Kashti, O. (2015), Israeli government's apathy is killing foreign workers' children, *Ha'aretz* newspaper, 31 March, available online at www.haaretz.com/opinion/.premium-1.649736.

Katz, M. B. (1989), *The Undeserving Poor*, New York: Pantheon Books.

Kochhar, R., R. Ruro and S. Tafoya (2005), *The New Latino South*, Washington, DC: Pew Hispanic Center.

Kovacs, J. (2003), Transplants for illegals igniting US firestorm, *World Net Daily*, available online at www.wnd.com/2003/03/17606.

Lancet (2008), Migrant health: what are doctors' leaders doing? *Lancet*, **371**, 178.

Larchanché, S. (2012), Intangible obstacles: health implications of stigmatization, structural violence, and fear among undocumented immigrants in France, *Social Science & Medicine*, **74**(6), 858–863.

Lawrance, B. N. (2012), Humanitarian claims and expert testimonies, *Ghana Studies*, **15/16**, 251–286.

Lipsky, M. (1980), *Street-Level Bureaucracy*, New York: Russell Sage Foundation.

Lynch, J. and S. E. Gollust (2010), *Playing Fair: Fairness Beliefs and Health Policy Preferences in the United States*, Robert Wood Johnson Foundation Working Paper Series (WP-47).

Malkin, M. (2003), *America: Medical Welcome Mat to the World*, available online at www.vdare.com/articles/america-medical-welcome-mat-to-the-world.

Marrow, H. (2011), Deserving to a point: undocumented immigrants in San Francisco's universal access healthcare model, *Social Science & Medicine*, **74**(6), 846–854.

Marrow, H. and T. Joseph (2015), Excluded and frozen out: unauthorised immigrants' (non) access to care after US health care reform, *Journal of Ethnic and Migration Studies*, **41**(14), 2253–2273.

Mesila Aid and Information Center (2006), *Annual Activity Report*, Tel Aviv: Mesila Aid and Information Center.

Mesila Aid and Information Center (2015), *Summer 2015 at Mesila*, Tel Aviv: Mesila Aid and Information Center.

Morgen, S. and J. Maskovsky (2003), The anthropology of welfare 'reform', *Annual Review of Anthropology*, 32, 315–338.
Newton, L. (2005), It is not a question of being anti-immigration, in A. Schneider and H. Ingram (eds.), *Deserving and Entitled*, Albany, NY: SUNY Press.
Ngai, M. M. (2004), *Impossible Subjects*, Princeton, NJ: Princeton University Press.
Office of the State Comptroller (2013), *Annual Report*, available online at http://old.mevaker.gov.il/serve/contentTree.asp?bookid=644&id=196&contentid=&parentcid=undefined&sw=1920&hw=1010.
Oliverio-Lauderdale, D. (2014), *Contradictions and Exclusions: An Ethnographic Study of African Im/migrants' Right to Health in Italy*, MA Thesis in Anthropology, University of British Columbia.
Olsen, J. A., J. Richardson, P. Dolan, and P. Menzel (2003), The moral relevance of personal characteristics in setting health care priorities, *Social Science & Medicine*, 57, 1163–1172.
Portes, A., P. Fernández-Kelly and D. Light (2012), Life on the edge: immigrants confront the American health system, *Ethnic and Racial Studies*, **35**(1), 3–22.
Quesada, J., L. K. Hart and P. Bourgois (2011), Structural vulnerability and health, *Medical Anthropology*, **30**(4), 339–362.
Rylko-Bauer, B. and P. Farmer (2002), Managed care or managed inequality? A call for critiques of market-based medicine, *Medical Anthropology Quarterly*, 16(4), 476–502.
Sales, R. (2002), The deserving and the undeserving? Refugees, asylum seekers and welfare in Britain, *Critical Social Policy*, **22**(3), 456–478.
Schneider, A. L. and H. M. Ingram (2005), *Deserving and Entitled: Social Constructions and Public Policy*, Albany, NY: SUNY Press.
Scott, C. (2008), Belief in a just world, *Hastings Center Report*, **38**(1), 16–19.
Stumpf, J. P. (2006), The crimmigration crisis, *American University Law Review*, **56**, 367.
Ticktin, M. (2011), *Casualties of Care*, Berkeley, CA: University of California Press.
Tiedje, K. and D. J. Plevak (2014), Medical humanitarianism in the United States, *Social Science & Medicine*, **120**, 360–367.
van Oorschot, W. (2000), Who should get what, and why? On deservingness criteria and the conditionality of solidarity among the public, *Policy & Politics*, **28**(1), 33–48.
van Oorschot, W. (2006), Making the difference in social Europe, *Journal of European Social Policy*, **16**(1), 23–42.
Vanthuyne, K., F. Meloni, M. Ruiz-Casares, C. Rousseau and A. Ricard-Guay (2013), Health workers' perceptions of access to care for children and pregnant women with precarious immigration status, *Social Science & Medicine*, **93**, 78–85.
Verkuyten, M. (2004), Emotional reactions to and support for immigrant policies, *Social Justice Research*, **17**(3), 293–314.
Viladrich, A. (2012), Beyond welfare reform: reframing undocumented immigrants' entitlement to health care in the United States, *Social Science & Medicine*, **74**(6), 822–829.
Vilnai, O. (2015a), Three infants died this month because of harsh conditions in daycares for children of asylum seekers, *Ha'aretz* newspaper, 25 February, available online at www.haaretz.co.il/news/orly/.premium-1.2573759.
Vilnai, O. (2015b), Four-month old infant dies in daycare for children of asylum seekers in South Tel Aviv, *Ha'aretz* newspaper, 29 March, available online at www.haaretz.co.il/news/education/.premium-1.2601973.
Vilnai, O. (2015c), Another infant dies in the 'child warehouses' in South Tel Aviv, the fifth in two months, *Ha'aretz* newspaper, 30 March, available online at www.haaretz.co.il/news/education/1.2602929.
Wailoo, K., J. Livingston and P. Guarnaccia (eds.) (2006) *A Death Retold: Jesica Santillan, the Bungled Transplant, and Paradoxes of Medical Citizenship,* Chapel Hill, NC: University of North Carolina Press.
Watters, C. (2007), Refugees at Europe's borders: the moral economy of care, *Transcultural Psychiatry*, **44**, 394–417.
Will, J. A. (1993), The dimensions of poverty: public perceptions of the deserving poor, *Social Science Research*, 22, 312–332.

Willen, S. S. (2010), Citizens, 'real' others, and 'other' others, in N. De Genova and N. Peutz (eds.), *The Deportation Regime*, Durham, NC: Duke University Press, pp. 262–294.
Willen, S. S. (2011), Do 'illegal' migrants have a 'right to health'? Engaging ethical theory as social practice at a Tel Aviv open clinic, *Medical Anthropology Quarterly*, **45**(3), 303–330.
Willen, S. S. (2012a), How is health-related 'deservingness' reckoned? *Social Science & Medicine*, **74**(6), 812–821.
Willen, S. S. (ed.) (2012b), Special issue—migration, 'illegality', and health: mapping embodied vulnerability and debating health-related deservingness, *Social Science & Medicine*, **74**(6), 805–811.
Willen, S. S. (2015), Lightning rods in the local moral economy: debating unauthorized migrants' deservingness in Israel, *International Migration*, **53**(3), 70–86.
WHO Commission on Social Determinants of Health (2008), *Closing the Gap in a Generation: Health Equity Through Action on the Social Determinants of Health*, Geneva: World Health Organization.
Yarris, K. and H. Castañeda (eds.) (2015), Special issue—discourses of displacement and deservingness: interrogating distinctions between 'economic' and 'forced' migration, *International Migration*, **53**(3), 64–69.
Yoo, G.J. (2002), Constructing deservingness, *Journal of Aging and Social Policy*, **13**, 17–34.
Yoo, G. J. (2008), Immigrants and welfare: policy constructions of deservingness, *Journal of Immigrant & Refugee Studies*, **6**(4), 490–507.

7 International health worker migration: issues of ethics, human rights and health equity

Vivien Runnels, Corinne Packer and Ronald Labonté

BACKGROUND

Health worker migration has been described as a major reason for, and contributor to, shortages of health workers, particularly in low- and middle-income countries (O'Brien and Gostin 2011; WHO, 2006). The *World Health Report* (WHO, 2006) estimated a global health workforce of about 59 million and a shortage of 4.3 million workers (midwives, nurses and physicians) in 2006. This figure has since been updated by the Global Health Workforce Alliance and the World Health Organization, which estimate a global shortage of 7.2 million health workers, with 83 countries facing a health worker crisis (Campbell et al. 2013). Given the evidence-based adage that health workers save lives, long-term projections of a global deficit of approximately 12.9 million skilled health professionals by the year 2035 are of major concern.

Shortages in the global health workforce are closely related to the unequal distribution of health workers, meaning how health-based human resources are located or distributed in relation to need. All countries require a health workforce to be sufficient in size and skills and properly located geographically to respond effectively to their populations' health-care needs. Many low-income countries have very high burdens of disease and low health worker density (WHO, 2006). This combination suggests that significant proportions of their populations have little, poor or no access to healthcare.

As O'Brien and Gostin (2011: 16) remark, '[n]ot only are there inadequate numbers of health workers . . . [and] a much greater burden of disease . . . [but also] scarce resources'. This creates a vicious cycle of health decline, as inevitably, the disease burden grows when there are so few human and other resources available to respond to the existing health problems.' They paint the picture with grave figures from sub-Saharan Africa, with '10% of the world's population, 24% of the world's disease burden, 3% of the world's health care workers, and less than 1% of the world health's expenditures' (O'Brien and Gostin 2011: 16).

Many high-income countries with lower burdens of disease have a higher density of health workers but in a context where population expectations and health systems organization create both high demand and domestic maldistribution, leading to a real or perceived health worker shortage. The European Commission forecasts Europe will have a shortage of 1 million health professionals by 2020. If long-term care and auxiliary professions are taken into account, this figure rises to 2 million (European Commission 2012: 5). Health Workforce Australia projects a 27 per cent shortage of nurses in the country by 2025 (HWA 2012: iii), while the US estimates it will have a shortfall of 21 per cent of nurses (HRSA 2014: 2) and 46,000–90,000 physicians by the same year (IHS 2015: v). Researchers and governmental and intergovernmental health human resources task forces have summarized the causes of these shortages in high-income countries. They include increases in life expectancy and subsequent demand for elderly care; insufficient training and recruitment of new health professionals; and burnout of existing health workers (O'Brien and Gostin 2011; WHO 2006).

Why some countries lack (or perceive that they lack) sufficient human resources for health is an important and often political question. But when countries that can least afford to lose health workers experience staff shortages associated with the international migration of health workers, it becomes a global ethical issue. This is especially so when émigré health workers move to higher-income countries that have lower disease burdens and greater capacity to build their own health workforce and address their own problems of shortages or maldistribution. Sometimes described as a 'perverse subsidy' (WHO 2006: 101), 'source' countries lose their public investments in training or support, while 'destination' countries save on foregone training costs. According to Mensah et al. (2005), for example, the UK government saved some £103 million alone from the employment of 293 doctors and 1,021 nurses from Ghana in 2004.

The movement of healthcare workers from poorer source countries to benefit richer destination countries is ethically challenging because such movement generally exacerbates health inequities in source countries, i.e., it makes healthcare less readily available to (at least) some of their citizens. Health equity, defined as '[t]he absence of disparities in health (and in its key social determinants) that are systematically associated with social advantage/disadvantage' (Braveman and Gruskin 2003: 12), has become a normative global standard for adjudicating the fairness or social justice of health systems (Whitehead 1992; Sen 2002; Goddard and Smith 2002).

WHO IS ETHICALLY RESPONSIBLE FOR SHORTAGES OF HEALTH WORKERS?

Modern globalization, which is highly flavoured by the politics, policies and economics of neoliberalism – that is, an unconditional support for the operation of free markets – has been shown to have contributed to the creation of a highly unequal and unfair world with both short- and long-term implications for reducing global health inequities (WHO Commission on Social Determinants of Health 2008; Schrecker and Bambra, 2015).

The conditions for skilled health worker migration have been facilitated by systems and processes associated with globalization, be it social, political or economic in nature. These include the liberalization and integration of trade, enhanced air travel, rapid international transfers of funds and international investments, communications through cellular telephone technology and the internet, and dual citizenship, all of which have enabled the mobility of workers, both temporary and permanent. Increased knowledge of labour market trends and employment opportunities in other countries, and the influence of diasporic communities that encourage mobility through word-of-mouth are other reasons cited for health worker migration (Runnels et al. 2010). For instance, in the year 2000, it was estimated that 65,000 African-born physicians and 70,000 African-born nurses worked in developed countries. Viewed from another perspective, this meant that one-fifth of all African-born physicians and one-tenth of African-born nurses practised their profession, or another form of work, overseas at that time. Occupational diaspora are created as word of success and employment opportunities spreads to family and former colleagues (Clemens and Pettersson 2007).

Theoretical underpinnings for health worker migration largely draw from a classic 'push/pull' dichotomy. Health workers are either 'pushed' out from source countries as a result of under-resourced health systems, dangerous working and poor living conditions, poor remuneration or a simple lack of employment opportunities and government encouragement to migrate; or 'pulled' to destination countries. Pull factors include employment opportunities, better working conditions and remuneration, better quality of life and, for some (especially those who consider their migration to be temporary), the ability to earn money that can be remitted back home to extended families, or for investment purposes (Packer et al. 2009: 222). In this complex of push and pull factors, active recruitment is not even required to entice health workers to leave their countries (Poppe et al. 2014). The global context smooths the way for health worker migration and mobility, neither of which are particularly new, but both of which have risen in global health policy importance over recent decades.

HUMAN RIGHTS IMPLICATIONS

Health worker migration is not only an ethical issue but also a human rights issue. Do rich nations that recruit health workers from poorer countries violate human rights they have committed to uphold? Or do health workers, like all other individuals, simply have the freedom to seek migration and move to countries that are willing to accept them?

Inadequately Protected Rights in Source Countries Leads to Migration

The Universal Declaration of Human Rights (UDHR) (UN 1994a) recognizes in Article 23(1) that individuals have the right to work, to free choice of employment, fair working conditions and protection against unemployment. Importantly, it links these rights and conditions to health, noting in Article 25(1) that '[e]veryone has the right to a standard of living adequate for the health and well-being of himself and of his family'. The literature on push factors consistently advances that health workers leave their countries because their fundamental rights to work, to an adequate standard of living and to security are not being protected. For instance, a survey of reasons to migrate cited by university students in six southern African countries revealed cost of living, inability to find a relevant job, lack of prospects for professional advancement, low income and personal and family security to be the most important factors (Crush et al. 2005). The prospect of significantly higher pay in rich countries acts as a considerable pull to address or compensate for these lacunae (Thomas 2006; Hagopian et al. 2005).

Health workers in poorer countries, *if* they are able to obtain work and *if* they are paid on a regular and commensurate basis, arguably are better able to support themselves and their families. In reality, however, health workers (nurses often more so than physicians) frequently face insufficient job opportunities, precarious employment, irregular or delayed payment of salaries, and/or low wages, which consequently make for a persistent struggle to sustain an adequate standard of living. Moreover, in many source countries, individuals cannot depend on an adequate social security system to support them in the event of unemployment, illness or retirement (O'Brien and Gostin 2011; WHO 2006). Inevitably, health workers (as with other individuals fortunate enough to have the means) consider migration as a solution.

Compounding their struggle to obtain an adequate standard of living and just and favourable working conditions is the threat to personal security that individuals face in less developed source countries. Both the UDHR and the International Covenant on Civil and Political Rights

(UN 1994b) stipulate that states must ensure that everyone has the right to security of person, recognizing the absence of security as an obstacle to the enjoyment of many other rights, such as the right to freedom of movement, to personal integrity and to freedom from violence. While health worker migrants do not necessarily articulate the reasons for migration relative to violations of their human rights, many may seek to migrate primarily because of concerns related to lack of or threats to human rights, including their own and their family and children's safety and security, at home and in the workplace (Labonté et al. 2015).

The health worker migration literature indicates strongly that movement from underdeveloped to developed countries will only begin to diminish when the root causes of health worker migration that include push/pull factors are addressed (Bidwell et al. 2014; Kline, 2003: Mejia et al. 1979). Back in 1994, the Cairo Declaration and Program of Action – adopted at the International Conference on Population and Development – described the complexity at hand: 'The long-term manageability of international migration hinges on making the option to remain in one's country a viable one for all people.' However, it also recognizes that to make this option viable, 'countries of origin and countries of destination must cooperate' (UN 1994b).

The Human Rights Obligations of Destination Countries

What then are the human rights based obligations of destination (recipient) countries, such as Western European countries, Canada, the US, Australia and New Zealand? Another human rights treaty – the International Covenant on Economic, Social and Cultural Rights (ICESCR) – provides in Article 12 for the right to health. This treaty provision obligates states to *respect* the right to health in other countries. Their actions or negotiations should not diminish the abilities of other countries to fulfil their own obligations under Article 12. A former UN Special Rapporteur on the Right to the Highest Attainable Standard of Health addressed what this means with regard to health workers (UNGA 2005: para. 61) specifying that:

> [D]eveloped countries should ensure that their human resource policies do not jeopardize the right to health in developing countries. If a developed country actively recruits health professionals from a developing country that is suffering from a shortage of health professionals in such a manner that the recruitment reduces the developing country's capacity to fulfill the right to health obligations it owes its citizens, the developed country is *prima facie* in breach of its human rights responsibility of international assistance and cooperation in the context of the right to health.

State parties to the ICESCR are also obligated to *protect* against infringements of this right by third parties such as corporations, by ensuring that third parties over whom they have legal or political influence respect the enjoyment of this right in other countries. This obligation should prevent health authorities in destination countries from using the services of recruiting agencies in developing countries with a shortage of health professionals. By this logic, both active and passive recruitment of foreign health workers by destination countries, whether by public health authorities or private recruitment firms in these countries, constitutes a violation of the right to health by destination countries, because the relocation of health workers adversely impacts source country health systems. The failure of wealthier destination countries to be self-reliant in domestic health human resources creates a pull on healthcare workers from source countries, thus undermining the ability of source countries to protect the right to health of their citizens.

Finally, countries that have ratified the ICESCR treaty are required to *fulfil* to the best of their abilities the progressive realization of rights therein, including the right to health. This includes an obligation on wealthier countries to help poorer countries meet their obligations under the right to health through, for example, international assistance and cooperation. Former UN Special Rapporteur Paul Hunt adds that it is fundamentally disingenuous to provide overseas development assistance, debt relief and other forms of aid with one hand while simultaneously taking health professionals trained at the expense of developing countries with the other. 'Recipient and other developed countries must therefore address their own inadequate production and retention of health professionals, adhere to ethical recruitment principles, help strengthen health systems in source countries and promote macro-economic policies consistent with human rights' (UNGA 2005: para. 64).

So Whose Right to Health Prevails?

Bueno de Mesquita and Gordon (2005) have recommendations for both source and destination countries to reduce threats to the rights discussed above. For source countries, they include allocating health budgets commensurate with their needs, and strengthening their public health systems, including better human resources planning. For destination countries, they include increasing their budgets for healthcare as well as international aid. While these appear fairly simplistic, they provide an easy reference point by which to begin tackling the impacts of health worker migration.

POLICIES FOR ETHICAL CONDUCT IN HEALTH WORKER RECRUITMENT AND MIGRATION

In addition to human rights instruments, we may also draw from policies and codes of conduct. A number of codes of conduct have been designed and adopted to help regulate health worker migration, promote the ethical recruitment of health workers and protect national health systems. These codes offer a type of ethical counterbalance to largely unregulated processes of migration. The WHO Global Code of Practice on the International Recruitment of Health Personnel, for example, is a multilateral agreement put in place to prevent unethical recruitment globally. It is important in that it raises awareness of the harms arising from health worker migration. The WHO Code remains a voluntary code. While placing limits on country (and recruiter) behaviour, it can be interpreted as opposing freedom of individual movement by placing restrictions on 'active' recruitment that facilitates mobility. Another problem results from the lack of an enforcement mechanism, despite the fact that the WHO Code covers the widest possible range of employers in both the public and private sectors, and includes NGOs, professional associations and regional health authorities. In short, the WHO Code represents 'just one instrument that is not in itself a sufficient policy response to the complexities of health worker migration' (Yeates and Pillinger 2013: 35–36).

Regional and bilateral agreements between specific source and destination countries also exist and may be more successful as the commitment is stronger and oversight more manageable. A good example of this, still as imperfect as it may be, is the Southern African Development Community (SADC) Treaty 1992 and Protocol on the Facilitation of Movement of Persons, signed in 2005, which both facilitates and restricts legal movement of persons in the region (Tjadens et al., 2013). Although the Protocol is not yet in force (too few member states have ratified it to date), South Africa issued a policy statement stating that 'recruitment of *individual* applicants from identified developing countries, in particular from another SADC country, will not be endorsed by the Department' (Department of Health 2006). South Africa is not just a source country for health workers, but also a destination country. In the 2000s, almost a quarter of physicians in South Africa were foreign-trained, the majority of whom worked in rural and remote areas (Sanders and Lloyd 2005).

MORAL COUNTERCLAIMS TO HEALTH WORKER MIGRATION AND SHORTAGES

In the case of migration of health workers, developed destination countries make gains. There are also some benefits to source countries that include remittances, transfer of knowledge and new skills gained on return migration. These benefits are argued as 'moral counterclaims' (Shah 2010: 4) and can be an exchange, recompense or equalizing factor for the losses that source countries experience. Remittances, in particular are extremely important for the economies of some countries, and have also been considered as a complement to development aid (ILO 2014; Packer et al. 2010; Ouaked 2002). Sent by migrants to communities and families, remittances may be used in part for healthcare purposes (money used to purchase healthcare; build community health centres; improve shelter, etc.) (Frank et al. 2009; Ratha 2011; Mercer et al. 2008). Transfer of knowledge and new skills gained by source countries on return migration are also claimed as important benefits.

In contrast, however, the healthcare systems of many developing countries are in a state of collapse or provide services that are out of reach of the poorest, clearly showing that healthcare across countries is anything but equitable (McCoy et al. 2006), and that moral counterclaims often have little to no benefit in reality. Health worker migration results in shortages of workers to deliver basic (primary) healthcare in countries already facing high disease burdens and limited health coverage, and unable to carry out universal preventive care programmes such as immunization, and primary healthcare. Box 7.1 presents some examples from an empirical study (Tomblin-Murphy et al. 2016) of how health worker migration from Jamaica leads to health inequity.

Ethical Issues Related to Gender in Health Worker Migration

Migrant health workers, like migrants in general, have been shown to experience an increase in vulnerability, including changes in their 'legal' relationship with both source and destination countries; loss of personal resources, social capital, power and human and legal rights (Bustamente 2010; George 2007). At the same time, health worker migration can bring benefits to individuals and families including improved status, greater autonomy and the ability to remit to families at home. However, while female nurses globally form the dominant health worker migrant group (Brush and Sochalski 2007), migration theory has generally disregarded gender (Carling 2005), although more recent research has acknowledged that differences exist between men and women in terms of motivations, norms and risks when it comes to migration (Curran and Saguy 2013).

BOX 7.1 HEALTH EQUITY IMPACTS OF HEALTH WORKER MIGRATION FROM JAMAICA

Jamaica (in the context of the Caribbean) has one of the highest emigration rates in the world, mostly to the US. Jamaica's health workers report their low income and the high cost of living as top-ranked reasons for leaving (Tomblin-Murphy et al. 2013: 10). Return challenges included adjusting to a lower salary (relative to the cost of living), poorer infrastructure, equipment and supplies, and being treated with hostility or disrespect as a result of having migrated. Some examples of health equity impacts of such migration are as follows (italicized).

- Loss of senior and experienced health professionals to migration, *depriving the health sector of valuable leadership and experience*.
- A reported shortage of nursing educators (some losses associated with migration), *affecting the quality of training* that nursing students receive (World Bank 2009).

  'We have lost a whole generation of nurses. Our records show that every health facility lose their qualified staff on a continuous basis, so at this time there are a few seniors at the top and the bottom is filled with juniors. We have lost the middle. . . .Tutors are short. So are the nurse managers as those who coach and mentor the nurses' (Tomblin-Murphy et al. forthcoming).

- Leaving the country financially worse off due to *lost public investments in education* (Yan 2006; Jones et al. 2009).
- Reduced supply of nurses *negatively affects the implementation of care and prevention strategies* for a large portion of the population. This is reported to have been particularly detrimental to those affected by the HIV/AIDS virus (Salmon et al. 2007).
- Shortage of nurses linked to the *fall in immunization coverage* for poliomyelitis, and diphtheria, pertussis and tetanus (DPT) in Jamaica in the late 1990s and early 2000s (HECORA 2008).
- Challenges associated with recruiting and retaining health professionals: *increased costs for recruitment and retention*.

Less-developed source countries, such as India and the Philippines, have also seen a rapid growth in the number of educational programmes designed to teach nursing care in international contexts, to help ensure nurses are able and ready to migrate and work abroad. However such training is often designed to capitalize on the recruitment of female nurse trainees for specific markets. Findings from our research in India, for instance, suggested that male nurses only trained for specific roles (such as psychiatric nursing), while female nurses were expected to carry out intimate personal care, also considered to be 'dirty' work in some cultures in the Middle East where female migrant Indian nurses are employed (Nair 2012; Walton-Roberts and Runnels, in process).

More recent thinking about the feminization of labour, (and nursing is a highly feminized profession), has brought attention to the vulnerabilities and exploitation of migrants in general, but more so those experienced by women including those in the health workforce such as deskilling, racial intolerance and discrimination (Kofman and Raghuram 2006; Ball 2004; Piper, 2003). In order to avoid rights abuses and other gender-related negative impacts, migration policy in general and health worker migration policy in particular can benefit from sex/gender analysis, something that the WHO Global Code of Practice on the International Recruitment of Health Personnel has, to this point in time, failed to incorporate.

Deskilling

Émigré health workers are frequently deskilled or underemployed in destination countries, representing a net loss to the global health workforce (McNeil-Walsh 2008). The migration of nurses that results in their working in fields other than nursing (including personal care work) can lead to their downward mobility or deskilling. Migrating health workers from the Philippines, for instance, become private sector care workers in the United States and other destination countries particularly for childcare, elder care and other types of long-term care and living.

Globalization, Privatization and Health Worker Migration

Lastly, we return to the global context of our chapter. Emphasis on free markets has facilitated the privatization of healthcare and the growth of multinational enterprises that are increasing their penetration of healthcare systems that previously had been largely under public financing and provision. Private healthcare, in turn, may promote health worker migration, encouraging the movement of public sector health workers to the private sector where jobs are more plentiful and lucrative. A typical pattern arises with physicians and nurses based in rural and poor areas moving to cities for better working conditions and environments; and urban-based physicians and nurses moving from the critically under-equipped and under-funded public sector to the private sector (Gerein et al., 2006). These processes of privatization and marketization in health services, with their implications for health worker migration, have their origin in the structural adjustment programs of the World Bank and International Monetary Fund of the 1980s and 1990s, which in large measure continue to today (Ruckert et al. 2015; Labonté 2014; Labonté and Stuckler 2015).

FUTURE DIRECTIONS AND CONCLUSIONS

Ethical policy in general assumes the prevention of new harms and the means or remedies to redress 'old' harms. In the case of health worker migration and associated shortages, ethical policy includes expanding a notion of harm that specifies reducing health inequities for populations regardless of their national or geographic location.

Implications for undertaking future research and building global policy for health worker migration, ethical responses and health equity are numerous. Primarily there is a need for specifying the impacts of privatized healthcare and health worker migration on ethics and health equity. According to Grieshaber-Otto and Sinclair (2004: 155), imbalances in the international system that give far greater priority to commercial and investor rights than to basic human rights, such as the right to health, must be corrected. Given the increased international privatization of healthcare, one might reasonably expect more in the way of global socially responsible corporate policy statements, but structures to monitor these policies, like the WHO Global Code, require careful crafting, consistent application and monitoring, and some form of penalty (even if only 'naming and shaming') for non-compliance. Governments, at a minimum, should be raising awareness and encouraging private sector responsibility for citizens' health and social outcomes.

The migration of health workers remains a concern for many source countries. However, greater threats to health equity may be in store. The migration of health workers is now becoming highly associated with private healthcare labour markets, and privatization can divert limited public resources to the private sector, amplifying health inequity. Factors that lie *outside* the public health sector (and the reach of domestic governments), in spite of possible harmful implications, can have critical impacts on health worker migration and associated shortages with implications for health equity. There is a flip side to health worker migration; instead of health workers from low- and middle-income countries moving abroad to take up jobs in the understaffed healthcare sectors of Western countries, Western patients facing long queues for care are increasingly moving to obtain treatment swiftly and economically in lesser developed countries (Labonté et al. 2013). The gold rush to primarily private medical tourism has providers in low- and middle-income countries attempting to capitalize on what they perceive to be an unfilled demand from the wealthier and demographically ageing North, some of whom are expatriates returning to countries of origin for healthcare (Labonté et al. 2013; Ormond, Chapter 26 this volume). A phenomenon associated with medical tourism in developing countries is a new form of health worker migration where doctors and nurses leave the public health system to work in the lucrative private hospitals established in their countries for medical tourists, further contributing domestically to health inequity (Labonté et al. 2013).

In sum, as one international agency representative recently interviewed, deftly concluded: 'Migration of health professionals is at the junction of the right to mobility, right to health and right to decent work . . . It is about finding an acceptable compromise between the rights and obligations of migrant workers, employers and governments based on sound research findings.'

REFERENCES

Ball, R. E. (2004), Divergent development, racialized rights: globalized labour markets and the trade of nurses – the case of the Philippines, *Women's Studies International Forum*, **27**(2), 119–133.

Bidwell, P., P. Laxmikanth, C. Blacklock, G. Hayward, M. Willcox, W. Peersman, S. Moosa and D. Mant (2014), Security and skills: the two key issues in health worker migration, *Global Health Action*, **7**, 24194.

Braveman, P. and S. Gruskin (2003), Defining equity in health, *Journal of Epidemiology & Community Health*, **57**, 254–258.

Brush, B. L. and J. Sochalski (2007), International nurse migration: lessons from the Philippines, *Policy, Politics & Nursing Practice*, **8**(1), 37–46.

Bueno de Mesquita, J. B. and M. Gordon (2005), *The International Migration of Health Workers: A Human Rights Analysis*, London: Medact.

Bustamente, J. A. (2010), Extreme vulnerability of migrants: the cases of the United States and Mexico, *Georgetown Immigration Law Journal*, **24**, 565–583.

Campbell, J., G. Dussault, J. Buchan, F. Pozo-Martin, M. Guerra Arias, C. Leone and G. Cometto (2013), *A Universal Truth: No Health Without a Workforce. Forum Report, Third Global Forum on Human Resources for Health, Recife, Brazil*, Geneva: Global Health Workforce Alliance and World Health Organization.

Carling, J. (2005), *Gender Dimensions of International Migration*, Global Migration Perspectives No. 35, Geneva: Global Commission on International Migration.

Clemens M. A. and G. Pettersson (2007), *New Data on African Health Professionals Abroad*, Working Paper Number 95, Washington, DC: Centre for Global Development, available online at www.cgdev.org/sites/default/files/9267_file_CGDWP95_Feb_2007.pdf.

Crush, J., W. Pendleton and D. S. Tevera (2005), *Degrees of Uncertainty: Students and the Brain Drain in Southern Africa*, Pretoria: Africa Institute of South Africa.

Curran S. R. and A. C. Saguy (2013), Migration and cultural change: a role for gender and social networks? *Journal of International Women's Studies*, **2**(3), 54–77.

Dahlgren, G. (2014), Why public health services? Experiences from profit-driven health care reforms in Sweden, *International Journal of Health Services*, **44**, 507–524.

Department of Health, South Africa (2006), *Foreign Workforce Management Programme National Department of Health, Republic of South Africa Policy: Recruitment and Employment of Foreign Health Professionals in the Republic of South Africa*, Pretoria: Department of Health, available online at www.equinetafrica.org/bibl/docs/GOVhres310108.pdf.

European Commission (2012), *Commission Staff Working Document on an Action Plan for the EU Health Workforce*, Strasbourg, 18 April, SWD(2012) 93 Final, available online at http://ec.europa.eu/health/workforce/docs/staff_working_doc_healthcare_workforce_en.pdf.

Frank, R., O. Palma-Coca, J. Rauda-Esquivel, G. Olaiz-Fernández, C. Díaz-Olavarrieta and

D. Acevedo-García (2009), The relationship between remittances and health care provision in Mexico, *American Journal of Public Health*, **99**(7), 1227–1231.
George, A. (2007), *Human Resources for Health: A Gender Analysis*, background paper prepared for the Women and Gender Equity Knowledge Network and the Health Systems Knowledge Network of the WHO Commission on Social Determinants of Health, available online at www.who.int/social_determinants/resources/human_resources_for_health_wgkn_2007.pdf.
Gerein, N., A. Green and S. Pearson (2006), The implications of shortages of health professionals for maternal health in sub-Saharan Africa, *Reproductive Health Matters*, **14**, 40–50.
Goddard, M. and P. Smith (2002), Equity of access to health care services: theory and evidence from the UK, *Social Science & Medicine*, **53**, 1149–1162.
Grieshaber-Otto, J. and S. Sinclair (2004), *Bad Medicine: Trade Treaties, Privatization and Health Care Reform in Canada*, Ottawa: Canadian Centre for Policy Alternatives.
Hagopian, A., A. Ofosu, A. Fatusi, R. Biritwum, A. Essel, L.G. Hart, and C. Watts (2005), The flight of physicians from West Africa: views of African physicians and implications for policy, *Social Science & Medicine*, **61**(8), 1750–1760.
HECORA (2008), *Draft Report Strategic Plan on Health and Related Social Services in the CARICOM*, available online at www.caricom.org/jsp/single_market/services_regime/concept_paper_health.pdf.
HRSA (2014), *US Department of Health and Human Services, Health Resources and Services Administration, National Center for Health Workforce Analysis: The Future of the Nursing Workforce: National- and State-Level Projections, 2012–2025*, Rockville, MD, available online at http://bhpr.hrsa.gov/healthworkforce/supplydemand/nursing/workforceprojections/nursingprojections.pdf.
HWA (2012), *Health Workforce 2025: Doctors, Nurses and Midwives, Volume 1*, available online at www.hwa.gov.au/sites/uploads/FinalReport_Volume1_FINAL-20120424.pdf.
IHS (2015), *The Complexities of Physician Supply and Demand: Projections from 2013 to 2025*, prepared for the Association of American Medical Colleges, Washington, DC: Association of American Medical Colleges.
ILO (2014), *Helping Migrants Make the Most of their Money*, available online at www.ilo.org/global/about-the-ilo/newsroom/features/WCMS_327092/lang--en/index.htm.
Jones, A., A. Bifulco and J. Gabe (2009), Caribbean nurses migrating to the UK: a gender focused literature review, *International Nursing Review*, **56**(3), 285–290.
Kline, D. (2003), Push and pull factors in international nurse migration, *Journal of Nursing Scholarship*, **35**(2), 107–111.
Kofman, E. and P. Raghuram (2006), Gender and global labour migrations: incorporating skilled workers, *Antipode*, **38**(2), 282–303.
Labonté, R. (2014), The global health agenda and shrinking policy spaces in the post-crisis landscape, in L. Jacobs, and D. Drache (eds.), *Linking Global Trade and Human Rights: New Policy Spaces in Hard Economic Times*, Cambridge: Cambridge University Press.
Labonté, R. and D. Stuckler (2015), The rise of neoliberalism: how bad economics imperils health and what to do about it, *Journal of Epidemiology and Community Health*, **0**, 1–7.
Labonté, R., V. Runnels, C. Packer and R. Deonandan (eds.) (2013), Travelling Well: Essays in Medical Tourism, Ottawa: Institute of Population Health, University of Ottawa, available online at www.globalhealthequity.ca/content/travelling-well-essays-medical-tourism.
Labonté, R., D. Sanders, T. Mathole, J. Crush, A. Chikanda, Y. Dambisya, V. Runnels, C. Packer, A. MacKenzie, G. Tomblin Murphy and I Bourgeault (2015), Health worker migration from South Africa: causes, consequences and policy responses, *Human Resources for Health*, **13**:92.
McCoy, D., R. Labonté and J. Orbinski (2006), Mobilising the Canadian public health community around a global health advocacy agenda, *Canadian Journal of Public Health*, **97**, 142–144.
McNeil-Walsh, C. (2008), Migrant nurses and the experience of skill: South African nurses in the UK health care sector, in J. Connell (ed.), *The International Migration of Health Workers*, New York: Routledge.

Mejia, A., H. Pizurk and E. Royston (1979), *Physician and Nurse Migration: Analysis and Policy Implications: Report of a WHO Study*, Geneva: World Health Organization.
Mensah, K., M. Mackintosh and L. Henry (2005), *The 'Skills Drain' of Health Professionals from the Developing World: A Framework for Policy Formulation.* London: Medact.
Mercer, C., B. Page, and M. Evans (2008), *Development and the African Diaspora: Place and the Politics of Home*, London: Zed Books.
Nair, S. (2012), *Moving with the Times: Gender, Status and Migration of Nurses in India*, India: Routledge.
O'Brien, P. and L. O. Gostin (2011), *Health Worker Shortages and Global Justice*, New York: Milbank Memorial Fund.
Ouaked, S. (2002), Transatlantic roundtable on high-skilled migration and sending countries issues, *International Migration*, **40**(4), 153–166.
Packer, C., R. Labonté and V. Runnels (2009), Globalization and the cross-border flow of health workers, in R. Labonté, T. Schrecker, C. Packer and V. Runnels (eds.), *Globalization and Health: Pathways, Evidence and Policy*, New York: Routledge, pp. 213–234.
Packer, C., V. Runnels and R. Labonté (2010), Does the migration of health workers bring benefits to the countries they leave behind? Impacts on health via wealth and knowledge transfers, in R. Shah (ed.), *The International Migration of Health Workers: Ethics, Rights and Justice*, Basingstoke: Palgrave Macmillan, pp. 44–61.
Piper, N. (2003), Feminization of labor migration as violence against women: international, regional and local nongovernmental organization responses in Asia, *Violence against Women*, **9**(6), 723–745.
Poppe, A., E. Jirovsky, C. Blacklock, P. Laxmikanth, S. Moosa, J. De Maeseneer, R. Kutalek and W. Peersman (2014), Why sub-Saharan African health workers migrate to European countries that do not actively recruit: a qualitative study post-migration, *Global Health Action*, **7**.
Ratha, D. (2011), *Leveraging Migration for Africa: Remittances, Skills, and Investments*, Washington, DC: World Bank.
Ruckert, A., R. Labonté and R. H. Parker (2015), Global healthcare policy and the austerity agenda, in E. Kuhlmann, R. Blank, I. Bourgeault and C. Wendt (eds.), *The Palgrave International Handbook of Healthcare Policy and Governance*, New York: Palgrave Macmillan, pp. 37–53.
Runnels, V., C. Packer and R. Labonté (2010), *Recruiting Internationally-Trained Health Human Resources: Practices and Perceptions of Canadian Health Organization Recruiters*, Ottawa: Globalization and Health Equity Research Unit, available online at www.globalhealthequity.ca/webfm_send/194.
Salmon, M., J. Yan, H. Hewitt and V. Guisinger (2007), Managed migration: the Caribbean approach to addressing nursing services capacity, *Health Services Research*, **42**, 1354–1372.
Sanders, D. and B. Lloyd (2005), Human resources: international context, in P. Ijumba and P. Barron (eds.), *South African Health Review 2005*. Durban: Health Systems Trust, pp. 76–87.
Schrecker, T. and C. Bambra (2015), *How Politics Makes Us Sick*, Basingstoke: Palgrave Macmillan.
Sen, A. (2002), Why health equity? *Health Economics*, **11**, 659–666.
Shah, R. (2010), The international migration of health workers: ethics, rights and justice, in R. Shah (ed.), *The International Migration of Health Workers: Ethics, Rights and Justice*, Basingstoke: Palgrave Macmillan.
Thomas, P. (2006), The international migration of Indian nurses, *International Nursing Review*, **53**(4), 277–283.
Tjadens, F., C. Weilandt and J. Eckert (2013), *Mobility of Health Professionals: Health Systems, Work Conditions, Patterns of Health Workers' Mobility, and Implications for Policy Makers*, Berlin and Heidelberg: Springer-Verlag.
Tomblin Murphy, G., A. MacKenzie, R. Palmer, B. Waysome, J. Guy-Walker, A. Elliott Rose and R. Labonté (2013), *Source Country Perspectives on the Migration of Health*

Personnel: A Report from the Literature, available online at www.healthworkermigration.com/images/stories/Jamaica%20Executive%20Summary.pdf.

Tomblin Murphy, G., A. Mackenzie, B. Waysome, J. Guy-Walker, R. Palmer, A. Rose, J. Rigby, I. Bourgeault and R. Labonté (2016), A mixed-methods study of health worker migration from Jamaica, *Human Resources for Health*, **14** (Suppl 1): 36.

UN (1994a), *Human Rights: A Compilation of International Instruments*, Volume I (First Part, Universal Declaration of Human Rights.

UN (1994b), *Report of the International Conference on Population and Development*, Cairo, 5–13 September 1994, UN doc. A/CONF.171/3, 18 October 1994.

UNGA (2008), *Promotion and Protection of all Human Rights, Civil, Political, Economic, Social and Cultural Rights: Report of the Special Rapporteur on the Right of Everyone to the Enjoyment of the Highest Attainable Standard of Physical and Mental Health*, United Nations Human Rights Council, seventh session, agenda item 3, available online at www.who.int/medicines/areas/human_rights/A_HRC_7_11.pdf.

Walton-Roberts, M. and V. Runnels (unpublished), *Out of India: Processes, Profiles and Policies Informing the Global Migration of Indian Nurses*.

Whitehead, M. (1992), The concepts and principles of equity and health, *International Journal of Health Services*, **22**, 429–445.

WHO (2006), *The World Health Report 2006: Working Together for Health*, Geneva: WHO.

WHO Commission on Social Determinants of Health (2008), *Closing the Gap in a Generation*, Geneva: World Health Organization, available online at www.who.int/social_determinants/final_report/csdh_finalreport_2008.pdf.

World Bank (2009), *The Nurse Labor and Education Markets in the English-Speaking CARICOM: Issues and Options for Reform*, available online at http://siteresources.worldbank.org/INTJAMAICA/Resources/The_Nurse_Labor_Education_Market_Eng.pdf.

Yan J. (2006), Health services delivery: reframing policies for global nursing migration in North America – a Caribbean perspective, *Policy, Politics and Nursing Practice*, supplement to **7**(3), 71S–75S.

Yeates, N. and J. Pillinger (2013), *Human Resources for Health Migration: Global Policy Responses, Initiatives, and Emerging Issues*, Milton Keynes: Open University.

8 Migration control and children's access to healthcare

Marry-Anne Karlsen

INTRODUCTION

In September 2015, pictures of the three-year-old boy Alan Kurdi's lifeless body on a Turkish beach made global headlines, the boy becoming a symbol for the human tragedy unfolding on the shores of the Mediterranean and the plight of the many migrants who attempt to enter Europe irregularly. The powerful impact of these photos in Europe can also be understood in light of the special position children and childhood has gained in Western societies and discourses. Being associated with purity and innocence as well as vulnerability, children have come to be considered both particularly needing and deserving of state protection (Giner 2007). The special position of children is perhaps best exemplified by the United Nations Convention on the Rights of the Child (UNCRC). This convention establishes both the principle that the best interests of the child shall be a primary consideration in all actions concerning children (Article 3) and the principle of non-discrimination, i.e., that party states shall respect and ensure the rights to each child within their jurisdiction without discrimination of any kind (Article 2).

Yet, despite such a seemingly 'child-friendly' policy context, children without state authorization to enter or remain on state territory are increasingly negatively impacted by states' attempts to manage and control unwanted migration, as was tragically illustrated by the case of Alan Kurdi. In Europe, these efforts progressively comprise, in addition to stricter external border control, restriction of access to welfare services, including healthcare (Bendixsen et al. 2015; Lahav and Guiraudon 2000). Hence, recent studies have pointed out how migrant children find themselves at the intersection between two opposing governmental rationalities; the exclusive migration control rationality, based on welfare restrictions and detention, and the inclusive child policy rationality, based on acknowledging children's particular rights to be recognized, protected and cared for (Giner 2007; Watters 2007a; Eastmond and Ascher 2011).

Caught in the tension between states' commitments to protecting children and their desire to limit unwanted migration, the treatment of migrant children has become a highly complex and controversial policy issue for governments in many European welfare states. More fundamentally, the presence of children without the legal right to stay challenges the idea of the child as a universal category beyond national state politics and interests (Vitus and Lidén 2010; Bhabha 2009). This raises troubling questions about how and when a child is not a child that should be cared for, and how the decision on the exception to the norm is made. Understanding the implications of these opposing rationalities is important in terms of law and policy, but also for how policy is translated into daily, situated practice on the ground level.

In this chapter, I examine how the tension between the nation-state's interest in controlling its borders and the universalized rights of children as enshrined in the UNCRC are negotiated in the encounter between healthcare service providers and 'irregular' migrant children with complex health needs in Norway. Generally, the term 'irregular migrant' refers to people who have entered the country without the required documents or remained after their visa has expired or their asylum application been rejected. In Norway, irregular migrant children are to a large extent assumed to be rejected asylum-seekers (Zhang 2008). In July 2011, a new healthcare regulation was implemented in Norway that restricted irregular migrants' access to healthcare. The restrictions on irregular migrant children's access to healthcare represented a significant shift in policy that did not receive public attention. According to the regulation, children (i.e., persons under the age of 18) without legal right to stay are entitled to necessary primary and specialist healthcare, but are not entitled to be part of the general practitioner scheme[1] or receive support for transportation to treatment facilities. Furthermore, and of particular importance here, the regulation states that these children have the right to necessary healthcare 'unless concern for the child dictates that assistance should not be provided'.[2] Hence, important questions are raised concerning the circumstances in which healthcare should not be provided due to this 'concern for the child'.

In this chapter, I will make three main arguments. First, that the ambiguous relationship between universal rights claims and their application in particular cases serve, in this case, a restrictive immigration policy by obscuring responsibility and controversy in official policy. Indeed, while the vulnerable child's position as a moral touchstone in society makes it difficult for policymakers to blatantly disregard irregular migrant children's rights and needs, the decision to include or exclude the children from healthcare is being delegated onto healthcare providers and their 'professional judgements', thus depoliticizing the sensitive question of healthcare to migrant children who are present within the state's borders without authorization. Second, by drawing the territorial and temporal rationality of migration control into medical evaluation, healthcare providers are reconfigured, not only as border guards, but also into what Butler (2004) calls 'petty sovereigns'. Petty sovereigns are professionals who use discretionary power, and who have important say on matters of life and death, but who are 'agents deployed by tactics of power they do not control' (Butler 2004: 65). In this sense, petty sovereigns are agents who often do not recognize the full impact of the work they do, 'but perform their acts unilaterally and with enormous consequence' (Butler 2004: 65). As a result, which is my third argument, healthcare providers are faced with ethical and practical dilemmas that medical humanitarianism, resting on a separation of medicine and politics, does not adequately address.

The chapter builds on material collected through ethnographic fieldwork undertaken in Norway between 2011 and 2014. In the course of this fieldwork I interviewed a wide range of healthcare providers, NGOs and irregular migrants. I also followed some irregular migrants over time, in the sense of having multiple encounters and conversations with them, accompanying them in their various daily activities, including on occasions to doctor's and lawyer's appointments, receiving access to their medical records, and correspondence with the immigration authorities, and talking to healthcare workers with whom they were in contact. One of those I followed closely over these years was Hind, a young girl with extensive medical needs.[3] To explore how 'concern for the child' was translated into practice, I will unpack her case, and that of Adam Dzortov, a similar case that for a short period gained extensive media cover in 2014. First, however, it is useful to briefly consider how sovereignty, rights and discretion have been theorized and what the concept of petty sovereignty can add to the analysis.

STATE SOVEREIGNTY AND THE RIGHT TO HEALTHCARE

Migrant irregularity is first and foremost a juridical status that entails a social relation to a state (De Genova 2002). The concept of irregular, or more precisely irregularized, migration is intimately tied to the system of sovereign nation-states and the sovereign prerogative of denying membership. Due to their particular position as formally excluded, but physically present within the state's territory, irregular migrants have gained a central position in political and academic discussions concerning the relationship between state sovereignty and rights. Is there a conflict between the rights of a nation to sovereignty and the rights of an individual to basic human rights?

In regard to these discussions, research on irregular migration has been highly influenced by Hannah Arendt's (1968) famous notion of 'the right to have rights'. The condition of access to universal rights is seen here not as universal but as resting in an exclusive and particular concept of national citizenship. As irregular migrants are deprived of the fundamental right of political membership, they can be understood as 'absolutely rightless' even though they may have access to some civic and social rights (Parekh 2004: 45). Even though irregular migrant children in many respects are more privileged than adults in the same situation, this also applies to them, illustrating how children's 'inalienable' rights depend on the willingness of a sovereign to enforce them. As such, the situation of irregular migrant children's rights in various countries could best be described as one of 'inconsistent universalism', where they are at certain times included in the universal notion of 'children', whereas in others the ambivalence surrounding them leads to situations in which they have rights that are different from those of other children (Sinha and Uppal 2009; Vitus and Lidén 2010).

Debates about migrant rights can also, as argued by Linda Bosniak (2007: 397), be characterized as debates about how far into the territory the border can come. By this, Bosniak suggests that borders can be conceptual as well as geographical, with the border, conceived as a regulatory sphere, following the migrants in their everyday life, providing a background set of rules that structure the relationships that they have in the states in which they reside (Bosniak 1991; Coutin 2003). This concept of borders draws attention to the proliferation of new actors involved in migration control. As such, it raises questions concerning not only the significance of legal status on children's capacity to access healthcare, but also the practical and ethical implications for service providers delegated the task of preserving and protecting states' territoriality. One of my arguments in this chapter, is that healthcare providers are not only reconfigured as border guards patrolling the (welfare) state borders, but are becoming petty sovereigns defining the threshold of exclusion in their everyday encounters with irregularized migrant children. Hence, what is at stake is not only the question of universal versus particular law, as noted by Arendt, but the passage from general law to concrete case, and the role of professional discretionary judgements in this passage. To understand the concept of petty sovereigns borrowed from Judith Butler (2004), and my usage of it here, it is necessary to look closer at the notion of sovereign decisionism.

PETTY SOVEREIGNTY AND DISCRETIONARY JUDGEMENTS

Butler's notion of petty sovereigns builds on a definition of sovereignty as a decision on the exception initially proposed by Carl Schmitt and later elaborated by Giorgio Agamben (1998, 2005). In this definition, rather than understanding sovereignty as the rule of law within a territory, sovereignty is seen as an extra-legal power that asserts itself in a decision on when exceptions to the law apply. In this sense, sovereignty not only defines the inside/outside of the state in terms of the territorial borders between nation-states, but through a decision that positions some lives outside of law's recognition and protection (Agamben 1998). For the purpose of this chapter, the interesting question thus becomes how such a decision on the exception is made and what the significance of this is for irregular migrant children's access to healthcare.

There are two aspects of Agamben's (re)theorization of sovereignty that are of particular relevance in approaching this question. First, to Agamben (1998, 2005), the decision on the exception does not only occur in a state of crisis, the context in which it is primarily associated, but has become a technique of government related to the rise of the regulatory state.[4] Hence, according to Agamben (2005), modern rule increasingly takes place through executive decrees that have the force of law but not its form. Such decrees are constituted with reference to the particular society it claims to regulate and not with respect to a set of universal principles. To Agamben, the problem with this is that the normative aspect of law can be obliterated and contradicted with impunity by a government that still claims to be applying the law (Agamben 2005: 87). In respect to the theme of this chapter, Agamben's claim draws attention to how states can maintain to adhere to the UNCRC, while at the same time perforating its application with executive discretion.

Second, the sovereign decision on the exception is not only reserved for the parliament, or government, but can be devolved onto administrative layers and street-level bureaucrats, including healthcare providers (Agamben 1998: 143; Dean 2007). This draws attention to how human discretion involves a sovereign suspension of law because law, as Agamben (2005) notes, cannot recognize singularities. However, in Butler's view, the bureaucrats that enact the exceptionalism of the state in their everyday practice are not true sovereigns. Instead, to her, petty sovereignty is the effect, not the cause, of the suspension of law. Hence, the exception is a mechanism that heightens discretionary power.

Both the blurring of law and exception and the transfer of the sovereign decision is, I suggest, central to the management of irregular migration in Norway. For instance, decision by executive decree, rather than law by the parliament, is rampant in the government of irregular migrants in Norway (Karlsen 2015b). Irregular migrants' access to welfare is thus mainly governed through regulations, circulars and letters issued by state departments that primarily restrict their rights in relation to legal residents without any comprehensive parliamentarian debate on these migrants', including children's, access to welfare (Søvig 2013). Legal scholars have thus questioned the legal basis of these decrees both in relation to due process and human rights obligations (Andersen 2014; Süssmann 2015). My concern here, however, is the implications of delegating the decision to include or exclude irregular migrant children from healthcare onto healthcare providers and their 'professional judgements'. I propose that this is a move that serves to depoliticize the sensitive question of healthcare to irregular migrant children.

I understand depoliticization here in line with Burnham (2014: 189) as the process of placing 'at one remove the politically contested character of governing'. This definition sees depoliticization, not as absence of politics, but as a tool of government through which blame, responsibility and the transaction costs of policymaking are reassigned (Foster et al. 2014). Depoliticization can also, in line with Brown (2009: 15), be understood to involve removing a political phenomenon from comprehension of its historical emergence and from a recognition of the powers that produce and contour it. This can be achieved for instance by recasting issues such as migration as a security or humanitarian rather than as a 'political' problem (Aradau 2004). Central to both depoliticization and exceptional politics is that it makes it harder for citizens and migrants to challenge the state's exclusionary practices related to migration control. On this note, I will turn to the cases of Hind and Adam.

Hind

Hind was a young primary school girl whom I met during the early stage of my fieldwork and who was in need of extensive surgery. Her condition was rare, but not necessarily lethal. Children left untreated could survive into adulthood, but morbidity was severe and the condition posed significant physical, functional, social and psychological burdens on patients and families. It was also a condition that was challenging to manage for healthcare providers, and would in normal circumstances be treated with surgery from a very early age, with lifelong follow-up care. However, upon learning that she and her family had received the 'final decision' to their asylum application,[5] the surgeon who had initially examined her was no longer willing to go through with complicated procedures.

Hind and her family had received the so-called final rejection in 2009 and when I met them their stay was no longer considered legal. They had, however, remained living in an asylum reception centre, working on various appeals and trying to get surgery for Hind.[6] About a year after I met her, Hind's condition started to worsen. She complained of pain, making it difficult for the parents to carry out the daily care necessary to keep her condition under control. Not able to help, the local doctors kept pushing the surgeon to see her again, at least to see if something could be done to ease her pain. After several attempts and months, Dr Johan, the surgeon, finally agreed to see her.

Over the years that I followed Hind and her family, Dr Johan had grown to become the villain in this story and the parents directed a lot of their anger of being rejected both by the immigration authorities and by the hospital at him. As the parents saw it, he was the main obstacle to both Hind's medical treatment and to their residence aspirations. Dr Johan, however, when I finally met him, was clearly uncomfortable with being the villain. In the medical appointment with Hind's parents, he tried to explain that it was not that he did not want to help them. He very much sympathized with their situation, he said, and he 'did not judge them' for trying to stay. His main dilemma, as he laid it out, was that the best medical option for Hind varied, depending on whether she would be deported or allowed to stay. If he performed the same surgery as he would for legal residents, and Hind was deported and left without proper medical follow-up, her situation could become fatal. Dr Johan could perform another type of surgery that would be less risky in case of deportation, but that would have a less satisfactory result in terms of life quality for Hind, and could entail more rounds of surgery to rectify this if she were ultimately allowed to stay. To Dr Johan this was therefore not only a question of whether Hind had a right to healthcare, but whether treatment would be 'medically safe' in her case due to the risk of deportation. Dr Johan found this to be a very difficult decision to make, and one that was difficult for the parents to respond to. Dr Johan had first appealed to his superiors who initially, in agreement with him, decided not to do anything as they believed that Hind would shortly leave the country having received the 'final decision'. Years later, with no change in Hind's legal situation, still rejected but not deported, and with her health situation worsening, the doctors decided they had to do something. Again, Dr Johan appealed to his superiors to make what he found to be a very difficult medical decision. In the end, they decided to go for the medically less optimal, but possibly safer surgical option in case of deportation.

Adam

Adam was a nine-year-old boy who, as with Hind, was in need of extensive surgery. Adam's spine was crooked and spinal pressures on his lungs made it difficult for him to breathe. According to Adam's doctors, his spine was so curved that it could not be corrected in a single operation. This meant that he would need follow-up, in the form of regular operations as long as he was growing. Without the operations, he would become disabled and most likely die young. However, as in Hind's case, surgery was initially denied by the hospital as he and his family had received the 'final rejection' to their asylum application in 2012.

In June 2014, his doctors, relieved of their doctor–patient confidentiality by Adam's parents, were interviewed by the Christian newspaper *Vårt Land*. In this interview, one of his doctors, Arild Egge, chief surgeon at the neurosurgical department at Oslo University Hospital (OUS) was quoted as saying: 'If law can trump medicine in this case, it is shocking.' He continued: 'As doctors, it is our duty to save lives and health. Adam's condition is life-threatening. Here we see that the system is speaking with two tongues. Had we failed to treat another patient in this way [i.e., not performing surgery], we would have been held legally responsible for not doing anything' (Huseby 2014a).

Egge's statement was followed up on by Adam's attending doctor, Rolf Riise, who stated that 'Adam's critical condition puts us as doctors in a huge ethical dilemma. On the one hand, we have a duty to help – and we have full opportunity to treat him. On the other hand, we are not allowed to operate on him now because of his unresolved asylum seeker status' (Huseby 2014a). As the quotes illustrate, the doctors in this case saw the law as preventing them from doing what they thought was medically right.

Adam's story was quickly picked up by most of the major media in Norway through an article by a news agency with the headline: 'Terminally ill nine-year-old does not get help because of his asylum-seeker status' (NTB 2014). Many news channels followed up with different individual articles published online. Svein Aarseth, head of the Council for Medical Ethics in the Medical Association, was one of those interviewed, stating that the doctors would not be doing anything 'illegal' if they chose to operate on Adam because, as he specified, 'it is still not illegal to help anyone in Norway – fortunately' (Huseby 2014b). Within hours, the hospital retracted their decision and the following statement was made by Olav Røise, head of the Clinic for Surgery and Neuroscience (OUS):

> We see now that we have interpreted the regulation too strictly. As the patient's future possibility to obtain follow-up with us had not been resolved, our

> original decision was based on that. However, since the patient is under 18 years of age, he is entitled to treatment on par with other patients who are presently in Norway. We find, therefore, that our responsibility is to provide healthcare to the patient.
>
> (Huseby 2014c)

Within 15 days from the story breaking in the media, Adam had his first surgery. Røise, who was the one ultimately responsible for both decisions in Adam's case (first refusing, then allowing surgery), explained in a later interview that it was the last sentence of the healthcare regulation that had been difficult to interpret. 'The sentence can be understood as both a "yes" and a "no" to healthcare', Røise explained, referring to the exception implied in the sentence 'unless concern for the child dictate that assistance should not be provided' (Huseby, 2014d). Yet, unlike Hind's doctors, Adam's doctors, as soon as it was clarified that the law was no obstacle to surgery, made no reservation to the treatment they provided him. This despite the question of what was considered medically essential follow-up care remained uncertain in both cases, and would remain uncertain as long as the children continued to be deportable.

Hind and Adam's cases are interesting to compare both for their similarities and differences. At the heart of both cases is the tension between children's right to healthcare and states' prerogative to define membership, but also how medical and migration control concerns should be assessed in the medical decision. The cases are also difficult precisely because they are children. On the one hand, their position as particularly needing and deserving of state protection makes it controversial to deny them treatment due to immigration concerns. On the other hand, treating the complicated conditions is particularly difficult because they are children whose bodies are growing and changing. The different approaches by the doctors in question, however, draw attention to how medical solutions become mixed with moral and legal concerns. In the following section, I will turn to examining the legal context in more detail.

IN WHOSE INTERESTS? OBSCURING RESPONSIBILITY AND CONTROVERSY IN POLICY

According to Agamben (1998: 57), one of the paradoxes of the exception as a technique of government lies in the fact that it becomes 'impossible to distinguish transgression of the law from execution of the law, such that what violates a rule and what conforms to it coincide without any remainder'. Hence, the issue is not only that law is suspended, but that fact and law are completely confused. Røise's comment above, that the clause in the healthcare regulation could be understood as both a 'yes' and a 'no' to healthcare, seems to point to exactly such an experience of legal indeterminacy. As Hind and Adam's cases showed, both denying and granting treatment at various stages in their contact with healthcare providers did not contradict 'the law', and nor did treating Hind differently than other children with similar conditions. In this case, I suggest, the healthcare regulation can be seen as an administrative decree that blurs the concept of children's universal right to healthcare by making this a question of 'professional judgement' *and* at the same time drawing the territorial and temporal rationality of migration control into the medical evaluation in terms of deciding a course of treatment.

To understand how this regulation draws the territorial and temporal rationality of migration control into the medical evaluation it is necessary to look closer at how 'concern for the child' is defined. At first glance, it may look like a reference to 'the best interests of the child' in line with the UNCRC. In Norway, the implementation of the UNCRC in the 2003 Norwegian Human Rights Act means that all national legislation affecting children has to be reconstructed in line with both the framework and specific articles of the Convention. In the UNCRC, states recognize not only that 'the best interests of the child shall be a primary consideration', but also 'the right of the child to the enjoyment of the highest attainable standard of health' and the states commit to making every effort to ensure that no child is deprived of his or her right of access to such healthcare services' (Article 24).

However, as the background documents and guidelines to the healthcare regulation make clear, this is not what the clause refers to. In the initial proposal from the Ministry of Health and Care Services, irregular migrant children such as Hind and Adam were to be entitled to healthcare unless 'special circumstances after a specific assessment suggest that healthcare should not be granted' (Ministry of Health and Care Services 2010). By this complicated sentence, the Ministry intended that, when deciding whether healthcare should be provided, due attention should be given to the fact that the child was in the country illegally and required to leave shortly. The Ministry specified two ways these concerns should be part of the medical evaluation. First, if treatment could be postponed without significant consequences until the child had left the country, the child would not be entitled to healthcare in Norway. Second, treatment requiring prolonged follow-up care should only be initiated if it was deemed medically necessary that treatment was started quickly (Ministry of Health and Care Services 2010). 'Special circumstances' thus referred to considerations or concerns related to migration control and not the children's medical needs.

When the proposal for the regulation was submitted for public consultation in 2010, it was the subject of strong criticism from among others, the Norwegian Medical Association (2010), the Norwegian Ombudsman for Children (2010) and Save the Children, Norway (2010). The critics were concerned that the proposal was not consistent with the UNCRC. They also raised the more pragmatic concern that it would be difficult for healthcare providers to determine realistically how long the child would be in the country, thus risking situations where children would be denied treatment, or treatment would be unnecessarily deferred, because healthcare providers assumed the child was going to leave but they did not. This happened, for example, in the case of Hind where, as noted earlier, the doctors initially decided not to do anything as they believed she would leave after having received the 'final decision'.

Nonetheless, the criticism raised was taken into consideration by the Ministry in the sense that they changed the wording from 'special circumstances' to 'concern for the child'. Still, the clause primarily continues to stipulate that treatment should not interfere with state efforts to deport the child (Karlsen, R., 2015). This is made clear in a circular issued by the Ministry of Health and Care Services in December 2011. Here, 'concern for the child' is clarified by the following definition: 'This will be a professional evaluation, and may for example include cases where healthcare professionals have definite knowledge that the child is about to leave the country, and it would be irresponsible to start a treatment that cannot be completed' (Rundskriv I-5 2011). It was, as seen above, the question of not being able to complete treatment due to the possibility of deportation that caused trouble for Hind and Adam. In both cases, the treatment was available and accorded to children with legal residency. Yet, in both cases the doctors' initial interpretation was that as long as they were deportable, and necessary medical follow-up was not guaranteed in Norway or in their country of origin, 'it would be irresponsible' to start treatment. Hence, the answer to the question of when healthcare should not be provided due to 'concern for the child' became as long as the child can be deported. The dilemma, however, is that, as long as a child is irregular, deportation will remain a possibility. In Hind and Adam's cases, the decision not to perform surgery became increasingly difficult to sustain medically as the children remained in the country. Still, as seen in Hind's case, even though the doctors eventually decided to act, these concerns made them opt for the compromise of a medically less optimal solution.

Adam and Hind's cases raise two central and interrelated questions: (1) what does the legal indeterminacy actually do? And (2) if the law does not prevent doctors treating irregular migrant children, why are they not necessarily treated as other children? In regard to the first question, I suggest, that the undecidable relationship between law and exceptions and the delegation of the decision to healthcare providers, primarily served to obscure responsibility and controversy in official policy. While the doctors felt restrained by law from acting, as seen in Adam's case, representatives of the government confronted with difficult cases by the media could, and would, refer to it as being the healthcare providers' decision. This was, for example, the political response in Adam's case. After his story received broad media coverage, the Minister of Health and Care Services, Bent Høie, specified that the government's position was that all children residing in Norway, 'as a general rule', should be entitled to necessary healthcare and that children's best interests should be a 'primary consideration'. Hence, he stated: 'Current regulations do not prevent children who are in the situation that was featured in *Vårt Land* on June 10, from getting the help that doctors deem necessary' (Bjåen, 2014). Yet, what the Minister actually clarifies is, in line with the regulation, that the decision to deny or grant treatment is deferred to the doctors' discretionary judgements. So, whereas the media coverage in Adam's case may have contributed to him getting surgery, no actual changes were made to the regulation.[7] In this sense, healthcare professionals have, in Butler's words, become designated sovereigns with extraordinary power. Yet, as I will now turn to in order to address the second question posed above, 'they do not fully control the aims that animate their actions' (Butler 2004: 62).

WHOSE DECISION? SOVEREIGN POWER AND EXPERT DISCRETION

> 'You know,' Hind's uncle who was there as an interpreter intercepted, 'if the surgeon would just start the operations, she would probably be allowed to stay at least until it is over.' To this Doctor Olav responded, 'It is not the doctor's job to decide your destiny,' before he added, more consolatory, 'but I will see what I can do.'
>
> Field note excerpt (my translation).

In this short field note excerpt from one of Hind's medical appointments, Hind's uncle indicates to the doctor that the surgeon could potentially exercise a form of sovereign power by just instigating treatment, making deportation practically or morally impossible for the immigration authorities. As noted above, a question that arises from the analysis so far is, if both denying and granting treatment did not contradict the law, why did Hind and Adam not receive the same medical treatment as children with the same conditions and legal residency? Healthcare providers are after all considered to have – and see themselves as having – a commitment to relieving suffering and maximizing the quality of life for service users (Grimen 2009). This commitment, as well as non-discrimination, is part of every health professional's code of ethics.

Hospital structures and management forms could, beside a legal ban, potentially represent formal structures that limit doctors' scope of actions. Like other bureaucratic organizations, hospitals have a hierarchy. Decisions are therefore not only up to the individual professional, and can, for instance, be overturned by economic considerations by managers. Literature on irregular migrants' informal incorporation in service provision has suggested that those in more service-oriented roles with a high degree of face-to-face contact with patients are more lenient and willing to provide care than those in more regulatory-oriented roles of higher-level administrators and utilization managers, whose primary responsibility is to maintain their organizations' fiscal survival (Marrow 2012; Van der Leun 2006).Yet, although these issues came up in my study, it did not adequately explain why healthcare providers would not initiate treatment. In Hind and Adam's cases, it was not a conflict between the doctors and management regarding the course of action. Instead, as seen in Hind's case, it was the surgeon who appealed to his superiors to make the decision as he found it to be too challenging for him to make alone.[8]

I propose that the main answer to the question is not found in coercively enforced constraints, but rather in more decentralized and diffused forms of power relations that regulate and discipline conduct. These forms of power do not, as Foucault (2003) notes, work through punishment but through normalization, where the norm acts as a continuous regulatory and corrective mechanism through which individuals and populations internalize what is demanded or expected of them. Although discretionary decisions on the exception are always to some extent arbitrary and sovereign, they are also, as Dean (2007) suggests, caught within normalizing frames that govern conduct. These may derive from more general social norms about gender, class, race, etc. In this study, professional codes of ethics and knowledge represented important normalizing frames that came into contradiction with 'the law' represented by the healthcare regulation, complicating the decision on the exception. Yet, part of the answer can still be found in the way law has acquired a regulating and disciplining role under governmentality (Rose and Valverde 1998; Ewald 1990). In this case, the regulation shaping healthcare according to the norms of citizenship, establishes the child with legal residency as the norm and thus legal status as a criterion for judgement. As such, the regulation establishes expectations about the conduct of experts that encourage self-regulation, in this case by making legal status part of their deliberation. Furthermore, the legal indeterminacy can also be said to have surveillance effect. As seen in Adam's case, the healthcare regulation initially discouraged healthcare providers from providing healthcare for fear of acting against the law.

In the following, I will focus on what I see as two other related explanatory factors. First, I suggest that the lack of familiarity with and knowledge of migration and migration policy was one of the main reasons healthcare providers were reluctant to act. The healthcare providers did not feel that they had the necessary expertise to make the decision they were required to make, such as means to know or evaluate how long the child would stay or if they would get treatment if deported. Second, as healthcare providers, at least in theory, had no influence over the question of residency, they could never be sure they would be able to finish the treatment. Hence, while their power to deny treatment was absolute, their ability to grant treatment was experienced as circumscribed and conditioned by decisions made by the immigration authorities. In light of these uncertainties, not acting became the safer option.

The idea of doctors as exercising a sovereign-based power over patients' bodies is not new. Modern government relies to a large extent on the institutionalization and exercise of expert knowledge, and medical sovereignty has been tied to doctors' exclusive and legitimate right to define medical reality and claim authority over issues defined by them as medical rather than caused, for example, by social inequalities (Lupton 2012). What is special here is that the healthcare regulation delegates responsibility to decide whether treatment should be given or not based on migration concerns and not just medical reasons. As such, doctors are being delegated the power of decision in areas where they do not have, or do not themselves experience that they have, state-sanctioned, socially accepted and ascribed exclusive knowledge and competence, in this case in immigration policy.

What constitutes medical knowledge, however, is not always clear. The pervasive role of clinical discretion in medical practice has long been recognized by medical ethicists and anthropologists, noting, for instance, how what constitutes 'medical necessity' or 'life-threatening' in particular cases can vary, and may be impacted by a range of factors including gendered and racial prejudices, institutional arrangements and so on (Bloche 2001; Ticktin 2011).

What counts as medical knowledge is also changing. In the past decades, research has shown how a neoliberal modernization agenda has signalled a shift from reflective clinical practice to scientific-bureaucratic medicine whereby medical practice and knowledge becomes rationalized and standardized (Harrison 2002). Ong, in her work on refugee medicine in the US, describes how clinicians, constrained by a market-driven healthcare system, have 'their gaze on their patients distracted by an eye on the bottom line' (Ong 2003: 92). Paraphrasing Ong, it could here be argued that the doctors' gaze on their patients is being distracted by an eye on the territorial border. However, there is a significant difference to the introduction of a cost–benefit perspective in medical practice. While hospitals have acquired financial expertise in management, they still do not have expertise, routines or capacities in evaluating migration concerns (i.e., means of acquiring necessary information about healthcare availability in the countries of origin, or how long patients would remain in the country). In this sense, healthcare providers were made to make unilateral decisions of potentially enormous consequence, without knowing, or being able to evaluate, the potential impact of them. Taking immigration concerns into consideration before instigating treatment still challenges established understandings of what clinical knowledge and professional ethics is and particularly what should count as medically significant and relevant information.

Hind and Adam's cases also illustrate the quandary arising from the medical decision being separated from the decision on legal residency. In Norway, there is no formal system for how medical claims in asylum cases should be assessed. Reports are generally written by regular healthcare professionals requested by the patients themselves and not by some specially appointed experts who issue medical statements in immigration cases. In this respect, Norway differs from, for instance, France where specific state-appointed healthcare professionals are involved both in assessing cases as well as writing land reports and categorizing illnesses that can provide the basis for temporary or permanent residence permits (Ticktin 2011). In my study, healthcare providers frequently expressed feelings that their expert views were ignored by the immigration authorities, questioning the authorities' competence in doing so (Karlsen 2015b). Adam's doctors were among those who felt their professional opinions were ignored. They were convinced that adequate medical help would not be available to him in his country of origin, despite the immigration authorities' assurances that it was, and even testified as expert witnesses in a court case for Adam and his family that they lost a few months before his health situation was exposed in the media (Huseby 2014e).

Nonetheless, as suggested by Hind's uncle, doctors could still potentially exercise a form of sovereign power by just instigating treatment. For example, when the doctors in Adam's case initiated surgery, they arguably bound him to a healthcare system of a certain type and standard. This surgery inserted growing rods along his spine that needed to be lengthened every six months to keep up with Adam's growth. He would also need close and continuous follow up in case of complications, which in these cases are not uncommon. Yet, what is a sovereign decision cannot necessarily be known in advance, and in these cases the outcome often remains uncertain. A year after surgery Adam's fate was still undecided. When Adam appealed his case to the immigration appeal board (UNE) after surgery, he was only given a temporary and conditional permit of one year to receive treatment. Although this could be renewed, it still meant that Adam and his doctors would have to cope with uncertainty. In their response, UNE recognized the strong humanitarian concerns in Adam's case, but insisted that the concern for 'health migration' weighed more than 'the best interest of the child'. According to them, 'it was clear' that the family's motive from the beginning was 'better and free healthcare', and as such it constituted 'an abuse of the asylum institute' (Jensen et al. 2014). Hind, on the other hand, was granted residency shortly after surgery. The permit, however, was not granted for medical reasons, but because Hind's 'affiliation to the Realm' was seen to outweigh migration concerns, as she had lived in Norway for six years. This was in line with political signals in a new White Paper that made children's integration into Norwegian society a key issue in evaluating residency on humanitarian grounds (Ministry of Justice and the Police 2012). Also, on the plus side, the acceptance letter from UNE noted that the family's identity had been substantiated and that by staying in a reception centre, it was clear they had not tried to hide from deportation.

The different treatment of Hind and Adam indicates some of the arbitrariness and entanglements regarding questions of deservingness and entitlement in asylum questions that have been noted in other European contexts (Fassin 2012), and how this affects children despite their special position in Western discourse and the discourse of international conventions (Eastmond and Ascher 2011). The different approaches by Hind and Adam's doctors, I suggest, also illustrate how the blurriness of the border between medical views and political and moral views on immigration and deservingness can impact medical evaluations. While Adam's doctors actively supported him in his asylum appeal, Hind's doctors were less willing to support her. Dr Johan, in conversation with Hind's family and me, brought up the fear of 'medical migration', in addition to his 'purely' medical doubts of the best course of action. Although he did not accuse Hind's family directly of medical migration, he elaborated examples of cases he had heard, seeing these as valid concerns the government had and that he felt obliged to take into consideration. In the discussion he also brought up Hind's country of origin. The medical care Hind needed was available in theory, as far as he knew, so the question was to a larger extent if it would be available to her for economic reasons. To Dr Johan, this seemed to complicate the question of deservingness, as he suggested that the decision would have been easier to make if she had been from a country 'such as Somalia or Afghanistan' where it was clearer that such medical expertise did not exist. Hind's case thus indicates how what has been called a 'culture of disbelief' (Watters 2007b) surrounding the category of asylum-seekers in Europe also becomes part of the medical encounter.

BORDERS, POLITICS AND MEDICINE

So far, I have described what I see as an attempt to depoliticize the sensitive question of healthcare to irregular migrant children by devolving the responsibility onto healthcare providers and their expert discretion. However, from the perspective of the healthcare providers I was in contact with during fieldwork, both those involved in Adam and Hind's cases and others, the requirement to take migration control concerns into consideration was predominantly experienced as a political interference in medical practice (Karlsen 2015a). For instance, Røise, the clinic director in Adam's case, argued against the exceptional clause in the healthcare regulation, stating that: 'If the sentence was removed from the regulation, there would be no grounds for doubt. It would make us doctors independent of political considerations and allow us to do what we should: let medical considerations decide' (Huseby 2014d). Others, such as Dr Hans, a paediatrician unrelated to the cases elaborated here, but with similar experiences, put it more broadly 'there has to be a clear separation between immigration regulation and healthcare policy. [. . .] When the die has been cast and the migrants are here, it can't be up to the healthcare services to get them out.'

The position of calling for a clear distinction between the right to healthcare and the right to stay was also adopted by the Norwegian Medical Association (2010), and has been a central tactic employed by healthcare providers challenging the state's attempts to manage and control unwanted migration through welfare restrictions in Norway and elsewhere (Karlsen 2015b; Castañeda 2013: Gottlieb et al. 2012). The separation between the right to healthcare and immigration policy was, for instance, used to justify and defuse criticism against volunteer-run healthcare centres for irregular migrants (see Ottesen et al. 2015). As Trygve Nordby, the secretary general of the Norwegian Red Cross explained when the organization launched their initiative to provide healthcare services to irregular migrants: 'We do not dispute the sovereign prerogative to decide who should have legal residence in a country. This is only a matter of safeguarding basic needs and basic rights' (Norwegian Red Cross 2007: 6).

The importance of this approach for creating a space for the provision of healthcare to irregular migrants and for pushing the political issue of their healthcare rights should not be underestimated. In this last section, however, I wish to draw attention to the limitation of separating medicine and politics as a response to the challenges that Hind and Adam's cases bring forth. The separation rests to a large extent on casting the issue of healthcare to irregular migrants as one of medical humanitarianism rather than as a 'political question'. It thus contributes, I suggest, to depoliticizing the issue by removing it 'from a recognition of the powers that produce [it]' (Brown 2009: 15) and limits the scope of action or advocacy by permitting intervention in welfare but not migration issues. However, the problem is, as Ticktin (2011: 123), exploring the role of medicine in immigration policies in France, appropriately remarks, that to truly exist outside politics as an irregular migrant 'is an impossible proposition, not least because the classification of "undocumented" or "illegal" is political'.

The separation between humanitarianism and politics is a central part of Agamben's critique of modern rule. To him, the problem is that this separation is ultimately based on a faulty notion that it is possible to separate the biological or 'bare life' of the individual from wider political questions. Thus, by relying on the political/humanitarian divide, humanitarian actors entrench a state sovereignty that is responsible for the very social suffering that they aim to minimize (Agamben 1998). Similarly, critical anthropological literature on medical humanitarianism, has pointed out how humanitarianism helps build legitimacy for states' exclusionary policies and their retreat from responsibility for service provision to irregular migrants (Ticktin 2006; Castañeda 2011). In addition, humanitarian actions are justified by references to suffering and compassion rather than rights. An increased emphasis on deservingness and moral worth is arguably the flip-side of a politics of compassion (Fassin 2012).

Within discourses of 'health-related deservingness' (Willen 2012; this volume), the innocent and valuable child tends to have a particularly privileged position (Ticktin 2011). Still, the dilemma of separating biological and political life is also the one faced by Hind and Adam's doctors. It could be easy to dismiss Dr Johan's concerns concerning 'medical safety', reducing them to his political views on migration. However, Hind and Adam's cases illustrate the difficulty of separating medical concerns from legal status. The paradox of the humanitarian/political separation was particularly obvious in Hind's case. While in contrast to Adam, Hind's doctors were, as mentioned, reluctant to get involved in her attempts to get residency. Hind's parents struggled to get medical reports for their appeals and none of the doctors were willing to talk to the media when the parents considered that option. Yet, most of them did try to provide whatever medical care they could within the biomedical framework, shy of surgery. At one point, Hind was even sent to a psychologist to learn pain management. The psychologist ended it after a few sessions, however, noting that the somatic situation was so serious that psychological treatment alone would not relieve the pain, yet also warning that the risk of additional psychological conditions was severe if nothing was done.

Hind and Adam, with their complicated somatic conditions, represent in many ways distinct, but not unique, cases where the tension between medicine and migration control intensifies. Many of the same dilemmas, such as the difficulties of providing continuity of care and dealing with health issues that were seen as related to a social and legal situation rather than a medical one, appeared in less complex cases as well, and in adult cases. This frequently led to what the healthcare providers in my study described as an orientation of medical practice to the 'here and now', rather than fully curing or caring for the patient. For the healthcare providers, this reorientation was not primarily due to the healthcare regulation, but due to the insecurity inscribed into the medical encounter by the possibility of patients suddenly disappearing (Karlsen 2015b). As such, it was framed by the wider sociopolitical condition of migrant illegality and deportability (De Genova 2002: Willen 2007). It is also, I suggest, the condition of migrant deportability that makes it challenging to treat children with complex health needs 'outside of politics'.

CONCLUSION

In this chapter I have examined how the tension between a state's interest in controlling its borders and its commitments to protecting children is negotiated in the encounter between healthcare service providers and irregular migrant children with complex health needs. Despite children's special position as particularly needing and being deserving of state's protection as enshrined in the UNCRC, irregular migrant children are increasingly negatively impacted by the attempts of many Western countries to manage and control unwanted migration. While Alan Kurdi's lifeless body on a Turkish beach tragically illustrated the potential harm of stricter external border control, Hind and Adam's cases outlined in this chapter draws attention to the challenges raised by an increased interaction between migration control and welfare policy.

Norway is in this regard an interesting but not unique case. While, the notion that the state is a guarantor of children's welfare has long been entrenched in the public mind (Vitus and Lidén 2010), the Norwegian authorities were able to limit irregular migrant children's access to healthcare in 2011, a significant shift in policy that went largely unnoticed. In this chapter I have argued that this was to a large extent accomplished by depoliticizing the sensitive question of irregular migrant children's right to healthcare by devolving responsibility for the decision to exclude them to professional discretion. For healthcare providers, this presented them with significant ethical and practical dilemmas. However, as I have argued, calling for a clear division between medicine and politics does not provide a sufficient answer to these dilemmas. To sum up, the Norwegian case highlights, I suggest, how the treatment of irregular migrant children, caught in the tension between states' commitments to protecting children and their desire to limit unwanted migration, becomes not only a complex and urgent question for policymakers, but also frontline service providers.

NOTES

1. Norway has a universal, public healthcare system that is financed by the country's tax revenues and a national insurance scheme mandatory for all legal residents. The responsibilities for healthcare services are divided between state and municipal levels. Primary healthcare (including general practitioners and nursing care) is a municipal responsibility and is based on a list system with regular general practitioners (GPs). Everyone who is registered in the Population Register as a resident in a municipality is entitled to be registered as a patient with a primary doctor. Irregular migrants cannot be registered here. As GPs are responsible for all initial assessment, investigation and treatment of patients, they have a key role in the healthcare system. Access to secondary care is based on referral by a GP.
2. All translation of public documents in Norwegian and quotes from fieldwork data is made by the author.
3. Due to strong privacy concerns when doing research with irregular migrants, I have, in addition to anonymizing names, altered what I considered non-essential information.
4. Agamben draws here on Foucault's (2007) notion of governmentality. Governmentality refers broadly to the way in which political power manages and regulates populations through a diffuse set of strategies and tactics that involves both state and non-state institutions, discourses and knowledges. Governmentality, as Butler (2004) remarks, denotes an operation of power that is extra-legal, even as it can and does return to law as a field of tactical operations.
5. In the Norwegian system, the Directorate of Immigration (UDI) makes the initial decision in asylum cases. In case the UDI rejects an application, it can be appealed to an independent appeal board called UNE. If UNE rejects the appeal, it is referred to as 'the final decision'. If the rejected asylum-seeker fails to leave before the departure date set for him/her, his/her stay is generally no longer considered legal.
6. Rejected asylum-seekers are still offered accommodation through the asylum reception system, but they receive less economic support than asylum-seekers whose application is still under evaluation.
7. That doctors could deny treatment was, for instance, confirmed by a case brought before the county governor in Oslo (as the appellate authority) in 2014. Here, the county governor concluded that irregular migrant children had the right to healthcare,

but that complicated surgery could be denied based on the sentence in the regulation ('unless concern for the child') and the legal requirement that treatment should be 'medically safe' (Specialist Health Services Act, 1999, §2-2).

8. Hospitals in Norway are organized into five regional health enterprises owned by the state. These enterprises provide decentralized management and delegation of financial responsibility at the same time that the Minister of Health, in theory, can instruct the regional health authorities and overturn board decisions.

REFERENCES

Agamben, G. (1998), *Homo Sacer: Sovereign Power and Bare Life*, Stanford: Stanford University Press.

Agamben, G. (2005), *State of Exception*, Chicago: University of Chicago Press.

Andersen, N. W. (2014), Den nasjonale reguleringen av retten og plikten til å yte nødhjelp til personer med ulovlig opphold i Norge – analysert ut fra et rettssikkerhetsperspektiv, *Nordisk socialrättslig tidskrift*, **9**(10), 31–77.

Aradau, C. (2004), The perverse politics of four-letter words: Risk and pity in the securitisation of human trafficking, *Millennium-Journal of International Studies*, **33**(2), 251–277.

Arendt, H. (1968), *The Origins of Totalitarianism*, New York: Harcourt, Brace & World.

Bendixsen, S., C. M. Jacobsen and K. H, Søvig (eds.) (2015), *Eksepsjonell velferd? Irregulære migranter i det norske velferdssamfunnet*, Oslo: Gyldendal Norsk Forlag.

Bhabha, J. (2009), Arendt's children: do today's migrant children have a right to have rights? *Human Rights Quarterly*, **31**(2), 410–451.

Bjåen, B.K. (2014), Barn som oppholder seg ulovlig i Norge skal få helsehjelp, *Vårt Land*, 20 June, available online at www.vl.no/barn-som-opp-holder-seg-ulovlig-i-norge-skal-f%C3%A5-helse-hjelp-1.85889.

Bloche, M. G. (2001), Race and discretion in American medicine, *Yale Journal of Health Policy, Law, and Ethics*, **1**(1), 95–132.

Bosniak, L. (1991), Human rights, state sovereignty and the protection of undocumented migrants under the International Migrant Workers Convention, *International Migration Review*, **25**(4), 737–770.

Bosniak, L. (2007), Being here: ethical territoriality and the rights of immigrants, *Theoretical Inquiries in Law*, **8**(2), 389–410.

Brown, W. (2009), *Regulating Aversion: Tolerance in the Age of Identity and Empire*, Princeton, NJ: Princeton University Press.

Burnham, P. (2014), Depoliticisation: economic crisis and political management, *Policy & Politics*, **42**(2), 189–206.

Butler, J. (2004), *Precarious Life: The Powers of Mourning and Violence*, London: Verso.

Castañeda, H. (2011), 'Medical humanitarianism and physicians' organized efforts to provide aid to unauthorized migrants in Germany', *Human Organization*, **70**(1), 1–10.

Castañeda, H. (2013), Medical aid as protest: acts of citizenship for unauthorized im/migrants and refugees, *Citizenship Studies*, **17**(2), 227–240.

Coutin, S. B. (2003), *Legalizing Moves: Salvadoran Immigrants' Struggle for US Residency*, Ann Arbor: University of Michigan Press.

De Genova, N. (2002), Migrant 'illegality' and deportability in everyday life, *Annual Review of Anthropology*, **31**(1), 419–447.

Dean, M. (2007), *Governing Societies: Political Perspectives on Domestic and International Rule*, Maidenhead: Open University Press.

Eastmond, M. and H. Ascher (2011), In the best interest of the child? The politics of vulnerability and negotiations for asylum in Sweden, *Journal of Ethnic and Migration Studies*, **37**(8), 1185–1200.

Ewald, F. (1990), Norms, discipline, and the law, *Representations*, **30**(1), 138–161.

Fassin, D. (2012), *Humanitarian Reason: A Moral History of the Present Times*, Berkeley, CA: University of California Press.

Foster, E. A., P. Kerr and C. Byrne (2014), Rolling back to roll forward: depoliticisation and the extension of government, *Policy & Politics*, **42**(2), 225–241.

Foucault, M. (2003) *Society Must Be Defended: Lectures at the Collège de France, 1975–76*, New York: Picador.

Foucault, M. (2007), *Security, Territory, Population: Lectures at the Collège de France, 1977–78*, Basingstoke and New York: Palgrave Macmillan.

Giner, C. (2007), The politics of childhood and asylum in the UK, *Children & Society*, **21**(4), 249–260.

Gottlieb, N., D. Filc and N. Davidovitch (2012), Medical humanitarianism, human rights and political advocacy: the case of the Israeli Open Clinic, *Social Science & Medicine*, **74**(6), 839–845.

Grimen, H. (2009), Power, trust, and risk, *Medical Anthropology Quarterly*, **23**(1), 16–33.

Harrison, S. (2002), New Labour, modernisation and the medical labour process, *Journal of Social Policy*, **31**(3), 465–485.

Healthcare Regulation (2011), *Forskrift om rett til helse- og omsorgstjenester til personer uten fast opphold i riket*, 16 December, no. 1255; previously *Forskrift om endring av forskrift 1. desember 2000 nr. 1208 om prioritering av helsetjenester, rett til nødvendig helsehjelp fra spesialisthelsetjenesten, rett til behandling i utlandet og om klagenemnd (prioriteringsforskriften)*, 30 June.

Huseby, V. B. (2014a), Hvis jussen kan trumfe medisinen, er det sjokkerende, *Vårt Land*, 10 June, available online at www.vl.no/samfunn/hvis-jussen-kan-trumfe-medisinener-det-sjokkerende-1.85289.

Huseby, V. B. (2014b), Legene kunne operert Adam, *Vårt Land*, 10 June, available online at www.vl.no/samfunn/legene-kunne-operert-adam-1.85305.

Huseby, V. B. (2014c), Sykehuset snur – Adam får operasjon, *Vårt Land*, 10 June, available online at www.vl.no/samfunn/sykehuset-snur-adam-f%C3%A5r-operasjon-1.85316.

Huseby, V. B. (2014d), Vil fjerne all tvil om helsehjelp til personer uten lovlig opphold, *Vårt Land*, 27 June, available online at www.vl.no/mobile/samfunn/vil-fjerne-all-tvil-om-helsehjelp-til-personer-uten-lovlig-opphold-1.86216.

Huseby, V. B. (2014e), Leger føler seg overkjørt av UNE, *Vårt Land*, 13 June, available online at www.vl.no/samfunn/leger-føler-seg-overkjørt-av-une-1.85456.

Jensen, R., H. Seferowicz and K. Turkerud, (2014), Adam (9) får operasjon likevel, *NrK*, 10 June, available online at www.nrk.no/ostlandssendingen/adam-_9_-far-operasjon-likevel-1.11768120.

Karlsen, M-A. (2015a), Når helsevesenet blir en del av migrasjonskontrollen – etiske og praktiske dilemmaer for helsepersonell, in S. K. Bendixsen, C. M. Jacobsen and K. H. Søvig (eds.), *Eksepsjonell velferd? Irregulære migranter i det norske velferdssamfunnet*, Oslo: Gyldendal Norsk Forlag, pp. 126–143.

Karlsen, M.-A. (2015b), *Precarious Inclusion: Irregular Migration, Practices of Care, and State B/ordering in Norway*, PhD thesis, University of Bergen.

Karlsen, R. (2015), Irregulære barns rett til helsehjelp i norge, in S. K. Bendixsen, C. M. Jacobsen and K. H. Søvig (eds.), *Eksepsjonell velferd? Irregulære migranter i det norske velferdssamfunnet*, Oslo: Gyldendal Norsk Forlag, pp. 88–106.

Lahav, G. and V. Guiraudon, (2000), Comparative perspectives on border control: away from the border and outside the state, in P. Andreas and T. Snyder (eds.), *The Wall Around the West: State Borders and Immigration Controls in North America and Europe*, Lanham, MD: Rowman and Littlefield, pp. 55–77.

Lupton, D. (2012), *Medicine as Culture: Illness, Disease and the Body*, London: Sage.

Marrow, H. B. (2012), The power of local autonomy: expanding health care to unauthorized immigrants in San Francisco, *Ethnic and Racial Studies*, **35**(1), 72–87.

Ministry of Health and Care Services (2010), *Høringsnotat: Endring av prioriteringsforskriften – Helsehjelp til personer som oppholder seg ulovlig i landet*, Oslo: Helse- og omsorgsdepartementet.

Ministry of Justice and the Police (2012), *Barn på flukt*, Meld. St. 27 (2011–2012). Oslo: Justis- og politidepartementet.

Norwegian Medical Association (Den norske legeforening) (2010), *Høringsuttalelser til endring av prioriteringsforskriften – Helsehjelp til personer som oppholder seg ulovlig i landet.*

Norwegian Ombudsman for Children (Barneombudet) (2010), *Høringsuttalelser til endring av prioriteringsforskriften – Helsehjelp til personer som oppholder seg ulovlig i landet.*

Norwegian Red Cross (2007), *Årsrapport 2007*, available online at www.rodekors.no/nyheter/rapportsenter/rapporter.

NTB (2014), Dødssyk niåring får ikke hjelp på grunn av asylsøkerstatus, *NRK*, 10 June, available online at www.nrk.no/norge/dodssyk-gutt-far-ikke-hjelp-1.11767035.

Ong, A. (2003), *Buddha is Hiding Refugees, Citizenship, the New America*, Berkeley, CA: University of California Press.

Ottesen, S. H., F. Eick and P. K. Hilden (2015), Erfaringer fra helsesenteret for papirløse migranter, in S. K. Bendixsen, C. M. Jacobsen and K. H. Søvig (eds.), *Eksepsjonell velferd? Irregulære migranter i det norske velferdssamfunnet*, Oslo: Gyldendal Norsk Forlag, pp. 144–162.

Parekh, S. (2004), A meaningful place in the world: Hannah Arendt on the nature of human rights, *Journal of Human Rights*, **3**(1), 41–52.

Patient Right's Act (1999), *Lov om pasient- og brukerrettigheter (pasient- og brukerrettighetsloven)*, 2 July, no. 63.

Rose, N. and M. Valverde (1998), Governed by law? *Social & Legal Studies*, **7**(4), 541–551.

Rundskriv I-5 (2011), *Om helsehjelp til personer uten fast opphold i riket og personer uten lovlig opphold*, Oslo: Helse- og omsorgsdepartementet.

Save the Children (Redd Barna) (2010), *Høringsuttalelser til endring av prioriteringsforskriften – Helsehjelp til personer som oppholder seg ulovlig i landet.*

Salter, M. (2008), When the exception becomes the rule: borders, sovereignty, and citizenship, *Citizenship Studies*, **12**(4), 365–380.

Sinha, S. and S. Uppal (2009), 'Lesser youth? Particular universalisms and young separated migrants in East London, *Journal of Youth Studies*, **12**(3), 257–273.

Social Services Act (2009), *Lov om sosiale tjenester i arbeids- og velferdsforvaltningen*, 18 December, no. 131.

Søvig, K. H. (2013), Hvorfor nekte, eller gi, irregulære immigranter tilgang til velferdsytelser? in Ø. Rasmussen, S. Eskeland Schütz and K.H. Søvig (eds.), *Undring og erkjennelse*, Bergen: Fagbokforlaget, pp. 705–717.

Süssmann, A. (2015), Dronning i grenseland? Et menneskerettslig perspektiv på forskrift om rett til helse og omsorgstjenester til personer uten fast opphold i riket, in S. K. Bendixsen, C. M. Jacobsen and K. H. Søvig, (eds.), *Eksepsjonell velferd? Irregulære migranter i det norske velferdssamfunnet*, Oslo: Gyldendal Norsk Forlag, pp. 66–87.

Ticktin, M. (2006), Where ethics and politics meet: the violence of humanitarianism in France, *American Ethnologist*, **33**(1), pp. 33–49.

Ticktin, M. (2011), *Casualties of Care: Immigration and the Politics of Humanitarianism in France*, Berkeley, CA: University of California Press.

Van der Leun, Joanne (2006), Excluding illegal migrants in the Netherlands: between national policies and local implementation, *West European Politics*, **29**(2), 310–326.

Vitus, K. and H. Lidén (2010), The status of the asylum-seeking child in Norway and Denmark: comparing discourses, politics and practices, *Journal of Refugee Studies*, **23**(1), 62–81.

Watters, C. (2007a), *Refugee Children: Towards the Next Horizon*, Abingdon: Routledge.

Watters, C. (2007b), Refugees at Europe's borders: the moral economy of care, *Transcultural psychiatry*, **44**(3), 394–417.

Willen, S. (2007), Toward a critical phenomenology of 'illegality': state power, criminalization, and abjectivity among undocumented migrant workers in Tel Aviv, Israel, *International Migration*, **45**(3), 8–38.

Willen, S. (2012), Migration, 'illegality', and health: mapping embodied vulnerability and debating health-related deservingness, *Social Science & Medicine*, **74**(6), 805–811.
Zhang, L-C. (2008), *Developing Methods for Determining the Number of Unauthorized Foreigners in Norway*, Oslo – Kongsvinger: Statistics Norway/Division for Statistical Methods and Standards.

9 Socio-spatial dimensions of healthcare for newly arrived migrants

Anne-Cécile Hoyez with Felicity Thomas

INTRODUCTION

This chapter aims at analysing the social and spatial dimensions of health and healthcare access for newly arrived migrants in France. Reports and analyses produced on health inequalities since the end of the 1990s have questioned the continuum of healthcare available to migrants within the wider context of their everyday lives (Chauvin et al. 2014; Thomas and Gideon 2013). Indeed, research emphasises that immigration policies that impose forms of regulation and control on immigrants and their access to social service provision, alongside the precarious nature of life as a newly arrived migrant, means that they are more likely than those who are more established and have more secure immigration status to be subject to staying (at worst) outside of the health system and/or (at best) confined within specific channels of healthcare access. In France, however, national-level policies relating to 'universalism' support the notion that all are entitled to healthcare regardless of background. Drawing on research undertaken in Rennes, this chapter examines how national-level policies are negotiated within, and impact on, local-level administration and action relating to migrant healthcare. The chapter examines the lived-experiences of migrants as they struggle to secure the basic requirements of daily living and examines the motivations and challenges faced by health professionals seeking to support them within a wider and, at times, contradictory political environment.

IMPLEMENTING NATIONAL POLICY AT THE LOCAL LEVEL

Since the beginning of the century, there has been a collective position towards controlling, regulating and restricting the arrival of immigrants across the countries of the European Union. However, it is important to recognise the diverse social, political and economic contexts that face migrants located within different European nations. France, for example, has long upheld the principle of 'universalism', in which each and every citizen has universal access to the same fundamental rights regardless of race, gender, religion or nationality and 'could be said to hold one of the most liberal and progressive healthcare system in the world' (Larchanché 2012: 858). Within this guiding principle, French institutions have a strong sense of *unicité* (oneness/uniqueness), meaning that the Republic is undividable and that citizens should not be categorised into distinct groups on the basis of race or ethnicity in the national census, in surveys or in statistics generated in France. Public policies are also guided by a strong sense of equality in the national territory and in each territorial unit that composes it. Yet despite the rhetoric of *unicité* that underpins French policy, in practice, regular debate takes place over the extent to which a focus on universalism obscures the very real discrimination and inequality experienced by migrants in France (see Simon 2008; Larchanché 2012).

Indeed, despite the principal of universalism, in reality the main national objective to control immigration and reduce the number of immigrants appears to take precedence over all other sectoral policies. There is clear evidence, for example, that access to healthcare is prioritised towards French nationals and immigrants with stable residence permits, while many migrants are left at the margins of universal health coverage (Izambert 2010). Under such circumstances, the imperative of controlling immigration collides with the imperative of universal access to fundamental rights for immigrants and, in turn, impacts at a local level on the aim and scope of a range of health and social care initiatives (Franco-British Working Group on Migration, Health and Wellbeing, 2009).

At the same time as France remains a very centralised state, the ways in which national-level policies are translated, taken up and implemented at local levels can vary widely across the country, and be influenced by the discretionary working practices of key decision-makers and service providers. Under such circumstances, principles of universalism are influenced not only by wider political agendas relating to immigration control, but by fairly wide interpretation at more localised levels (d'Halluin and Hoyez 2012). Drawing on in-depth qualitative research undertaken in and around the city of Rennes, this chapter examines the spatial dimensions of social determinants of health, and examines how national level principles of universalism are being 'reinterpreted' at a local level by health professionals working in a changing institutional context in which health policies are increasingly bound up with wider debates around immigration control. Focusing on the lived experiences of migrants, alongside the perspectives of health professionals, the chapter examines how workable humanitarian responses are initiated, developed and legitimised by health providers in response to the difficult daily circumstances facing migrants in the region.

THE SOCIAL AND POLITICAL CONTEXTS OF HEALTHCARE ACCESS FOR MIGRANTS

In the domain of healthcare rights in France, the arrival of the Couverture Maladie Universelle (CMU)[1] and the Assistance Medicale d'Etat (AME)[2] in 1999 allowed the regulation of administrative access to healthcare for populations facing socioeconomic difficulties (CMU) and for populations living in an 'irregular' situation (AME). Despite their good intentions, placing people into these categories has contributed to their marginalisation and stigmatisation (Maille and Toulier, 2009). In consequence, since the beginning of the 2000s, research in anthropology and in the sociology of health have shed light on the emergence of representations that give way to processes of stigmatisation and discrimination toward immigrant populations: Estelle Carde describes in detail these processes in terms of discrimination (see Carde, 2006, 2007), while others have undertaken quantitative research on the origins and trajectories of immigrant populations in France to assess how difficulties identified in immigrant populations' access to healthcare are linked to wider circumstances such as residential and economic instability (Simon et al. 2010; Cognet and Hamel 2012).

Two important statements must be emphasised regarding newly arrived migrants in France. First, administrative issues relating to factors such as legal status and health insurance mean that healthcare provision only starts to become 'coordinated' once migrants have stabilised their immigration status; and, second, the complexities and stresses of the asylum process mean that many migrants only start to think about their health and their access to healthcare once they have sorted out their immigration and housing situation (Bergeon and Hoyez, 2015; Franco-British Working Group on Migration, Health and Wellbeing, 2009). Even then, the fear surrounding recrimination or arrest, particularly among illegal or undocumented migrants can dissuade people from approaching healthcare providers (Cognet et al. 2009). This means that delays in accessing formal service provision characterise migrants' healthcare pathways (Médecins du Monde, 2009), and that overuse of the few (usually voluntary sector) structures that are specifically dedicated to newly arrived migrants is common (Hoyez 2011; Warin 2013).

Linguistic difficulties also enter into consideration: competency with the French language is important when a person has to deal with administrative staff and healthcare professionals. These difficulties, when they exist, can adversely impact both a patient's explanation of their ill-health and their understanding of a diagnosis or of the doctor's recommendations (Cognet and Montgomery 2007). Negative representations of migrants fuelled by popular media and policy can also have important repercussions on healthcare pathways and/or delay health seeking. For example, some patients in our research were reluctant to frequent medical centres dedicated to immigrants for fear of being seen as a potential carrier of an infectious disease. We have also observed that some practitioners tend to categorise immigrant patients as 'different', and to introduce an 'alterity bias' in the healthcare relationship considering them first as 'immigrants' (which generally involves depreciative representations of this population and a loss of quality in the follow-up of the person) and not as 'patients'.

While the 'official' delivery of healthcare in France (as in much of Europe) is achieved through static outlets (i.e., a healthcare provider based in a fixed location), newly arrived migrants in France face considerable economic and logistical barriers moving into and around cities in order to access conventional outlets of healthcare. Such circumstances are likely to account, in part at least, to poor health outcomes, and an ongoing reliance on distanced or transnational networks to access medical information.

SPACE AND MOBILITY

An examination of healthcare pathways for immigrants demonstrates how multiple difficulties within daily life impact on healthcare experiences. Many of these difficulties arise because of the precarious economic situation many migrants find themselves in, and as a result of this, their reliance on the often poorly funded and targeted services provided to them. Accommodation, for example, is often unstable, resulting in migrants being transferred from place to place at frequent intervals. At the same time, migrants experience constraints travelling to multiple locations in order to access their basic needs such as food, clothes and administrative papers. Likewise, while migrants may qualify for social support via mechanisms such as the CMU and AME, the process of activating these rights may prove extremely difficult when this requires soliciting different desks in different administrative institutions (e.g., immigration, social services, health services), particularly when this is likely to take second precedence to more basic everyday needs such as securing food. Thus while access to healthcare is reduced or hindered for all precarious populations (Chauvin and Parizot 2005; Parizot 2003; Rode 2009), fieldwork in Rennes found that for immigrants, healthcare is often delayed or not taken-up at all because of the accumulation of daily constraints linked to their status as immigrants, and that this, in turn, has extremely adverse implications for psychological wellbeing. Interviews led with newly arrived immigrants in Rennes and other areas of Brittany allow insight into the ways in which socioeconomic determinants and local contexts of health provision are combined and come into play for migrants seeking to access healthcare. These kinds of daily difficulties faced by migrants were frequently discussed during the fieldwork as the following examples demonstrate:

> Natalia comes from an Eastern European country. She arrived in France at the age of 18, after spending time in various countries seeking healthcare for a life-threatening disease. She is accommodated by the authorities in an asylum-seeker shelter located 30km away from Rennes (she had no choice in the location), in an apartment she shares with people from different nationalities. Her health condition requires regular monitoring at Rennes University Hospital and a medical centre where she relies on the support of an interpreter. She is very satisfied with the medical and social care she receives. However, to get to Rennes, she must take a bus that passes only once per hour and takes 40 minutes to reach the centre of the city. She must then use a subway or bus to take her to the place of consultation. In the small town where she lives, her activities are limited to going to the church or the pharmacy; she does not know anyone in this area and few opportunities exist to meet with local people. The few compatriots she knows are based in Rennes. However, her health condition limits her trips there to medical consultations, meaning that her opportunities for social interaction and support are extremely limited.

Tariq comes from the Indian subcontinent. He fled his country with his wife and daughter after two murder attempts against him. Initially supported by an asylum-seekers' shelter in the Paris region, the family was then moved by the authorities to the Rennes area. They are accommodated in a house in the countryside, without walking access to any basic service. For food, they retrieve a package from an NGO, for mail they depend on the Red Cross, for clothes on another NGO and for the regular healthcare consultations required for Tariq's baby, they depend on the University Hospital. To reach Rennes, they have to walk 20 minutes to a bus stop. It runs every hour between 9am and 5pm and takes 25 minutes to reach the centre of Rennes. French people living in this area do it by choice and have access to private transport. Because most of them rely on getting to Rennes for work, they have a much wider range of options available to them for accessing basic services such as food and local health provision. Because of their immigration status, Tariq's family, however, must rely on public transport to Rennes and then take a number of bus or subway journeys within the city to get to the various places where they are able to access food, clothes or honour a medical consultation. While Tariq and his wife are very satisfied with the medical care they receive, the geographical and social isolation they experience are an ongoing source of anguish that has resulted in them needing to receive psychiatric treatment. Tariq described their accommodation, saying that 'For my baby, this house is not good. There is no [mother and child welfare], there is no transportation services, there is no grocery services, there is no pharmacy, there is no taxi. There is nothing. [. . .] This is jungle, you understand "jungle"? There are only farm houses. Cattle farm, goat farm, horse farm. We are not dogs, we are less than dogs.' He went to describe his daily experience as an asylum-seeker in France, saying, 'We are very happy with the medication matters but we are not satisfied with the human rights, with the refugee system, with the place where they sent us. In this kind of place, they have to send the bachelor people, not those having family. Not sending people like us, with small baby, all alone in jungle [. . .] They [social workers] told me "This is a very nice place for the French people!" I say "I'm not a French. I'm a Pakistani". In Pakistan, we are not used to live in the jungles. I am a city man. I am not a villager.'

Research on migrant health and wellbeing has highlighted the importance of social resources such as compatriot networks, formal and informal associations (Pian 2012). Others have recognised the range of spatial resources that can be mobilised for health, in particular, resources that are multi-localised; for example, networks constituted of individuals and/or organisations in diasporic systems that provide access to treatments and social support (Ma Mung 1999; Thomas 2010). While not undermining the value of such resources, the two examples above highlight how the everyday circumstances of precarity facing many migrants can make basic daily survival an all-consuming occupation.

LOCAL HEALTHCARE INITIATIVES

Despite the kinds of constraints discussed above, local initiatives are taking an increasingly important and dynamic role in supporting the healthcare of precarious populations in France (Skinner and Fleuret 2011; Hassenteufel et al. 1998). These initiatives are diverse, vary considerably from place to place, and are often run by NGOs such as Médecins du Monde. In Rennes, a number of such organisations have been set up to support immigrants, following a local tendency of mobilisation towards marginalised migrant populations.[3] However, following a decision by the government in the 1990s to leave decisions over follow-up care for HIV-positive patients to the medico-social field, a group of doctors in Rennes decided to create a medical centre with an 'associative' rather than a 'public health' status, specifically dedicated to supporting immigrants. They did this at their own discretion after observing that immigrant patients (being HIV-positive or not) were being marginalised in public health service access. The doctors were able to do this by using their legitimacy and standing as 'health professionals' and 'infectious disease specialists' to convince the necessary regulating institutions to found them.

A key part of the work of these doctors lies in their recognition of the interrelationship between good healthcare, residential stability and access to basic services. In other words, they recognise that migrants are more likely to access healthcare effectively once their other basic needs – for example, accommodation – have been stabilised. At the same time, they recognise that by accessing migrant populations via outreach work, they can then use the legitimacy and power afforded by their status to be able to set in motion a range of actions that can enable migrants to access more stable accommodation. The following section draws on interviews undertaken with these health professionals working with immigrants in Rennes to examine their motivations, and to explore how they make and legitimise radical and often controversial short-term arrangements to provide immediate healthcare to precarious migrant groups in order to support longer-term goals that ensure that France's universalist principles are upheld.

Research on professionals working with patients in precarious situations reveals the multiple outreach actions targeted towards specific populations. These practices are not really new: they are well-known in the domain of social work, particularly in actions against addictions (e.g., alcoholism, drug addiction). However, it is a practice that comes in different types of interventions meant to reach out towards a population identified, usually, as precarious. This practice implies that professionals should go where the person is located: in the street, but also in other areas such as schools, hospitals, social centres and prisons (Roche 2007). Roaming, mobile medical teams or inter-institutional liaison teams are some of the arrangements put in place for this purpose. In the fieldwork in Rennes, we encountered many such practices in the actions undertaken with newly arrived immigrants, whether in the street or in unstable housing such as shelters for asylum-seekers or informal squats. The outreach therefore involves 'going to' the spaces frequented by targeted populations while also attempting to reduce the distance in power relations and social interactions between professionals and patients. Indeed, this intervention is not only made to find and assist people *in situ*, but also to create what Mellier (2006: 153) calls 'interactional opportunities', a notion mobilised mainly in the field of social work and psychology to describe the action of professionals working with people facing complex challenges in everyday life (such as homeless people) to provide specific and personalised interactions. A healthcare professional who decides to make visits to patients in the street or in a squat therefore creates these 'interactional opportunities' not only because s/he meets patients in non-standard places of living, but also because their presence here overcomes issues of power-relations that may be present in more conventional healthcare settings.

Interviews undertaken with doctors in Rennes revealed insights into their motivations and experiences in providing this kind of outreach work,

Interviewer: Where and how do you see patients?

Doctor: There are two types of people we see. There are asylum-seekers, the classics, who are orientated towards us either by an association or by the platform for asylum-seekers . . . Regardless . . . But those, we see. There are asylum-seekers we will never see [in the formal healthcare system] because they are living in squats. And then there are others especially those who have not gone through the platform for asylum-seekers, who are 'undocumented'. And those, if you do not go looking for them, you will not see them. In addition they are scared. Hence the need [for us] to go to the squat: it is to go fishing for people we do not see. [. . .] It's made for that, that approach: to reach people who do not come. This is fishing, anything else. It is really fishing.

Interviewer: And you become mobile?

Doctor: This is essential. Practicing medicine cannot be done [with] the butt on a chair. Well, not for me.

Interviewer: But that means setting up a mobile team?

Doctor: Yes, but this is a transitional mobility. We cannot do medicine in a squat. I consider it difficult. We can do it, but it's more of 'bricolage' [piecing together different approaches]. What would be interesting is to see if we can bring people living in squats here, because here we have the equipment, we have interpreters. [. . .] So the aim is to take these people, to get them here, provide them appointment, with be a doctor, a social worker, a nurse, an interpreter.

The outreach practice described can therefore be seen as representing an innovative attempt to help build trust with precarious populations so that over time, they will start to more readily use and engage with the formal healthcare system.

However, these kinds of actions also need to be understood within the broader context in which health professionals practise in France. Professionals who take it upon themselves to implement such actions are relatively uncommon,[4] and while their actions may be heralded by some as innovative humanitarianism, they may also be regarded with suspicion or work unsupported, even by others within their own profession. They also face a more fundamental problem within the wider political context: namely, that by providing targeted support to distinct populations they encourage a process that endorses a 'differential' vision of access to public services. This can be seen as problematic in France, where implementing and negotiating special channels to promote or support a distinct category of the population over others can be seen as contravening the requirements of universalism. It is an argument often faced in France, by funders, public policy and health professionals whose ethics are based – at least in principle – on strict equality between all people.

Because the outreach approach differentiates between different populations, doctors involved have had to mobilise strong arguments to legitimise their actions, both to other health professionals and their institutions as well as to policy regulators more widely. Very often under such circumstances, an argument that posits migrants as a potential threat to public health is invoked. However, for most doctors in Rennes, this kind of approach is deeply unsatisfactory because by implying that migrants pose an inherent health risk to the general population, they risk invoking further discrimination against them. In the fieldwork undertaken in Rennes, an alternative narrative was observed in which doctors drew on the widely heralded value of multi-sectoral working to evoke what is widely deemed as an innovative, 'modern' and uncontroversial response to local concerns.

One public health professional working with the Agence Régionale de Santé (Regional Health Agency), for example, explained how under the system of universal ethics that framed public health services it was not possible to be seen to be giving precedence to migrants, even when their health issues were clearly not always being met. However, they explained how the 'proactive', multidisciplinary approach taken by the doctors provided a practical, innovative and workable 'solution' without compromising the position and impartiality of the health service. Indeed, the ambiguous positioning of the doctors as outreach workers was considered a real bonus to the health system because it provided a form of flexible and ad hoc working that enabled the project to succeed 'without institutionalising and without creating [the] heavy structures' that characterised so much of their more conventional work.

The doctors therefore invest in the social and spatial interstices of precariousness – that is to say, they follow an approach that places them 'in-between': between medicine and social work, and between healthcare places such as the street, the home and the healthcare centre. In this way, they have been able to develop targeted and mobile activities while respecting the wider common framework of their professional practice. Yet despite this framing of their outreach work, the ongoing insecurity of funding and support and the potential clash with principals of universalism mean that doctors are continually required to craft their narratives in a way that enables them to legitimise and secure funding for their work.

CONCLUSION

This chapter has emphasised the precarious nature of the daily lives of newly arrived migrants in France, and has demonstrated the difficulties that many people face in accessing basic service provision from multiple locations in and around the city. While the material used in this chapter is taken from fieldwork led in France (Hoyez 2015), parallels can be drawn with situations in other European countries (see, for example, Chauvin et al. 2014) where migrants' access to healthcare is constrained by the impacts of immigration policies on their daily lives. Indeed, even if the right to health is recognised, and even in a country like France, which is widely heralded for having progressive 'universal' healthcare policies, the political nature of immigration has meant that in reality, migrants find it extremely difficult to access their fundamental human rights. The precedence given to immigration control undermines the principle of universalism and universal health coverage in France and in so doing, renders a form of socially structured illegitimacy on certain categories of immigrants, especially undocumented migrants and those waiting for asylum claims to be assessed (Larchanché 2012).

As this chapter has demonstrated, such circumstances point to the importance of understanding both the daily realities of newly arrived migrants, and the perspectives and experiences of those seeking to support them. This means moving understandings of migrant health and wellbeing beyond the static conceptualisations of healthcare and healthcare delivery that tend to be encompassed within macro-scale policy, to consider the role of more localised responses to supporting precarious populations. In Rennes, the 'invention' of outreach practices to find and treat the 'invisible' have been enabled because of the commitment and humanity of a group of dedicated health professionals, and their willingness to seek ways of legitimising their actions within the institutions that guide their profession. At a regional and national scale, the actions they undertake to support precarious populations can induce different difficulties that require them to juggle the different demands and expectations of different audiences (the government, the general public, the target population) in order to legitimise and gain ongoing support for their actions. Such insights highlight the profusion of innovative modes of action that are built at the margins of the health system and demonstrate the need to pay more critical attention to the ways that the territorialisation of action to support precarious migrant populations can oscillate between the paradoxes and ambiguities of national-level policy and its implementation within specific local situations.

NOTES

1. Couverture Maladie Universelle – state health insurance for people on low incomes.
2. Assistance Médicale d'Etat – state health assistance for people in irregular situations.
3. Some would say that Brittany has a long tradition of welcoming and helping minorities as the region is historically sensitive to the issues of minorities due to the unstable links between the French state and local governments between the sixteenth and the twentieth century (until the end of the 1970s there were still Breton nationalism movements); others would say that the region has politically always been stable, voting largely for 'Christian socialism' (leftist Christian) parties, which have a tendency to valorise actions towards the oppressed.
4. In the Rennes area, there are only 15 doctors who have chosen to provide this form of outreach work to migrants.

REFERENCES

Bergeon, C. and A. C. Hoyez (2015), Etre migrant et vivre en squat, *L'Espace Politique*, available online at http|://espacepolitique.revues.org/3517.

Carde, E. (2006), *Les discriminations selon l'origine dans l'accès aux soins. Etude en France métropolitaine et en Guyane Française*, Le Kremlin-Bicêtre, Val-de-Marne, Université de Paris-Sud.

Carde, E. (2007), Les discriminations selon l'origine dans l'accès aux soins, *Santé Publique*, **2**, 99–109.

Chauvin, P. and I. Parizot (2005), *Santé et recours aux soins des populations vulnérables*, Paris: INSERM.

Chauvin, P., N. Simonnot, C. Douay and F. Vanbiervliet (2014), *Access to Healthcare for People Facing Multiple Vulnerability Factors in 27 Cities Across 10 Countries: Report on the Social and Medical Data Gathered in 2013 in Eight European Countries, Turkey and Canada*, Paris: International Network of Médecins du Monde.

Cognet, M. and C. Hamel (2012), Santé des migrants en France: l'effet des discriminations liées à l'origine et au sexe, *Revue Européenne des Migrations Internationales*, **28**(2), 11–34.

Cognet, M. and C. Montgomery (2007), *Ethique de l'altérité. La question de la culture dans le champ de la santé et des services sociaux*, Québec.

Cognet, M., C. Gabarro and E. Adam-Vezina (2009), Entre droit aux soins et qualité des soins, *Hommes et Migrations*, available online at www.hommes-et-migrations.fr/index.php?/numeros/sante-et-droits-des-etranger-realites-et-enjeux/5725-entre-droit-aux-soins-et-qualite-des-soins.

d'Halluin, E. and A.C. Hoyez (2012), L'initiative associative et les reconfigurations locales des dispositifs d'accès aux soins pour les migrants primo-arrivants, *Humanitaire*, **33**, available online at http://humanitaire.revues.org/1407.

Franco-British Working Group on Migration, Health and Wellbeing (2009), Health, well-being and immigrant populations in France and Britain, *International Journal of Migration, Health and Social Care*, **5**(4), 4–19.

Hassenteufel, P., B. Le Bihan-Youinou, P. Loncle and A. Vion (1998), L'émergence problématique d'une nouvelle santé publique. Forums d'action publique et coalitions de projets à Rennes et à Brest, in D. Fassin (ed.), *Figures urbaines de la santé publique. Enquête sur les expériences locales*, Paris: La découverte.

Hoyez, A. C. (2011), L'accès aux soins des migrants en France et la 'culture de l'initiative locale'. Une analyse des contextes locaux à l'épreuve des orientations nationales, *Cybergeo: European Journal of Geography*, available online at http://cybergeo.revues.org/24796.

Hoyez, A. C. (2015), Territoires, mobilités et santé: comment composer et penser une offre de soins pour les populations migrantes en situation précaire? *Revue Francophone sur la Santé et les Territoires*, available online at http://rfst.hypotheses.org.

Izambert, C. (2010), 30 ans de régressions dans l'accès aux soins, *Plein Droit*, **86**, available online at www.gisti.org/spip.php?article2102.

Larchanché, S. (2012), Intangible obstacles: health implications of stigmatization, structural violence, and fear among undocumented immigrants in France, *Social Science and Medicine*, **74**, 858–863.

Maille, D. and A. Toulier (2009), Les dix ans de la CMU, *Hommes et Migrations*, **1282**, available online at www.hommes-et-migrations.fr/index.php?id=5716.

Ma Mung, E. (1999), La dispersion comme ressource, *Cultures & Conflits*, **33–34**, available online at http://conflits.revues.org/index225.html.

Médecins du Monde (2009), *L'accès aux soins: un droit non respecté en Europe*, Paris: Médecins du Monde.

Mellier, D. (2006), Précarité psychique et dispositifs d'intervention clinique, *Pratiques Psychologiques*, **12**(2), 145–155.

Parizot, I. (2003), *Soigner les exclus*, Paris: Presses Universitaires de France.

Pian, A. (2012), De l'accès aux soins aux 'trajectoires du mourir'. Les étrangers atteints de cancer face aux contraintes administratives, *Revue Européenne des Migrations Internationales*, **28**(2), 101–127.

Roche, P. (2007), Les défis de la proximité dans le champ professionnel, *Nouvelle revue de psychosociologie*, **3**(1), 63–82.

Rode, A. (2009), L'émergence du non-recours aux soins des populations précaires: entre droit aux soins et devoirs de soins, *Lien social et politique*, **61**, 149–158.

Simon, P. (2008), The choice of ignorance: the debate on ethnic and racial statistics in France, *French Politics, Culture & Society*, **26**(1), 7–31.

Simon, P., C. Beauchemin and C. Hamel (2010), Trajectoires et Origines : enquête sur la diversité des populations en France. Premiers résultats, *Documents de Travail*, no.168, Paris: INED.

Skinner, M. W. and S. Fleuret (2011), Health geography's voluntary turn: a view from western France, *Health & Place*, **17**(1), 33–41.

Thomas, F. (2010), Transnational health and treatment networks: meaning, value and place in health seeking amongst southern African migrants in London, *Health & Place*, **16**(3), 606–612.

Thomas, F. and J. Gideon (2013), *Migration, Health and Inequality*, London: Zed Books.

Warin, P. (2013), L'accès aux soins des populations vulnérables, *Colloque 'Accès aux soins des plus démunis'*, Paris, France.

PART IV

VULNERABILITY AND PRECARITY

10 The health and wellbeing of survival migrants

Katherine Vasey, Lenore Manderson and Louise Newman

INTRODUCTION

The global dynamics of displacement in the twenty-first century are characterized by economic and political crises, natural and human disasters, protracted wars and civil strife, demographic and environmental changes, and human rights violations. More than 1.5 billion people live in countries that are blighted by such crises, conflicts and repeated cycles of violence. One-third of the world's poor live in failed states, post-conflict settings or in countries where conflict continues, where basic human needs may not be met. By 2018, the number of people living under such conditions is likely to have increased to one-half, and by 2030 as many as two-thirds of poor people may live in these circumstances (Chandy et al. 2013). Humanitarian and survival migration, as a consequence, has increased dramatically in recent decades, as we explore below. By the end of 2013, 51 million people had been forcibly displaced as a result of persecution, conflict, violence or human rights violations (UNHCR 2014b). At the time of writing (2015), millions of people have been driven from their homes by conflict in the Syrian Arab Republic, Democratic Republic of the Congo, the Central African Republic, Mali and the border areas of South Sudan and Sudan, and the Ukraine. There is a growing humanitarian crisis in Nigeria and neighbouring Niger as tens of thousands of people flee Boko Haram attacks. People are also fleeing Libya, Somalia, Iran, Iraq, Afghanistan, Eritrea, West Papua, Vietnam, Myanmar (formerly Burma), China, Cambodia, Liberia, Mauritania, Sri Lanka, Burundi, Algeria and Angola. Unaccompanied children flee to the United States of America from Mexico, Guatemala, Honduras and El Salvador as a result of increased 'northern triangle' violence, poverty and family reunification, for fear of life and lack of livelihoods. Multiple circumstances therefore shape flight and the need to relocate.

While most displaced persons remain in their country of origin, forced migrants are increasingly relying on wider patterns of mobility, both regionally and globally (Zetter 2015). With this mobility comes massive inconsistency in the ways that migrants are treated in different countries, some survival migrants are offered asylum as refugees; others are rounded up, detained, and deported, often in brutal conditions. For example, as Andersson (2014) notes, in the US, irregular migrants are pushed through mass trials and deported back to Mexico far from their place of entry. In collectively pleading guilty to crossing illegally, they avoid a potentially long incarceration. In Israel, African migrants launched hunger strikes in the summer of 2014 in protest at their 'inhuman and unlimited' detention. In Australia, asylum-seekers arriving by boat are incarcerated in remote detention centres in Papua New Guinea and Nauru.

In this chapter we explore the concept of 'survival migration' to highlight the predicament in which many people around the world find themselves. Using examples from diverse settings, and drawing on our work in Australia and elsewhere, we present a broad overview of survival migration. For pragmatic reasons, we have divided this chapter in relation to the chronology of internal displacement through to permanent resettlement. However, the circumstances in which people leave their homes and seek sanctuary elsewhere varies greatly, and clean divisions between each stage – exit, transit, arrival and resettlement – cannot be assumed (Duvell 2012). As we discuss, each stage of the migratory process can be fraught with dangers, variability and unpredictability, high levels of risk and low levels of protection impacting upon people's access to livelihoods, safety and wellbeing.

DEFINING 'SURVIVAL MIGRATION'

As survival migrants move across boundaries and borders, they necessarily contend with global technologies – laws, regulations and law-enforcement bodies, at national and international levels – that seek to categorize their motivations for flight, so to define their legal status and rights as migrants. A refugee is defined under the Geneva Convention in relation to perceived and/or demonstrated persecution for reasons of race, nationality, membership of a particular social group, or political opinion, outside their country of origin (UNHCR 2005; Black 2003; Perrenoud 2000). Refugees and people who seek asylum are managed by nation-states, international humanitarian law and multilateral agencies as categories separate from each other. Many humanitarian migrants do not fit the criteria of the formal UN legal definition of a refugee, and how people are categorized varies from one country to another because not all countries accept this definition, and because of the variable interpretation of the validity of claims for sanctuary at national levels. Terms such as 'refugee' and 'asylum-seeker' also risk reifying the categories of people who are displaced, and the diverse circumstances and complex paths that lead people to relocate. Many 'forced migrants', including those displaced by environmental devastation or protracted civil conflict, are not formally recognized by the international protection regime (Castles 2003; Zetter 2015). In addition, some undocumented migrants and asylum-seekers are regarded as 'economic' migrants; their motivation to migrant may be due to extreme poverty, lack of any work, discrimination in finding employment or the circumstances under which they are employed. People in many countries labour under unsafe, violent, near slave-like conditions. Social factors including ethnicity and cultural affiliation influence where they are employed, under what conditions and whether or not they can change these. These latter migrants who have fled from environmental disaster, continued conflict, fear and terror, and economic violence are those who we include in our broader term 'survival migrants'. In essence, 'survival migrants' are all people who seek refuge in another state with the aim of survival (Betts 2013).

By the end of 2014, the number of internally displaced persons (IDPs) – forced migrants living in displacement within the borders of their own country – had grown to about 38 million (IDMC 2015). These figures fail to include less systematic patterns of internal displacement, including others migrating for survival, stranded migrants – including rejected asylum-seekers and those who fit with other categories of humanitarian migrants – including illegal, informal and unregistered migrants (with UNHCR), asylum-seekers, stateless persons and returnees, this last group returning either voluntarily or forcibly, at times because of human rights abuses in camps or countries of temporary resettlement. In addition, we include people subject to episodic and sustained physical violence and sexual violence (Theidon 2012), to populations subject to sporadic terror through raids on villages and the theft of goods, compounded by structural violence – as occurs, for example, in Burma (Skidmore 2004), and Uganda under the Lord's Resistance Army (Finnstrom 2003) – and nationalist violence, as experienced by Tamil workers in the highlands in Sri Lanka (see, for instance, Daniel (1997)). We include too people living in environments of intimidation and despotism, including those living under military rule, in settings of civil war and those subject to systemic everyday lack of liberty (in North Korea, for instance). This broad and extended definition allows for people fleeing from violent gangs, as occurs in parts of Central and South America in relation to the drug trade and protracted civil wars (Pine 2008); for people who cannot survive without moving either because of generalized state oppression combined with drought and the collapse of the state (Zimbabwe mid-2000s) or because of targeted discrimination as illustrated by the oppression of people according to sexuality, sexual and cultural identity, and occupation (Scorgie et al. 2013).

In this chapter, therefore, we use the term 'survival migrant' to refer to any person who is stateless, a refugee or asylum-seeker, or who for any other reason relocates out of fear of loss of life, livelihood, liberty, targeted persecution or torture, or who, on an everyday basis, is subject to harassment, confinement (within homes or villages, not in specific institutions), or is subject to discrimination at any and all levels of society for any reason (gender, ethnicity, sexuality or religion). The United Nations High Commissioner for Refugees (UNHCR) classifies many of these people as 'irregular' migrants or 'people of concern'. This classification emerges from juridical and administrative structures, which position people as either involuntary or volitional migrants. This affects their rights to healthcare, education, employment, housing and welfare assistance, and access to services. The ways in which people are categorized also affects their wellbeing during flight and resettlement, determining where they might go and stay; if they are to be registered in order to access basic health and educational services; if, indeed, any state is willing to take on responsibility for their welfare. These points are well-illustrated for people without papers, such as those from North Africa in France (Ticktin 2011) and those from Central America in the US (Holmes 2013).

INTERNAL DISPLACEMENT

Data collected by international agencies indicate that forced displacement predominantly occurs *within* the countries that are affected (Zetter 2015). By the end of 2014, 38 million people worldwide were forced to flee their homes and were living in displacement within the borders of their own country (IDMC 2015). People in these circumstances abandon their home environments and their places of habitual residence and rupture their social networks and economic livelihoods only when other strategies of survival have failed (Zetter 2015). The majority of forced migrants remain within their own national borders for numerous reasons – maintaining social networks, livelihoods and the fragments of a familiar environment, wanting to remain close to their origins in case return is conceivable, where protection and assistance may be provided by their governments (in some countries) or international humanitarian actors, or where they may lack the capacity or resources to move further afield (Zetter 2014).

The social, economic and human costs of war and internal displacement are profound. People find temporary accommodation with host families, or find their own accommodation for as long as their resources will permit, or end up resident in makeshift camps and scattered informal settlements, with significant security risks. In many such settings, safe access to food, water, shelter, medical care and other essentials is a daily struggle. Many displaced people, and others dependent on them, suffer from chronic disease and disability, and their continuing need for health, medical and welfare services following displacement occurs in addition to basic needs (Gammouh et al. 2015). In addition, the wounds of violence, persecution, homelessness and invisibility are often long-term and debilitating. Psychiatric disorders, including anxiety and depression, post-traumatic stress disorder, mental exhaustion and chronic fatigue, are experienced by many internally displaced people as well as external humanitarian migrants (Quosh et al. 2013).

Forced internal displacement may be short-lasting, but for many it involves much longer periods *in situ* and in protracted exile. When displacement is prolonged, people are often neglected, resulting in adverse social, cultural, economic and health impacts (Roberts et al. 2009; Gülsen et al. 2010). In addition, many people are displaced more than once in their lifetime, and the impact of recurrent flight on both migrants and local communities is severe. Each time people are displaced, they have to start life again somewhere new, and lose more of their assets, eroding their ability to cope and increasing their poverty, needs and vulnerability (IDMC 2015). The more often people are displaced, the more it is likely families are separated, making it difficult to maintain or establish support networks. Further, the capacity and goodwill of local communities to help and support internally displaced migrants shrinks over time and with every new wave of displacement, as access to jobs, livelihoods, land, education and health services also diminishes (Internal Displacement Monitoring Centre and Norwegian Refugee Council 2015). Internal displacement therefore imposes considerable economic and health burdens on displaced people and recipient communities, as exemplified within Syria in 2014–2015 (ACAPS 2015), and recurrently in South Africa, resulting in hostile attitudes and xenophobic attacks (ACMS 2009, 2010).

FLIGHT

Little is known about the experiences of displaced individuals en route to destination countries (Nakash et al. 2014), and few studies exist documenting the dangers asylum-seekers are exposed to during migration (Infante et al. 2012). The circumstances in which people leave their homes and seek sanctuary elsewhere varies greatly, and clean divisions between each stage – exit, transit, arrival, and resettlement – cannot be assumed (Duvell 2012). However, as we discuss below, each stage can be fraught with dangers, variability and unpredictability, high levels of risk and low levels of protection (Zetter 2014).

People tend to flee to the nearest location thought to be safe but if the danger is persistent and pervasive, they are forced to take long journeys into bordering countries and beyond. For most, there is little opportunity to plan the journey, and people flee with few possessions or personal documentation. Many have never had travel documents – they had not needed them – or their documents are destroyed intentionally or in the circumstances of flight. Others, assuming available time, may fake their ethnicity, occupation and other kinds of identification. People also make decisions about who will travel and who will stay behind, and some may send their children ahead alone. Others leave children and other family members behind, and family members may be separated or apprehended en route.

The most organized flights are those of families with some resources, able to pay for fares and, where necessary, for falsified documents, for legitimate or illegal journeys to other countries, such as to Europe or Australia. People often transit through territories where there is continued conflict, famine and political instability sometimes spanning decades in some instances. Journeys are also hazardous as a result of mode of transport – on foot, by boat, in truck containers and hiding in cars, taking risks during physical border crossings and in face of hostilities from border patrols. Reliance on smugglers, organized-crime groups and traffickers to facilitate movement by providing transportation, using fraudulent documents and bribes for border officials all expose migrants to extreme risks (Zetter 2015). Migrants in transit are more vulnerable, more exposed to human rights violations and lack adequate protection (Zetter 2014). Women and children are particularly vulnerable, at risk of abuse, exploitation, sexual violence, forced labour and trafficking (Dudley et al. 2012; Gerard and Pickering 2014). Thousands of migrants have died in poorly equipped and heavily laden boats travelling across the Mediterranean, the Gulf of Mexico, and the Indian Ocean (Fazel et al. 2014). For example, as many as 20,000 migrants and refugees may have lost their lives attempting to reach Europe via the Mediterranean Sea in the past 16 years (EMHRN 2014). UNHCR (2014a) estimates 3,000 died in 2014 alone. These figures constitute only a fraction of the unnamed lives lost on irregular and dangerous routes to safe countries. In addition to these deaths, others are killed or die from infectious disease, in childbirth or as infants, from uncontrolled pre-existing health problems or from injuries en route (IOM 2014).

LIFE IN TRANSIT COUNTRIES

Entry into bordering countries is often irregular or illegal, preventing access to basic protection. In addition, their entry makes it difficult to access refugee, asylum or temporary protection measures, even if they are eligible for these statuses. Many countries endeavour to systematically deny undocumented migrants access to these procedures or engage in forced deportation, returning the migrants to the conditions from which they fled (Zetter 2014). As a result, many survival migrants live in the shadows in transit countries. Evidence from Mexico, Yemen, Morocco and Tunisia shows that migrants may be stranded or trapped indefinitely in transit countries because of inadequate funds or documentation (Zetter 2015). This structural vulnerability has serious implications on their health and wellbeing, since such migrants lack access to emergency and routine health services (Cartwright and Manderson 2011).

Media representations of forced migrants tend to focus on those languishing in refugee camps in isolated areas. Many such camps do exist, the focus of the work of various international programmes and non-government organizations. However, the vast majority of survival migrants end up in cities, in informal housing and squatter settlements on their periphery, and in other towns (IFRC 2012; UNHCR 2012; Landau 2014). There are a number of reasons for this, despite the poor conditions and environmental hazards of informal settlements, and the lack of access to medical services and food support, processing assistance and protection that may be available in camps (Pantuliano et al. 2012). Many displaced people who flee from urban areas seek refuge in a similar environment, where economic opportunities are presumed to be greater for them (UNHCR 2011), and where there may be pre-existing family or economic networks (Gwatirisa and Manderson 2009). Some refugees may also see advantage in the anonymity of urban spaces, thus reducing potential threats from rival ethnic groups in exile, and minimising the risk of *refoulement*. These advantages are, as indicated above, offset by the substantial protection risks and increased vulnerability due to immigration laws and encampment policies, and are subject to harassment and exploitation (Landau 2014). As for internal migrants, survival migrants who have moved across borders and are living in urban settings are subject to violence, as a result of competition with local populations for scarce resources including food, housing and employment. The xenophobic attacks against migrants from central and southern African countries living in South Africa illustrate this (Misago and Monson 2010; ACMS 2009, 2010).

Although the health and wellbeing of those forcibly migrating to urban areas is not well documented (Steel et al. 2011a; Crisp et al. 2012), demographic and socioeconomic factors combine with the lack of legal status to increase vulnerabilities to impact on health and wellbeing (Zetter 2014). While infectious diseases are prevalent because of crowded conditions and work in high-risk occupations (IOM 2011), urban refugees appear to be particularly prone to developing non-communicable diseases (Amara and Aljunid 2014), arguably in relation to poor nutrition, stress and stress-related behaviours such as tobacco, drug and alcohol consumption.

CAMPS

Much of the existing research on the health and wellbeing of survival migrants has focused on people living in camps. Refugee camps may afford some with better services than they had left behind, by providing them with access to water, fuel, sanitation, personal security, and healthcare. Matthew Wilhelm-Solomon (2013), for example, illustrated that people with HIV in camps in northern Uganda are provided with antiretrovirals and nutritional supplements, which they would not have had in the areas from which they fled. But this specialized care is distributed in such a way as to make clear to everyone in the camp which people are HIV-positive: food rations are labelled differently; supplements are provided on different days. Further, although camps may provide assistance in delivery, emergency obstetric care, vaccinations and treatment for acute infections, this is not always sustainable. In protracted refugee situations, tens of thousands of people may move and so camps expand quickly, without the time or resources for external agencies to build the necessary infrastructure or to organize support for all arrivals. In such settings, people are at heightened risk of disease from poor hygiene and sanitation, lack of food and fuel, polluted water, limited shelter and inadequate medical staff, faculties and drugs (Steel et al. 2011a; Milner 2014). Governing agencies may not be able to meet basic requirements nor enable subsistence activities. Furthermore, livelihood activities outside camps and freedom of movement are usually discouraged, impacting on the mental and physical health of those living within them. In many cases, people do not seek medical attention outside of the camps, or may not have the financial resources in any case (Lori and Boyle 2015).

Migration facilitates the transmission of infectious disease either when infected people move into new settings, or when people move to areas where disease is already established, especially when new arrivals lack immunity to particular pathogens. Further, control and prevention services are rarely in place in refugee settings, and there are few resources to extend such activities to new populations. Some people may be treated on arrival at a camp, particularly for HIV and virulent infections such as TB, but the conditions of 'temporary' residences in camps and towns, including of multiple families living in small houses or tents, and more general crowding, increase the risks of all bacterial and viral infections. People's constant movement within and between countries also increases the probability of the introduction and transmission of and reinfection from communicable diseases (Mendelsohn et al. 2014; Sturrock et al. 2015). Inadequate surveillance methods and poor diagnostic capacity in camp clinics, problems in the procurement of drugs and other supplies, and the lack of public health services to support the delivery of care within camps further inhibit early detection and control of infections, leading to epidemic outbreaks (De Buck et al. 2015; Mahamud et al. 2012; Minetti et al. 2010).

Deprivation, isolation, lack of productivity, violence and uncertainty are all associated with intermediate and temporary migration, and in many cases, this results in a near-permanent sense of liminality, with constant fear, anxiety and stress (McGuire and Georges 2003). The situation of ongoing uncertainty and anxiety contributes to a state of psychological constriction and numbing. Louise Newman (pers. comm. 2015), for instance, has heard many people describe a sense of loss of self and loss of sense of a future – of becoming a 'ghost-like being' with no purpose. This is also impacted by ongoing experiences of fear and trauma common in many camps and limits the ability to engage with legal and review processes. The psychological mode of survival orientation, on a collective basis, dominates (Newman, pers. comm. 2015)

DETENTION

Many countries have adopted increasingly punitive measures to prevent migrants from making asylum claims through heightened border surveillance, outsourcing procedures for determining refugee status to other countries, and the incarceration of men, women and children in immigration detention facilities (Fazel et al. 2014). The controversial incarceration of 'unauthorised arrivals' in Australia has received much attention worldwide. Australia requires the mandatory detention of all unauthorized arrivals for an indefinite period, using remote detention facilities until resolution of their asylum claims (Human Rights and Equal Opportunity Commission 2008). The process of reviewing and determining immigration status in Australia can take between two and seven years. According to Philips (2011), between 70 and 97 per cent of asylum-seekers arriving by boat have been found to have valid refugee claims, with a final protection grant rate of 96–100 per cent for people from Afghanistan, Iran, Iraq and Burma. There is a scarcity of rigorous and reliable information about the occurrence, operation, and outcomes of immigration detention worldwide (Fazel et al. 2014). However, there is clear evidence that Australian immigration detention, especially long-term detention, is detrimental to physical health and mental health, in the short and long term (Newman et al. 2011, 2013a ; Dudley et al. 2012; Green and Eagar 2010; Steel et al. 2011b).

There is also significant documentation of the behavioural disturbances, riots, self-harm and suicidal behaviour reflecting detainee distress, frustration and despair in detention. Prolonged detention has a damaging effect on asylum-seekers' physical and mental health, especially among vulnerable groups such as torture and trauma survivors, children and unaccompanied minors. In addition, non-resolution of refugee status and uncertainty about the future emerge as major contributing factors for persistent anxiety, depression, increasing hopelessness and mental deterioration (Newman 2013). The limited evidence available also suggests that poor facilities are widespread (Fazel et al. 2014). For example, conditions on the remote islands of Nauru and Christmas Island are hot, humid and crowded. Asylum-seekers in Nauru live in unhygienic and overcrowded tents that leak and preclude privacy. The island is very small and much of it is uninhabitable following phosphate mining. There are problems with disposal of rubbish and sewage, and limited facilities for the collection of groundwater, with detainees and staff sometimes dependent on bottled water for drinking and washing, thus impacting upon their access to adequate amounts of clean water, sufficient showering and toilet amenities, and opportunities to wash clothes. The potential for the spread of communicable diseases is high in both places. People also experience the deterioration of physical health because of the lack of access to nutritious food, as everything is flown in and there are limited opportunities for asylum-seekers to grow their own produce (de Costa 2014).

Service provision and access to health and mental health services are also problematic because of limited infrastructure and substandard medical care (Newman 2013). A lack of sufficient health services is a common complaint in many immigration detention systems, affecting most dramatically pregnant women, children and people with existing conditions or experiences of torture and trauma. As closed, unregulated sites, detention centres have also been the sites of physical and sexual abuse and drug trafficking (Silverman and Nethery 2015).

A significant number of pregnant women have been detained on Christmas Island and Nauru, as well as in mainland Australian detention centres. In 2014, there were 304 women, 208 children aged under 17 years, and ten unaccompanied minors in detention on Nauru, and 128 women and 196 children, including 70 babies, in detention on Christmas Island (Children Out of Immigration Detention, n.d. ; Australian Human Rights Commission 2014). However, according to de Costa (2014), there is no obstetrician on either Christmas Island or Nauru, no paediatrician on Christmas Island and no paediatrician attached to the International Health and Medical Services (IHMS) on Nauru. The Christmas Island clinic is not equipped to deal with obstetric emergencies such as preterm labour (de Costa 2014). Detention facilities have been criticized for a lack of understanding of both cultural and gender issues (de Costa 2014). Louise Newman (pers. comm. 2015) has witnessed how the lack of provision of sanitary supplies or treatments for common gynaecological conditions are both humiliating for women and distressing. Women have described public queuing for supplies and lack of female medical and clinical staff and some have avoided treatment as a result (Milner 2014; de Costa 2014).

CHILDREN IN DETENTION

Documented cases of children held in detention are available for more than 60 countries (Fazel et al. 2014). The available evidence suggests that children are particularly vulnerable to the impact of detention in harsh conditions and develop significant psychological and emotional problems (Kronick et al. 2015; Newman et al. 2013b; Shehadeh et al. 2015). Many children have experienced trauma prior to their detention and then have parents who are themselves traumatized and depressed and impaired in their parenting as a result. Many children have little access to play education or health services and limited clinical services for trauma-related difficulties (Fazel et al. 2014). As noted above, prolonged uncertainty about personal safety and limited opportunity for resettlement contribute to toxic effects on children's mental, developmental, and physical health (Newman 2013; Newman et al. 2013a). Immigration detention can cause the development and maintenance of psychiatric difficulties, with children and adolescents in detention reporting increased rates of deliberate self-harm and suicidal behaviour, voluntary starvation, severe depression, sleep difficulties, somatic complaints, anxiety and post-traumatic stress reactions (Jensen et al. 2015; McGregor et al. 2015; Shehadeh et al. 2015). Reports are also common of poor nutritional access, regression in language development, bedwetting and social withdrawal in children. There are specific issues for infants born in detention who often have primary carers who themselves are depressed and emotionally unavailable. These infants show signs of developmental delay and failure to thrive, and they are particularly vulnerable to ongoing mental health and attachment difficulties (Australian Human Rights Commission 2014).

RESETTLEMENT

Less than 1 per cent of the world's refugees have the opportunity to be resettled (UNHCR Regional Office Canberra, n.d.). Only a small number of countries currently take part in UNHCR resettlement programmes. Countries in North America, Scandinavia, Australia and New Zealand accept a small number of refugees every year, and recently there has been an increase in the number of European and Latin American countries also involved in resettlement. Even so, resettlement is a solution for relatively few humanitarian and survival migrants, subject to the policies of accepting countries. These policies are shaped by assessments of occupational demand and judgements around the claims of some people but not others; that is, governments make decisions about accepting immigrants according to skill priorities and the structure of the local workforce, and whether or not the evidence offered for asylum fits specific criteria. In providing asylum, different countries have very different laws, procedures and ideas of worthiness that permit the granting of either permanent residence or temporary asylum. As part of the Australian humanitarian programme, since 1989 and to the present, women are accepted as immigrants provided they can prove that they are 'at risk'; that is, that they do not have the protection of a male relative, typically from the death or disappearance of their husband, brothers and father – they are judged to be especially vulnerable to gender-based violence as they lack a man to take care of them (Manderson et al. 1998). Miriam Ticktin (2011) illustrates how in France, people can claim ill-health in order to gain a temporary visa, with the option of legal residency after five years. Through such a claim, they have access to essential care, but this comes at a cost: family members cannot join them and they cannot work legally, and so are forced to work illegally or live on restricted allowances; in either case, in circumstances of continued deprivation. In Italy, in contrast, the right to a visa is determined not by ill-health as a *prima facie* case for care, but from proof of human rights abuses leading to their present unauthorized residence (Giordano 2014). In Giordano's account, sex workers from Africa applying for permission to stay must provide authorities with 'credible' accounts of forced migration, enslavement, violence and/or abuse.

On arrival in most countries of resettlement, services may be available in the short term, including for the provision of material support (language, housing, counselling, welfare payments and so on). Such practical concerns with settlement often disguise the psychosocial trauma experienced by forced migrants and other settlers, as well as disguising the health needs of people with pre-existing mental and physical health problems (Cavazos-Rehg et al. 2007). The impacts of trauma can be long-term and not fully described by the diagnosis of post-traumatic stress disorder. Chronic responses to trauma may persist even after permanent protection is granted and the lack of trauma resolution reflects the complex interplay of pre-existing vulnerability and issues on reworking a sense of identity as a 'survivor'. In addition, trauma-related mental health approaches are not always aware of cultural differences in the reaction and appraisal of trauma (Kinzie et al. 2012; Tempany 2009).

While many health problems derive from the experience of flight and resettlement, language dispossession and low socioeconomic status create the conditions for the development of chronic health problems through housing insecurity and overcrowding, poor nutrition and low-skilled and low paid work. In extreme cases, immigrants are exploited as workers, paid under-award wages and forced to work in poor conditions (Vasey and Manderson 2012). Meagan Wilson (pers. comm. 2015), for instance, has documented the dependence of Shan immigrants from Burma (Myanmar) to Thailand, where they often live and work in slave-like conditions, unable to complain because they are most likely to lose their jobs and to be apprehended and deported, rather than to be assisted out of bondage and freed of the risk of further violence and abuse. The reluctance of immigrants to question their circumstances, when they are without documents and vulnerable to deportation, is a global problem: Stephanie Larchanché (2012) similarly illustrates the difficulties for people without papers in France, for whom fear and suspicion, in the context of the country's restrictive immigration policies, limits their access to healthcare and so their rights to health.

Over time, the structural vulnerability of refugees, humanitarian and survival immigrants leads to high rates of chronic illness and disability, poor mental health and family disruption. For these as well as for pre-existing health problems, people face difficulties in accessing appropriate healthcare and in communicating with doctors and other professionals (Germov 2002; Takeuchi et al. 2002). Such people often have poor familiarity of how health, welfare and other services (e.g., housing assistance) operate, and have limited access to such services (Rousseau et al. 2008; Lindert et al. 2008; Haasen et al. 2008). This may be compounded by anxiety around state services and those provided by social support organizations operated by migrants themselves, because of fears of compromised confidentiality, exposure to authorities, and prejudices that reflect home country tensions. Lack of facility of the dominant language of a given country of resettlement may leave some migrants virtually unreachable by government, social or ethnic organizations and groups. For example, in Australia, people who are placed on temporary protection visas (TPV) often continued to experience post-traumatic stress disorder, chronic anxiety and depression, with pre-migration trauma compounded by their indeterminate status (Mansouri and Cauchi 2007). In addition, immigrants regardless of visa status report lower quality of care when they do access healthcare services compared to the average population (Murray and Skull 2005; Larson et al. 2001; Manderson and Allotey 2003; Allotey et al. 2003).

AGE AND GENDER

Women comprise a significant proportion of migrants, for all types of migration, for work, through flight with families, and as indicated above, as 'women at risk' (Manderson et al. 1998). Despite their diversity by age and motivation, considerable attention has been given to women migrants in relation to pregnancy and childbirth (Carolan 2010; Collins et al. 2011). This emphasis is for several reasons. Adults are more likely to migrate in reproductive age than when older, and so the needs of refugees and new immigrants, and parents, converge. Reproduction places demands on women's bodies, and the general health of women who conceive in flight or in detention camps is often compromised, so raising concerns also about foetal health and pregnancy outcome. Conventional and familiar practices around pregnancy, birth and infant feeding have the potential for conflict between women and the health services of settlement countries (Benza and Liamputtong 2014). There is, in addition, the risk of antenatal and postnatal depression among women in refugee settings and from new communities, especially those who have little social support in pregnancy and in the early months of parenting (O'Mahony et al. 2012; Tobin et al. 2015; O'Mahony and Donnelly 2013). The difficulties in diagnosing and managing this are compounded for people when communication is difficult, and the added stressors for new mothers whose own mother and others who might provide personal support are absent (Andajani-Sutjahjo et al. 2007; Small et al. 2002; Small and Lumley 2007; Armstrong and Small 2007).

Gender-based violence in flight, in transitional settings and in resettlement is rarely addressed, despite growing reporting of sexual violence and survival sex (Wirtz et al. 2014). But there is mounting awareness of the effects of 'warehousing' on women and men, and on gender relations within such environments (Black 1998; Feseha et al. 2012; Latif 2012).

Furthermore, in camps, health services routinely fail to meet women's needs, including in relation to maternal and child health, family planning, non-communicable and communicable diseases, malnutrition and reproductive and sexual health problems. Breastfeeding; gynaecological health problems; female genital surgery, infibulation and their affects; fistulas; and various bacterial and fungal infections all impact women's health in detention and subsequently. Gender relations limit access to reproductive health services, and both pre-migration and in transit, women have little support where they are subject to sexual violence (Byrskog et al. 2014).

The increasing feminization of migration also has implications for the emotional and psychological health of immigrant women. One such example is of women's migration from Oaxaca, Mexico (McGuire and Martin 2007). Women often arrive in the United States having left their children and other family members behind; opportunities to reunite with their children may be rare. At the same time, women who are left behind must also deal with the suffering of separation and persistent undercurrents of sorrow, particularly because of the uncertainty of being reunited with their partners and the constant need, for economic or political reasons, to separate again. Difficulties also arise as migrant women combine paid work and household responsibilities, regardless of age of children or household structure. Women are also vulnerable within immigrant households to gender-related and sexual violence from husbands and familiar others, partly reflecting the stressors on these families and the powerlessness of women to leave such conditions (Gagnon and Stewart 2014; Keygnaert et al. 2015; Woelz-Stirling et al. 1998, 2000).

The children of immigrants, both those who have migrated when young and those born after their parents' migration, are also vulnerable to mental health problems (Mace et al. 2014). Children and young people face the complex issue of dealing with trauma and, when migrating without parents, the loss of key support networks and the task of reworking their own sense of identity in a new cultural context. This need for both cultural identity and history as well as the new identity as a young person requires endless negotiation. Peer groups may reflect some broader community negative reactions to cultural difference resulting in bullying, discrimination and racism and young people may be alienated and angered as a result. Antisocial group membership and behaviour reflects a way of forging a new group identity and position of strength. Rates of depression and behavioural problems including school failure and alienation are common. Young asylum-seekers without family may be deeply traumatised; with the added burden of responsibility and worry about their homes and a desire to return and help their families. These young people may have limited ability to recover from their experiences in the face of lack of knowledge about family welfare (Majumder et al. 2015; Oppedal and Idsoe 2015; Ramel et al. 2015).

CONCLUSION

Forced and survival migrants experience various challenges in seeking safe spaces, including – due to the growing numbers of displaced people – the increasing restrictions around border protection and the securitization of asylum-seeking. Changing structures and processes of access to refuge impact on health and wellbeing. Not all people are able to move safely within countries and beyond borders. Those who can do so often risk their lives to survive. In drawing on the term 'survival migrant' (Betts 2013), above, we have highlighted the dilemmas for people created by the administrative categories of refugee and asylum-seekers. These categories and associated procedures fail to accommodate contemporary patterns of population mobility, and allow governments to dictate who is worthy, and who is not, of safety and survival.

The backgrounds of immigrants, the reasons for migrating and the capacity to resettle, vary for political, social, economic, cultural and personal reasons. Migration status is only one signpost of the need for protection, and the disadvantages, inequality and health costs of this. Multilateral agencies and high-income countries that accept humanitarian migrants need to revise and develop new comprehensive policies, programmes and services to respond to mobile populations who are displaced and are seeking resettlement. While countries continue to think through these needs in face of growing contemporary patterns of mobility, there is also a need for attention to individuals in the delivery of clinical services, and for further research on broad social interventions within and beyond the health sector.

REFERENCES

ACAPS (2015), *Syria Four Years On: No End in Sight. Mapping the Situation for Internally Displaced Syrians and Refugees After Four Years of Civil War*. Geneva: Assessment Capacities Project.

ACMS (2009), *Towards Tolerance, Law, and Dignity: Addressing Violence against Foreign Nationals in South Africa*. Johannesburg: IOM.

ACMS (2010), *May 2008 Violence Against Foreign Nationals in South Africa: Understanding Causes and Evaluating Responses*. Johannesburg: CoRMSA and ACMS.

Allotey, P., L. Manderson and D. Reidpath (2003), Addressing cultural and linguistic diversity in Australian health services, *Health Promotion Journal of Australia*, **13**, 29–33.

Amara, A. H. and S. M. Aljunid (2014), Noncommunicable diseases among urban refugees

and asylum-seekers in developing countries: a neglected health care need, *Globalization and Health*, **10**(24).
Andajani-Sutjahjo, S., L. Manderson and J. Astbury (2007), Complex emotions, complex problems: understanding the experiences of perinatal depression among new mothers in urban Indonesia, *Culture, Medicine & Psychiatry*, **31**(1), 101–122.
Andersson, R. (2014), Time and the migrant other: European border controls and the temporal economics of illegality, *American Anthropologist*, **116**, 1–15.
Armstrong, S. and R. Small (2007), Screening for postnatal depression: not a simple task, *Australian and New Zealand Journal of Public Health*, **31**, 57–61.
Australian Human Rights Commission (2014), *The Forgotten Children: National Inquiry into Children in Immigration Detention 2014*, Sydney: Australian Human Rights Commission.
Benza, S. and P. Liamputtong (2014), Pregnancy, childbirth and motherhood: a meta-synthesis of the lived experiences of immigrant women, *Midwifery*, **30**, 575–584.
Betts, A. (2013), *Survival Migration: Failed Governance and the Crisis of Displacement*, New York: Cornell University Press.
Black, M. (1998), Girls and war: an extra vulnerability, *People & the Planet*, **7**, 24–25.
Black, R. (2003), Breaking the convention: researching the 'illegal' migration of refugees to Europe, *Antipode*, **35**, 34–54.
Byrskog, U., P. Olsson, B. Essen and M. K. Allvin (2014), Violence and reproductive health preceding flight from war: accounts from Somali born women in Sweden, *BMC Public Health*, **14**, 892.
Carolan, M. (2010), Pregnancy health status of sub-Saharan refugee women who have resettled in developed countries: a review of the literature, *Midwifery*, **26**, 407–14.
Cartwright, E. and L. Manderson (2011), Diagnosing the structure: immigrant vulnerabilities in global perspective, *Medical Anthropology*, **30**(5), 451–453.
Castles, S. (2003), Towards a sociology of forced migration and social transformation, *Sociology*, **37**, 13–34.
Cavazos-Rehg, P. A., L. H. Zayas and E. L. Spitznagel (2007), Legal status, emotional wellbeing and subjective health status of Latino immigrants, *Journal of the National Medical Association*, **99**, 1126–1131.
Chandy, L., N. Ledlie and V Penciakova (2013), *The Final Countdown: Prospects for Ending Extreme Poverty by 2030*, Global Views Policy Paper 2013-04, Washington, DC: The Brookings Institution.
Children out of Immigration Detention (n.d.), Stats + report, available online at www.chilout.org/statsreports.
Collins, C. H., C. Zimmerman and L. M. Howard (2011), Refugee, asylum seeker, immigrant women and postnatal depression: rates and risk factors, *Archives of Women's Mental Health*, **14**, 3–11.
Crisp, J., T. Morris and H. Refstie (2012), Displacement in urban areas: new challenges, new partnerships, *Disasters*, **36**(S1).
Daniel, E. V. (1997), *Charred Lullabies: Chapters in an Anthropography of Violence*, Princeton, NJ: Princeton University Press.
De Buck, E., V. Borra, E. De Weerdt, A. Vande Veegaete and P. Vandekerckhove (2015), A Systematic review of the amount of water per person per day needed to prevent morbidity and mortality in (post-)disaster settings, *Plos One*, **10**.
de Costa, C. M. (2014), Antenatal care for asylum seeker women: is 'good enough' good enough? *Medical Journal of Australia*, **201**, 299–300.
Dudley, M., Z. Steel, S. Mares and L. Newman (2012), Children and young people in immigration detention, *Current Opinion in Psychiatry*, **25**, 285–292.
Duvell, F. (2012), Transit migration: a blurred and politicised concept, *Population, Space and Place*, **18**, 415–427.
EMHRN (2014), *Prioritising Border Control over Human Lives: Violations of the Rights of Migrants and Refugees at Sea (EMHRN Policy Brief, Euro-Mediterranean Human Rights Network*, Copenhagen: Euro-Mediterranean Human Rights Network.

Fazel, M., U. Karunakara and E. Newnhamemail (2014), Detention, denial, and death: migration hazards for refugee children, *The Lancet*, **2**.
Feseha, G., A. G. Mariam and M. Gerbaba (2012), Intimate partner physical violence among women in Shimelba refugee camp, northern Ethiopia, *Bmc Public Health*, **12**.
Finnstrom, S. (2003), *Living with Bad Surroundings: War and Existential Uncertainty in Acholiland, Northern Uganda*, Uppsala: Uppsala University Press.
Gagnon, A. J. and D. E. Stewart (2014), Resilience in international migrant women following violence associated with pregnancy, *Archives of Women's Mental Health*, **17**, 303–310.
Gammouh, O. S., A. M. Al-Smadi, L. I. Tawalbeh and L. S. Khoury (2015), Chronic Diseases, lack of medications, and depression among Syrian refugees in Jordan, 2013– 2014, *Preventing Chronic Disease*, **12**.
Gerard, A. F. and S. J. Pickering (2014), Gender, securitization and transit: refugee women and the journey to the EU, *Journal of Refugee Studies*, **27**, 338–359.
Germov, J. (2002), Class, health inequality, and social justice, in J. Germov (ed.), *Second Opinion: An Introduction to Health Sociology*, New York: Oxford University Press.
Giordano, C. (2014), *Migrants in Translation: Caring and the Logics of Difference in Contemporary Italy*, Berkeley, CA: University of California Press.
Green, J. P. and K. Eagar (2010), The health of people in Australian immigration detention centres, *The Medical Journal of Australia*, **192**, 65–70.
Gülsen, C., J. Knipscheer and R. Kleber (2010), The impact of forced migration on mental health: a comparative study on posttraumatic stress among internally displaced people and externally migrated Kurdish women, *Traumatology*, **16**, 109–116.
Gwatirisa, P. and L. Manderson (2009), Food insecurity and HIV/AIDS in low-income households in urban Zimbabwe, *Human Organization*, **68**.
Haasen, C., A. Agorastos, C. Demiralay and J. Reimer (2008), Access to mental health care: how can barriers for migrants be reduced? *European Psychiatry*, **23**, S4.
Holmes, S. M. (2013), *Fresh Fruit, Broken Bodies: Indigenous Mexican Farmworkers in the United States*, Berkeley, CA: University of California Press.
Human Rights and Equal Opportunity Commission (2008), *Immigration Detention Report: Summary of Observations Following Visits to Australia's Immigration Detention Facilities*, Sydney: Human Rights and Equal Opportunity Commission.
IDMC (2015), Global Overview 2015: People Internally Displaced by Conflict and Violence, Geneva: Internal Displacement Monitoring Centre.
IFRC (2012), *World Disasters Report 2012 Focus on Forced Migration and Displacement*, Geneva: IFRC.
Infante, C., A. J. Idrovo, M.S. Sánchez-Domínguez, S. Vinhas and T. González-Vázquez (2012), Violence committed against migrants in transit: experiences on the northern Mexican border', *Journal of Immigrant and Minority Health*, **14**, 449–459.
Internal Displacement Monitoring Centre and Norwegian Refugee Council (2015), *Global Overview 2015: People Internally Displaced by Conflict and Violence*, Geneva: Internal Displacement Monitoring Centre Norwegian Refugee Council.
IOM (2011), *An Analysis of Migration Health in Kenya: Healthy Migrants in Healthy Communities*, Nairobi: International Organization for Migration.
IOM (2014), *Fatal Journeys Tracking Lives Lost During Migration*, Geneva: International Organization for Migration.
Jensen, T. K., K. W. Fjermestad, L. Granly and N. H. Wilhelmsen (2015) 'Stressful life experiences and mental health problems among unaccompanied asylum-seeking children', *Clinical Child Psychology and Psychiatry*, **20**, 106–116.
Keygnaert, I., S. F. Dias, O. Degomme, W. Deville, P. Kennedy, A. Kovats, S. De Meyer, N. Vettenburg, K. Roelens and M. Temmerman (2015), Sexual and gender-based violence in the European asylum and reception sector: a perpetuum mobile? *European Journal of Public Health*, **25**, 90–96.
Kinzie, J. D., J. M. Kinzie, B. Sedighi, A. Woticha, H. Mohamed and C. Riley (2012), Prospective one-year treatment outcomes of tortured refugees: a psychiatric approach,

Torture: Quarterly Journal on Rehabilitation of Torture Victims and Prevention of Torture, **22**, 1–10.
Kronick, R., C. Rousseau and J. Cleveland (2015), Asylum-Seeking children's experiences of detention in Canada: a qualitative study, *American Journal of Orthopsychiatry*, **85**, 287–294.
Landau, L. (2014), Urban refugees and IDPs, in E. Fiddian-Qasmiyeh, G. Loescher, K. Long and N. Sigona (eds.), *The Oxford Handbook of Refugees and Forced Migration Studies*, Oxford: Oxford University Press.
Larchanché, S. (2012), Intangible obstacles: health implications of stigmatization, structural violence, and fear among undocumented immigrants in France, *Social Science & Medicine*, 74, 858–863.
Larson, A., I. Frkovic, M. van Kooten-Prasad and L. Manderson (2001), Mental health needs assessment in Australia's culturally diverse society, *Transcultural Psychiatry*, **38**, 335–350.
Latif, N. (2012), 'It was better during the war': narratives of everyday violence in a Palestinian refugee camp, *Feminist Review*, 24–40.
Lindert, J., A. Schouler-Ocak, A. Heinz and S. Priebe (2008), Mental health, health care utilisation of migrants in Europe, *European Psychiatry*, **23**, S14–S20.
Lori, J. R. and J. S. Boyle (2015), Forced migration: health and human rights issues among refugee populations, *Nursing Outlook*, **63**, 68–76.
Mace, A. O., S. Mulheron, C. Jones and S. Cherian (2014), Educational, developmental and psychological outcomes of resettled refugee children in Western Australia: a review of school of special educational needs: medical and mental health input, *Journal of Paediatrics and Child Health*, **50**, 985–992.
Mahamud, A. S., J. A. Ahmed, R. Nyoka, E. Auko, V. Kahi, J. Ndirangu, M. Nguhi, J. W. Burton, B. Z. Muhindo, R. F. Breiman and R. B. Eidex (2012), Epidemic cholera in Kakuma Refugee Camp, Kenya, 2009: the importance of sanitation and soap, *Journal of Infection in Developing Countries*, **6**, 234–241.
Majumder, P., M. O'Reilly, K. Karim and P. Vostanis (2015), 'This doctor, I not trust him, I'm not safe': the perceptions of mental health and services by unaccompanied refugee adolescents, *International Journal of Social Psychiatry*, **61**, 129–136.
Manderson, L. and P. Allotey (2003), Storytelling, marginality, and community in Australia: how immigrants position their difference in health care settings, *Medical Anthropology*, **22**, 1–21.
Manderson, L., M. Kelaher, M. Markovic and K. McManus (1998), A woman without a man is a woman at risk: women at risk in Australian humanitarian programs, *Journal of Refugee Studies*, 11, 267–283.
Mansouri, F. and S. Cauchi (2007), A psychological perspective on Australia's asylum policies, *International Migration*, **45**, 123–150.
McGregor, L. S., G. A. Melvin and L. K. Newman (2015), Differential accounts of refugee and resettlement experiences in youth with high and low levels of posttraumatic stress disorder (PTSD) symptomatology: a mixed-methods investigation, *American Journal of Orthopsychiatry*, **85**, 371–381.
McGuire, S. and J. Georges (2003), Undocumentedness and liminality as health variables, *Advances in Nursing Science*, **26**, 185–195.
McGuire, S. and K. Martin (2007), Fractured migrant families – paradoxes of hope and devastation, *Family & Community Health*, **30**, 178–188.
Mendelsohn, J. B., T. Rhodes, P. Spiegel, M. Schilperoord, J. W. Burton, S. Balasundaram, C. Wong and D. A. Ross (2014), Bounded agency in humanitarian settings: a qualitative study of adherence to antiretroviral therapy among refugees situated in Kenya and Malaysia', *Social Science & Medicine*, **120**, 387–395.
Milner, J. (2014), Protracted refugee situations, in E. Fiddian-Qasmiyeh, G. Loescher, K. Long and N. Sigona (eds.), *The Oxford Handbook of Refugee and Forced Migration Studies*, Oxford: Oxford University Press.
Minetti, A., O. Camelique, K. Hsa Thaw, S. Thi, W. Swaddiwudhipong, C. Hewison,

L. Pinoges, M. Bonnet and P. J. Guerin (2010), Tuberculosis treatment in a refugee and migrant population: 20 years of experience on the Thai–Burmese border, *International Journal of Tuberculosis and Lung Disease*, **14**, 1589–1595.
Misago, J. and T. Monson (2010), Non-nationals displaced in South Africa, *Forced Migration Review*, **34**, 62–64.
Murray, S. and S. Skull (2005), Hurdles to health: immigrant and refugee health care in Australia, *Australian Health Review*, **29**, 25–29.
Nakash, O., B. Langer, M. Nagar, S. Shoham, I. Lurie and N. Davidovitchref (2014), Exposure to traumatic experiences among asylum seekers from Eritrea and Sudan during migration to Israel, *Journal of Immigrant and Minority Health*, April.
Newman, L. (2013), Seeking asylum – trauma, mental health, and human rights: an Australian perspective, *Journal of Trauma & Dissociation*, **14**, 213–223.
Newman, L., N. Proctor and M. Dudley (2013a), Seeking asylum in Australia: immigration detention, human rights and mental health care, *Australasian Psychiatry*, **21**, 315–320.
Newman, L., N. Procter and M. Dudley (2011), Suicide and self-harm in immigration detention, *The Medical Journal of Australia*, **195**.
Newman, L., N. Proctor and M. Dudley (2013a), Seeking asylum in Australia: immigration detention, human rights and mental health care, *Australasian Psychiatry: Bulletin of Royal Australian and New Zealand College of Psychiatrists*, **21**, 315–320.
Newman, L., N. Proctor and M. Dudley (2013b), Seeking asylum in Australia: immigration detention, human rights and mental health care, *Australasian Psychiatry*, **21**, 315–320.
O'Mahony, J. M., and T. T. Donnelly (2013), How does gender influence immigrant and refugee women's postpartum depression help-seeking experiences? *Journal of Psychiatric and Mental Health Nursing*, **20**, 714–725.
O'Mahony, J. M., T. T. Donnelly, S. R. Bouchal and D. Este (2012), Barriers and facilitators of social supports for immigrant and refugee women coping with postpartum depression, *Advances in Nursing Science*, **35**, E42–E56.
Oppedal, B. and T. Idsoe (2015), The role of social support in the acculturation and mental health of unaccompanied minor asylum seekers, *Scandinavian Journal of Psychology*, 56, 203–211.
Pantuliano, S., V. Metcalfe, S. Haysom and E. Davey (2012), Urban vulnerability and displacement: a review of current issues, *Disasters*, **36**, 1–22.
Perrenoud, M. (2000), Switzerland and the international protection of refugees: from the First World War to the Geneva Convention (1914–1951), in V. Chetail and V. Gowlland-Debbas (eds.), *Switzerland and the International Protection of Refugees*, The Hague: Kluwer Law International, pp. 47–66.
Philips, J. (2011), *Asylum Seekers and Refugees: What Are the Facts?* Parliament of Australia, Department of Parliamentary Services, available online at www.aph.gov.au/binaries/library/pubs/bn/sp/asylumfacts.pdf.
Pine, A. (2008), *Working Hard, Drinking Hard: On Violence and Survival in Honduras* Berkeley, CA: University of California Press.
Quosh, C., L. Eloul and R. Ajlani (2013), Mental health of refugees and displaced persons in Syria and surrounding countries: a systematic review, *Intervention*, **11**, 276–294.
Ramel, B., J. Taljemark, A. Lindgren and B. A. Johansson (2015), Overrepresentation of unaccompanied refugee minors in inpatient psychiatric care, *SpringerPlus*, **4**, 131.
Roberts, B., F. Ocaka, J. Browne, T. Oyok, and E. Sondrop (2009), Factors associated with the health status of internally displaced persons in northern Uganda, *Journal of Epidemiology & Community Health*, **63**, 227–232.
Rousseau, C., S. ter Kuile, M. Munoz, L. Nadeau, M. J. Ouimet, L. Kirmayer, and F. Crepeau (2008), Health care access for refugees and immigrants with precarious status – public health and human right challenges, *Canadian Journal of Public Health-Revue Canadienne De Sante Publique*, **99**, 290–292.
Scorgie, F., K. Vasey, E. Harper, M. Richter, P. Nare, S. Maseko and M. F. Chersich (2013), Human rights abuses and collective resilience among sex workers in four African countries: a qualitative study, *Globalization and Health*, **9**.

Shehadeh, A., G. Loots, J. Vanderfaeillie and I. Derluyn (2015), The impact of parental detention on the psychological wellbeing of Palestinian children, *Plos One*, **10**, e0133347-e47.

Silverman, S. J. and A. Nethery (2015), Introduction: understanding immigration detention, in A. Nethery and S. J. Silverman (eds.), *Immigration Detention: The Migration of a Policy and Its Human Impact*, London: Routledge.

Skidmore, M. (2004), *Karaoke Fascism: Burma and the Politics of Fear*, Philadelphia, PA: University of Pennsylvania Press.

Small, R. and J. Lumley (2007), Reduction of maternal depression: much remains to be done, *Lancet*, **370**, 1593–1595.

Small, R., J. Yelland, J. Lumley, S. Brown and P. Liamputtong (2002), Immigrant women's views about care during labor and birth: an Australian study of Vietnamese, Turkish and Filipino women, *Birth*, **29**, 266–277.

Steel, Z., B. J Liddell, C. R. Bateman-Steel and A. B. Zwi (2011a), Global protection and the health impact of migration interception, *PloS Medicine*, **8**.

Steel, Z., S. Momartin, D. Silove, M. Coello, J. Aroche and K. W. Tay (2011b), Two year psychosocial and mental health outcomes for refugees subjected to restrictive or supportive immigration policies, *Social Science and Medicine*, **72**, 1149–1156.

Sturrock, H. J. W., K. W. Roberts, J. Wegbreit, C. Ohrt and R. D. Gosling (2015), Tackling Imported malaria: an elimination endgame, *American Journal of Tropical Medicine and Hygiene*, **93**, 139–144.

Takeuchi, D. T., C. A. Chun, F. Gong and H. Shen (2002), Cultural expressions of distress, *Health: An Interdisciplinary Journal for the Social Study of Health, Illness and Medicine*, **6**, 221–235.

Tempany, M. (2009), What research tells us about the mental health and psychosocial wellbeing of Sudanese refugees: a literature review, *Transcultural Psychiatry*, **46**, 300–315.

Theidon, K. (2012), *Intimate Enemies: Violence and Reconciliation in Peru*, Philadelphia, PA: University of Pennsylvania Press.

Ticktin, M. (2011), *Casualties of Care: Immigration and the Politics of Humanitarianism in France*, Berkeley, CA: University of California Press.

Tobin, C., P. Di Napoli and M. Wood-Gauthier (2015), Recognition of risk factors for postpartum depression in refugee and immigrant women: are current screening practices adequate? *Journal of Immigrant and Minority Health*, **17**, 1019–1024.

UNHCR (2005), *An Introduction to International Protection*, available online at www.hrea.org/erc/Library/display_doc.php?url.http%3A%2F%2Fwww.unhcr.org%2F3ae6bd5a0.html&;external.N.

UNHCR (2011), *The Benefits of Belonging: Local Integration Options and Opportunities for Host Countries, Communities and Refugees*, Geneva: UNHCR.

UNHCR (2012), *State of the World's Refugees: in Search of Solidarity*, Oxford: Oxford University Press.

UNHCR (2014a), On eve of Lampedusa disaster anniversary, UNHCR warns that irregular Mediterranean crossings becoming more deadly, UNHCR, available online at www.unhcr.org/542cfe899.html.

UNHCR (2014b), *UNHCR Global Trends 2013: War's Human Cost*, New York: UN High Commissioner for Refugees.

UNHCR Regional Office Canberra (n.d.), Resettlement, available online at http://unhcr.org.au/unhcr/index.php?option=com_content&view=article&id=139&Itemid=60.

Vasey, K. and L. Manderson (2012), Regionalizing immigration, health and inequality: Iraqi refugees in Australia, *Administrative Sciences*, **2**, 47–62.

Wilhelm-Solomon, M. (2013), The priest's soldiers: HIV therapies, health identities, and forced encampment in Northern Uganda, *Medical Anthropology*, **32**, 227–246.

Wirtz, A. L., K. Pham, N. Glass, S. Loochkartt, T. Kidane, D. Cuspoca, L. S. Rubenstein, S. Singh and A. Vu (2014), Gender-based violence in conflict and displacement: qualitative findings from displaced women in Colombia, *Conflict and Health*, **8**.

Woelz-Stirling, N., M. Kelaher and L. Manderson (1998), Power and the politics of

abuse: rethinking violence in Filipina-Australian marriages, *Health Care for Women International*, **19**.
Woelz-Stirling, N., L. Manderson, M. Kelaher and S. Gordon (2000), Marital conflict and finances among Filipinas in Australia, *International Journal of Intercultural Relations*, **24**, 791–805.
Zetter, R. (2014), *Protecting Forced Migrants: A State of the Art Report of Concepts, Challenges and Ways Forward*, Switzerland: Swiss Federal Commission on Migration.
Zetter, R. (2015), Protection in Crisis: Forced Migration and Protection in a Global Era, Washington, DC: Migration Policy Institute.

11 The health and wellbeing outcomes of former 'unaccompanied minors': shifting contours of vulnerability and precarity

Elaine Chase

INTRODUCTION

Institutional definitions of vulnerability and the governed responses to it have significant implications for young people in transition. This chapter considers the challenges to young people's wellbeing as they make the complex shift in status from the 'unaccompanied child' to that of 'adult' within immigration and social care systems. At this juncture, 'vulnerability' takes on very different economic, social and political meanings and associations. While young people may no longer meet the institutional criteria of the 'vulnerable child' (in need of care and protection), paradoxically they may become more vulnerable as they encounter multiple changes and uncertainties as young 'adults' with undetermined immigration status. Drawing on emerging themes from ongoing research, this chapter outlines the multiplicity of interacting factors influencing young people's wellbeing and vulnerability to adversity (Thomson 2011; Hardgrove et al. 2014). In doing so, it draws distinction between vulnerability, precariousness and precarity in the context of these young people's lives, arguing that refocusing the lens away from individualised factors and circumstances associated with vulnerability towards broader questions of precariousness and the politics of precarity forces a reconsideration of policies and practices that fundamentally determine young people's wellbeing outcomes.

YOUNG PEOPLE'S TRANSITIONS WITHIN AND WITHOUT IMMIGRATION CONTROL

Up until 2014, every year an average of 12,000 children under the age of 18 arrived in Europe from other parts of the world with no accompanying adult, becoming institutionally defined as 'unaccompanied asylum seeking children' (UASC) or, commonly, 'unaccompanied minors'. In the context of the refugee crisis in 2015, the number of unaccompanied minors arriving in Europe rose dramatically to over 88,000 (Eurostat,

2016). The number arriving in the UK has fluctuated widely over recent years – peaking at more than 4,000 in 2008; falling to just over 1,100 in 2012 and then rising again to almost 2,000 in 2014 with a further increase evident from data available for the first two quarters of 2015 (Chase and Allsopp 2013; Refugee Council 2015). Children and young people typically make the journey without accompanying adult family members via a third party, usually referred to as an 'agent', who receives a fee for their services. They come from many different countries in Africa, the Middle and Far East and countries bordering Europe; and for a variety of reasons including fleeing violence, persecution, poverty and political and climate instability. Once in the UK, children under the age of 18 usually come under the care of the local authority in which they first arrive. They are accommodated according to their age; those under 16 usually placed in foster care (subject to availability of foster care placements), while those over 16 are most often placed in semi-independent accommodation facilities where they are given additional support from a key worker and normally have a named social worker. The level and type of support provided across different local authorities is known to differ widely (Brownless and Finch 2010; Wilding 2015).

Aside from unaccompanied minors who come under the care of local authorities, other young people enter the UK out of sight of immigration control procedures and never claim asylum. For example, they may arrive under private fostering arrangements; may be trafficked into the UK or may actively avoid the lens of immigration control since they fear having their asylum claim rejected and the consequent possibility of forced return.

Much research has examined the health and wellbeing outcomes of the 'unaccompanied child', most notably with respect to their mental health (see, for example, Reed et al 2011; Fazel et al. 2012). Similarly, there has been a raft of policy responses to the circumstances of unaccompanied children who are variously defined and treated according to different categorisations of vulnerability and become eligible to commensurate forms of social care and support. Such support is, however, contingent on them being deemed eligible through the notoriously contentious processes of age assessment (Crawley 2007; ADCS 2015). Much less research attention has been paid to these young people's wellbeing outcomes as they make the transition from the status of 'child' to 'adult' (at the age of 18) within the immigration and asylum system.

Previous research with young people who have uncertain legal status has demonstrated how their sense of subjective wellbeing is inherently linked to the possibility of a viable future for themselves and others in their lives (Chase 2013a, 2013b; Chase and Allsopp 2013) and that when the likelihood of such a future is undermined, they may experience a profound sense of insecurity and compromised wellbeing. A fairly expansive literature, drawn primarily from the experiences of adult refugees, similarly demonstrates how most other aspects of their health and wellbeing, including access to basic needs such as shelter, food, healthcare and protection are also compromised when they become ineligible for ongoing welfare support (see other chapters in this volume). Yet there has been very limited research on the impact of immigration status on young people's wellbeing during the transition from the status of child to that of adult (Wade 2011; Barrie and Mendes 2011). Small-scale studies by non-governmental organisations (NGOs) have proved important in highlighting the barriers to young people in pursing or maintaining educational and employment trajectories as well as personal goals and relationships at this point of transition (Refugee Support Network 2012; Brighter Futures 2013; Gladwell and Elwyn 2012; Pinter 2012; Bloch 2013). These practical difficulties are known to be produced and reproduced by legal and social care structures that pattern the lives of young people and their access to services and support at key points in their chronological age (Allsopp and Chase 2014).

The failure of policy frameworks to adequately respond to the needs of young people during this transition to 'adulthood' has been previously noted (European Migration Network 2010; European Union Agency for Fundamental Rights 2011) but, as yet, the policy response has been largely muted. This is arguably because at this same transitional point, young people may lose their status as vulnerable children from an institutional and policy perspective and become, instead, absorbed into the corps of asylum-seeking and refugee adults. Whether or not this happens, and the extent to which they are able to access ongoing care provisions after the age of 18 has been demonstrated to be largely a question of luck (Chase 2013b; Wilding 2015). Yet, as will be argued below, this redefinition of – or assumed reduction in – vulnerability (or even 'invulnerability') at the point of transition to adulthood, paradoxically induces new forms of risk and potential harm for young people and raises important questions about the conceptual validity of vulnerability itself.

SITUATING VULNERABILITY

Although often considered synonymous, vulnerability and precariousness have some important theoretical differences (Gilson 2014). Vulnerability assumes a pervasive uncertainty and instability in life, encompassing the likelihood of destabilising alterations in general that may or may not have loss as an outcome. Chambers (1989) defines it as a state of being defenceless, insecure and exposed to shocks and stresses. Vulnerability with respect to young people is frequently associated with the somewhat slippery and vague (yet normatively deficit) transitory phase of 'adolescence', a time when such vulnerability is considered to be self-imposed – a result of taking risks or falling under the delusion of invulnerability; a stage when young people may actively render themselves a burden of vulnerability (Fischhoff et al., 2001).

Precariousness is arguably more profound, since it speaks to the tenuousness of existence and the potential of risk to life itself; 'while increased precariousness produces increased exposure to injury, violence and death, the consequences of vulnerability are indeterminate' (Gilson 2014: 25). The outcome of precariousness, therefore, is loss that may be physical (a loss of food or safety) or psychological (the loss of dignity, self-esteem, sense of agency, etc.). Much previous research attention has tended to focus on youth vulnerabilities (rather than on their precariousness) and with respect to very specific employment market or 'human capital' transitions (Furlong et al. 2003; Morrow 2013). 'Precarity' has similarly for the most part been understood in economic terms and captures the insecurity and instability of employment and the impact on lifestyle, livelihoods and wellbeing; the 'youth' *precariat* epitomising the core of young people who experience such instability over extended periods of time (Standing 2011).

Yet, precarity is not a neutral state but rather engages with the politics of loss and is helpfully defined by Butler (2009) as the 'politically induced' state of precariousness:

> '[P]recarity' designates that politically induced condition in which certain populations suffer from failing social and economic networks of support and become differentially exposed to injury, violence, and death . . . Precarity also characterizes that politically induced condition of maximized vulnerability and exposure for populations exposed to arbitrary state violence and to other forms of aggression that are not enacted by states and against which states do not offer adequate protection.
>
> (Butler 2009: ii)

Importantly, however, the state of precarity creates its own dynamics and has been defined as a condition not only of uncertainty and insecurity but also as a possible rallying point for resistance (Waite 2009; Allsopp and Gill forthcoming). So while the politically induced state of young people subject to immigration control undoubtedly pushes them to the brink of loss, there is always the possibility of them finding ways to counter the political power that renders them precarious in various ways – such as in relation to their ability to remain in the UK or continue to access publicly funded sources of support. However, resistance to such forms of instrumental power on the part of young people may in itself entail new threats and risks to self, health and wellbeing.

By drawing on examples of embodied precarity, in Butler's terms, this chapter illustrates the politically induced nature of precariousness for young people who previously arrived in the UK as unaccompanied children. These examples demonstrate that although young people do take risks in response to the structures and situations they encounter, they are not inherently vulnerable or precarious but are rendered so as a result of policies and practices that undermine and limit their possibilities and futures.

THE STUDY

Themes for this chapter are drawn from early stages of a three-year ESRC-funded research project: 'Becoming Adult: Young People's Conceptions of Futures and Wellbeing while Subject to Immigration Control in the UK'. Working with young people from four countries of origin (Afghanistan, Eritrea, Albania and Vietnam), the research examines the outcomes of children who arrived on their own in the UK as they experience the transition to adulthood over time. For the purposes of this chapter, I draw on some preliminary themes emerging from early analysis of findings with young people from Afghanistan and Eritrea and here examine the emerging theme of the shifting nature of precariousness.[1] The chapter highlights some of the individual, political and social factors – what Thomson (2011) has termed the 'dynamic mutuality' of factors – governing such precarity over time and young people's own responses to the causes of their precariousness.

PRECARITY OF CHILDHOOD

As noted earlier, young people seeking asylum alone in the UK end up here as a result of politically induced precariousness in one form or another, whether war, conflict, poverty, discrimination, persecution, denial of political freedoms or political voice. As noted elsewhere, while many have witnessed extreme atrocities and direct persecution, others have migrated, or their migration has been organised, to protect them from the likelihood of such adversities (Chase et al. 2008). Young men from Afghanistan, for example, typically describe the risks and dangers they face on a daily basis, including forced conscription by the Taliban (Schuster and Majidi 2014); while for young people from Eritrea, whether girls or boys, enforced recruitment into the military for indefinite periods of time and from a young age is what drives many to migrate (Bozzini 2011; Hirt and Mohammad 2013).

These forms of precarity in the countries from which they flee are often magnified by their journeys, young people frequently making reference to the extreme risks and dangers they have encountered and have had to cope with throughout the migratory process as they duck and dive borders that they are unable to cross legitimately due to lack of papers and documentation (Bloch et al. 2014) – a process that Iqbal, a young man from Afghanistan described as 'literally gambling your life'.

Those young people that refer to their childhoods in their countries of origin, frequently conjure the juxtaposition between norms surrounding daily life, risks and expectations back 'home' with the life they have experienced in the UK. In such widely different cultural, societal and economic contexts where there are equally widely different norms and expectations surrounding 'childhood' and 'adulthood', the distinction between the two phases in life is frequently blurred – as is commonly noted in the sociologies of childhood literature (Boyden 2003; Mayall 2004; Morrow and Vennam 2012). As Kahlil from Afghanistan explained:

> The thing with us is that we have been raised in difficult situations. Even if you are ten years old, we don't consider ourselves adults but we have developed those life skills in that tough life we had. It helps you to grow up quicker and mature quicker . . . It's probably different to people that have been raised or born here or somewhere else . . . but with us, it's . . . our parents wouldn't have let us come if they didn't know we are not adults. They know the life we have had, the tough life and that we could cope . . . at the same time, they want you to be safe . . . But they wouldn't let you come if they didn't know you were tough enough.

This exposure to the realities and dangers of life from a relatively young age may result in young people being perceived as older than their chronological age would suggest for a child having grown up in the UK. Young people often describe instances where their age has been disputed, not necessarily because of how old they appear but as a result of being perceived as not acting in age-appropriate ways. Hafiz, for example commented on why he believed his age was disputed soon after he arrived in the UK:

> And that's the reason why when I came here Social Services said, 'looking at you, looking at your body, looking at your face he [sic] doesn't look more than 13, but what you are saying . . . the answers you are giving, you looks even more than 15'.

Such perceptions by immigration officers, social workers, foster carers and other professionals fundamentally affect the ways in which young people are treated on arrival in the UK; dictating whether or not they receive the care and support they require and ultimately determine their wellbeing outcomes.

THE LOTTERY OF SECURITY OR ONGOING PRECARITY IN THE UK

Findings from our research so far confirm the serendipity of outcomes for young people that have emerged from earlier work (Chase 2013b). Whether or not young people are recognised and believed to be children create a whole set of risks, vulnerabilities and possibilities for their futures and wellbeing outcomes. At this juncture, young people frequently get torn between state mechanisms governing the provision of social welfare and support on the one hand and immigration control on the other, the latter epitomising politically induced precariousness. And while some young people may be forcibly excluded from provisions reserved for children, as noted above, others may choose not even to attempt to access such support because of fear of such exclusions and the possible repercussions of forced return.

These different levels of engagement with statutory systems and procedures soon after their arrival set young people along very different pathways – young people within the system are likely to receive at least some, if temporary, social care support such as accommodation, care, education and welfare security; whereas those excluded from or choosing not to engage with statutory systems and structures have no support from the very beginning of their arrival. In the latter case, there is an inherent precariousness for children and young people from the day they arrive; while in the former a period of security is frequently followed by rapid transition into uncertainty and insecurity, largely governed by chronological age (Allsopp and Chase 2014). The cusp of adulthood (institutionally at the age of 18) becomes in some respects, therefore, a point of convergence for these two different trajectories, and young people, irrespective of their route into the UK, may become more or less precarious at this point.

Fazil from Afghanistan, for example, spoke of how on arriving in the UK at the age of 14, he was never accepted as a child. As a result, he was immediately placed in a shared house with adults, and after one and half years received a letter of refusal for his asylum application from the Home Office. At that point his eligibility to any public-funded support ceased. He described how he survived initially with help from friends who shared food with him and sometimes gave him somewhere to stay. Over the years, however, he gradually lost contact with some friends while others were deported and his network of support dissolved. As a result, he spent a number of years on the streets with no access to social care or support. It was only through the involvement of a non-governmental organisation at the point at which he was 'appeal rights exhausted'[2] and on the brink of being forcibly returned to Afghanistan, that his case for asylum was reviewed and he was granted indefinite leave to remain (ILR) in the UK. When we spoke to Fazil, just a few months after this decision, he described how he felt stuck and unable to move forward with his life, despite now having his papers proving his status in the UK. He commented, 'papers don't give you hope . . . they only mean I am safe from the Taliban, or the police or badness . . . I can't just sit at home with a passport'. Fazil lamented the fact that he had never had a chance to have an education and that now, at the age of 24, it was too late to do all the things he had hoped for in the past. He commented, 'in year one, year two, I had hope and then it all goes . . . I lost trust in people . . . there was no humanity . . . now I feel it's too late for me – I can't learn now, my brain doesn't work . . . I have problems remembering'.

Similarly, Peter from Eritrea had his age disputed soon after his arrival in the UK and, as a result, has never had access to care and support from social services or any leaving care support. Until recently, his circumstances have been alleviated to some extent through the support of a charity (paying his bus fares to college and a small stipend for living expenses each week) meaning that despite this period of prolonged precariousness, he has been able to sustain his education at a local further education college. However, since he is now 23, Peter is no longer eligible to support from the charity and survives essentially on the goodwill of friends – this reliance on others' help is, he says, a constant source of embarrassment. Peter conforms to his obligation of having to sign on with the Home Office and is hoping that a fresh claim for asylum will enable him to make a life for himself in the UK. In the meantime he experiences a further dimension of liminality since, for young people from Eritrea, their situation is further complicated by the fact that, at the time of writing, they are not 'deportable' in the same way as young people from Afghanistan are considered to be. Current guidance in the UK suggests that the risks of return for young people to Eritrea mean that the government would be contravening the basic principle of non-refoulement by returning them. Peter, like many other young people we meet, therefore is at once protected from immediate enforced return from the UK but at the same time denied any viable future here.

THE RE-EMERGENCE OF PRECARITY

The majority of children arriving on their own in the UK do not meet the criteria for refugee status but are afforded discretionary leave for the period of time that they are children, provided that is that they are accepted as being the age they claim to be. At the age of 18, some continue to be eligible for government-funded leaving care support while their applications for further leave to remain in the UK are pending. Ultimately, it is the decision on such applications by the Home Office that dictate whether or not they are able to remain and build their lives in the UK.

In practice, therefore, the run up to the transition to 'adulthood' is demarcated in UK policy by a series of biologically defined age boundaries (16, 18 and 21) that are accompanied by differentiated rights and entitlements. While for immigration control purposes, adulthood begins at the age of 18 in the UK, for certain welfare entitlements this boundary is more fluid and young people may or may not be able to access support beyond the age of 18. Yet the rules and regulations are far from transparent (Chase 2013b; Chase and Allsopp 2013; Allsopp and Chase 2014), and may in fact constitute more of a 'lottery' of opportunity (Wilding 2015). As noted earlier, the disputed nature of this terrain is characterised by ubiquitous age assessment procedures (Dorling 2013; Crawley 2007), creating much confusion among young people who must grapple with Western concepts of chronological age and time and the limitations these impose on them. For those young people who never claim asylum in the UK, on turning 18, they may continue to live in the UK by whatever means they can without legal status or documentation (Bloch et al. 2014; Sigona and Hughes 2012). Once they turn 17½, most are unsure whether or not they will be able to remain in the UK and for how long. With no legal right to stay, they may be categorised as eligible for voluntary or forced return to countries of origin, although the practical challenges in deporting young people often render their futures more insecure (Gladwell and Elwyn 2012; Gibney 2008). For example, there are clear differences in the likelihood of forced return according to young people's country of origin – typically young people from Afghanistan are deemed to be more 'deportable' than other groups of young people such as Eritreans (although these potential outcomes can shift dramatically in tune with other geopolitical changes at different points in time). The uncertainties of these outcomes are likely to impact in profound ways on young people's conceptions of their futures and their subjective sense of wellbeing.

During this time of waiting, often for a number of years, young people speak not only about the re-emergence of a sense of insecurity (emphatically linked to their sense of subjective wellbeing) but also a sense of powerlessness to do anything about it. As the uncertainties about their futures re-emerge, they are faced with difficult decisions about whether or not to stay in touch with systems and structures that on the one hand provide often their only means of practical and financial support, but on the other impose systems of total control and, in the extreme, the risk of forced return. In an effort to shake off immigration surveillance and its inherent risk of removal, young people may at this point make the transition into illegality (Gonzales 2011).

Bashir spoke of his dilemma at the point when he became appeal rights exhausted and when he had to decide whether or not to maintain contact with the Home Office. At the same time, the rules and regulations had changed concerning applications for a fresh claim for asylum, meaning that in order to submit such a claim, people had to present themselves in person to an official at the Home Office, rather than submit their papers by post, which had previously been the case. This shift in institutional process, he was aware, rendered him more vulnerable to the vagaries of immigration control than the paper version of the application where he could maintain a degree of hiddenness and safety:

> I wanted to go and sign and submit my fresh application but I told my solicitor, 'if I get detained are you responsible? – can you do anything?' And she said, 'no . . . I cannot guarantee anything' And I said, 'so you are telling me that if I get detained, you can't do anything?'. . . and so I said, 'I am not going', I said 'if you've got any other way to send my fresh application through the post or whatever then do it . . . If you can't then I am not going to sign'. Because if you go . . . I wanted to go for the first few signs because there is very little chance to get detained in the first, second or third week to go for signing. But after that you will most likely be detained you know. . . . Because to me, if you are going to sign, you have got both sides – a positive and a negative. . . . I wasn't like strong enough to make that decision to say 'OK I am going to go for signing' – because I have seen so many of my friends that have been deported . . . so I just decided, 'I will stay and see whatever happens later on', but thinking that by yourself you are going to go into danger . . . obviously you are not going to do it. So that's it. . . I just quit.

The dynamics of precarity are complex here – Bashir weighed the pros and cons of 'signing on' – on the one hand, it would enable him to put in a fresh claim for asylum with the possibility of his case being accepted; but on the other, it laid him bare to the possibility of detention and forced return to Afghanistan.

ENFORCED RETURN AND NEW FORMS OF RISK AND PRECARITY

For those who are forcibly returned, there is scant information on their outcomes. However, an emerging body of evidence suggests that return renders many young people extremely vulnerable to a range of negative outcomes (Schuster and Majidi 2014; Gladwell and Elwyn 2012; Chase and Sigona 2016). Yet, while the politically induced state of precariousness for young people undoubtedly pushes them to the brink of loss, at the same time they are not routinely passive recipients of their 'lot', but find ways to counter the political power used to render them precarious. Examples above are implicit in the forms of support afforded by communities of young people, who have shared a similar trajectory with more successful refugee outcomes, to those who no longer are eligible to publicly funded sources of support – such examples abound in this research. But they are also evidenced by young people's actions and resistance to the extreme forms of precarity epitomised by enforced return.

We first met Majeed from Afghanistan when he was aged 24 and living 'black' (illegally) in a UK city where he had first arrived at the age of 16. Soon after his arrival, Majeed was age-assessed as being at least two years older than the age he claimed to be. He spoke of how the age assessment occurred in total contradiction to the response he had received from other adults working with him in the hostel/care centre that housed him when he first arrived. They had, he said, repeatedly made reference to how young he looked and how he should be being placed with a family.

At the age of 18, Majeed was deported back to Afghanistan. He spoke of how life in Afghanistan was untenable – there was no way of earning a living; people viewed him with suspicion and he was under constant pressure to join the Taliban. He felt unsafe and after just one and half months and encouraged by family and friends, he set off again to return to Europe via Pakistan. He spoke of how his journey from Calais to the UK took 15 attempts before he successfully boarded a lorry that brought him back to the UK. On arrival he made his way back to his network of friends in the city where he had spent his years as a teenager. At our first meeting, he described an extreme state of liminality, unable to move forward with his life and totally dependent on friends and networks for survival. Six months later, when we spoke again – nothing had changed – he was pretty much in the same place as he had been six months previously. He grappled with the pros and cons of making himself known to the authorities and making a fresh asylum claim. His greatest fear was to be sent back to Afghanistan, although he knew that the most likely scenario was return to Italy where he had acquired a temporary residence document during one of the stages of his lengthy journey. However, life in Italy, he felt was not sustainable either – he had no job, could not speak the language and was not eligible for any financial or other support.

The efforts made and risks endured by young people such as Majeed (and many others we have spoken to) to resist forces of power and control in these processes of migration are ultimate examples of resistance. Yet, while on the one hand temporarily 'safe' in the UK, any sense of viable future – intrinsically linked to a sense of wellbeing – for Majeed is currently thwarted. He exists as an invisible other, unable to make the normal sorts of choices and steps forward with his life that others of his age would be making as they transition towards adulthood. For others, forms of resistance have been even more extreme. Some young people we are in contact with, fearing a repeat of their forced removal from the UK, embark on even more complex journeys in search of sanctuary outside of Europe. In doing so, emerging evidence suggests that they may face further risks of prolonged limbo and uncertainty (including periods of immigration detention) as they search for 'any safe place' where they can imagine and live out a viable future for themselves.

THE LIMITS OF VULNERABILITY AS A CONCEPT

Butler's notion of the politically induced nature of precariousness is something experienced by young people over extended periods of time and so has temporal as well as geographical dimensions. Typically young people describe circumstances of their childhood imbued with precariousness, largely the result of geopolitical events and circumstances of which they have little understanding and over which they have no control.

Once in the UK, 'children' – provided they are accepted as such – normally experience a period of respite from these forms of precariousness (although they may remain 'vulnerable' as defined earlier to more generalised insecurities and uncertainties). Yet precarity re-emerges around the time that young people make the transition to adulthood, in institutional terms at 18 (or in a practical sense now at the age of 17½ years). At this point, a whole new set of legislative and political conditions and frameworks expose them to multiple forms of precariousness – including the likelihood of homelessness, destitution, termination of educational opportunities and no access to public funds, detention, forced removal and ultimate statelessness. In a subjective sense, precariousness takes on other forms – breakdown of friendships and relationships; becoming objectified by systems and structures that impose stigma and discrimination; portrayals of self as the Other/the outsider; difficulties in establishing a sense of belonging or firm identity – and being denied the ties and connections that have been established over many years (Carens 2009).

Within policy and political discourses surrounding migration, vulnerability and precariousness are frequently presented in neutral terms. Young people apparently face inherent difficulties or are exposed to risks and shocks that are considered to be either in the 'natural order of things' or are perceived to be self-inflicted. Yet in reality, just about all the difficulties, shocks and uncertainties described by young people are arguably generated by political decisions in one form or another – and across different social, political and geographical domains. Undoubtedly young people in the current study clearly make decisions that may be perceived as placing themselves at risk – but such risk-taking is bounded by the political, social and economic contexts that straightjacket the range of options they have and that curtail their aspirations and goals for a viable future.

Solidifying ideas about inherent vulnerability in discourses surrounding young people seeking asylum in the UK is itself a political process. In essence, it absolves governments and policymakers of the responsibility for causing or failing to respond to such precariousness other than relieving its symptoms at the point of crisis. Recognition that legislation, policies and practice decisions are not apolitical but in fact perpetuate these different forms of precarity has multiple implications.

Butler's notion of politically induced precariousness – that is precarity – is clearly evident from accounts of young people's own experiences of negotiating their pathway towards adulthood at a time when they have not managed to secure refugee status. As shown in the above examples, precarity – understood as imposed precariousness – at this stage in their lives takes on many different forms. What these examples also demonstrate is how young people make sense of and respond to such precarity with their own counter tactics (Allsopp and Chase 2014; Schuster and Majidi 2014). Policy perspectives and responses are often devised in relation to specific peoples deemed to be 'vulnerable' and that, as a result, demand a more specialised/targeted response. Social work practice, healthcare provision, public health initiatives and other facilities such as housing are frequently designed according to a matrix of needs assessment; prioritising concerns and then designing appropriate interventions accordingly. Much less is written or said about the imposed vulnerability by welfare systems and structures working in tandem with immigration control procedures that simultaneously respond to politically viable forms of 'vulnerability' in one space while reconstituting new forms of vulnerability in another.

There is nothing intrinsic about vulnerability – it is not a neutral state that requires a response by different providers – in the context of these young people's lives, it is politically induced, by implication requiring counter political responses on the part of all those charged with providing services and support. As evidenced from emerging themes from our current research, these dynamics of vulnerability, precariousness and precarity are played out at many different institutional, local, national and supranational levels. While some young people face the immediate precariousness of their immigration status, for example, others produce narratives of precarity, endured across time, geographical space (local, national and supranational) and in relation to multiple institutions and actors with which they are forced, by the nature of their journeys and transitions, to interact. These politics of 'precarity' and the dynamics of the responses to it are clearly fields that require further investigation and reflection.

An important postscript to Fazil's narrative above is that when we spoke to him again, six months after our initial meeting, life had got better. By then he recognised and had made full use of his secure immigration status; he had a job that he loved; he had got married and had made a number of other concrete steps forward with his life. He smiled and laughed and was beginning to imagine a future for himself and his wife once they could be permanently reunited. This is further testament to the dynamics not only of precarity but of the possibility to return from the losses and setbacks imposed by systems and structures of power that govern young people's lives, provided there is a political will to enable this.

NOTES

1. The study 'Becoming Adult' is funded by the Economic and Social Research Council. Further details of the study and its progress can be found at www.becomingadult.net.
2. 'Appeal rights exhausted' refers to when someone has been refused asylum or any form of temporary protection or whose leave to remain has expired (and an application to extend it refused), and they have exhausted all possibilities to appeal this decision.

REFERENCES

ADCS (2015), *Age Assessment Guidance: Guidance to Assist Social Workers and their Managers in Undertaking Age Assessments in England*, London: Association of Directors of Children's Services.

Allsopp, A. and E. Chase (2014), The tactics of time and status: young people's experiences of building futures while subject to immigration control in Britain, *Journal of Refugee Studies*, available online at http://jrs.oxfordjournals.org/content/early/2014/10/29/jrs.feu031.full.pdf+html.

Allsopp, J. and N. Gill (forthcoming), Beyond limbo: precariousness and the agency of young people seeking asylum in British tribunals, *Journal of Migration Studies*.

Barrie, L. and P. Mendes (2011), The experiences of unaccompanied asylum-seeking children in and leaving the out-of-home care system in the UK and Australia: a critical review of the literature, *International Social Work*, **54**(4), 485–503.

Bloch, A. (2013), The labour market experiences and strategies of young undocumented migrants, *Work, Employment and Society*, **27**(2), 272–287

Bloch, A., N. Sigona and R. Zetter (2014), *Sans Papiers: The Social and Economic Lives of Young Undocumented Migrants*, London: Pluto Press.

Bozzini, D. (2011), Low-tech state surveillance: the production of uncertainty among conscripts in Eritrea, *Surveillance and Society*, **9**(1/2), 93–113.

Boyden, J. (2003), Children under fire: challenging assumptions about children's resilience, *Children, Youth and Environments*, **13**, 1.

Brighter Futures (2013), *The Cost of Waiting*, London: Praxis.

Brownless, L. and N. Finch (2010), *Levelling the Playing Field: A UNICEF UK Report into Provision of Services to Unaccompanied or Separated Migrant Children in Three Local Authority Areas in England*, London: UNICEF.

Butler, J. (2009), *Performativity, Precarity and Sexual Politics*, available online at www.aibr.org/antropologia/04v03/criticos/040301b.pdf.

Carens, J. (2009), The case for amnesty: time erodes the state's right to deport, *Boston Review*, May/June.

Chambers, R. (1989), Editorial introduction: vulnerability, coping and policy, *Institute of Development Studies Bulletin*, **20**(2), 1–7.

Chase, E. (2013a), Security and subjective wellbeing: the experiences of unaccompanied young people seeking asylum in the UK, *Sociology of Health and Illness*, **35**(6): 358–372.

Chase, E. (2013b), In search of security: the mental health and rights of unaccompanied young people seeking asylum in the UK, in F. Thomas and J. Gideon (eds.), *Migration, Rights and Inequality*, London: Zed Books.

Chase, E. and J. Allsopp (2013), *'Future Citizens of the World'? The Contested Futures of Independent Young Migrants in Europe*, RSC Working Papers Series, Oxford: Refugee Studies Centre, available online at www.rsc.ox.ac.uk/files/publications/working-paper-series/wp97-future-citizens-of-the-world-2013.pdf.

Chase. E. and N. Sigona (2016), Lost in the world: young people shunted around a global asylum system, *The Conversation*, available online at http://theconversation.com/lost-in-the-world-the-young-people-shunted-around-a-global-asylum-system-55991.

Chase, E., A. Knight and J. Statham (2008) *The Emotional Wellbeing of Unaccompanied Young People Seeking Asylum in the UK*, London: BAAF.

Crawley, H. (2007), *When is a Child not a Child? Asylum, Age Disputes and the Process of Age Assessments*, London: ILPA.

Dorling, K. (2013), *Happy Birthday? Disputing the Age of Children in the Immigration System*, Essex: Coram Children's Legal Centre.

European Migration Network (2010), *Policies on Reception, Return and Integration Arrangements for, and Numbers of Unaccompanied Minors – an EU Comparative Study*, Brussels: European Migration Network.

European Union Agency for Fundamental Rights (2011), *Separated, Asylum-Seeking Children in European Union Member States: Comparative Report*, Luxembourg: European Union Agency for Fundamental Rights.

Eurostat (2016) Asylum applications considered to be unaccompanied minors by citizenship, age and sex Annual Data. Available at: http://ec.europa.eu/eurostat/web/products-datasets/-/migr_asyunaa.

Fazel, M., R. Reed, C. Panter-Brick and A. Stein (2012), The mental health of displaced and refugee children resettled in high-income countries: risk and protective factors, The Lancet, 379, 266–282.

Fischhoff, B., E. Nightingale and J. Innotta (eds.) (2001), *Adolescent Risk and Vulnerability: Concepts and Measurements*, Washington, DC: National Academy Press.

Furlong, A., F. Cartmel, A. Biggart, H. Sweeting and P. West (2003), *Youth Transitions: Patterns of Vulnerability and Processes of Social Inclusion*, Edinburgh: Central Research Unit, Scottish Executive.

Gibney, M. J. (2008), Asylum and the expansion of deportation in the United Kingdom, *Government and Opposition*, **43**(2), 146–167.
Gilson, E. (2014), *The Ethics of Vulnerability: A Feminist Analysis of Social Life and Practice*, Abingdon: Routledge.
Gladwell, C. and H. Elwyn (2012), *Broken Futures: Young Afghan Asylum Seekers in the UK and in their Country of Origin*, London: Refugee Support Network.
Gonzales, R. G. (2011), Learning to be illegal: undocumented youth and shifting legal contexts in the transition to adulthood, *American Sociological Review*, **76**(4), 602–619.
Hardgrove, A., K. Pells, J. Boyden and P. Dornan (2014), *Youth Vulnerabilities in Life Course Transitions. UNDP Human Development Report Office*, Occasional Paper, available online at http://hdr.undp.org/sites/default/files/hardgrove_boyden_hdr_2014.pdf.
Hirt, N. and A. Mohammad (2013), 'Dreams don't come true in Eritrea': anomie and family disintegration due to the structural militarization of society', *Journal of Modern African* Studies, **51**(1), 139–168.
Mayall, B. (2004), Sociologies of childhood, in M. Holborn (ed.), *Developments in Sociology: An Annual Review*, 20, 37–57.
Morrow, V. (2013), Troubling transitions: young people's experiences of growing up in poverty in rural Andhra Pradesh, India, *Journal of Youth Studies*, **16**(1), 86–100.
Morrow, V. and U. Vennam (2012), Children's responses to risk in agricultural work in Andhra Pradesh, India, *Development in Practice*, **22**(4), 549–561.
Pinter, I. (2012), *'I Don't Feel Human': Experiences of Destitution among Young Refugees and Migrants*, London: The Children's Society.
Reed, R., M. Fazel, L. Jones, C. Panter-Brick and A. Stein (2011), The mental health of refugee and internally displaced children Part I: a systematic review of risk and protective factors in children resettled in low and middle income countries, *Lancet*, *379*, 250–265.
Refugee Council (2015), *Children in the Asylum System*, London: Refugee Council.
Refugee Support Network (2012), *'I Just Want to Study': Access to Higher Education for Young Refugees*, London: Refugee Support Network.
Schuster, L. and N. Majidi (2014), Deportation stigma and re-migration, *Journal of Ethnic and Migration Studies*, **41**(4), 635–652.
Sigona, N. and V. Hughes (2012), *No Way Out, No Way In: Irregular Migrant Children and Families in the UK*, Oxford: COMPAS.
Standing, G. (2011), *The Precariat*, London: Bloomsbury Academic.
Thomson, R. (2011). *Unfolding Lives: Youth, Gender and Change*, Bristol: Policy Press.
Wade, J. (2011), Preparation and transition planning for unaccompanied asylum-seeking and refugee young people: a review of evidence in England, *Children and Youth Services Review*, **33**(12), 2424–2430.
Waite, L. (2009), A place and space for a critical geography of precarity? *Geography Compass*, **3**(1), 412–433.
Wilding, J. (2015), Asylum-seeker children face welfare lottery on arrival in Britain, *The Conversation*, September 24, available online at https://theconversation.com/revealed-asylum-seeker-children-face-welfare-lottery-on-arrival-in-britain-47864.

12 Human trafficking and health

Siân Oram

INTRODUCTION

Human trafficking is the recruitment and movement of people across and within international borders, by means such as force, fraud, deception, abduction and the abuse of vulnerability, for the purposes of exploitation (United Nations 2000). Exploitation takes a range of forms, including forced sex work, domestic servitude and forced labour in a diverse array of industries, including agriculture, construction, factories and fishing.

Human trafficking is recognised as a crime and as a significant violation of human rights that affects every country of the world. Efforts to estimate the scale of human trafficking are, however, impeded by both definitional and methodological problems. For example, although human trafficking and human smuggling are distinguished in law, in practice they may be difficult to disentangle and consensus is yet to be reached on how exploitative living and working conditions must be before a person can be considered to be a victim of human trafficking. The hidden nature of human trafficking and the reluctance or inability of many victims to come forward to seek help suggests that the problem is underreported, but the ratio of detected to undetected cases is unknown. The International Labour Organization estimated in 2012, however, that approximately 20.9 million people were victims of forced labour worldwide, including 4.5 million victims of forced sex work (International Labour Office 2012). More than half – an estimated 11.2 million – of the world's victims of trafficking are believed to be exploited in the Asia-Pacific region, with 3.7 million exploited in Africa, 1.7 million in Latin America and the Caribbean, 1.6 million in Central and South Eastern Europe, 1.5 million in developed economies and the European Union and 600,000 in the Middle East (International Labour Office 2012).

The dynamics of human trafficking – including, for example, the recruitment methods, travel arrangements and the types of exploitation and abuse – can vary substantially, including in relation to geographical location (Zimmerman 2007). Research suggests that individuals who are trafficked from South-East Europe for sexual exploitation, for example, are typically recruited by individuals who are known to them and who take advantage of desires to migrate and to earn higher salaries, using contracts and legal documentation to deflect concerns about exploitation (Surtees 2008a; US Department of State 2015). Traffickers move their victims within Albania and across Europe, typically operating as part of highly organised criminal gangs, and often subjecting their victims to high levels of violence and abuse. In Nigeria, individuals are typically trafficked from rural areas and, with respect to children and adolescents, traffickers take advantage of the widespread practice of young people being placed and fostered within extended family networks (UNICEF Nigeria 2007; US Department of State 2015). Traffickers promise jobs and study opportunities, taking up-front payments from families and exploiting their victims through forced sex work, domestic servitude and forced labour in settings as diverse as street vending, mining and quarrying, and manufacturing (US Department of State 2015). Common across victims' diverse experiences, however, is their loss of power and control (Zimmerman 2007).

Traffickers use a variety of techniques to control their victims, including the use of violence, threats, debt bonds, personal and intimate relationships and the manipulation of religious and spiritual beliefs. While trafficked, individuals are exposed to multiple health risks, including physical, sexual and psychological abuse, and of exploitative living and working conditions. Trafficked people may additionally experience a range of health risks both prior to trafficking and after their escape, and may have difficulties in accessing healthcare services that are appropriate to their needs. For example, prior to leaving home, victims of trafficking may have been sexually or physically abused by family members, partners, acquaintances and strangers. During travel to the destination location, victims may be exposed to further violence and may be forced to endure hazardous conditions. After escaping their traffickers, victims may be held in detention or deported, or may be required to recount their experiences during police or immigration interviews or court proceedings. This chapter details the major health risks and health needs commonly reported by trafficked people, and the obligations of states to respond.

HEALTH RISKS AND EXPERIENCES PRIOR TO TRAFFICKING

Numerous pre-trafficking factors may influence a person's health and, although empirical evidence is lacking, have been suggested to contribute to their vulnerability to exploitation (Zimmerman et al. 2011). These include experiences of interpersonal violence and abuse; exposure to conflict, political and economic instability, and natural disasters; poverty; lack of education; and pre-existing health problems (including mental health problems and learning difficulties) (Dottridge 2002, Zimmerman et al. 2003, 2011a; Nelson et al. 2004; World Health Organization 2005; Munro and Pritchard 2013). Particularly for women and children, the loss of fathers and familial protection – whether as a result of abandonment or bereavement – may jeopardise safety and financial security (Matthews 2015). Vulnerable individuals may be targeted by traffickers, who are often known to their victims as friends or relatives (Zimmerman et al. 2006; Fleisher et al. 2008; Surtees 2008b).

Exposure to violence and abuse predates many trafficked people's contact with their traffickers, and indeed may contribute to their decision to migrate and influence how they experience and respond to later health risks (Zimmerman et al. 2003). The prevalence of pre-trafficking violence reported in studies with women trafficked for forced sex work is comparable to some of the highest levels of violence against women reported anywhere in the world. The prevalence of childhood sexual abuse reported by the World Health Organization multi-country study on violence and women's health, for example, ranges from 1 per cent to 21 per cent, while the prevalence of adulthood violence ranges from 18.5 per cent to 75.8 per cent (Garcia-Moreno et al. 2006). In comparison, in a multi-country study of 207 women trafficked for forced sex work in Europe, one in seven reported having experienced sexual abuse before the age of 15 (Zimmerman et al. 2006). More than half reported that the perpetrator was a family member, and a quarter reported more than one perpetrator. Abuse since the age of 15 was also reported by a quarter of the women, with the majority of women reporting that abuse was perpetrated by an acquaintance or a stranger. Asked about experiences of physical violence, 60 per cent of women reported having been physically abused prior to having been trafficked.

Experiences of childhood sexual abuse, domestic abuse, sexual assault and other forms of violence may increase vulnerability to human trafficking, as people who are experiencing violence and abuse may be looking for an escape and be more likely to accept risks that they would otherwise refuse. Organisations working with trafficked people report that traffickers often target women and girls in dysfunctional and abusive homes and relationships (Zimmerman 2007). Traffickers may also use experiences of violence and abuse to psychologically manipulate and control their victims, taking advantage of feelings of low self-esteem, shame, guilt and higher risk-taking behaviours (Zimmerman 2007). Experiences of pre-trafficking violence also have significant implications for trafficked people's physical safety if they choose or are forced to return home. As childhood abuse can increase risk of post-traumatic stress disorder (PTSD) in adulthood and memories of early abuse can be reactivated by later similar traumas, experiences of pre-trafficking violence may also have significant implications for victims' mental health (Brewin et al. 2000). Indeed, survey research has suggested that experiences of childhood sexual abuse is a risk factor for diagnosed mental disorder among women survivors of human trafficking (Hossain et al. 2010; Abas et al. 2013).

HEALTH RISKS AND EXPERIENCES DURING TRAVEL AND TRANSIT

For many trafficked people, the realisation that they have been deceived into journeying with their traffickers occurs while travelling to their destination. Trafficked people may be subjected to threatened or actual violence while travelling, be physically confined, and have their travel and identity documents confiscated (Zimmerman et al. 2011). For others, however, the realisation that they have been deceived and are at risk from their traffickers will not occur until reaching their destination, or even for several months afterwards. Trafficked people may also encounter health risks as a result of their mode of travel. Many trafficked people undertake hazardous journeys to reach their destination, and may be at risk of serious harm through exposure to infectious disease, dehydration, drowning and suffocation (Zimmerman et al. 2011).

HEALTH RISKS AND EXPERIENCES DURING THE PERIOD OF EXPLOITATION

Trafficked people may experience multiple health risks during their exploitation, including experiences of physical and sexual violence, psychological abuse, material deprivation, confinement, poor living and working conditions, and coerced use of drugs and alcohol (Oram et al. 2012b). The tactics used by traffickers to control their victims severely limit victims' ability to predict or manage events that affect their health and safety, and have been compared to torture (Hossain et al. 2010; Organization for Security and Co-operation in Europe 2013). The effect of these abuses can be to disorient and isolate victims, to create fear, dependency, and helplessness, and to encourage guilt and self-blame.

Studies conducted with women and girls trafficked for forced sex work report high levels of physical and sexual violence (Oram et al. 2012b). Traffickers may use violence against their victims in order to threaten, coerce, humiliate, degrade or punish them. Many trafficked women and girls – including those trafficked for domestic servitude and for labour exploitation – suffer multiple rape and sexual abuse. For women trafficked for forced sex work, physical and sexual violence may be inflicted not only by their traffickers but also by their customers. Zimmerman's multi-country study of women trafficked for forced sex work in Europe found, for example, that 95 per cent of women reported having experienced either physical or sexual violence while trafficked (Zimmerman et al. 2006). High levels of violence have also been reported by studies conducted in India and South-East Asia. A qualitative analysis of case files of women and girls receiving support from an Indian NGO after being trafficked for forced sex work found that many women were raped upon initiation into sex work and were subjected to ongoing physical and sexual violence as a means of punishment and control (Gupta et al. 2009).

A number of studies have compared the risk of violence among women trafficked into forced sex work and non-trafficked sex workers. Three studies, conducted in India and Thailand, suggest that the risk of violence shortly after entry into sex work is significantly higher among trafficked women (Sarkar et al. 2008; Decker et al. 2011; Silverman et al. 2011). Studies that have measured overall experiences of workplace violence have reported mixed findings: two studies conducted in India and Thailand have found that the risk of any workplace violence was higher among trafficked women than among non-trafficked sex workers (Gupta et al. 2009; Decker et al. 2011), whereas two studies in Nicaragua and Israel have found no difference between the two groups (Cwikel et al. 2004; Decker et al. 2009).

Victims may also be subjected to sustained verbal abuse and humiliation, to threats of violence against themselves and their loved ones, and may be forced to witness the harm of others (Zimmerman et al. 2006). Reports from the UK and USA have also described how women may be forced to pose for pornographic pictures or be filmed in pornographic videos, which may be posted on the internet or kept by the traffickers, who may to threaten to send the materials to the victims' families if they do not comply with their demands (Raymond and Hughes 2001; Organization for Security and Co-operation in Europe 2013). Women trafficked for forced sex work may also be forced to use alcohol and drugs in order to make them more compliant, work longer hours, take on more customers and perform sexual acts to which they might otherwise object (Zimmerman et al. 2006; Organization for Security and Co-operation in Europe 2013). Women trafficked for forced sex work have reported being drugged prior to being raped, particularly when being sold or initiated into sex work (Derks 1997), while women forced to work as sex workers in bars may be required to make customers purchase drinks for them (Zimmerman et al. 2003). Trafficked men and women may also use drugs and alcohol even if not forced to do so, in order to cope with their situation.

Other psychological traumas inflicted on trafficked people include the control of victims' freedom of movement and access to basic resources. A multi-country study of women trafficked for forced sex work and domestic servitude found, for example, that 77 per cent reported they had never been free to go outside unaccompanied (Zimmerman et al. 2006), while restriction of movement was reported by 58.3 per cent of men, women and children trafficked in South-East Asia (Kiss et al. 2015). Traffickers may control how and whether their victims are able to meet their basic physiological needs, withholding access to food, water, toilet and washing facilities, clean clothing and sleep in order to punish, reward and manipulate. Similar to perpetrators of domestic violence, traffickers may create disequilibrium by alternating threats and abuse with apparent kindnesses (Hopper and Hidalgo 2006).

Further humiliation and control may be inflicted through the violation or manipulation of religious beliefs and taboos, including in parts of Africa traditional beliefs in witchcraft and Juju rituals (AFRUCA 2010; Organization for Security and Co-operation in Europe 2013). Victims may be forced by traffickers to swear oaths of allegiance and to participate in ritualised Juju ceremonies, and may fear repercussions – including physical and mental illness, infertility and death – if they break their vows by disobeying their traffickers or disclosing their experiences of abuse. These fears may make it extremely difficult for victims to seek help from support agencies and law enforcement authorities (AFRUCA 2010; Organization for Security and Co-operation in Europe 2013).

The poor working conditions and long working hours also pose risks to the physical and psychological wellbeing of many trafficked people, including men and women trafficked into numerous industries for the exploitation of their manual labour. Evidence on the health risks associated with trafficking for labour exploitation is limited, but it is likely that industry-specific health consequences of labour exploitation are predictable from normal occupational health risks (Zimmerman and Borland 2009). Two examples are provided below, drawing on evidence on occupational risks in two industries into which many thousands of men are trafficked for labour exploitation: construction and fishing.

Construction workers are at increased risk of numerous health problems, including musculoskeletal problems arising from repetitive bending and lifting; respiratory and dermatological problems resulting from exposure to chemicals and dust; and injuries and death including from falls and falling equipment (OSHA 2012). Similarly, workers in the fishing industry face a range of occupational risks, including injuries from fishing equipment and knives; falls on deck or into the sea; sleep deprivation; hypothermia, frostbite, dehydration and heat-related illnesses; and death from drowning (Norrish and Cryer 1990; Driscoll et al. 1994; Matheson et al. 2001). In both these industries, and elsewhere, the poor working conditions to which trafficked people are forcibly subjected – including longer working hours, lack of personal protective equipment and poorer training, and prolonged exposure to extremes of heat or cold – are likely to intensify these risks, increasing the risk of accident, injury and infection (Oram and Zimmerman 2008; Kiss et al. 2015). A high proportion of people trafficked for labour exploitation also report having inadequate food and water and may consequently suffer from weight loss, malnutrition, weakness and lethargy (Turner-Moss et al. 2014, Kiss et al. 2015).

Finally, trafficked people may be forced to live in cramped, overcrowded and unsanitary conditions, often living at their working site or in substandard accommodation provided by their traffickers. Such conditions may increase the risk of infectious diseases such as tuberculosis and scabies and in combination with poor access to healthcare services can lead to the onset or exacerbation of wound and gastrointestinal infections (Organization for Security and Co-operation in Europe 2013). Conversely, trafficked people may be held in isolation from others, with their traffickers and customers providing their only contact with the outside world (Zimmerman et al. 2006).

HEALTH RISKS IN THE POST-TRAFFICKING PERIOD

Trafficked people often experience a range of stressors and health risks after escaping their abusers. Many will not come forward to seek help as a result of not self-identifying as victims of crime or because of fears of prosecution, deportation, and police corruption (United Nations Economic and Social Commission for Asia and the Pacific 2003, United Nations Office on Drugs and Crime and United Nations Global Initiative to Fight Human Trafficking 2009, Baldwin et al. 2011). Others may be detained as illegal immigrants and prosecuted for illegal entry and for other crimes, including sex work. Conditions in detention facilities may be overcrowded, unhygienic, and violent, and access to healthcare potentially limited. Trafficked people who agree –or are compelled – to testify against their traffickers as part of criminal proceedings may risk retribution and may be re-traumatised as a result of recounting their experiences of abuse (Pearson 2002), and should be provided with support and protection as vulnerable witnesses. Trafficked people claiming asylum or other immigration protections may similarly experience extreme stress during the ensuing months – or even years – of legal and financial insecurity. In both criminal and immigration proceedings, being aggressively questioned and disbelieved can be psychologically devastating to victims. Finally, in the absence of safe return procedures, trafficked people who are returned to their countries of origin may be at risk of harm, including re-trafficking (Zimmerman et al. 2006).

HEALTH OUTCOMES

Physical Health

Trafficked people may experience a range of physical injuries and health problems as a result of physical and sexual violence (Organization for Security and Co-operation in Europe 2013). Dental injuries resulting from blows to the face and mouth may include broken or missing teeth, contusions, fractures and dislocations, and may contribute to difficulties speaking, eating and drinking. Beatings may result in abrasions, bruises, fractures, scars, damage to tendons and ligaments, damage to internal organs and both specific and generalised pain. Scarring may also result from being stabbed, cut, scratched, scalded or burned with cigarettes, hot liquids or chemicals, or from being tied with ropes, chains or handcuffs (Zimmerman et al. 2006; Organization for Security and Co-operation in Europe 2013). Disfigurement and injury may also arise from cosmetic ill-treatment, including forced use of skin lightening creams, breast augmentation and tattoos. Head injuries are common and may lead to a variety of symptoms, including headaches, dizziness, nausea, blurred vision, fatigue, altered sleep patterns, altered mood and behaviour, memory and cognitive problems and episodes of collapse (Decker et al. 2009). Violence and injuries may also compound older injuries from abuses suffered prior to trafficking.

Studies on the health consequences of human trafficking have predominantly been conducted with women trafficked for forced sex work and who are in contact with post-trafficking support services having escaped their traffickers. These studies have demonstrated that women suffer from a wide range of physical symptoms in the post-trafficking period, including constitutional, neurological, musculoskeletal and gastrointestinal symptoms. Across a range of studies, the most commonly reported physical symptoms include headaches, fatigue, memory problems, dizziness, back pain, stomach pain and dental pain (Oram et al. 2012a). Less is known about the physical health consequences of trafficking for forced labour. However, a recent study conducted in Cambodia, Thailand and Vietnam surveyed male and female survivors within the first two weeks of entering into support services (Kiss et al. 2015). A high proportion of men, the majority of whom had been trafficked into the fishing industry or into factory labour, reported physical violence and poor living conditions. More than 60 per cent screened positive for depression, more than 40 per cent for PTSD and over a fifth reported symptoms such as headache, fatigue, weight loss and memory problems.

Pain may be caused by violence and injuries experienced prior to and during trafficking or may be psychological in origin; somatisation is common among victims of violence, including human trafficking (Organization for Security and Co-operation in Europe 2013). Headache, tiredness, dizziness, nausea, bowel problems, chest pain and back pain are common psychosomatic symptoms and can be further exacerbated by stress and anxiety (United Nations High Commissioner for Human Rights 2004). Trafficked people may also be vulnerable to psychosomatic disorders (physical diseases such as stomach ulcers, high blood pressure, eczema and psoriasis that are caused or made worse by psychological factors). Many of these symptoms may adversely affect cognitive functioning, hindering ability to recall and recount traumatic experiences (Brewin 2007; Zimmerman 2007). This may negatively impact assessments of credibility made, for example, by law enforcement and immigration personnel, who may mistakenly infer that individuals are being uncooperative or untruthful (Herlihy et al. 2002, 2012). The consistency and quality of memories of events contribute significantly to appraisals of credibility within criminal and immigration proceedings. Yet, studies have demonstrated the disruptive effects of trauma on memory and that traumatic memories are often fragmented, disordered, and incomplete, with particular loss of peripheral detail (Brewin 2007). Such studies suggest that trafficked people may be unable to recall, for example, peripheral details such as travel arrangements, names or addresses, or be able to provide descriptions of clothing, rooms or vehicles (UNODC and UNGIFT 2009). It is also common for memories to alter over time, particularly in relation to highly emotional events (Herlihy et al. 2002).

Longitudinal data on physical health recovery are limited. However, a multi-country study of women trafficked for forced sex work in Europe showed that the proportion of women reporting 12 or more concurrent physical health symptoms reduced from 57 per cent at 0–14 days after entering into services to 7 per cent at 28–56 days (Zimmerman et al. 2006). Such findings highlight the need for immediate post-trafficking medical assistance that attends to urgent health problems (including acute pain, injuries and infections) and to basic care needs (including safety, rest and nutrition). Once addressed, access to comprehensive assessment and treatment is required to address the complex array of symptoms suffered by trafficked women.

Mental Health

Several studies have demonstrated a high prevalence of mental health problems among men and women trafficked for labour and forced sex work. The majority of this research focuses on depression and PTSD. Symptoms of depression may include feeling sad or irritable most of the time; loss of pleasure or interest in things that used to be enjoyed; fatigue; feeling restless or slowed down; difficulties sleeping or over-sleeping; significant weight loss or gain; difficulties concentrating, remembering or making decisions; and feelings of worthlessness or excessive guilt (World Health Organization 1992). People with depression may also have thoughts of self-harm or of suicide. PTSD is a psychiatric disorder that can occur in people who have witnessed or experienced a traumatic event that involved 'actual or threatened death or serious injury, or a threat to the physical integrity of the self or others' and that evoked 'intense fear, helplessness or horror'. PTSD typically develops within the first three months after a traumatic event, although can develop much later, and causes people to continue to have intense and disturbing feelings about their experiences. Symptoms of PTSD include involuntary memories, dreams and flashbacks of the traumatic event; avoidance of people, places, activities and situations that bring back distressing memories of the event; negative thoughts and feelings about oneself and others and feelings of detachment from others; and irritable or self-destructive behaviour, problems with concentrating or sleeping or exaggerated startle responses (World Health Organization 1992). Human trafficking has also been described as a form of complex trauma, defined as trauma that occurs 'repeatedly and cumulatively, usually over a period of time and within specific relationships and contexts' (Courtois 2004). Exposure to complex trauma has been suggested to result in a particular post-traumatic response that is characterised by disturbances in emotional regulation, greater rates of dissociation and somatisation, difficulties trusting or forming intimate relationships with other people and changes in the victim's self-image and concept of the aggressor (Herman 1992; Pearlman 2001; Courtois 2004). Consensus on the distinctiveness of a 'Complex-PTSD' diagnosis is, however, lacking, and research to investigate the phenomenology of the traumatic response in trafficked people is, however, yet to be conducted.

Risk of mental health problems may be increased by experiencing violence either prior to or during trafficking and by longer duration of exploitation. Women who are trafficked for longer periods of time may experience more episodes of physical and sexual violence and suffer from prolonged exposure to psychological entrapment, physical restrictions, loss of control, and hopelessness (Abas et al. 2013). There is emerging evidence to suggest that post-trafficking factors – including levels of social support and unmet social needs – are significant in predicting risk of mental health problems. This is consistent with meta-analyses that have found that post-trauma social support independently predicts risk of PTSD (Brewin et al. 2000), and with studies of asylum seekers showing that post-migration stressors are associated with mental disorder (Silove et al. 2000; Laban et al. 2004). Previous research has also demonstrated that poor social support and life difficulties are perpetuating factors for chronic depression (Brown and Harris 1978; Broadhead and Abas 1998). High levels of mental health symptoms are likely to make it difficult for victims to engage in normal daily activities, including employment, education and caring for family. Symptoms are also likely to hinder the ability of victims to cooperate with law enforcement and immigration service personnel.

SEXUAL AND REPRODUCTIVE HEALTH

Sexual violence causes sexual and reproductive health problems through trauma to the reproductive tract, increased transmission of infections into the bloodstream following trauma and immune system depression (Campbell et al. 2002). Sexual violence may also increase the risk of sexual and reproductive health problems by reducing women's ability to protect themselves through condom use (Campbell et al. 2002; Jewkes et al. 2002). Women trafficked for forced sex work often find that their ability to negotiate condom use is limited and at the discretion of their traffickers and clients. Women whose freedom of movement and access to cash is limited may find that they are unable to purchase condoms or traffickers and brothel owners may charge women inflated prices for condoms and add the costs to their debts (Zimmerman et al. 2003). Women who are able to use condoms with customers may not be able to use them with their traffickers, and may not use them consistently between oral, vaginal and anal sex. Women may also agree to provide unprotected sex or other high-risk acts if they are able to charge more for doing so and pay off their debts more quickly. Women may also be forced to work through their menses, which is associated with a higher rate of sexually transmitted infection (Tanfer and Aral 1996; Aral 2001; Kalichman and Simbayi 2004), and may be experienced as a further form of humiliation and degradation.

Evidence on the sexual and reproductive health problems experienced by trafficked women is, however, limited. A systematic review identified five studies reporting on the prevalence of HIV infection among women trafficked for forced sex work in India and Nepal (Oram et al. 2012b). As risk and prevalence depends on the prevalence and patterns of infection in the areas of exploitation, the findings of these studies are unlikely to be more widely generalisable. Four studies reported serological test results extracted from the case files of women in contact with post-trafficking shelters, finding that the prevalence of HIV ranged from 23 per cent to 46 per cent. A fifth study surveyed brothel-based trafficked women in India, and reported a prevalence of 13 per cent. Risk factors associated with HIV in these studies of trafficked women include younger age when trafficked and longer duration of exploitation. Younger victims may be more biologically vulnerable to infection, and may also have poorer knowledge of risk of infection and appropriate protection methods, and may also be less able to negotiate the use of condoms (Silverman et al. 2007). Five studies reported on the prevalence of self-reported symptoms of sexually transmitted infections, which ranged from 6 per cent to 66 per cent (Oram et al. 2012b).

Left untreated, sexually transmitted infections can result in pelvic inflammatory disease; damage to the reproductive tract, kidney, and bladder; cervical cancer; miscarriage; and infertility. Support for trafficked people should include prompt access to testing for sexually transmitted infection, and appropriate treatment and counselling. People who have suffered anal rape may also require treatment for constipation, pain or bleeding as a result of their injuries (Organization for Security and Co-operation in Europe 2013). Anecdotal evidence suggests a high prevalence of pregnancy and cases of unsafe abortion among women trafficked for forced sex work and other forms of exploitation. Access to maternity and termination of pregnancy services must also be provided to trafficked women in line with guidelines on supporting victims of sexual violence.

RESPONDING TO THE HEALTH NEEDS OF TRAFFICKED PEOPLE

Although the availability, configuration, and cost of healthcare services may vary between countries, there are a limited number of scenarios by which trafficked people may present to services and a number of common barriers to accessing care (Zimmerman and Borland 2009). Trafficked people may access healthcare services while they are still being exploited, when they have recently escaped the trafficking situation, or after they have been out of the trafficking situation for some time. They may be known to the healthcare professional and others involved in their care as a victim of trafficking, or the healthcare professional may notice indicators of abuse and exploitation that make them suspect that the person has experienced trafficking. A trafficked person attending for healthcare may, for example, present with physical or psychological symptoms of trauma, with illnesses or injuries associated with poor living and working conditions, and seem fearful and mistrusting. They may be working in an industry that is commonly associated with trafficking and exploitation, have migrated locally or internationally, and be unable to give a clear account of where they are living or how they arrived in the area (Zimmerman and Borland 2009). Yet, during their exploitation and after their escape, many trafficked people will face multiple barriers to accessing appropriate healthcare services.

During the time they are exploited, trafficked people may be prevented by their abusers from accessing healthcare services, or may be accompanied to medical appointments to prevent disclosures of abuse. Trafficked patients who are able to access healthcare services without being accompanied by their trafficker may have been instructed about what to tell healthcare professionals and may be reluctant to disclose their experiences of abuse because of fear, shame and feelings of hopelessness (Zimmerman and Borland 2009). Research in the USA has also documented cases in which traffickers had personal or family relationships with healthcare professionals, minimising the possibility that a healthcare encounter could be used to escape abuse (Baldwin et al. 2011). The same research found cases of traffickers adding healthcare charges to victims' debts (Baldwin et al. 2011). The actual or perceived cost of healthcare may also create a barrier to accessing care after a trafficked person has escaped exploitation, as might difficulties speaking the local language and unfamiliarity with local healthcare systems.

Trafficked people's immigration status may create an additional barrier to accessing healthcare, both during the time they are exploited and after their escape, despite the specific protection for trafficked people's health rights provided by a number of international and regional instruments. The United Nations Optional Protocol on the Prevention, Suppression and Punishment of Trafficked Persons, Especially Women and Children (United Nations 2000), which as of 2015 had been signed by 117 countries, predominantly focuses on the investigation and prosecution of cases of human trafficking but nonetheless states that signatories should consider implementing measures to provide for the 'physical, psychological and social recovery' of trafficked people, including the provision of counselling and medical, psychological and material assistance. In 2005, the Council of Europe Convention on Action against Trafficking in Human Beings required signatory states to provide 'emergency medical treatment' to trafficked people and to ensure that necessary but non-emergency medical treatment is provided to 'victims [who are] lawfully resident within [a signatory state's] territory who do not have adequate resources and need such help' (Council of Europe 2005). Six years later, the European Union Framework Directive 2011/36 went further, by requiring states to provide 'necessary treatment [and] psychological assistance' to trafficked people and to 'attend to victims with special needs, where those needs derive, in particular, from whether they are pregnant, their health, a disability, a mental or psychological disorder they have, or a serious form of psychological, physical, or sexual violence they have suffered' (European Union 2011). Framework Directive 2011/36 additionally required states to establish procedures to identify and provide support to trafficked people. A number of other international and regional legal instruments provide more generally for the health rights of trafficked people. The general health rights of all persons, regardless of residence status, are emphasised by the International Convention on Economic, Social and Cultural Rights (ICESCR) (United Nations 1966), the European Social Charter (ESC) (Council of Europe 1961) and the Charter of Fundamental Rights of the European Union (European Union 2000). Trafficked people are specifically named as a group to whom the ICESCR applies within General Comment 20 (United Nations 2009). The rights of migrants to healthcare and other protections are also provided for by the United Nations International Convention on the Protection of the Rights of All Migrant Workers and Members of their Families (United Nations 1990), which as of 2015 had been signed by 38 countries.

International guidelines on supporting trafficked people also recommend the implementation of victim-centred national and international referral mechanisms to ensure the provision of coordinated support for trafficked people and the introduction of 'recovery and reflection periods' (Kröger et al. 2004; Oram et al. 2011). Recovery and reflection periods provide trafficked people with time to access crisis-stage support and consider their participation in procedures – including police and immigration proceedings – that could have implications for their health and wellbeing. To date, however, health services have been poorly integrated into national referral mechanisms and evidence-based guidance on referring and caring for trafficked people within health settings remains limited (Oram 2011). Commonly cited examples of good practice, however, include ensuring that patients are seen privately (even where the person accompanying them claims to be a friend or relative), providing access to independent and qualified interpreters, and developing trust by ensuring confidentiality and maintaining a non-judgemental and sympathetic manner (Yakushko 2009; Zimmerman and Borland 2009; Dovydaitis 2010). Physical, sexual and mental healthcare should be appropriate to individual victims' gender, age and culture, and should address both acute and longer-term health needs, including counselling and treatment for sexually transmitted infections, HIV/AIDS, tuberculosis, substance abuse and physical and psychological trauma. The effectiveness of psychological interventions in promoting the recovery of trafficked people is unknown (Abas et al. 2013). However, interventions will need to take account of the prolonged abuse experienced during – and often prior to – trafficking, and care professionals are likely to need to work to stabilise physical and psychological health and to address social needs before commencing trauma-focused psychological therapies. Psychological stabilisation may include re-establishing trust with other people, learning techniques to cope with dissociation and to regulate emotions, and the treatment of depression, including through the use of antidepressants in moderate to severe cases (Abas et al. 2013). Evidence-based therapeutic treatment options for PTSD include cognitive behavioural therapy, narrative exposure therapy and eye movement desensitisation and reprocessing (Rauch and Cahill 2003), but require that survivors are ready to talk about the traumas they have experienced.

CONCLUSIONS

Despite more than a decade of policy, media and academic attention to human trafficking and widespread recognition of the violence and abuse experienced by many trafficked people, evidence on the health needs of trafficked people remains limited. The little research that has been conducted to date concerns the health risks and consequences of the trafficking of women for forced sex work. The majority of this research has been conducted in South and South-East Asia, with fewer studies conducted elsewhere. Findings relating to occupational injuries and infectious diseases – including sexually transmitted infections – are likely to be less generalisable than findings on the prevalence of non-specific physical symptoms such as headache and back pain and of mental health problems. Evidence on the health needs of women trafficked for other forms of exploitation, of trafficked men and of trafficked children is extremely scarce. Virtually nothing is known about the long-term health needs of trafficked people or about the factors that contribute to trafficked people's physical and psychological recovery, and despite a number of studies demonstrating a high burden of poor mental health among women trafficked for forced sex work, psychological interventions to support recovery are yet to be tested. Given the loss of power and control that characterises trafficking, many similarities can be drawn between the experiences of trafficked people and those of survivors of torture and of domestic violence. In seeking to provide support for trafficked people, policymakers, providers and researchers should look to best practice with these other abused and marginalised populations.

REFERENCES

Abas, M., N. V. Ostrovschi, M. Prince, V. I. Gorceag, C. Trigub and S. Oram (2013), Risk factors for mental disorders in women survivors of human trafficking: a historical cohort study, *BMC Psychiatry*, **13**(1), 1–11.

AFRUCA (2010), *Breaking the Cycle of Fear: Witchcraft, Juju and Safeguarding Victims of Human Trafficking*, London: AFRUCA.

Aral, S. O. (2001), Sexually transmitted diseases: magnitude, determinants and consequences, *International Journal of STD & AIDS*, **12**(4), 211–215.

Baldwin, S. B., D. P. Eisenman, J. N. Sayles, G. Ryan and K. S. Chuang (2011), Identification of human trafficking victims in health care settings, *Health and Human Rights: An International Journal*, **13**(1), e36–e49.

Brewin, C. R. (2007), Autobiographical memory for trauma: update on four controversies, *Memory*, **15**(3), 227–248.

Brewin, C. R., B. Andrews, and J. D. Valentine (2000), Meta-analysis of risk factors for posttraumatic stress disorder in trauma-exposed adults, *Journal of Consulting and Clinical Psychology*, **68**(5), 748–766.

Broadhead, J. and M. Abas (1998), Life events, difficulties and depression among women in an urban setting in Zimbabwe, *Psychological Medicine*, **28**(1), 29–38.

Brown, G. W. and T. Harris (1978), Social origins of depression: a reply, *Psychological Medicine*, **8**(4), 577–588.

Campbell, J. C., A. S. Jones, J. Dienemann, J. Kub, J. Schollenberger, P. O'Campo, A. C. Gielen and C. Wynne (2002), Intimate partner violence and physical health consequences, *Archives of Women's Mental Health*, **162**(10), 1157–1163.

Council of Europe. (1961), *European Social Charter*, 529 U.N.T.S. 89 Art 13. (1961).

Council of Europe (2005), *Council of Europe Convention on Action against Trafficking in Human Beings and its Explanatory Report*, Warsaw 16V 2005, Council of Europe.

Courtois, C. A. (2004), Complex trauma, complex reactions: assessment and treatment, *Psychotherapy: Theory, Research, Practice, Training*, **41**(4), 412–425.

Cwikel, J., B. Chudakov, M. Paikin, K. Agmon and R. Belmaker (2004), Trafficked female sex workers awaiting deportation: comparison with brothel workers, *Archives of Women's Mental Health*, **7**(4), 243–249.

Decker, M. R., K. P. Mack, J. J. Barrows and J. G. Silverman (2009), Sex trafficking, violence victimization, and condom use among prostituted women in Nicaragua, *International Journal of Gynecology & Obstetrics*, **107**(2), 151–152.

Decker, M. R., H. L. McCauley, D. Phuengsamran, S. Janyam and J.G. Silverman (2011), Sex trafficking, sexual risk, sexually transmitted infection and reproductive health among female sex workers in Thailand, *Journal of Epidemiology and Community Health*, **65**(4), 334–339.

Derks, A. (1997), *Trafficking of Cambodian Women and Children to Thailand*, Geneva: Center for Advanced Study and IOM International Organization for Migration.

Dottridge, D. (2002), Trafficking in children in West and Central Africa, *Gender & Development*, **10**(1), 38–49.

Dovydaitis, T. (2010), Human trafficking: the role of the health care provider, *Journal of Midwifery & Women's Health*, **55**(5), 462–467.

Driscoll, T. R., G. Ansari, J. E. Harrison, M. S. Frommer and E. A. Ruck (1994), Traumatic work related fatalities in commercial fishermen in Australia, *Occupational and Environmental Medicine*, **51**(9), 612–616.

European Union (2000), Charter of Fundamental Rights of the European Union, 2000/C 364/01, Art. 35.

European Union (2011), Directive 2011/36/EU of the European Parliament and of the Council of 5 April 2011 on Preventing and Combating Trafficking in Human Beings and Protecting its Victims, and Replacing Council Framework Decision 2002/629/JHA, 15 April 2011, 2011/36/EU, available online at www.refworld.org/docid/50ec1e172.html.

Fleisher, M., R. Johnston and I. Alon (2008), *Eastern Africa: Research Assessment and Baseline Information in Tanzania, Kenya, Uganda, and Burundi*, Geneva: International Organization for Migration.

Garcia-Moreno, C., H. A. Jansen, M. Ellsberg, L. Heise and C.H. Watts (2006), Prevalence of intimate partner violence: findings from the WHO multi-country study on women's health and domestic violence, *The Lancet*, **368**(9543), 1260–1269.

Gupta, J., A. Raj, M.R. Decker, E. Reed and J. G. Silverman (2009), HIV vulnerabilities of sex-trafficked Indian women and girls, *International Journal of Gynecology and Obstetrics*, **107**(1), 30–34.

Herlihy, J., P. Scragg and S. Turner (2002), Discrepancies in autobiographical memories – implications for the assessment of asylum seekers: repeated interviews study, *BMJ*, **324**(7333), 324–327.

Herlihy, J., L. Jobson and S. Turner (2012), Just tell us what happened to you: autobiographical memory and seeking asylum, *Applied Cognitive Psychology*, **26**(5), 661–676.

Herman, J. L. (1992), Complex PTSD: a syndrome in survivors of prolonged and repeated trauma, *Journal of Traumatic Stress*, **5**(3), 377–391.

Hopper, E. and J. Hidalgo (2006), Invisible chains: psychological coercion of human trafficking victims, *Intercultural Human Rights Law Review*, **1**, 185–209.

Hossain, M., C. Zimmerman, M. Abas, M. Light and C. Watts (2010), The relationship of trauma to mental disorders among trafficked and sexually exploited girls and women, *American Journal of Public Health*, **100**(12), 2442–2449.

International Labour Office (2012), *ILO Global Estimate of Forced Labour: Results and Methodology*, Geneva: International Labour Office.

Jewkes, R., P. Sen and C. Garcia-Moreno (2002), Sexual violence, in E. Krug, L. L. Dahlberg, J. A. Mercy, A. B. Zwi and R. Lozano (eds.), *World Report on Violence and Health*, Geneva: World Health Organization, pp. 147–181.

Kalichman, S. C. and L. C. Simbayi (2004), Sexual exposure to blood and increased risks for heterosexual HIV transmission in Cape Town, South Africa, *African Journal of Reproductive Health*, **8**(2), 55–58.

Kiss, L., N. Pocock, V. Naisanguansri, S. Soksreymom, B. Dickson, D. Thuy, J. Koehler, K. Sirisup, N. Pongrungsee, V. Nguyen, R. Borland, P. Dhavan and C. Zimmerman (2015), Health of men, women, and children in post-trafficking services in Cambodia, Thailand, and Vietnam: an observational cross-sectional study, *Lancet Global Health*, **3**, e157–e164.

Kröger, T., J. Malkič and B. H. Uhl (2004), *National Referral Mechanisms: Joining Efforts to Protect the Rights of Trafficked Persons: A Practical Handbook*, Warsaw: OSCE Office for Democratic Institutions and Human Rights.

Laban, C. J., H. B. Gernaat, I. H. Komproe, B. A. Schreuders and J. T. De Jong (2004), Impact of a long asylum procedure on the prevalence of psychiatric disorders in Iraqi asylum seekers in the Netherlands, *The Journal of Nervous and Mental Disease*, **192**(12), 843–851.

Matheson, C., S. Morrison, E. Murphy, T. Lawrie, L. Ritchie and C. Bond (2001), The health of fishermen in the catching sector of the fishing industry: a gap analysis, *Occupational Medicine*, **51**(5), 305–311.

Matthews, E. (2015), *No Way Home: The Exploitation and Abuse of Children in Ukraine's Orphanages*, Washington, DC: Disability Rights International.

Munro, G. and C. Pritchard (2013), *Support Needs of Male Victims of Human Trafficking: Research Findings*, London: Salvation Army.

Nelson, S., J. Guthrie and P. Sumner Coffey (2004), *Literature Review and Analysis Related to Human Trafficking in Post-Conflict Situations*, Washington, DC: USAID.

Norrish, A. E. and P. C. Cryer (1990), Work related injury in New Zealand commercial fishermen, *British Journal of Industrial Medicine*, **47**(11), 726–732.
Oram, S.L. (2011), *Human Trafficking and Health in UK Public Policy*, PhD thesis, London School of Hygiene & Tropical Medicine.
Oram, S. and C. Zimmerman (2008), The health of persons trafficked for forced labour, *IOM Global Eye on Trafficking*, **4**, 4.
Oram, S., C. Zimmerman, B. Adams and J. Busza (2011), International law, national policy-making, and the health of trafficked people in the UK, *Health and Human Rights*, **13**(2), 7–12.
Oram, S., N. V. Ostrovschi, V. I. Gorceag, M. A. Hotineanu, L. Gorceag, C. Trigub and M. Abas (2012a), Physical health symptoms reported by trafficked women receiving post-trafficking support in Moldova: prevalence, severity and associated factors, *BMC Women's Health*, **12**(20).
Oram, S., H. Stöckl, J. Busza, L.M. Howard and C. Zimmerman (2012b), Prevalence and risk of violence and the physical, mental and sexual health problems associated with human trafficking: systematic review, *PLOS Medicine*, **9**(5): e1001224.
Organization for Security and Co-operation in Europe (2013), *Trafficking in Human Beings Amounting to Torture and other Forms of Ill-treatment*, Vienna: Office of the Special Representative and Co-ordinator for Combating Trafficking in Human Beings in partnership with the Ludwig Boltzmann Institute of Human Rights and the Helen Bamber Foundation.
OSHA (2012), *Health Hazards in Construction Workbook: Construction Safety Council*, Hillside, IL: Construction Safety Council.
Pearlman, L. A. (2001), Treatment of persons with complex PTSD and other trauma-related disruptions of the self, in J. P. Wilson, M. J. Friedman and J. D. Lindy (eds.), *Treating Psychological Trauma and PTSD*, New York: Guildford Press, pp. 205–236.
Pearson, E. (2002), Half-hearted protection: what does victim protection really mean for victims of trafficking in Europe? *Gender & Development*, **10**(1), 56–59.
Rauch, S. A. and S. P. Cahill (2003), Treatment and prevention of posttraumatic stress disorder, *Primary Psychiatry*, **10**(8), 60–65.
Raymond, J. G. and D. M. Hughes (2001), *Sex Trafficking of Women in the United States: International and Domestic Trends*, Washington, DC: US Department of Justice.
Sarkar, K., B. Bal, R. Mukherjee, S. Chakraborty, S. Saha, A. Ghosh and S. Parsons (2008), Sex-trafficking, violence, negotiating skill, and HIV infection in brothel-based sex workers of eastern India, adjoining Nepal, Bhutan, and Bangladesh, *Journal of Health, Population and Nutrition*, **26**(2), 223–231.
Silove, D., S. Ekblad and R. Molica (2000), The rights of the severely mentally ill in post-conflict societies, *The Lancet*, **355**, 1548.
Silverman, J. G., M. R. Decker, J. Gupta, A. Maheshwari, B. M. Willis and A. Raj (2007), HIV prevalence and predictors of infection in sex-trafficked Nepalese girls and women, *JAMA*, **298**(5), 536–542.
Silverman, J. G., A. Raj, D. M. Cheng, M. R. Decker, S. Coleman, C. Bridden, M. Pardeshi, N. Saggurti and J. H. Samet (2011), Sex trafficking and initiation-related violence, alcohol use, and HIV risk among HIV-infected female sex workers in Mumbai, India, *Journal of Infectious Diseases*, **204**(S5), S1229–S1234.
Surtees, R. (2008a), Traffickers and trafficking in Southern and Eastern Europe: considering the other side of human trafficking, *European Journal of Criminology*, **5**(1), 39–68.
Surtees, R. (2008b), *Trafficking of Men – a Trend Less Considered: The Case of Belarus and Ukraine*, Geneva: International Organization for Migration.
Tanfer, K. and S. O. Aral (1996), Sexual intercourse during menstruation and self-reported sexually transmitted disease history among women, *Sexually Transmitted Diseases*, **23**(5), 395–401.
Turner-Moss, E., C. Zimmerman, L. Howard and S. Oram (2014), Labour exploitation and health: a case series of men and women seeking post-trafficking services, *Journal of Immigrant and Minority Health*, **16**, 473–480.

UNICEF Nigeria (2007), *Information Sheet: Child Trafficking*, available online at www.unicef.org/wcaro/WCARO_Nigeria_Factsheets_ChildTrafficking.pdf.

United Nations (1966), International Covenant on Economic, Social and Cultural Rights (ICESCR), G.A. Res. 2200A (XXI).

United Nations (1990), Convention on the Protection of the Rights of All Migrant Workers and Members of their Families, G.A., Res 45/158.

United Nations (2000), Optional Protocol to Prevent, Suppress and Punish Trafficking in Persons, Especially Women and Children, Supplementing the United Nations Convention Against Transnational Organized Crime, G.A. Res. 55/25(2000).

United Nations (2009), Committee on Economic, Social and Cultural Rights, General Comment No. 20, Nondiscrimination in economic, social and cultural rights (Article 2), UN Doc. No. E/C.12/GC/20.

United Nations Economic and Social Commission for Asia and the Pacific (2003), *Combating Human Trafficking in Asia: A Resource Guide to International and Regional Legal Instruments, Political Commitments and Recommended Practices*, Bangkok: United Nations.

United Nations High Commissioner for Human Rights (2004), *The Istanbul Protocol: Manual on the Effective Investigation and Documentation of Torture and Other Cruel, Inhuman or Degrading Treatment or Punishment*, Geneva: United Nations High Commissioner for Human Rights.

UNODC and UNGIFT (2009), *Anti-Human Trafficking Manual for Criminal Justice Practitioners*, New York: United Nations.

US Department of State (2015), *Trafficking in Persons Report*, Washington, DC: US Department of State.

World Health Organization (1992), *The ICD-10 Classification of Mental and Behavioural Disorders: Clinical Description and Diagnostic Guidelines*, Geneva: World Health Organization.

World Health Organization (2005), *Violence and Disasters*, Geneva: World Health Organization.

Yakushko, O. (2009), Human trafficking: a review for mental health professionals, *International Journal for the Advancement of Counselling*, **31**(3), 158–167.

Zimmerman, C. (2007), *Trafficking in Women: The Health of Women in Post-Trafficking Services in Europe who were Trafficked into Prostitution or Sexually Abused as Domestic Labourers*, PhD thesis, University of London.

Zimmerman, C. and R. Borland (2009), *Caring for Trafficked Persons: Guidance for Health Providers*, Geneva: International Organisation for Migration, London School of Hygiene and Tropical Medicine, and the United Nations Global Initiative to Fight Trafficking.

Zimmerman, C., K. Yun, C. Watts, I. Shvab, L. Trappolin, M. Treppete, F. Bimbi, S. Jiraporn, L. Beci and M. Albrecht (2003), *The Health Risks and Consequences of Trafficking in Women and Adolescents: Findings from a European Study*, London: London School of Hygiene & Tropical Medicine.

Zimmerman, C., M. Hossain, K. Yun, B. Roche, L. Morison and C. Watts (2006), *Stolen Smiles: The Physical and Psychological Health Consequences of Women and Adolescents Trafficked in Europe*, London: London School of Hygiene & Tropical Medicine.

Zimmerman, C., M. Hossain and C. Watts (2011), Human trafficking and health: A conceptual model to inform policy, intervention and research, *Social Science & Medicine*, **73**(2): 327–335.

13 Migrating to work at what cost? The cumulative health consequences of contemporary labour migration

Stephanie Mayell and Janet McLaughlin

INTRODUCTION

Migrant labour has become a major component of the global economy, integrated across various sectors, industries and national contexts. The migrant workers in these positions come from a variety of countries and sociocultural backgrounds, and possess varying levels of education and training. Both men and women migrate for work, although the types of jobs available to them can be highly gendered based on labour market preferences. Most migrant workers share in common the motivation to find decent employment and secure livelihoods, choosing labour migration as the best alternative of those available to them. Others are forced to leave their homes due to famine, extreme poverty, environmental degradation, natural disasters, trafficking or other reasons. In such instances, labour may have not been their primary motivation to migrate, yet they still may work in their place of destination. Some international migrant workers participate in transnational labour programmes or have temporary work permits, while others work in countries where they do not have legal permission to reside and/or work. Whatever the circumstances, the conditions associated with labour migration may increase health vulnerabilities for migrant workers throughout the migration process, although these vary considerably based on migrants' level/sector of empowerment, and factors such as legal and socioeconomic status, as well as available labour, health and social protections.

This chapter begins with a broad sketch of contemporary transnational labour migration, and proceeds to explore the health vulnerabilities faced by migrant workers during each stage of the migratory process (pre-departure, travel, destination, interception and return), based on a review of international literature. The local conditions and environment at the place of origin influences the health of migrant workers throughout all stages of the migratory process, and many pre-departure health issues continue to affect workers after their arrival at their destination (Gushulak and MacPherson 2011). In destination countries, migrant workers are structurally vulnerable to occupational health and safety risks, and often these risks can vary according to level of skill and socioeconomic status (Benach et al. 2011; Sargeant and Tucker 2009). Migrant workers return to their countries of origin in a variety of ways, and the health status of migrant workers upon return is influenced by the cumulative exposure to risk factors and social determinants of health throughout the migratory process (Davies et al. 2011).

The second section of the chapter discusses the case study of workers from Mexico and the Caribbean who labour in Canadian agriculture. Following the various stages of migration, we detail how these workers experience health risks and implications at each phase of their migration journey. The findings and analysis are based on our primary research with this population, including a decade of ethnographic and survey-based study (McLaughlin) and more than two years of clinical-based observations, participant observation and interview-based research (Mayell).

CONTEMPORARY MIGRANT WORKERS: DEFINITIONS, NUMBERS AND INTERNATIONAL PROTECTIONS

In this chapter, a *migrant worker* is generally understood to be a person who leaves his or her region of birth or permanent residence in order to find employment in another country. Although the term 'migrant worker' often refers to a transnational worker, it is also applicable in reference to a person who engages in labour migration within the borders of their home country, as in the case of rural-to-urban labour migration in China (see Qu and Zhao 2011; Wen and Hanley 2015). Notably, international organizations and instruments, such as the United Nations (UN) and the International Labour Organization (ILO), define 'migrant worker' differently.

The UN sought to address the human rights of migrant workers in its 1990 International Convention on the Protection of the Rights of All Migrant Workers and Members of Their Families. The Convention's primary objective is to protect migrant workers and their families from exploitation and the violation of their human rights. The Convention defines a migrant worker as: 'a person who is engaged or has been engaged in a remunerated activity in a State of which he or she is not a national'. The Convention was entered into force in July 2003 after the threshold of 20 ratifying countries was reached. To this day, only 48 countries – mainly migrant-sending rather than destination states – have ratified it.

The ILO, the UN's specialized labour agency, considers a migrant worker to be: 'a person who migrates from one country to another with a view to being employed otherwise than on his own account and includes any person regularly admitted as a migrant for employment' (ILO 1949). The predominant difference between these two definitions is that the UN includes self-employed workers, but the ILO instruments related to migrant workers' protection do not include such persons (IOM 2004). Both the UN and ILO consider only transnational migrant workers (those working between states) in their definitions.

Because various international organizations work with different definitions of 'migrant worker', and use different terms (such as 'economic migrant'), it is difficult to source the number of migrant workers in the world today. And, despite the fact that the vast majority of workers return home after seasonal or temporary employment, precise measures on circular temporary migration are lacking (Lucas 2008). Since 1990, the Population Division of the United Nations' Department of Economic and Social Affairs (UN-DESA) has been tracking the number of international migrants worldwide, defined as 'people living in a country or area other than the one in which they were born', while the ILO compiles data only on the number of migrants who are journeying for work (UN-DESA 2013a).

In 2013, the UN estimated there to be 232 million international migrants worldwide (UN-DESA 2013a). The ILO reported that more than 50 per cent of these migrants were economically active (in the labour market), a figure projected to be closer to 90 per cent if the workers' family members are also counted (ILO 2013). In 2013, women accounted for nearly half (48 per cent) of the international migrant population, and many were migrating independently for low-skill labour opportunities (ILO 2013; UN-DESA 2013a). At present, it is estimated that 21 million people are in forced labour and being trafficked globally (ILO 2015b).

In 2012, the United Nations convened a Conference on Sustainable Development (Rio+20) with the goal that member states would launch development processes aimed at recognizing a set of sustainable development goals. One of the targets identified by the UN's Working Group on Sustainable Development Goals includes a target (Target 8.8) on 'protecting labour rights and promoting safe and secure working environments of all workers, including migrant workers, particularly women migrants, and those in precarious employment' (UN-DESA 2015). In order to measure Target 8.8, the ILO has advanced a number of tentative indicators intended to promote decent work for migrant workers, including indicators on international labour standards, employment, wages and working conditions, skills and qualifications recognition, social security coverage, reducing the costs related to recruitment, and social dialogue (ILO 2015a).

TYPES OF MIGRANT WORKERS

There are a variety of conditions under which people legally migrate for work, both across and within national borders. The movement of transnational migrant workers is generally regulated and facilitated by labour agreements, such as bilateral agreements and memoranda of understanding. All bilateral labour agreements share three common objectives that overlap with the three areas laid out by the ILO in its *Multilateral Framework on Labour Migration*: effective governance of labour migration flows, protection of migrant workers and promotion of the development benefits of migration (ILO 2006; Wickramasekara 2015). Despite these explicit goals, the efficacy of such programmes to protect migrant workers' human and labour rights is questionable (Cholewinski 2015).

The classification of migrant work is typically based on the duration of activities, as well as the conditions of admission and stay that are outlined in the regulatory framework of receiving countries (IOM 2004). Contemporary types of migrant workers include: *contract migrant workers*, who are working in a country other than their own under contractual limitations regarding period of employment; *established migrant workers*, who are granted permanent residency and the ability to work unimpeded after many years of return employment to a host country; *highly skilled migrant workers*, whose skills subject them to preferential treatment regarding admission and fewer restrictions regarding employment; *project-tied workers*, who are admitted into a country for a defined duration solely to work on a project carried out in that country by his or her employer; *seasonal migrant workers*, who are transnationally employed for part of the year due to the seasonal nature of the work; and *temporary migrant workers*, who are admitted into a country to work for a limited duration in a specific occupation or job but may change employers and have their work permits renewed without leaving the country of employment (IOM 2004).

In addition, millions of people every year attempt to migrate illegally in order to find employment, while others may enter countries legally but then stay past visas or work without proper authorization. Such people are sometimes referred to as 'irregular' or 'unauthorized' workers, or 'workers with precarious immigration status' (see Goldring and Landolt 2013). *Irregular migrants* are 'individuals who enter a country, often in search of employment, without the required documents or permits, or who overstay the authorized length of stay in the country' (Zimmerman et al. 2011). Migrating for work outside of the regulatory frameworks of sending or receiving countries predisposes such workers to myriad health vulnerabilities (IOM 2009). One major challenge for such workers is that they often fear accessing public services such as police protections and healthcare due to their precarious status and fear of deportation. Undocumented workers are especially vulnerable to abuse, and women in particular are at risk for sexual violence, human trafficking and sexual exploitation (Davies et al. 2011; IOM 2009).

Unfortunately, there is no authoritative source specifically focusing on global trends and numbers on irregular migration at the global level. In 2010, the International Organization for Migration (IOM) estimated that approximately 10–15 per cent of the world's then 214 million international migrants were undocumented (IOM 2010). The United States maintains statistics on the number of undocumented workers in its labour economy, and in 2013 there were an estimated 11.1 million undocumented workers present (PICUM 2013). In 2007, the Organisation for Economic Co-operation and Development (OECD) estimated that 10 to 15 per cent of Europe's 56 million migrants were undocumented (OECD 2012).

Some individuals are forced to migrate against their will, and these workers are referred to as 'trafficked persons', 'forced migrants', 'unfree labourers' or 'forced labourers' (see Strauss 2012). Trafficked persons are individuals who are tricked or forced into situations in which their labour or bodies are exploited, and trafficking can occur across international borders or within national borders (Zimmerman et al. 2011).

The ILO estimated that in 2012 there were 21 million trafficked persons worldwide: 18.7 million (90 per cent) of whom were exploited in the private economy – 4.5 million (22 per cent) were victims of forced sexual exploitation; 14.2 million (68 per cent) were victims of forced labour exploitation in economic activities such as agriculture, construction, domestic work and manufacturing – and the remaining 2.2 million (10 per cent) were in state-imposed forms of forced labour under conditions that contravene ILO standards on the subject (ILO 2012). Women and girls are particularly vulnerable to trafficking and they represent the greater share of total forced labour: 11.4 million victims (55 per cent), as compared to 9.5 million (45 per cent) men and boys (ILO 2012).

GLOBAL LABOUR MIGRATION FLOWS

Global economic inequalities have been primary drivers of labour migration flows for more than a century. When considering the movement of migrant workers around the world, it is analytically convenient to divide the world into two general regions: the *Global North* and *Global South*. The Global North is the region comprised of the countries or regions statistically classified as economically developed, whereas the Global South is comprised of countries or regions classified as economically developing. High levels of poverty and unemployment in the Global South motivate many people to seek employment elsewhere ('push factor'), while demographic and economic transitions in the countries of the Global North have increased their demand for (primarily) unskilled, low-paid labour ('pull factor').

ORIGINS AND DESTINATIONS

The majority of migrant workers worldwide come from countries located in the Global South. In 2013, an estimated 71 per cent of the world's 232 million international migrants originated from the South (UN-DESA 2013b). In recent decades, South–South migration has become as common as South–North migration: in 2013, approximately 82 million migrants originated from and were residing in the South (UN-DESA 2013b). Although South–South migration is the largest migration category, South–North migration continues to be the main driver of global migration trends (UN-DESA 2013b).

Regionally, in 2013 there were 136 million migrants residing in the Global North and 96 million residing in the Global South (see Figure 13.1). Europe and Asia combined hosted approximately two-thirds of all international migrants worldwide in 2013, with 72 million residing in Europe and 71 million in Asia (see Figure 13.2).

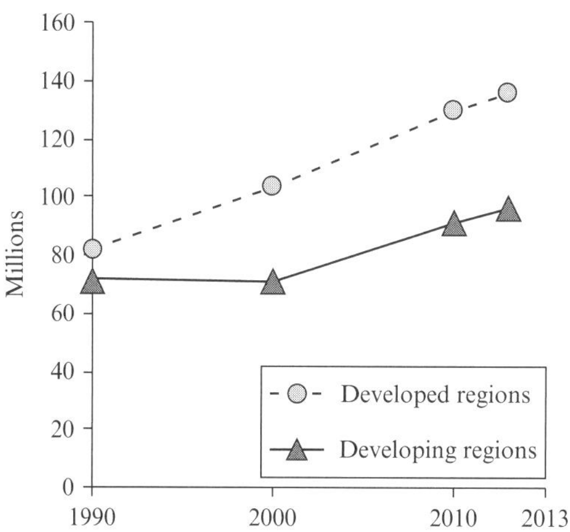

Figure 13.1 International migrants, 1990–2013 (millions)

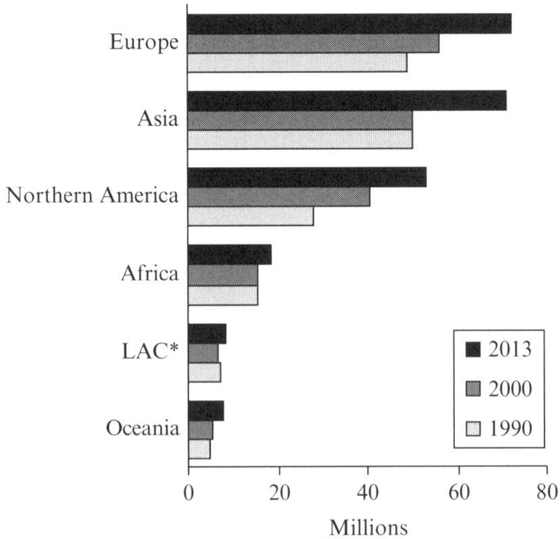

Figure 13.2 International migrants by major area, 1990, 2000 and 2013

INDUSTRIES

Migrant workers fill jobs in various sectors of the global economy. In the North, migrant workers are predominantly found in the agricultural, food processing and construction sectors, working semi- or low-skilled jobs in the manufacturing sector, and working in low-wage service positions (Benach et al. 2011). The international hotel, catering and tourism sector relies on temporary and seasonal labour, and although the experiences of migrant workers in the hotel industry vary greatly according to country, culture and context, these workers are disproportionately likely to remain in low-skilled and lower-paid positions, face particular vulnerabilities in terms of health and safety, and are more likely to be involved in workplace accidents (Baum 2012).

Female migrant workers employed in the North primarily work in retail, domestic work, and consumer services (Benach et al. 2011). The feminization of migration throughout the developing world is a predominant characteristic of the twenty-first century, epitomized by the domestic work sector (see Piper 2013; Romero et al. 2014). Over recent decades, the demand for domestic services by private households across the North has been steadily increasing, making domestic work the largest occupation group among migrant women, accounting for 20 per cent of all economically active migrant women (Gallotti 2009; Piper 2013).

Migrant women working in the South are frequently employed in the garment industry, where they face sexual abuse, experience barriers to freedom of movement and generally are not able to acquire leading positions (see Ansell et al. 2015; CCC 2009). Women crossing borders to work also experience particularly complex challenges in terms of managing their responsibilities to their children and natal families (Pearson and Kusakabe 2012). Some women who migrate for work, however, report certain benefits beyond income, such as distance from patriarchal social relations, increased independence, and escape from conjugal conflicts and familial tensions (Bélanger and Rahman 2013).

HEALTH CONSIDERATIONS ACROSS THE PHASES OF LABOUR MIGRATION

Labour migration influences health at both the individual and population levels. Generally, the health of migrant workers varies along the lines of socioeconomic status, education and skill levels, and language skills (Sargeant and Tucker 2009). The health status of migrant workers moving between developed countries in the North differs significantly from that of workers who migrate from the South to work in the North, insofar as unskilled workers from countries in the South are more vulnerable to occupational health and safety risks (Sargeant and Tucker 2009). Workers migrating from the South generally have fewer employment options and are more likely to be in a restricted employment situation. For these reasons, they are often concerned with appeasing their employers to secure their jobs. Consequently, they are willing to work long hours and are less empowered to advocate for their rights. This situation predisposes these workers to an increased risk of work injury, illness or disablement (Richardson et al. 2003).

The health of migrant workers fluctuates throughout the migratory process; thus it is important to examine migrant worker health at each stage of their journey. This chapter adopts the framework advanced by health researchers in a recent series of publications exploring the intersections of migration and health (Zimmerman et al. 2011). The five phases of labour migration are: pre-departure, travel, destination, interception and return (Figure 13.3). Migrant workers are vulnerable to multi-staged and cumulative health vulnerabilities throughout the migratory process, including occupational health risks, injuries, poor mental health, diabetes mellitus, certain communicable diseases and maternal and child health problems (Sargeant and Tucker 2009; Rechel et al. 2013; Zimmerman et al. 2011). To follow, the health impacts associated with each phase are explored.

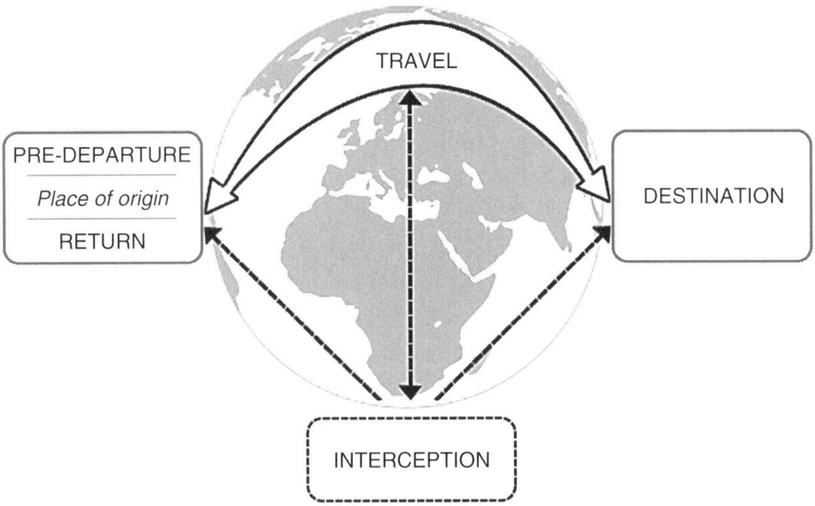

Source: Zimmerman et al. 2011.

Figure 13.3 Migration phases framework

PRE-DEPARTURE PHASE

The pre-departure phase is the time before migrant workers leave their place of origin, when they prepare for their migratory journey. There are some indications that those seeking migrant work may be generally among those in the population with relatively good levels of health and fitness. There are compelling reasons for this phenomenon. For example, some migrant worker programmes and destination countries screen for medical conditions (including HIV and pregnancy) in this phase; thus prospective workers with medical problems or limitations may be eliminated from participation (Qureshi 2013). Likewise, those considering perilous migration journeys (for example, across the US–Mexico border via a river or desert) or contemplating work in industries with major physical demands (such as agriculture and construction) may be deterred from such opportunities if they are in poor health.

The health characteristics of pre-departure migrant workers vary according to disparities in the determinants of health at both the individual and societal levels (Gushulak and MacPherson 2011). The determinants of health during this stage affect both existing and future health outcomes of migrant workers. These determinants include: geographically disparate disease epidemics and pathogens, biological and inherited characteristics, environmental factors, sociocultural practices, and political and personal circumstances (Gushulak and MacPherson 2011; Zimmerman et al. 2011).

For trafficked persons, this is the phase when criminal acts may begin, such as kidnappings, illegal border crossings and, for women and children, sexual violence. As a result, forced labourers are particularly vulnerable to trauma during this phase, which in turn negatively impacts their psychological and physical health throughout their ordeal (Zimmerman et al. 2011).

TRAVEL PHASE

The travel phase encompasses the period of time when migrant workers are between their country of origin and their destination or interception location, and could include multiple locations where the individuals stop for long or short periods of time. From a global public health perspective, this is the phase during which pathogens could be carried across different zones of disease prevalence and instigate changes in international and local transmissible disease epidemiology, as in the case of malaria among migrants moving between different African countries (Lynch and Roper 2011; Zimmerman et al. 2011).

For undocumented workers or trafficked persons, health influences during this phase are generally determined by the mode of transportation and circumstances of migration. For example, every year many Mexican migrants die from heat exposure on their journey across the desert into the United States, thus prompting several health education and support initiatives in US–Mexico border towns (Forster-Cox et al. 2010; Sapkota et al. 2006). Likewise, Central American migrants travelling through or to Mexico face risks of assault and robbery along migrant corridors. In recent years, the number of undocumented migrants travelling by boat across the Mediterranean to the EU has been steadily increasing, giving rise to a 'Mediterranean migrant crisis'. This phenomenon is characterized by overcrowded boats that are in poor condition, which in turn has resulted in many deaths caused by boats sinking or capsizing (Kassar and Dourgnon 2014). Between 2012 and 2013, approximately 460 undocumented migrants died while crossing the Mediterranean Sea, and in August 2015 a boat sank off the coast of Libya killing nearly 200 (Kassar and Dourgnon 2014; Kingsley 2015).

On the other end of the spectrum, for workers flying directly between their origin and destination, the travel phase may be reasonably short and involve minimal risk. In general, migrants with higher levels of socioeconomic status and those with legal contracts are more likely to travel under safe, direct and regularized conditions with minimal health risks, while poor and undocumented workers are more likely to face hazards during their journeys.

DESTINATION PHASE

This phase is marked by arrival at the destination country or region. In receiving countries, the arrival of migrant workers has implications for both public health and healthcare.

Migrant workers' health outcomes in destination countries are influenced by a variety of social determinants, including socioeconomic status, education and skill levels, work environments and degree of exploitation. Although high-skilled workers may suffer some health risks in destination countries, they often receive greater protections and benefits, whereas workers in low-skilled positions often fill dangerous, undesirable jobs characterized by precariousness, long hours, low pay and fewer protections (Benach et al. 2011; Sargeant and Tucker 2009). In fact, even when they are overqualified, migrant workers often serve as the low-skill labour force, and as such they fill the '3-D' jobs (dangerous, dirty and demanding) that are known to contribute to health disparities (Benach et al. 2011; Fernández and Ortega 2008; Quandt et al. 2013). Moreover, migrant workers in low-skilled positions regularly experience discrimination, exploitation and social isolation in destination countries (Benach et al 2011).

Many of the health issues facing migrant workers in receiving countries are related to occupational injuries. Few migrant workers receive the medical treatments they are entitled to, while the majority obtain no treatment at all (Benach et al. 2011; Sargeant and Tucker 2009). Beyond workplace injuries, migrant workers suffer a number of social problems, including social exclusion, fear of reprisals for demanding better working conditions, lack of health and safety training, linguistic barriers that minimize the effectiveness of training, concealing their need for medical care from employers, lack of knowledge regarding their rights as workers and difficulty accessing care and compensation when injured (Benach et al. 2011; McLaughlin and Hennebry 2013; McLaughlin et al. 2014b). Migrant workers' unstable working conditions and social isolation puts them at an increased risk of poor mental health outcomes, including anxiety, chronic stress and depression (Georges et al. 2013; Hovey and Magaña 2002; Mayell 2016; Mysyk et al. 2008). Moreover, their housing quality in destination countries predisposes them to poor sleep quality, which in turn places workers at increased risk for job injury as well as myriad mental and physical health consequences (Sandberg et al. 2014).

In destination countries, migrant workers face multiple barriers to accessing medical care, including: lack of transportation, insurance, and sick leave; fear or threat of wage or job loss; language barriers between workers and healthcare providers; and limitations in clinic hours of operation (Arcury and Quandt 2007; Hansen and Donohoe 2003; Moldovan 2015; Preibisch and Hennebry 2011; Hennebry et al. 2015). Communication with healthcare professionals is often further limited by illiteracy, and literacy barriers partly explain why the majority of migrant workers seek treatment for acute rather than chronic conditions or preventative services (Hansen and Donohoe 2003).

Women face added vulnerabilities in destination countries, as they are at increased risk of facing harassment and sexual exploitation. Women working irregular jobs are at an elevated risk of falling victim to smuggling by migration agents, criminal organizations or sex traffickers, which has a deleterious effect on their physical and mental health (Benach et al. 2011). Pregnant women who migrate for labour are at risk for negative pregnancy outcomes (Bollini et al. 2009). Children born to migrant workers are often excluded from the healthcare and education systems in destination countries, which in turn gives rise to poor physical and mental health outcomes (Martin et al. 1996; Yeoh and Lam 2007). Some receiving countries conduct mandatory pregnancy testing; for example, female migrant workers in Singapore and Taiwan are required to undergo pregnancy tests every six months and will be repatriated if they become pregnant (Constable 2013; Tseng and Wang 2011). Undocumented workers and trafficked persons are likewise vulnerable, and their social invisibility and abusive working and living conditions in destination countries predisposes such persons to enduring negative physical and psychological health outcomes (Zimmerman et al. 2011).

INTERCEPTION PHASE

This phase applies to undocumented workers and forced labourers, and is characterized first by interception by the authorities, followed by situations of temporary detention or interim residence. Interception strategies are often linked to immigration control policies used by states. Such policies are designed to stop the movements of undocumented workers, and they generally have negative or punitive implications (Steel et al. 2011; Zimmerman et al. 2011). The practice of confining workers under threat of persecution has a deleterious impact on their health and wellbeing (Steel et al. 2011).

RETURN PHASE

This migratory journey is complete when workers return to their place of origin. The health of returning migrant workers is largely determined by the cumulative exposure to social determinants of health and risk factors throughout the migratory process, and these vulnerabilities are exacerbated by the general conditions surrounding migration (Davies et al. 2011). Some of the determinants of health faced by returning workers include: reasons for migrating, type of travel, legal status and length of stay (Davies et al. 2010, 2011).

The mode of return is associated with health risks that directly impact health outcomes of migrant workers during and following their return. Workers who return through legal channels following a formal temporary migration are subject to fewer risks than those who return irregularly. Undocumented workers who migrate for informal work outside the regulatory norms of the sending, transit and receiving countries are at an increased risk for poor health outcomes, and they present challenges to health systems (Davies et al. 2011). Undocumented workers may travel clandestinely, which increases health consequences, including dehydration, physical injury or exposure to communicable diseases (IOM 2009).

Trafficked persons often experience a range of abuse, deprivation and violence, which results in serious physical and mental health consequences that persist long after their ordeal ends (Davies et al. 2011). Such persons who return home after suffering serious abuse may sustain elevated levels of distress, or psychiatric morbidity (Hossain et al. 2010).

Migrant workers returning to low-resource settings with life-threatening, disabling or chronic health concerns that require ongoing or high-tech treatment may have difficulty identifying or affording adequate care (Zimmerman et al. 2011). In fact, migrant workers with life-threatening conditions are often repatriated under conditions that do not adhere to human rights principles, which in turn places these workers at risk for long-term morbidity or mortality (Davies et al. 2011; Zimmerman et al. 2011). For some migrant workers, however, their remittances and remuneration help them afford a healthier lifestyle and improved healthcare for themselves and their families (Zimmerman et al. 2011).

CASE STUDY: MIGRANT WORKERS IN CANADIAN AGRICULTURE

With a population of just over 35 million (2014), Canada has the 19th highest level of gross national income per capita in the world – $51,690 as of 2014 (World Bank 2015). Like the United States and other advanced capitalist countries in the Global North, Canada has grown highly dependent on the use of migrant workers to support a flexible, globally competitive economy. This trend has been particularly evident in low-skilled, low-paid, high demand sectors such as agriculture and domestic work, in which few Canadians are willing to work under prevailing labour market conditions. Given its geographic location (sharing an international border only with another advanced Global North economy, the United States), undocumented migration is less common in Canada than it is in other countries that share borders (e.g., United States/Mexico) or small waterways (e.g., Southern Europe/Northern Africa) between richer and poorer regions, conditions which encourage higher levels of clandestine migration.

In this context, the Canadian government has worked to expeditiously and efficiently facilitate the movement of international migrants into various sectors of the economy through managed migration schemes, particularly its Temporary Foreign Worker Program (TFWP), which has various streams for skill levels and sectors, each with its own restrictions and guidelines. In this way, the Canadian government has appeased businesses' desire for low-paid, flexible and reliable labour, while limiting the potential of these migrants to gain citizenship by putting in place a strict 'point system' under which few low-skilled migrants can qualify (see Faraday 2012; Sharma 2006). As of 2012 there were approximately half a million temporary foreign workers (TFWs) across the country, a threefold increase in just ten years (see Curry 2014; Faraday 2012). With some exceptions in mainly high-skilled sectors, most of these workers come from the Global South, with top source countries including the Philippines, Mexico, the United States, India, Jamaica and Guatemala (Curry 2014).

While the use of the TFWP has exploded across various sectors of the economy over the past decade, this chapter will focus on one of the longest-standing groups of migrants: those who take part in the Seasonal Agricultural Workers Program (SAWP). Initiated as a pilot project between Jamaica and Canada in 1966, the SAWP has continually expanded and now includes about 40,000 workers migrating under bilateral contracts with Mexico and other Commonwealth Caribbean countries, including Trinidad and Tobago, Barbados and the Organization for Eastern Caribbean States (ESDC 2015). The SAWP is unique from other streams within the TFWP that employ workers in positions of up to four years at a time, as it is intended to be a seasonal, and often circular, migration programme. Workers are brought to work under contracts of between six weeks and eight months per year, after which they must return to their countries of origin. Upon the invitation or positive evaluation of employers, many workers return for successive years or even decades in a row, effectively living their lives as transnationals between two countries – spending winters with their families in their countries of citizenship, and the remainder of the year working 'temporarily' in Canada, their country of employment. Migrants are not permitted to bring families to Canada with them, nor are they typically allowed to visit families during their period of employment. This arrangement of constant movement between places of citizenship and employment and continual family separations generates unique risks and outcomes for migrants' mental and physical health; unsurprisingly, it is also difficult for migrant families, contributing to mental health concerns among spouses and children as well (McLaughlin 2009).

Under the SAWP, employers retain absolute control over their workforce compositions, as they may request specific nationalities and genders. This system results in shifting labour force compositions over time, and also the placement of workers in racialized and gendered tasks. For example, men are favoured for most physically demanding agricultural tasks, but women are often selected for specific 'delicate' tasks such as handling and packing soft fruit (e.g., peaches, grapes) or flowers (Preibisch and Binford 2007; McLaughlin 2010). As a result, only 3–4 per cent of requested workers are women. Similarly, Caribbean men appear to be favoured for crops such as tobacco, while Mexican men are preferred for work in greenhouses. As crops have shifted over time, with rising numbers of greenhouses, for example, so too have nationalities, resulting in more Mexican workers in place of those from the Caribbean. While overtly discriminatory, this system also generates a constant sense of pressure, precarity and competition among workers, who feel as though their jobs are always at risk of being replaced by either workers from the same nationality or others, and also works to undermine inter-group solidarity and resistance (Preibisch and Binford 2007; McLaughlin 2009, 2010).

In the pre-departure phase, pre-existing social determinants of health issues related primarily to low socioeconomic status – including low incomes, food precarity, low education levels and poor housing – place these workers at higher risks of health concerns. Notwithstanding these vulnerabilities, SAWP migrants normally begin their migration journeys as young, healthy adults. Given that employment prospects are bleak for many citizens of participating countries, there is a good deal of competition among prospective workers to enter the programme, and SAWP recruiters can take their pick based on a number of considerations, including health and physical stamina. Thorough medical exams that take place as part of recruitment and screening procedures ensure that selected applicants are fit for intense agricultural work and have no major health issues that may impact their ability to work or cause a drain on the health-care system (McLaughlin 2010). Thus, during the pre-departure phase, SAWP migrants tend to be in good health. The same remains true during the travel phase, in which workers are organized and transported by airplane and ground transportation from their point of departure to their destination farm, facing minimal risks along the journey. Accordingly, the SAWP does a good job of mitigating health risks both to migrant and destination populations during these first two migration phases. Indeed, the promise of safe, regularized travel is a major draw to the SAWP among prospective Mexican workers, as the US border has become increasingly perilous. These protections are a major advantage of legalized and government controlled labour migration programmes.

The health needs of workers are not as well protected in subsequent phases, however, particularly the destination and return phases. In fact, the Canadian government and society has largely neglected the health risks and needs of these workers for most of the decades of their employment. Throughout the programme's history, SAWP migrants have had legal access to workers' compensation and have been provided with free, legal access to 'universal' provincial healthcare services, the same as any Canadian citizen who may seek a doctor or hospital services without payment. These measures had been considered sufficient to manage their health needs. Over the past decade, however, a growing body of research as well as community groups have begun to recognize the unique and magnified health concerns of this population, and the challenges they face to access healthcare and related services even when given legal rights (Hennebry et al. 2015; McLaughlin and Hennebry 2015).

Living and working away from their families, in conditions under which they have very little control, and in societies in which they lack social support and integration, SAWP workers face a variety of risks related to their precarious, demanding and often dangerous employment, living and working conditions (Hennebry et al. 2015; McLaughlin et al. 2014a). Agriculture is among Canada's most dangerous industries, and farm workers face regular exposures to dust, chemicals, insects, machines, dangerous/sharp tools, farm vehicles and climactic extremes, as well as tasks that require continual bending and lifting, often without sufficient training or protective equipment (McLaughlin et al. 2014a). Workplace health and safety protections and regimes remain elusive for many workers, who are reluctant to raise concerns or make complaints for fear of angering employers and compromising their employment relationship (McLaughlin et al. 2014a; McLaughlin and Hennebry 2015). In this context, SAWP workers report high levels of health concerns, in particular related to musculoskeletal, skin, eye, respiratory, and gastrointestinal systems (Mayell et al. 2015; McLaughlin and Tew forthcoming). Women migrants face compounded risks of sexual and gender-based harassment and aggression, unwanted pregnancies and other sexual and reproductive concerns, while men, also living in highly masculinized environments, sometimes experience pressure to engage with sex workers (Edmunds et al. 2011; McLaughlin 2008, 2009; Narushima et al. 2015). All workers face numerous risks to their mental health related to the low-control, high-stress nature of their employment and repeated, prolonged family separations (Mayell 2016; McLaughlin 2009; Mysyk et al. 2008). Although living quarters are subject to pre-arrival health inspections, in practice they are often over-crowded and unsanitary (Hennebry et al. 2012; McLaughlin 2009).

While it is certainly commendable that Canada affords SAWP migrants legal access to healthcare services, there are numerous barriers that inhibit their full use in practice. For example, migrant workers' limited free hours on weekends and late evenings generally do not align with rural clinics' operating hours, nor can migrants – who are normally isolated on the rural properties of their employers – easily access transportation to seek care in town centres. Workers are reluctant to take time off work to seek care due to concerns over losing pay or angering employers (Hennebry et al. 2015). Workers also face barriers related to delays in receiving their insurance cards and information about their rights, as well as language and/or literacy barriers that prohibit effective communication during clinical encounters. Thus, migrants are often left at the mercy of their employers to mediate and facilitate access to healthcare, but they are often reluctant to disclose health concerns, for fear that this could negatively impact their prospects of future employment. For these and other reasons, many workers facing illness and injury often feel unable to benefit from the medical care and insurance programmes legally available to them (Hennebry et al. 2015; McLaughlin and Tew forthcoming; Pysklywec et al. 2011).

In recognition of the practical barriers to accessing health services faced by SAWP workers, in 2014 the Migrant Agricultural Workers Program (MAWP) was launched in the two regions of the province of Ontario with the highest concentrations of SAWP workers. This pilot programme was designed to mitigate practical barriers through the provision of walk-in style primary care clinics and community outreach. To this end, the clinics are situated in accessible locations frequented by SAWP migrants, operate at hours that coincide with the general days off in each region and offer Spanish translation services on-site. Many of the SAWP workers that visit the clinics suffer from musculoskeletal issues (back, neck, knees), gastrointestinal concerns, skin rashes and infections or eye injuries, and when surveyed many of these workers express that were it not for the migrant worker clinic, they would have gone without healthcare (Mayell et al. 2015). Other reasons workers sought care at the clinics included management of Type II diabetes and blood pressure, STI screening, prescription renewals and referrals to specialists for follow-up care. This programme also engages SAWP workers in health promotion education through community outreach and workshops that focus on topics such as occupational health and safety, mental health, nutrition and sexual health. Many of the workers expressed sincere gratitude for the clinics and workshops, often stating that in previous years they suffered while working in Canada without healthcare or community outreach. The MAWP is an example of a specialized healthcare model that is bolstered by community support, and the success of the clinics in both regions indicates the need for expansion of such initiatives to other agricultural regions in Canada (Mayell et al. 2015).

This effort, while laudable, only benefits a small proportion of migrant workers across the country, and its impacts are limited by the structural constraints of migrant employment. When workers do become sick or injured and are no longer able to work, they are normally fired and deported, a unique phenomenon in which illness, job loss and deportability are equated (see Orkin et al. 2014). In some cases, injured or sick workers prefer to stay in Canada, even if their work permits have expired, in the hopes that they can receive superior medical care than might be available in their countries of origin. For such workers, they may then lose their legal status and be subjected to the precarious circumstances associated with the interception phase, in which they may be hiding from authorities or being forced to return against their will (see McLaughlin and Hennebry 2013).The majority of workers, however, comply with the programme structure as intended, and acquiesce to managed repatriation when they are no longer able to work. Residing in employer-owned housing, many such workers see no alternative but to return, since they have nowhere else to live, no other income source and lose access to healthcare upon termination of their work permits.

The return phase for injured and ill workers also offers few, if any, supports. While some injured workers may be able to access long-term workers' compensation benefits, many others suffer the long-term consequences of illness or injury without access to benefits or other supports (McLaughlin 2009; McLaughlin et al. 2014b). Like many other bilateral migration programmes, the SAWP has failed to set up long-term or transborder health insurance, despite the fact that workers pay Canadian taxes and various programme administration fees that include supplementary insurance packages equivalent to travel insurance. Once workers are returned from Canada, they no longer have access to these healthcare services. This is a major shortcoming of the SAWP that has serious implications for workers facing long-term injuries and illnesses. Consequences for workers and their families can be devastating, especially when workers are no longer able to earn an income to support their families, and live with chronic pain, physical and/or mental limitations.

CONCLUSION

Despite migrant workers' centrality in the contemporary global economy, and the increasing international instruments aimed at recognizing and protecting their rights, their health considerations have been largely neglected in both policy and practice. As this chapter has shown, migrant workers face a variety of health risks across each stage of their journeys, although these risks and their outcomes vary considerably based on factors such as socioeconomic and legal status and gender. The case study of migrant agricultural workers in Canada illustrates the fluctuating health of workers throughout the migration process. Like many workers employed in low-skilled positions, these workers are structurally vulnerable and often experience poor health outcomes that result from the cumulative exposure to risk factors and the social determinants of health. While civil society and medical groups have begun to support the needs of migrants in specific localities, these efforts only scratch the surface, and their efficacy is limited by the structural precariousness embedded in migration systems like the SAWP. Recognizing the tremendous contributions that migrant workers make to various national economies, it is incumbent upon the international community, as well as sending and receiving states, to take greater responsibility for ensuring migrants' health is protected across all phases of their journeys.

REFERENCES

Ansell, N., S. Tsoeu and F. Hajdu (2015), Women's changing domestic responsibilities in neoliberal Africa: a relational time-space analysis of Lesotho's garment industry, *Gender, Place and Culture*, **22**(3), 363–382.

Arcury, T. and S. Quandt (2007), Delivery of Health Services to migrant and seasonal farmworkers, *Annual Review of Public Health*, **28**(1), 345–363.

Baum, T. (2012), *Migrant Workers in the International Hotel Industry*, paper presented International Labour Office, International Migration Branch, Sectoral Activities Department, Geneva: ILO.

Bélanger, D. and M. Rahman, (2013), Migrating against all the odds: international labour migration of Bangladeshi women, *Current Sociology*, **61**(3), 356–373.

Benach, J., C. Muntaner, C. Delclos, M. Menendez,and C. Ronquillo (2011), Migration and 'low-skilled' workers in destination countries, *PLOS Medicine*, **8**(6), e1001043.

Bollini, P., S. Pampallona, P. Wanner and B. Kupelnick (2009), Pregnancy outcome of migrant women and integration policy: a systematic review of the international literature, *Social Science and Medicine*, **68**(3), 452–461.

CCC (2009), *False Promises: Migrant Workers in the Global Garment Industry*, Clean Clothes Campaign discussion paper, Amsterdam.

Cholewinski, R. (2015), Evaluating bilateral labour migration agreements in the light of human and labour rights, in M. Panizzon, G. Zürcher and E. Fornalé (eds.), *The Palgrave Handbook of International Labour Migration: Law and Policy*, Basingstoke: Palgrave, pp. 231–252.

Constable, N. (2013), Migrant workers, legal tactics, and fragile family formations in Hong Kong, *Oñati Socio-Legal Series*, **3**(6), 1004–1022.

Curry, B. (2014), Everything you need to know about temporary foreign workers, *The Globe and Mail*, June, available online at www.theglobeandmail.com/news/politics/temporary-foreign-workers-everything-you-need-to-know/article18363279.

Davies, A. A., A. Basten and C. Frattini (2010), Migration: a social determinant of the migrants' health, *EuroHealth*, **16**(1), 10–12.

Davies, A. A., R. M. Borland, C. Blake and H. E. West (2011), The dynamics of health and return migration, *PLOS Medicine*, **8**(6), e1001046.

Edmunds, K., H. Berman, T. Basok, M. Ford-Gilboe and C. Forchuk, (2011), The health of women temporary agricultural workers in Canada: a critical review of the literature, *Canadian Journal of Nursing Research*, **43**(4), 68–91.

EDSC (2015), *Labour Market Opinions: Annual Statistics*, Employment and Social Development Canada, available online at http://www.esdc.gc.ca/en/reports/foreign_workers/2014/lmia_annual_statistics/agricultural.page?

Faraday, F. (2012), *Made in Canada: How the Law Constructs Migrant Workers' Insecurity*, Metcalfe Foundation Report, September.

Fernández, C. and C. Ortega (2008), Labor market assimilation of recent immigrants in Spain, *Spanish Economic Review*, **10**(2), 83–107.

Forster-Cox, S. C., T. Mangadu, B. Jacquez and L. Fullerton (2010), The Environmental Health/Home Safety Education Project: a successful and practical US–Mexico border initiative, *Health Promotion Practice*, **11**, 325–331.

Gallotti, M. (2009), *The Gender Dimension of Domestic Work in Western Europe*, International Migration Programme Paper 96, Geneva: International Labour Office.

Georges, A., T. Alterman, S. Gabbard, R. Shen, J. Nakamoto, D. J. Carroll and C. Muntaner (2013), Depression, social factors, and farmworker healthcare utilization, *Journal of Rural Health*, **29**, s7–s16.

Goldring, L. and P. Landolt (eds.) (2013), *Producing and Negotiating Non-citizenship: Precarious Legal Status in Canada*, Toronto: University of Toronto Press.

Gushulak, B. D. and D. W. MacPherson, (2011), Health aspects of the pre-departure phase of migration, *PLOS Medicine*, **8**(5), e1001035.

Hansen, E. and M. Donohoe (2003), Health issues of migrant and seasonal farmworkers, *Journal of Health Care for the Poor and Underserved*, **14**(2), 153–164.

Hennebry, J., K. Preibisch and J. McLaughlin (2012), *Health Across Borders – Health Status, Risks and Care among Transnational Migrant Farm Workers in Ontario*, Ontario: CERIS, the Ontario Metropolis Centre, Research Summary, February.

Hennebry, J., J. McLaughlin and K. Preibisch, (2015), Out of the loop: (in)access to health care for migrant workers in Canada, *Journal of International Migration and Immigration*, published online 14 January 2015.

Hossain, M., C. Zimmerman, M. Abas, M. Light and C. Watts (2010), The relationship of trauma to mental disorders among trafficked and sexually exploited girls and women, *American Journal of Public Health*, **100**, 2442–2449.

Hovey, J. D. and C. G. Magaña (2002), Exploring the mental health of Mexican migrant farm workers in the Midwest: psychosocial predictors of psychological distress and suggestions for prevention and treatment, *Journal of Psychology*, **136**(5), 493–513.

ILO (1949), *Migration for Employment Convention (Revised), 1949 (No. 97)*, Geneva: International Labour Organization.

ILO (2006), *ILO Multilateral Framework on Labour Migration: Non-Binding Principles and Guidelines for a Rights-Based Approach to Labour Migration*, Geneva: International Labour Organization.

ILO (2012), *ILO Global Estimate of Forced Labour: Results and Methodology*, Special Action Programme to Combat Forced Labour (SAP-FL), Geneva: International Labour Organization.

ILO (2013), *Mainstreaming of Migration in Development Policy and Integrating Migration in the Post-2015 UN Development Agenda*, Background Note, available online at www.ilo.org/wcmsp5/groups/public/---ed_protect/---protrav/---migrant/documents/genericdocument/wcms_220084.pdf.

ILO (2015a), *Promoting Decent Work for Migrant Workers*, paper presented at the Global Forum on Migration and Development in Geneva, Switzerland, 5 February 2015.

ILO (2015b), *The Fair Recruitment Initiative: Fostering Fair Recruitment Practices, Preventing Human Trafficking and Reducing the Costs of Labour Migration*, brochure issued in March 2015.

IOM (2004), Migration and Labour, Section 2.6, in *Essentials of Migration Management: A Guide for Policy Makers and Practitioners*, Geneva, Switzerland: International Organization for Migration.

IOM (2009), *Migrants' Needs and Vulnerabilities in the Limpopo Province, Republic of South Africa*, Report on Phase Two, February–March 2009, Pretoria: International Organization for Migration.

IOM (2010), World Migration Report 2010: The Future of Migration: Building Capacitates for Change, available online http://publications.iom.int/system/files/pdf/wmr_2010_english.pdf.

IOM (2014), *World Migration Report 2013: Migrant Wellbeing and Development*, Geneva: International Organization for Migration.

Kassar, H. and P. Dourgon (2014), The big crossing: illegal boat migrants in the Mediterranean, *European Journal of Public Health*, **24**(1), 11–15.

Kingsley, P. (2015), Migrant crisis: up to 200 dead after boat carrying refugees sinks off Libya, *Guardian*, 28 August, available online at www.theguardian.com/world/2015/aug/27/at-least-30-dead-after-boat-carrying-migrants-sinks-in-mediterranean.

Lucas, R. E. B. (2008), International labor migration in a globalizing economy, *Trade, Equity, and Development Program*, **92**, July, Carnegie Endowment for International Peace.

Lynch, C. and C. Roper (2011), The transit phase of migration: circulation of Malaria and its multidrug-resistant forms in Africa, *PLOS Medicine*, **8**(5): e1001040.

Martin, S. L., J. B. Kupersmidt and K. S. M. Harter (1996), Children of farm laborers: utilization of services for mental health, *Community Mental Health Journal*, **32**(4), 327–340.

Mayell, S. (2016), *Up-rooted Lives, Deep-rooted Memories: Stress and Resilience among Jamaican Agricultural Workers in Southern Ontario*, master's thesis, McMaster University.

Mayell, S., J. McLaughlin and M. Tew (2015), *Migrant Agricultural Workers and Canada's 'Not So Universal' Health Care System: Lessons Learned from an Effort to Improve Access to Health Care in the Province of Ontario*, paper presented at the International Congress on Rural Health, Lodi, Italy, 9 September.

McLaughlin, J. (2008), Gender, health and mobility: health concerns of women migrant farm workers in Canada, *Health Studies*, **7**(8), Paper 1.

McLaughlin, J. (2009), *Trouble in Our Fields: Health and Human Rights among Mexican and Caribbean Migrant Farm Workers in Canada*, dissertation, University of Toronto.

McLaughlin, J. (2010), Classifying the 'ideal migrant worker': Mexican and Jamaican transnational farmworkers in Canada, *Focaal*, **57**, 79–94.

McLaughlin, J. and J. Hennebry, (2013), Pathways to precarity: structural vulnerabilities and lived consequences for migrant farmworkers in Canada, in L. Goldring and P. Landolt (eds.), *Producing and Negotiating Non-Citizenship: Precarious Legal Status in Canada*, Toronto, ON: University of Toronto Press, pp. 176–190.

McLaughlin, J. and J. Hennebry (2015), Managed into the margins: examining citizenship and human rights of migrant workers in Canada, in R. E. Howard-Hassmann and M. Walton-Roberts (eds.), *The Human Right to Citizenship: A Slippery Concept*, Philadelphia,: University of Pennsylvania Press.

McLaughlin, J. and M. Tew (forthcoming), Migrant farm worker health care: unique strategies for a unique population, in N. Arya and T. Piggott (eds.), *Pursuing Health: Intervening to Improve Health Care of Underserved Populations in Canada*, Edmonton: Athabasca University Press.

McLaughlin, J., J. Hennebry and T. Haines (2014a), Paper versus practice: occupational health and safety protections and realities for temporary foreign agricultural workers in Ontario, *Perspectives interdisciplinaires sur le travail et la santé*, **16**(2), 2–17.

McLaughlin, J., J. Hennebry, D. Cole and G. Williams, (2014b), The migrant farmworker health journey: stages and strategies', *IMRC Policy Points*, International Migration Research Centre, Waterloo, ON.

Moldovan, A. (2015), Labour relations in Canada in light of provincial cleavages for migrant farm workers, *Glendon Journal of International Studies*, **8**(2), 1–26.

Mysyk, A., M. England and J. A. A. Gallegos (2008), Nerves as embodied metaphor in the Canada–Mexico seasonal agricultural workers program, *Medical Anthropology*, **27**(4), 383–404.

Narushima, M., J. McLaughlin and J. Barrett-Greene (2015), Needs, risks, and context in sexual health among temporary foreign migrant farmworkers in Canada: a pilot study with Mexican and Caribbean workers, *Journal of Immigrant and Minority Health*, 1–8.

OECD (2012), *International Migration Outlook 2012*, Paris: OECD Publishing, available online at www.npdata.be/BuG/165-NV-A-migratie/0ECD-Migration-Outlook-2012.pdf.

Orkin, A., M. Lay, J. McLaughlin, M. Schwandt and D. Cole (2014), Medical repatriation of migrant farm workers in Ontario: a descriptive analysis, *Canadian Medical Association Open Access Journal*, **2**(3), e192–e198.

Pearson, R. and K. Kusakabe (2012), Who cares? Gender, reproduction and care chains of Burmese migrant workers in Thailand, *Feminist Economics*, **18**(2), 149–175.

PICUM (2013), *PICUM Submission to the UN Committee on the Protection of the Rights of All Migrant Workers and Members of their Families*, presented at Day of General Discussion on the role of migration statistics for treaty reporting and migration policies, Geneva: Platform for International Cooperation on Undocumented Migrants.

Piper, N. (2013), *Contributions of Migrant Domestic Workers to Sustainable Development*, Bangkok: United Nations Entity for Gender Equality and the Empowerment of Women.

Preibisch, K. and L. Binford (2007), Interrogating racialized global labour supply: an exploration of the racial/national replacement of foreign agricultural workers in Canada, *Canadian Review of Sociology*, **44**(1), 5–36.

Preibisch, K. and J. Hennebry (2011), Temporary migration, chronic effects: the health of international migrant workers in Canada, *CMAJ*, **183**(9), 1033–1038.

Pysklywec, M., J. McLaughlin, M. Tew and T. Haines (2011), Doctors within borders: meeting the health care needs of migrant farm workers in Canada, *Canadian Medical Association Journal*, **183**, 1039–1042.

Qu, Z. and Z. Zhao (2011), *Evolution of the Chinese Rural–Urban Migrant Labor Market from 2002 to 2007*, discussion paper no. 5421 presented at the Institute for the Study of Labor (IZA), Bonn, January 2011.

Quandt, S. A., A. E. Arcury-Quandt, E. J. Lawlor, L. Carrillo, A. J. Marín, J. G. Grzywacz and T. A. Arcury (2013), 3-D jobs and health disparities: the health implications of Latino chicken catchers' working conditions, *American Journal of Industrial Medicine*, **56**, 206–215.

Qureshi, A. (2013), Structural violence and the state: HIV and labour migration from Pakistan to the Persian Gulf, *Anthropology and Medicine*, **20**(3), 209–220.

Rechel, B., P. Mladovsky, D. Ingleby, J. P. Mackenbach and M. McKee (2013), Migration and health in an increasingly diverse Europe, *The Lancet*, **381**, 1235–1245.

Richardson, G. E., P. L. Jenkins, T. Slingerland, C. Mason, M. Miles and J. J. May (2003), Occupational injury and illness among migrant and seasonal farmworkers in New York

State and Pennsylvania, 1997–1999: pilot study of a new surveillance method, *American Journal of Industrial Medicine*, **44**, 37–45.
Romero, M., V. Preston and W. Giles (2014), Care work in a globalizing world, in M. Romero, V. Preston and W. Giles (eds.), *When Care Goes Global: Locating the Social Relations of Domestic Work*, Surrey: Ashgate.
Sandberg, J. C. with J. W. Talton, S. A. Quandt, H. Chen, M. Weir, W. R. Doumani, A. B. Chatterjee and T. A. Arcury (2014), Association between housing quality and individual health characteristics among Latino farmworkers, *Journal of Immigrant Minority Health*, **16**, 365–272.
Sapkota, S., H. W. Khol, J. Gilchrist, J. McAuliffe, B. Parks, B. England, T. Flood. C. M. Sewell, D. Perrotta, M. Escobedo, C. E. Stern, D. Zane and K. B. Nolte (2006), Unauthorized border crossings and migrant deaths: Arizona, New Mexico, and El Paso, Texas, 2002–2003, *American Journal of Public Health*, **96**(7), 1282–1287.
Sargeant, M. and E. Tucker (2009), *Layers of Vulnerability in Occupational Health and Safety for Migrant Workers: Case Studies from Canada and the United Kingdom*, Comparative Research in Law & Political Economy, Research Paper No.8/2009.
Sharma, N. (2006), *Home Economics: Nationalism and the Making of 'Migrant Workers' in Canada*, Toronto: University of Toronto Press.
Steel, Z., B. J. Liddell, C. R. Bateman-Steel and A. B. Zwi (2011), Global protection and the health impact of migration interception, *PLOS Medicine*, **8**(6), e1001038.
Strauss, K. (2012), Coerced, forced and unfree labour: geographies of exploitation in contemporary labour markets, *Geography Compass*, **6**(3), 137–148.
Tseng, Y-F. and H-Z. Wang (2011), Governing migrant workers at a distance: managing the temporary status of guestworkers in Taiwan, *International Migration*, **51**(4), 1–19.
UN-DESA (2013a), The number of international migrants worldwide reaches 232 million, **2013**(2), 1–4, United Nations Department of Economic and Social Affairs.
UN-DESA (2013b), International migration 2013: migrants by origin and destination, **2013**(3), 1–4, United Nations Department of Economic and Social Affairs.
UN-DESA (2015), *Open Working Group Proposal for Sustainable Development Goals*, available online at https://sustainabledevelopment.un.org/focussdgs.html.
Wen, Y. and J. Hanley (2015), Rural-to-urban migration, family resilience, and policy framework for social support in China, *Asian Social Work and Policy Review*, **9**(1), 18–28.
Wickramasekara, P. (2015), *Bilateral Agreements and Memoranda of Understanding on Migration of Low Skilled Workers: A Review*, report prepared for the Labour Migration Branch, International Labour Organization, Geneva: ILO.
World Bank (2015), *Gross National Income Per Capita 2014, Atlas Method and PPP*, available online at http://databank.worldbank.org/data/download/GNIPC.pdf.
Yeoh, B. S. A. and T. Lam (2007), The cost of (im)mobility: children left behind and children who migrate with a parent, in *Perspective on Gender and Migration*, Bangkok: United Nations, pp. 120–149.
Zimmerman, C., L. Kiss and M. Hossain (2011), Migration and health: a framework for 21st century policy-making, *PLOS Medicine*, **8**(5), e1001034.

14 Occupational health and safety of migrant workers

Alison Reid

INTRODUCTION

The aim of this chapter is to examine the occupational health and safety (OH&S) of migrant workers and, where possible, to compare outcomes with native-born populations. I will start with an examination of the broad trends in international labour migration in recent years, and examine the determinants of occupational health and safety and how they differ between migrant and native-born workers. This will be followed by an examination of exposure to specific workplace hazards, namely carcinogens, workplace injustice, skill mismatch and work-related fatal and non-fatal accidents and injuries, where possible, comparing rates between migrant and native-born workers. I will conclude with a discussion of the Layers of Vulnerability framework that explains the reasons why migrants have differential occupational health and safety than native-born workers.

Of today's 232 million international migrants, half are estimated to be economically active, highlighting the importance of work and the quest for decent work as a driver of migration (International Organization for Migration 2013). Sargeant and Tucker (2009) define migrant workers as those workers who have a legal right to enter and work; those who have entered and are working but who do not have a legal right to work; temporary workers whose right to stay is time delimited, and foreign workers who have a right to stay but have not yet obtained permanent status (Sargeant and Tucker 2009). Other commonly used terms include: 'immigrant workers', those who migrate to another country for permanent residence; 'foreign-born workers', those not born in the country in which they are living and working (Loh and Richardson 2004); 'minority workers', those workers who differ from the majority population by race or ethnicity; and 'visible minority workers', those who are from minority racial groups phenotypically different to the majority population (e.g., in Canada, Asian, black and Aboriginal are visible minority groups compared with whites) (Breslin et al. 2006). In this chapter I will refer to 'migrant workers' as a generic term to cover all of the above definitions.

Globally, the majority of migrant workers are young and unskilled and do the '3-D' jobs: dirty, dangerous and difficult (Schenker 2008). In many destination countries, migrants tend to work in jobs in agriculture, construction, food processing and in semi-skilled or low-skilled manufacturing and low-paid service sector jobs (Benach et al. 2011), while many migrant women still work predominantly in 'cooking, caring and cleaning' sectors (Raijman et al. 2003). Industries such as agriculture, construction and transport have traditionally been the source of most work-related accidents, injuries and exposure to workplace hazards (Bonauto et al. 2006; Safe Work Australia 2014). In the United States, the term 'job ghetto' has been coined to describe the phenomena of minority workers being relegated to jobs with a disproportionate exposure to workplace hazards (Loomis and Richardson 1998).

More recently there has been an increasing trend among some countries (e.g., Australia and Canada) to focus on the recruitment of skilled workers. Migration of tertiary educated workers to OECD countries increased by more than 70 per cent between 2000 and 2010, with 17 per cent arriving in the past five years. This increase was largely driven by migrants from Asia, with India, China and the Philippines accounting for one-fifth of all tertiary-educated immigrants in OECD countries (OECD and UN 2013). These highly skilled workers tend to work as information communication and technology professionals, health workers and engineers (Australian Bureau of Statistics 2009; Dunnewijk 2008). Migrant workers therefore tend to cluster at the bottom and top of their destination-country occupational hierarchies, and occupational health and safety conditions vary greatly among these workers.

DETERMINANTS OF OCCUPATIONAL HEALTH AND SAFETY (OH&S)

A range of factors at the macro-level (e.g., labour market and employment conditions), the level of the organisation and the job, as well as characteristics of the migrant can influence occupational health and safety in the workplace (Landsbergis et al. 2014). This next section describes these determinants of OH&S, how they impact on worker health and safety, and how they have been found to differ between migrant and native-born workers.

MACRO-LEVEL DETERMINANTS

Legislation, regulation and enforcement of occupational health and safety standards are macro-level determinants that play an important role in protecting the health and safety of migrant workers. The Gulf Cooperation Council region (Kuwait, Bahrain, Oman, Qatar, Saudi Arabia and the United Arab Emirates) is the most popular region for temporary migrant workers (Malit and Al Youha 2013). In many of these countries, migrant workers are covered by employment laws distinct to those that apply to their own nationals. This exposes the migrants to occupational health and safety abuses including non-payment of salaries, restrictions on freedom to organise and collectively bargain and exploitative working conditions (Malit and Al Youha 2013). For example, Kuwait has three types of employment law: (1) the Kuwait Public Sector Law, (2) the Oil Sector Law and (3) the Private Sector Labour Law. Migrant workers in Kuwait are covered only by the Private Sector Labour Law, irrespective of which industry they work in (Boocock et al. 2011). A similar system exists in the United Arab Emirates (UAE) and Qatar, where migrant workers are covered by the Kafala Sponsorship system (Crepeau 2014). This system links a work permit to a sponsor, often the employer. Therefore changing jobs or obtaining an exit visa is not possible without permission from the sponsor, thus increasing a migrant's vulnerability to exploitation. Additionally, migrant workers in this region are typically taken on by private recruitment agents, who often exploit the workers by charging large fees and so encouraging debt bondage (Agunias 2010).

However, domestic workers (largely female) who make up 19 per cent of the migrant labour force in Kuwait, were specifically excluded from a new Private Sector Labour Law introduced in 2010 to improve the wages and working conditions of migrant workers, meaning that they tend to have even poorer protections than other migrant workers (Boocock et al. 2011). The situation is similar in the UAE and Qatar where domestic workers are covered by the Ministry of the Interior while other foreign-born workers are covered by the Ministry of Labour (Malit and Al Youha 2013). This system has implications for reporting occupational health and safety complaints because domestic workers can only lodge complaints against their employer through the Department of Immigration, who may then forward the complaint on to either the police or labour hire agents (Boocock et al. 2011; Malit and Al Youha 2013).

Differential enforcement of occupational health and safety regulations and policies in specific industries may have a greater impact on migrant than native-born workers. For example, farms that employ fewer than ten workers in several US states are exempt from Occupational Safety and Health Administration (OSHA) regulations. Recent work has shown higher worker fatality rates in those states that observe this exemption than in states that do not (Somervell and Conway 2011). This is likely to impact most on foreign-born workers, as 78 per cent of US farmworkers were born outside of the United States (JBS International 2012). Equally, the suspension of wage policies and occupational health and safety regulations during the clean-up after hurricanes Katrina and Rita mostly impacted Hispanic day labourers (Delp et al. 2009; Pastor et al. 2006).

PRECARIOUS WORK AND PRECARIOUS STATUS AS A DETERMINANT OF OCCUPATIONAL HEALTH AND SAFETY

'Precarious' work is an employment condition that developed, globally, as a result of deregulation of the labour market and employer/labour market demand for flexible employment practices. Precarious workers have been found to have higher work-related injury rates and reduced knowledge about OH&S regulation and practice, and they are less likely than workers with full-time, permanent jobs with job security, paid leave and other employee benefits to complain about their working conditions or to seek legal protection or redress (Benavides et al. 2006; Quinlan et al. 2001). Temporary workers employed on casual contracts or through labour hire contractors or agencies are less likely to be entitled to work benefits such as sick pay or paid holidays (McDowell et al. 2009) and reports of underpayment or non-payment of wages are not uncommon (Underhill and Rimmer 2015). Precarious work has also been associated with increased risks of psychological distress and ill-health (Virtanen et al. 2005) and physical ill health (Benavides et al. 2000).

Migration for some workers is synonymous with precarious work (Woolfson and Likic-Brboric 2008). In the United Kingdom, for example, the increase in precarious work has been linked to the increase in the number of economic migrants following the expansion of the European Union in 2004 (McDowell et al. 2009). Low-skilled service jobs in hotels and restaurants, employing up to 60 per cent of foreign-born workers in London, are among the most 'precarious' types of jobs (Dyer et al. 2011). Similarly in Spain, the prevalence of employment precariousness among Spanish-born workers was 45.2 per cent compared with 77.1 per cent among foreign-born workers (Vives et al. 2011).

Many migrants are employed on contracts or in temporary jobs, but another group of migrants come to a country on a temporary working visa. These migrants are particularly vulnerable to workplace exploitation, which may be exacerbated as a result of their visa status, where in many cases their right of stay is dependent on their employer (Preibisch 2010). Reports of underpayment of wages – particularly those who were paid for piecework where the piece rate was set too low – and non-payment of wages were common complaints among temporary migrants working in the horticulture industry in Australia (Underhill and Rimmer 2015). Similar findings have been reported from other countries and across a range of industries (Anderson 2010; Fudge and MacPhail 2009; Lowell 2001; Mares 2005; Potter and Hamilton 2014). As a condition of their visa, in some cases the employer must provide accommodation for temporary migrants. Reports of unsanitary, overcrowded, unventilated and dilapidated housing are not uncommon (Preibisch and Hennebry 2011).

A further dimension of precariousness is that of the irregular or undocumented migrant, those migrants who do not have the requisite documents to work legally in the receiving country. Overall, research examining the OH&S of this group of workers is limited because of the difficulties involved in reaching this largely hidden group of workers. However, statistics from Australia report that undocumented workers tend to work in agriculture, forestry, fishing, construction and accommodation and food services (Clibborn 2015). Similarly, in Canada, undocumented workers are based in construction, hospitality, manufacturing or as domestics, such as cleaners, cooks and housekeepers (Magalhaes et al. 2010), industries in which the work is often seasonal and part-time, therefore increasing their precariousness. Undocumented workers are excluded from employment laws in Australia, the United Kingdom and Ireland, but some European countries and Canada and the United States permit varying degrees of employment rights (Clibborn 2015). Seeking redress against workplace exploitation is unlikely to occur because of the risk of deportation (McKay et al. 2009).

Reports from several sources show that undocumented workers are at risk of workplace abuse and exploitation. Undocumented migrant farmworkers in California, for example, were more likely to work for a farm labour contractor rather than directly for a grower, were less likely to be aware of workers' compensation schemes and were more likely to use *raiteros* (informal and often expensive drivers) for transportation to and from worksites (Villarejo et al. 2010). Undocumented Latino workers in Cincinnati and Santa Fe conveyed a reluctance to report unsafe conditions or injuries at work for fear of deportation (Flynn et al. 2015). In Australia, a government inquiry to examine the effectiveness of the Migration Amendment Act reported that undocumented workers were 'underpaid, misled about what they are doing, undernourished, beaten and threatened' (Howells 2011). Similarly, young undocumented workers working in the UK reported disparities in working conditions and pay between themselves and documented co-workers, and susceptibility to employer and gang-master abuse (Bloch 2013; Wilkinson 2014). However documentation status was not found to influence either work tasks or exposure to hazards directly among household service workers in Spain (Ahonen et al. 2009).

WORK ORGANISATION AND JOB LEVEL DETERMINANTS OF OCCUPATIONAL HEALTH AND SAFETY

Features of work organisation and job specific characteristics have been associated with work-related injury and illness and hazard exposure. Increased risk of injury has been associated with long working hours (Dembe et al. 2005), shift work (Horwitz and McCall 2004), effort–reward imbalance (the combination of low rewards at work and high effort) (Siegrist 1996; Rugulies and Krause 2008) and job strain (the combination of high demand and low control at work) (Karasek 1979; Kim et al. 2009). Similarly the number of employees is an important factor for adverse OH&S outcomes. Small to medium-size enterprises (SMEs) (often defined as having fewer than 20 employees) have consistently shown more work-related accidents and injury fatalities and more ergonomic, physical and chemical exposures than larger enterprises (Sørensen et al. 2007). Factors related to the specific job or tasks that can increase the risk of occupational injury and illness include exposure to hazards such as psychosocial or ergonomic or chemical hazards, or loud noise. For example, working at high speed, undertaking continuous repetitive work or carrying heavy loads have been associated with musculoskeletal disorders (Punnett and Wegman 2004).

Work from several countries has reported disparities in work organisation and employment arrangements between migrant, foreign and native-born workers. In Europe, working conditions and employment arrangements were shown to differ between migrant and native-born populations (Ronda Pérez et al. 2012). Male manual migrant workers self-reported the most exposure to negative working conditions of all the groups (migrant/non-migrant/male/female/manual/non-manual). Their prevalence of exposure, presented as a prevalence ratio adjusted for age, education and industrial sector with 95 per cent confidence intervals (aPR, 95%CI), was higher for eight of 11 negative working conditions compared with non-migrants. Non-manual migrant males and females were exposed to more negative working arrangements, such as shift work (aPR 1.66, 95%CI 1.27–2.17) and (aPR 1.61, 95%CI 1.29–2.01) respectively and variable start and finish times (aPR 1.17, 95%CI 1.04–1.32) and (aPR 1.10, 95%CI 1.01–1.19) for males and females respectively. Manual migrant females had greater exposure to carrying or lifting heavy loads and adverse employment arrangements such as not having a contract (aPR 2.94, 95%CI 2.07–4.10), and not being free to decide days off or holidays (aPR 1.25, 95%CI 1.07–1.48) (Ronda Pérez et al. 2012).

However, a similar study from Spain reported a lower prevalence of self-reported exposure to occupational health risks (physical load, safety risks, chemicals/physical agents and psychosocial factors) among male and female manual migrant workers than native-born workers. Twenty exposures were assessed and are presented as odds ratios with 95%CI (aOR, 95%CI) adjusted for age, education and contract type to show the relationship between OH&S risk and migration status. Only standing for many hours a day (aOR 1.92, 95%CI 1.20–3.07) and working cutting objects (aOR 1.62, 95%CI 1.02–2.57) were increased among non-manual migrant male and female workers respectively, compared with Spanish-born workers (Ronda et al. 2013). Different perceptions of self-reported exposure among migrant and Spanish-born workers may explain this finding.

An unequal distribution of OH&S risks has been observed among migrant compared with Canadian-born workers. Measures of immigration status (e.g., length of time in Canada, visible minority status, mother tongue) were associated with five of six OH&S risk factors examined (e.g., working in small workplaces or in a physically demanding occupation). In particular, immigrants who had lived in Canada for less than 21 years were less likely to belong to a union and more likely to work in a workplace with fewer than 20 employees. Visible minorities were more likely to work shift work and to have non-permanent employment than Canadian-born workers. Adjustment for industry did not attenuate the relationships and in some cases marginally increased the risks associated with immigration characteristics. This suggests that the higher exposure to occupational health and safety risks among immigrants is not due solely to the industry they work in but also due to other factors that position immigrants in jobs that contain more OH&S risks (Smith and Mustard 2010). Similarly, an examination of working arrangements between foreign and native-born workers in Australia found that foreign-born workers were more likely to work without paid leave entitlements (16.2 per cent versus 13.8 per cent), on a contract or a fixed term (9.7 per cent versus 8.5 per cent), and to work shift work (15.6 per cent versus 12.7 per cent) compared with Australian-born workers (Reid et al. 2014).

The most common complaint among immigrant workers in Chicago attending an Interfaith Workers' Rights Centre was their failure to get paid for their scheduled hours or overtime. This condition in many cases stemmed from the way the workers were employed, often on a verbal contract and so when lesser wages were received, they could not produce written proof of agreement (de Castro et al. 2006). Similar reports emerge from the United Kingdom where migrants across the country reported routinely working overtime, sometimes without extra payment and mostly without being paid an overtime premium. Working hours were often reported in excess of 60 hours per week in agriculture, hotels and catering, and processing and packaging, and some workers reported getting less than the national minimum for holidays or not knowing their holiday entitlements (McKay et al. 2006). Research in Spain also found that female migrant household service workers reported an inability to take breaks or sick or personal time because of work-time constraints (Ahonen et al. 2009).

INDIVIDUAL-LEVEL MIGRANT WORKER DETERMINANTS OF OCCUPATIONAL HEALTH AND SAFETY

Attributes of the migrant worker can also impact on their practice and understanding of occupational health and safety. Lack of proficiency in speaking the dominant language in the receiving country, for example, can be a determinant for exposure to negative working conditions and employment arrangements. Among recent migrants to Canada, those who came on a family class or refugee visa, and those with less English proficiency were statistically significantly more likely to be employed in more physically demanding occupations two and four years after migrating than skilled migrants (Smith et al. 2009a). Similarly, limited-English-proficient foreign-born Hispanic men in the United States were found to receive significantly higher compensating wages, because they were working in unsafe jobs, than their English fluent counterparts (Dávila et al. 2011). Other work from Canada examined the mechanisms between lack of language proficiency and disparities in occupational health and safety. Lack of language proficiency affected workers' ability to understand and communicate information and limited their supporting relationships that can affect work and health (Premji et al. 2008).

Beliefs about work and safety and the use of personal protective equipment (PPE) have been reported to differ by cultural background (Reid et al. 2014). Among Latino roofers working in the United States, for example, productivity was favoured over safety, and use of PPE was limited if it reduced productivity or was uncomfortable to use. Participants felt that they needed to work fast in order to secure more work, which improved their job security (Arcury et al. 2014). However, a review of the literature examining national culture and safety in the oil and gas industry found that proximal influences such as management commitment to safety were more influential on workforce behaviour than national values (Mearns and Yule 2009). Precarious work and the demands of production as well as cultural factors were shown to impact on foreign-born workers in Australia reporting OH&S incidents. Understanding and practice of OH&S in Australia differed by community integration and cohesiveness, duration of residence, type of job, skill level and level of education (Reid et al. 2014).

In summary, determinants of OH&S can differ among migrant and native-born workers at macro-level, at the level of work organisation and job- and individual-level characteristics that influence the OH&S outcomes of migrant workers.

EXPOSURE TO WORKPLACE HAZARDS

This next section examines specific workplace exposures, namely exposure to carcinogens, workplace injustice and skill mismatch and how they may differ between migrant and native-born workers.

Carcinogens

Occupational cancers (e.g., mesothelioma, lung and bladder cancers) are cancers caused by exposure to carcinogens at work and are therefore largely preventable. Carcinogens are chemical (e.g., pesticides or diesel exhaust), physical (e.g., asbestos or radiation) or organisational (e.g., shift work) exposures that increase the incidence of malignant neoplasms. In general, little is known about the risk of occupational cancer among migrant workers (Zahm and Blair 1993). Similarly, little is known about the prevalence of exposure to workplace carcinogens among workers and less is known for migrant workers or whether the prevalence of exposure differs between migrant and native-born workers. Nonetheless, some work has been undertaken to examine the prevalence of exposure to carcinogens at work and whether this differs by migration status.

An examination of exposure to chemical and physical agents among migrant and Spanish-born workers in Spain found no difference in self-reported exposure between manual workers, male and female. However male, non-manual migrant workers reported a twofold non-statistically significant risk of inhaling dust, smoke and toxic, noxious gases (Ronda et al. 2013). Foreign-born workers in the United States, however, had a lower prevalence of self-reported exposure to dusts and chemicals than US-born workers (Quinn et al. 2007). Other work has examined the prevalence of exposure by race or ethnic status. For example, Maori workers in New Zealand self-reported greater exposure to dusts (OR 2.04, 95%CI 1.03–4.06) after adjusting for age and matching on occupation compared with European-ancestry New Zealanders (Eng et al. 2011).

These studies suffer from several limitations that make interpreting their findings difficult. Most of these studies ask participants to self-report their exposure to carcinogens at work. This is a limitation because it assumes the participant has a high level of knowledge about carcinogens and their means of exposure that may be unrealistic (McGuire et al. 1998). Also, the perception of exposure to carcinogens has been shown to vary by ethnicity (Macias 2015; Vaughan and Nordenstam 1991), suggesting that exposure reporting may be under- or overestimated in some groups. Another limitation is that many studies require their participants to speak the dominant language in order to participate in the study, therefore possibly excluding those most at risk of exposure and underestimating the prevalence of exposure (Premji and Krause 2010).

CASE STUDY

One study (Boyle et al. 2015a) attempted to address these limitations. In 2013, telephone interviews were conducted with 749 ethnic minority workers (EM-AWES) (210 (28 per cent) Arabic,[1] 232 (31 per cent) Vietnamese and 307 (41 per cent) Chinese workers, aged 18–65 years) residing in the cities of Perth, Melbourne or Sydney, Australia. The telephone numbers of surnames most likely to fit the populations of interest were selected from a list purchased from a commercial survey sampling firm, and a random sample was selected from these numbers. Participants could complete the interview in English, Arabic, Vietnamese, Mandarin or Cantonese. Questions sought basic demographic information, job title and tasks undertaken in their current occupation, which was used to determine whether they were potentially exposed to any of 38 predetermined workplace carcinogens, such as asbestos, lead, diesel engine exhaust and polycyclic aromatic hydrocarbons (Fernandez et al. 2012). The interview was terminated if the participant's job was designated as not exposed to any of the predetermined carcinogens. The remaining participants were asked questions about the specific tasks they do in their current job, the frequency of those tasks, how they were performed and whether any protective measures were taken. The questions relate to tasks performed by participants and not exposure to chemicals, so information bias is limited and participants do not self-report their exposure. Based on the answers to the questions, participants were classified as unexposed, possibly or probably exposed to each of the 38 carcinogens.

Thirty-two per cent of the EM-AWES participants were assessed as being probably exposed to at least one of the 38 carcinogens. More Arabs (38.6 per cent) than Chinese (31.0 per cent) or Vietnamese (27.4 per cent) were exposed and more men (41.5 per cent) than women (19.3 per cent). The most common exposure among men was to solar ultraviolet radiation (20.6 per cent), environmental tobacco smoke (17.3 per cent), diesel engine exhaust (15.1 per cent) and silica (9.6 per cent). Among women, the most common exposures were environmental tobacco smoke (6.9 per cent), polycyclic aromatic hydrocarbons (4.5 per cent), ionising radiation (3.9 per cent) and solar ultraviolet radiation (3.3 per cent) (Boyle et al. 2015a).

The prevalence of exposure to carcinogens among the ethnic minority workers was compared with that of a subset of English-speaking Australian-born workers, also residing in the cities of Perth, Melbourne and Sydney (n = 952). This study (the Australian Workplace Exposure Study – AWES) was conducted in 2012 and used the same methodology as that used in the EM-AWES described here, except that participants could only complete the interview in English and therefore had to have sufficient English ability to complete the interview by telephone (Carey et al. 2014).

Compared with the English-speaking Australian-born workers, the prevalence of overall exposure was slightly higher among the ethnic minority workers (31.6 per cent versus 29.7 per cent), although the difference was only statistically significantly greater among the Arabs (38.6 per cent). After adjusting for occupation, Arab and Vietnamese participants were more likely to be exposed to silica and Chinese participants more likely to be exposed to polycyclic aromatic hydrocarbons than English-speaking Australian-born workers. However, exposure to solar ultraviolet radiation was lower among Chinese and Vietnamese participants and exposure to diesel engine exhaust and benzene was lower among Chinese participants than English-speaking Australian-born participants. A possible explanation for these differences is that workers in the same occupations conduct different tasks and carcinogen exposure is likely to differ between tasks, i.e., for silica exposure the Arabic and Vietnamese workers may be doing the 'dirtier tasks' than the English-speaking Australian-born workers. Insufficient sample size in this study prevented the examination of whether tasks within occupations varied by ethnic minority status (Boyle et al. 2015a).

Twenty-six per cent of participants opted to complete the telephone interview in a language other than English (LOTE) (Arabic 29.5 per cent, Chinese 31.6 per cent and Vietnamese 16.4 per cent). Prevalence of exposure was statistically significantly higher among participants who interviewed in a LOTE (39.6 per cent) compared with those who interviewed in English (28.8 per cent). The prevalence of exposure to the five most common carcinogens (solar ultraviolet radiation, environmental tobacco smoke, diesel engine exhaust, polycyclic aromatic hydrocarbons and silica) was higher among participants who interviewed in a LOTE compared with those who interviewed in English. Results from the regression modelling showed that without adjusting for occupation, those who interviewed in a LOTE were 20 per cent more likely to be exposed to a workplace carcinogen (RR=1.19, 95%CI 0.94–1.52). After adjusting for occupation the estimate attenuated (RR=1.08, 95%CI 0.86–1.36), suggesting that workers who were interviewed in a LOTE were working in different jobs, that were possibly lower skilled and more hazardous than those who were interviewed in English. Excluding those who chose to be interviewed in a LOTE would have underestimated the prevalence of exposure to workplace carcinogens by 8.9 per cent (Boyle et al. 2015b). This study highlights the importance of examining carcinogens among and between different ethnic groups and the necessity of offering multilingual interviewing when researching migrants and ethnic minority groups.

WORKPLACE INJUSTICE AND SKILL MISMATCH

Collectively racism, discrimination, harassment, abuse or bullying that occur in the workplace are referred to as 'workplace injustice' (Okechukwu et al. 2014). Considerable research has been undertaken to examine workplace injustice among specific racial groups – for example, Hispanic and African-American workers in the United States (Krieger et al. 2006) – but few have examined the experience of migrants or immigrants specifically in the workplace. The effect of workplace injustice may be greater among migrant and immigrant workers because they are generally resident in their host country for reasons of work and economy and have often invested considerable resources in the migration process. Workplace injustice can occur before the worker gets a job in their host country. Labour stratification segregates workers into lower jobs based on their ethnicity (job ghettos) (Loomis and Richardson 1998). In the same vein, several studies have shown that employers fail to interview applicants from specific ethnic backgrounds, thereby discriminating against applicants for certain types of jobs (Okechukwu et al. 2014). In Australia, for example, a Chinese applicant had to submit 64 per cent more applications to get the same number of interviews as a Caucasian Australian applicant (Berman 2008; Booth et al. 2012). Recent immigrants to Australia reported leaving off non-Australian work experience from their applications, not stating qualifications obtained in their home countries and anglicising their names in order to get a job interview (Kosny et al. 2016). Parallel findings were found among recent migrants to Spain who reported a social division of work between themselves and Spanish-born workers where immigrants were limited to applying for jobs in construction, hotels and restaurants, domestic service and agriculture (Agudelo-Suárez et al. 2009).

Workplace injustice once an immigrant worker has obtained a job can take many different forms. Indigenous farmworkers in the United States (those immigrants from Mexico who speak Triqui or Mixteco rather than Spanish), for example, were restricted to working in more physically taxing roles and were consequently more exposed to adverse weather conditions and pesticides than non-Indigenous farmworkers (Holmes 2006, 2011). Similarly immigrant workers in Germany (first- and second-generation migrants) were exposed to more psychosocial stressors but similar levels of task stressors as German workers (Hoppe 2011). Migrant workers in England reported discrimination that took the form of name-calling and harassment by supervisors and co-workers and their allocation to the worst shifts and denial of favourable terms and conditions granted to local workers (McKay et al. 2006). Meanwhile Nepalese construction workers in Hong Kong reported more incidents of racist name-calling and jokes than Pakistani and other minority worker groups (Kwok Wai Wong and Lin 2014).

Workplace injustice has also been shown to impact on the OH&S of workers. Among Latino poultry processors in the United States, abusive power relations based on ethnicity, immigration status and rank were the basis for occupational injuries and illnesses, particularly among women. Specifically, retaliatory supervision was associated with increased odds of neck and back pain for men and women and increased odds of arm and hand pain, lower body pain, eye problems and injury or illness for women (Marín et al. 2009). Among Chinese and white workers in Toronto, disparities in exposure to adverse working conditions was more pronounced among Chinese women (Premji and Lewchuk 2014). Similarly, when the supervisor valued work safety, the use of job-appropriate personal protective equipment (PPE) was significantly greater among Latino poultry processing workers compared with those whose supervisor placed less value in safety at work (Arcury et al. 2012). It is unclear whether workplace injustice impacts on the reporting and challenging of poor working conditions among migrant workers.

Skill or qualification mismatch or underutilisation (e.g., working in a job for which you are overqualified) also constitutes a workplace hazard (Sauter et al. 1999).The International Organization for Migration (IOM) recognises this as a particular problem for highly qualified migrant women, many of whom work in professions linked to social reproduction (health, education and culture), whose skills are less transferable between countries. Therefore qualified women are often unable to apply their skills and are pushed into lower-skilled employment (Mollard and Umar 2012). In Australia, an examination of three longitudinal cohort studies of recent migrants reported that between 36 and 49 per cent of participants used their skills in their current job sometimes/rarely or never up to 42 months after arrival in Australia. This finding was associated with poorer mental health as measured by the General Health Questionnaire (e.g., depression, anxiety somatic symptoms and social withdrawal (Reid 2012). Similar findings were reported among recent migrants to Canada (Chen et al. 2010; Shetterly et al. 1996). As well as poor mental health outcomes, working in mismatched jobs may also increase exposure to occupational health and safety risks. In the United Kingdom, for example, migrant workers reported being offered potentially dangerous jobs such as scaffolders without the experience or qualifications to undertake the work (McKay et al. 2006).

WORK-RELATED FATAL AND NON-FATAL ACCIDENTS AND INJURIES

Examining rates of work-related injuries (WRI) and injury fatalities has been the most common method to study differences between migrant and foreign and native-born workers. Administrative data is often used for this examination, such as the US Bureau of Labor Statistics Census of Occupational Fatalities (Byler 2013; Loh and Richardson 2004; Sincavage 2005) or national death records (Reid et al. 2015) and hospital admissions or trauma data (Forst et al. 2010; Friedman and Forst 2008; McGreevy et al. 2010; Reid et al. 2015), or compensation claim records (Premji et al. 2010; Tiagi 2015). A range of national surveys (e.g., labour force surveys, community health surveys) have also been examined (Reid et al. 2014; Salvatore et al. 2013; Smith and Mustard 2009; Zhang et al. 2009). All of these data sources have inherent limitations when comparing work-related injuries between migrant and native-born workers. Migrant and foreign-born workers may be less likely to claim compensation than native-born workers as has been shown from work undertaken in Canada (Smith et al. 2009b), and so are likely to be underrepresented in compensation statistics. Also, compensation and accident statistics in many countries do not tend to capture claimant nationality (Guldenmund et al. 2013). Because of the precarious nature of many migrants' work, they are less likely to be included in official surveys or databases. Likewise, occupational injuries are often not the main focus of national surveys or, if they are, numbers may be small. Similarly migrants form a small proportion of a nationally representative survey and so again numbers are likely to be small limiting the possibility of examining these issues (Reid et al. 2014).

Nevertheless, despite the wide range of data sources used, increased risks of work-related injury and fatalities in migrants and foreign-born workers (compared with native-born workers) have been reported from a range of countries. In particular a higher rate of work-related fatalities has been reported among Hispanic and Latino workers in the United States compared with native-born workers working in a range of occupations and industries (Forst et al. 2010). With deindustrialisation, work-related fatalities decreased by 45 per cent among all workers in the United States between 1980 and 1996 (Loomis et al. 2004). In contrast, they increased from 4.3 to 5.7 per 100,000 among foreign-born workers and most of this increase was observed in Hispanic and Latino workers (Loh and Richardson 2004). An update using the same data showed that fatality rates for the years 2006–2008 were higher among Hispanic and Latino workers (4.8 per 100,000) compared with all workers (4.0 per 100,000) and in particular fatality rates were higher among foreign-born Hispanic and Latino workers (5.7 per 100,000) than native-born Hispanic and Latino workers (3.6 per 100,000) (Byler 2013). Hispanic migrants largely work in the high-risk industries of agriculture, construction and transport (Schenker 2010).

Comparison of work-related injury (WRI) rates among other ethnic group workers and native-born US workers is less clear. Non-fatal WRI rates between 1997 and 2005 were lower among foreign-born workers (50 per 10,000) in the US compared with native-born workers (89 per 10,000) (Zhang et al. 2009). However, only medically consulted injuries were included in this report and 35 per cent of foreign-born were uninsured compared with 12.5 per cent of US-born workers. Therefore WRI is likely to be underestimated among the foreign-born. Other work examining the Census of Fatal Occupational Injuries found that overall, fatal WRI were lower among Asian native (1.65 per 100,000) and foreign-born (2.85 per 100,000) workers compared with non-Asian foreign (5.38 per 100,000) and native-born (4.03 per 100,000) workers between 1997 and 2003. However, the workplace homicide rate was considerably higher among Asian foreign-born (1.38 per 100,000) workers compared with non-Asian native (0.37 per 100,000) and foreign-born (0.94 per 100,000) workers (Sincavage 2005).

Higher rates of fatal and non-fatal injury rates among migrant workers compared with native-born workers have been shown from work undertaken in other countries. Work examining the 2003 and 2005 Canadian

Community Health Surveys showed that immigrants who arrived in the previous five years had an increased risk of work-related injuries that required hospital admission, but a lower rate of activity limiting injuries overall than Canadian-born workers (Smith and Mustard 2009). Work-related injuries were significantly higher among immigrants to Italy (OR 1.82, 95%CI 1.53–2.16) than Italian-born males (Salvatore et al. 2013), and foreign-born workers, male (RR 3.9, 95%CI 3.9–3.9; RR 4.4, 95%CI 3.9–5.1) and female (RR 5.4, 95%CI 5.4-5.56; RR 6.0, 95%CI 3.6-9.6) had higher rates of fatal and non-fatal WRI respectively, compared with Spanish-born workers (Ahonen and Benavides 2006).

Migration of workers to developing countries is also associated with an excess risk of work-related injuries. Among foreign-born workers in Qatar, for example, rates of work-related non-fatal injuries per 100,000 workers ranged from 84.3 among 'Others', 46.2 for Nepalese workers, 23.0 among Indian workers, 16.3 among Filipino to 4.84 among Qatari workers (Al-Thani et al. 2015).

In contrast, more recent work from Canada examined compensation claims data and found no difference in occupational injury rates between immigrant and Canadian-born workers and in contrast found that newly arrived migrants had lower work-related injuries compared with the Canadian-born (Tiagi 2015). Similarly, recent work examining work-related injury fatalities and admissions to hospital found lower rates among foreign-born workers compared with Australian-born workers (Reid et al. 2015).

DISCUSSION AND CONCLUSION

Migrant, immigrant, foreign-born workers often have differential exposure to the determinants of occupational health and safety than native-born workers, which impacts detrimentally on their exposure to workplace hazards and work-related fatal and non-fatal accidents and injuries. The Layers of Vulnerability framework (hereafter referred to as the 'framework') explains why this may be the case (Sargeant and Tucker 2009). The framework is composed of layers of macro- and meso-level OH&S risk factors that have been shown to explain the observed disparities in working conditions that exist among and between migrant workers and native-born workers. *Layer 1* consists of OH&S risk factors that are specific to migration. This includes such things as the legal status of the migrant in the receiving country, whether legal status is tied to an employment contract or the role and practice of recruitment agents. As shown above, access to work rights and protections varies by legal status across countries, and where a migrant has full legal status they may be reluctant to enforce those rights. For example, migrant workers with undocumented migration status and precarious work are very vulnerable to this risk factor, but so too are those workers whose right of stay is contingent on a contract with one employer. Similarly, the way that migrants are recruited can impact on their OH&S vulnerabilities. Those who are indebted to a recruitment agent or employer because of excessive fees paid to obtain their job may be reluctant to complain about adverse working conditions. In contrast, some countries – for example, the Philippines – license recruitment agents and provide a regulatory role to ensure that migrant workers are protected from illegal recruitment and abuse (O'Neil 2004). *Layer 2* consists of OH&S risk factors specific to the migrant worker. This layer includes such factors as socioeconomic conditions in the home country or their education and skill levels and receiving-country language proficiency. Workers from poor countries are less likely to enforce their work rights but may also try to boost their earnings in the receiving country by working long hours and taking risks, because they are unable to return to a comparable job in their own country. Less-educated and lower-skilled workers have fewer labour market opportunities, they may not have received OH&S training, may be unaware of their OH&S rights and entitlements and may have little control over the demands placed on them at work. In the same vein, migrant workers who are not proficient in the dominant language may be less likely to receive OH&S training, be unable to read warning signs and instructions or learn about their legal rights. For example, a humanitarian migrant, who has skills and qualifications from his own country, but who has poor English-language skills and has pressure to send remittances back to his family, may be more inclined to work long hours to maximise his income in a job in which he does not use his skills and qualifications, where he may increase his risk of incurring a work-related injury (Dembe et al. 2005). *Layer 3* consists of OH&S factors related to the receiving country. This includes such factors as the sectors in which the migrant workers are employed, or the socioeconomic conditions in the receiving country or the workers social inclusion/exclusion. In practice, large organisations are less hazardous than small or medium-size enterprises and some industries and occupations are more hazardous than others. Therefore, the industry, occupation and firm where a migrant is employed can influence their vulnerability. As discussed above, migrants can be segregated into the more hazardous jobs or jobs with a higher level of compensated risk (Premji et al. 2010). In contrast, a worker who migrated independently as a skilled migrant, who is working for a large employer and whose migration status is not dependent on that employer, would have few OH&S vulnerabilities.

The Layers of Vulnerability framework therefore recognises the heterogeneity of migrant work and helps to explain why migrant workers experience different degrees of OH&S vulnerabilities, leading to differential occupational health and safety compared with native-born workers. Additionally the framework identifies those migrants who are most vulnerable to OH&S risks. This information can be used to develop, strengthen and enforce legislation and regulation at the national and international level to ensure that the work rights and protections of the most vulnerable migrant workers are equal to those of native-born workers.

NOTE

1. Arabic refers to people who self-identified as having an Arabic language speaking ancestry. Most study participants in this group were born in Australia (26 per cent), Lebanon (26 per cent), Egypt (7 per cent), Iraq (9 per cent), Sudan (5 per cent), Syria (4 per cent) and Saudi Arabia (3 per cent) and other countries in the Middle East.

REFERENCES

Agudelo-Suárez, A., D. Gil-González, E. Ronda-Pérez, V. Porthé, G. Paramio-Pérez, A. M. García and Garí, A. (2009), Discrimination, work and health in immigrant populations in Spain, *Social Science & Medicine*, **68**(10), 1866–1874.

Agunias, D. V. (2010), Migration's Middlemen: Regulating Recruitment Agencies in the Philippines-United Emirates Corridor, Migration Policy Institute, available online at www.migrationpolicy.org/research/migrations-middlemen-regulating-recruitment-agencies-philippines-united-arab-emirates.

Ahonen, E. and F. G. Benavides (2006), Risk of fatal and non-fatal occupational injury in foreign workers in Spain, *Journal of Epidemiology & Community Health*, **60**(5), 424–426.

Ahonen, E., M. J. López Jacob, M. L. Vázquez, V. Porthé, D. Gil González, A. M. García, C. Ruiz Frutos, J. Benach, and F. G. Benavides (2009), Invisible work, unseen hazards: the health of women immigrant household service workers in Spain, *American Journal of Industrial Medicine*, **53**(4), 405–416.

Al-Thani, H., A. El-Menyar, R. Consunji, A. Mekkodathil, R. Peralta, K. A. Allen and A. A. Hyder (2015), Epidemiology of occupational injuries by nationality in Qatar: evidence for focused occupational safety programmes, *Injury*, **46**(9), 1806–1813.

Anderson, B. (2010), Migration, immigration controls and the fashioning of precarious workers, *Work, Employment & Society*, **24**(2), 300–317.

Arcury, T. A., J. G. Grzywacz, A. M. Anderson, D. C. Mora, L. Carrillo, H. Chen and S. A. Quandt (2012), Personal protective equipment and work safety climate among Latino poultry processing workers in Western North Carolina, USA, *International Journal of Occupational and Environmental Health*, **18**(4), 320–328.

Arcury, T. A., P. Summers, L. Carrillo, J. G. Grzywacz, S. A. Quandt and T. H. Mills (2014), Occupational safety beliefs among Latino residential roofing workers, *American Journal of Industrial Medicine*, **57**(6), 718–725.

Australian Bureau of Statistics (2009), *Perspectives on Migrants: Skilled Migrants*, available online at www.abs.gov.au/AUSSTATS/abs@.nsf/Lookup/3416.0Main+Features32009.

Benach, J., C. Muntaner, C. Delclos, M. Menéndez and C. Ronquillo (2011), Migration and 'low-skilled' workers in destination countries, *PLOS Medicine*, **8**(6), 775.

Benavides, F. G., J. Benach, A. V. Diez-Roux and C. Roman (2000), How do types of employment relate to health indicators? Findings from the Second European Survey on Working Conditions, *Journal of Epidemiology and Community Health*, **54**(7), 494–501.

Benavides, F. G., J. Benach, C. Muntaner, G. L. Delclos, N. Catot and M. Amable (2006), Associations between temporary employment and occupational injury: what are the mechanisms? *Occupational and Environmental Medicine*, **63**(6), 416–421.

Berman, G. (2008), *Harnessing Diversity: Addressing Racial and Religious Discrimination in Employment*, Melbourne: Victorian Equal Opportunity & Human Rights Commission.

Bloch, A. (2013), The labour market experiences and strategies of young undocumented migrants, *Work, Employment & Society*, **27**(2), 272–287.

Bonauto, D., B. Silverstein, D. Adams and M. Foley (2006), Prioritizing industries for occupational injury and illness prevention and research, Washington State Workers' compensation claims, 1999–2003, *Journal of Occupational and Environmental Medicine*, **48**(8), 840–851.

Boocock, M., S. Jamieson, Z. Hannif, R. Lamare, F. Lamm, C. Martin, N. McDonnell, C. Robertson, P. Schweder and B. Shulruf (2011), Occupational health and safety of migrant workers: an international concern, in M. Sargeant and M. Giovannone (eds.), *Vulnerable Workers: Health, Safety and Well-Being*, London: Gower, pp. 121–144.

Booth, A. L., A. Leigh and E. Varganova (2012), Does ethnic discrimination vary across minority groups? Evidence from a field experiment, *Oxford Bulletin of Economics and Statistics*, **74**(4), 547–573.

Boyle, T., R. N. Carey, D. C. Glass, S. Peters, L. Fritschi and A. Reid (2015a), Prevalence of occupational exposure to carcinogens among workers of Arabic, Chinese and Vietnamese ancestry in Australia, *American Journal of Industrial Medicine*, **58**(9), 923–932.

Boyle, T., R. N. Carey, S. Peters, D. C. Glass, L. Fritschi and A. Reid (2015b), Demographic and occupational differences between ethnic minority workers who did and did not complete the telephone survey in English, *Annals of Occupational Hygiene*, **59**(7), 862–871.

Breslin, F. C., P. Smith, C. Mustard and R. Zhao (2006), Young people and work injuries: an examination of jurisdictional variation within Canada, *Injury Prevention*, **12**(2), 105–110.

Byler, C. G. (2013), Hispanic/Latino fatal occupational injury rates, *Monthly Labor Review*, **136**, 14.

Carey, R. N., T. R. Driscoll, S. Peters, D. C. Glass, A. Reid, G. Benke and L. Fritschi (2014), Estimated prevalence of exposure to occupational carcinogens in Australia (2011–2012), *Occupational and Environmental Medicine*, **71**(1), 55–62.

Chen, C., P. Smith and C. Mustard (2010), The prevalence of over-qualification and its association with health status among occupationally active new immigrants to Canada, *Ethnicity & Health*, **15**(6), 601–619.

Clibborn, S. (2015), Why undocumented immigrant workers should have workplace rights, *The Economic and Labour Relations Review*, **26**(3), 465–473.

Crepeau, F. (2014), *Report of the Special Rapporteur on the human rights of migrants. Addendum: Mission to Qatar*, United Nations General Assembly.

Dávila, A., M. T. Mora and R. González (2011), English-language proficiency and occupational risk among Hispanic immigrant men in the United States, *Industrial Relations: A Journal of Economy and Society*, **50**(2), 263–296.

de Castro, A. B., K. Fujishiro, E. Sweitzer and J. Oliva (2006), How immigrant workers experience workplace problems: a qualitative study, *Archives of Environmental & Occupational Health*, **61**(6), 249–258.

Delp, L., L. Podolsky and T. Aguilar (2009), Risk amid recovery: occupational health and safety of Latino day laborers in the aftermath of the Gulf Coast hurricanes, *Organization & Environment*, **22**(4), 479–490.

Dembe, A. E., J. B. Erickson, R. G. Delbos and S. M. Banks (2005), The impact of overtime and long work hours on occupational injuries and illnesses: new evidence from the United States, *Occupational and Environmental Medicine*, **62**(9), 588–597.

Dunnewijk, T. (2008), *Global Migration of the Highly Skilled: A Tentative and Quantitative Approach*, UNU-MERIT Working Paper Series, Maastricht: United Nations University.

Dyer, S., L. McDowell and A. Batnitzky (2011), Migrant work, precarious work–life balance: what the experiences of migrant workers in the service sector in Greater London tell us about the adult worker model, *Gender, Place & Culture*, **18**(5), 685–700.

Eng, A., A. Mannetje, L. Ellison-Loschmann, D. McLean, S. Cheng and N. Pearce (2011), Ethnic differences in patterns of occupational exposure in New Zealand, *American Journal of Industrial Medicine*, **54**(5), 410–418.

Fernandez, R. C., T. R. Driscoll, D. C. Glass, D. Vallance, A. Reid, G. Benke and L. Fritschi (2012), A priority list of occupational carcinogenic agents for preventative action in Australia, *Australia and New Zealand Journal of Public Health*, **36**(2), 111–115.

Flynn, M. A., D. E. Eggerth and C. J. Jacobson (2015), Undocumented status as a social determinant of occupational safety and health: the workers' perspective, *American Journal of Industrial Medicine*, **58**(11), 1127–1137.

Forst, L., S. Avila, S. Anozie and R. Rubin (2010), Traumatic occupational injuries in Hispanic and foreign born workers, *American Journal of Industrial Medicine*, **53**(4), 344–351.

Friedman, L. S. and L. Forst (2008), Ethnic disparities in traumatic occupational injury, *Journal of Occupational and Environmental Medicine*, **50**(3), 350–358.

Fudge, J. and F. MacPhail (2009), The temporary foreign worker program in Canada: low-skilled workers as an extreme form of flexible labour, *Comparative Labor Law and Policy Journal*, **31**, 101–139.

Guldenmund, F., B. Cleal and K. Mearns (2013), An exploratory study of migrant workers and safety in three European countries, *Safety Science*, **52**, 92–99.

Holmes, S. M. (2006), An ethnographic study of the social context of migrant health in the United States, *PLOS Medicine*, **3**(10), e448.

Holmes, S. M. (2011), Structural vulnerability and hierarchies of ethnicity and citizenship on the farm, *Medical Anthropology*, **30**(4), 425–449.

Hoppe, A. (2011), Psychosocial working conditions and well-being among immigrant and German low-wage workers, *Journal of Occupational Health Psychology*, **16**(2), 187.

Horwitz, I. B. and B. P. McCall (2004), The impact of shift work on the risk and severity of injuries for hospital employees: an analysis using Oregon workers' compensation data, *Occupational Medicine*, **54**(8), 556–563.

Howells, S. (2011), *Report of the 2010 Review of the Migration Amendment (Employer Sanctions) Act 2007, Prepared for the Minister for Immigration and Citizenship*, Canberra: Government of Australia.

International Organization for Migration (2013) *Labour Migration*, available online at www.iom.int/cms/en/sites/iom/home/what-we-do/labour-migration.html.

JBS International (2012) National Agricultural Workers Study Data Tables, Secondary National Agricultural Workers Study Data Tables.

Karasek, R. A. (1979), Job Demands, job decision latitude, and mental strain: implications for job redesign, *Administrative Science Quarterly*, **24**(2), 285–308.

Kim, H. C., J. Y. Min, K. B. Min and S. G. Park (2009), Job strain and the risk for occupational injury in small-to medium-sized manufacturing enterprises: a prospective study of 1,209 Korean employees, *American Journal of Industrial Medicine*, **52**(4), 322–330.

Kosny, A., I. Santos and A. Reid (2016), Employment in a 'land of opportunity'? Immigrants' experiences of racism and discrimination in the Australian workplace, *Journal of International Migration and Integration*.

Krieger, N., P. D. Waterman, C. Hartman, L. M. Bates, A. M. Stoddard, M. M. Quinn, G. Sorensen and E. M. Barbeau (2006), Social hazards on the job: workplace abuse, sexual harassment, and racial discrimination – a study of black, Latino, and white low-income women and men workers in the United States, *International Journal of Health Services*, **36**(1), 51–85.

Kwok Wai Wong, J. and A. Lin (2014), Construction workplace discrimination: experiences

of ethnic minority operatives in Hong Kong construction sites, *Engineering, Construction and Architectural Management*, **21**(4), 403–420.
Landsbergis, P. A., J. G. Grzywacz and A. D. LaMontagne (2014), Work organization, job insecurity, and occupational health disparities, *American Journal of Industrial Medicine*, **57**(5), 495–515.
Loh, K. and S. Richardson (2004), Foreign-born workers: trends in fatal occupational injuries, 1996–2001, *Monthly Labor Review*, **127**, 42.
Loomis, D. and D. Richardson (1998), Race and the risk of fatal injury at work, *American Journal of Public Health*, **88**(1), 40–44.
Loomis, D., D. B. Richardson, J. F. Bena and A. J. Bailer (2004), Deindustrialisation and the long term decline in fatal occupational injuries, *Occupational and Environmental Medicine*, **61**(7), 616–621.
Lowell, B. L. (2001), Skilled temporary and permanent immigrants in the United States, *Population Research and Policy Review*, **20**(1–2), 33–58.
Macias, T. (2015), Environmental risk perception among race and ethnic groups in the United States, *Ethnicities*, 15 March.
Magalhaes, L., C. Carrasco and D. Gastaldo (2010), Undocumented migrants in Canada: a scope literature review on health, access to services, and working conditions, *Journal of Immigrant and Minority Health*, **12**(1), 132–151.
Malit, F. T. and A. Al Youha (2013) *Labor Migration in the United Arab Emirates: Challenges and Responses*, available online at www.migrationpolicy.org/article/labor-migration-united-arab-emirates-challenges-and-responses.
Mares, P. (2005), *Seasonal Migrant Labour: A Boon for Australian Country Towns?* Paper presented at the 2nd Future of Australia's Country Towns Conference, Bendigo, Victoria, July 11–13.
Marín, A. J., J. G. Grzywacz, T. A. Arcury, L. Carrillo, M. L. Coates and S. A. Quandt (2009), Evidence of organizational injustice in poultry processing plants: possible effects on occupational health and safety among Latino workers in North Carolina, *American Journal of Industrial Medicine*, **52**(1), 37–48.
McDowell, L., A. Batnitzky and S. Dyer (2009), Precarious work and economic migration: emerging immigrant divisions of labour in Greater London's service sector, *International Journal of Urban and Regional Research*, **33**(1), 3–25.
McGreevy, K., D. Lefkowitz, D. Valiante and S. Lipsitz (2010), Utilizing hospital discharge data (HD) to compare fatal and non-fatal work-related injuries among Hispanic workers in New Jersey, *American Journal of Industrial Medicine*, **53**(2), 146–152.
McGuire, V., L. M. Nelson, T. D. Koepsell, H. Checkoway and W. Longstreth (1998), Assessment of occupational exposures in community-based case-control studies, *Annual Review of Public Health*, **19**(1), 35–53.
McKay, S., M. Craw and D. Chopra (2006), *Migrant Workers in England and Wales: An Assessment of Migrant Worker Health and Safety Risks*, Health and Safety Executive.
McKay, S., E. Markova, A. Paraskevopoulou and T. Wright (2009), *The Relationship Between Migration Status and Employment Outcomes*, Undocumented Workers Transitions Report.
Mearns, K. and S. Yule (2009), The role of national culture in determining safety performance: challenges for the global oil and gas industry, *Safety Science*, **47**(6), 777–785.
Mollard, B. and S. Umar (2012), Gender, migration and deskilling: a broad review of the literature, in *Crushed Hopes: Underemployment and Deskilling among Skilled Migrant Women*, Geneva: International Organization for Migration, pp. 9–29.
OECD and UN (2013) *World Migration in Figures: A Joint Contribution by UN-DESA and the OECD to the United Nations High-Level Dialogue on Migration and Development*, 3–4 October 2013.
Okechukwu, C. A., K. Souza, K. D. Davis and A. B. de Castro (2014), Discrimination, harassment, abuse, and bullying in the workplace: contribution of workplace injustice to occupational health disparities, *American Journal of Industrial Medicine*, **57**(5), 573–586.

O'Neil, K. (2004), Labor export as government policy: the case of the Philippines, *Migration Information Source*, **1**.
Pastor, M., R. D. Bullard, J. K. Boyce, A. Fothergill, R. Morello-Frosch and B. Wright (2006), *In the Wake of the Storm: Environment, Disaster and Race after Katrina*, New York: Russell Sage Foundation, available online at www.e-education.psu.edu.geog882/files/file/in_the_wake_of_the_storm.pdf.
Potter, M. and J. Hamilton (2014), Picking on vulnerable migrants: precarity and the mushroom industry in Northern Ireland, *Work, Employment & Society*, **28**(3), 390–406.
Preibisch, K. (2010), Pick-your-own labor: migrant workers and flexibility in Canadian agriculture, *International Migration Review*, **44**(2), 404–441.
Preibisch, K. and J. Hennebry (2011), Temporary migration, chronic effects: the health of international migrant workers in Canada, *Canadian Medical Association Journal*, **183**(9), 1033–1038.
Premji, S. and N. Krause (2010), Disparities by ethnicity, language, and immigrant status in occupational health experiences among Las Vegas hotel room cleaners, *American Journal of Industrial Medicine*, **53**(10), 960–975.
Premji, S. and W. Lewchuk (2014), Racialized and gendered disparities in occupational exposures among Chinese and white workers in Toronto, *Ethnicity & Health*, **19**(5), 512–528.
Premji, S., K. Messing and K. Lippel (2008), Broken English, broken bones? Mechanisms linking language proficiency and occupational health in a Montreal garment factory, *International Journal of Health Services*, **38**(1), 1–19.
Premji, S., P. Duguay, K. Messing and K. Lippel (2010), Are immigrants, ethnic and linguistic minorities over-represented in jobs with a high level of compensated risk? Results from a Montréal, Canada study using census and workers' compensation data, *American Journal of Industrial Medicine*, **53**(9), 875–885.
Punnett, L. and D. H. Wegman (2004), Work-related musculoskeletal disorders: the epidemiologic evidence and the debate, *Journal of Electromyography and Kinesiology*, **14**(1), 13–23.
Quinlan, M., C. Mayhew and P. Bohle (2001), The global expansion of precarious employment, work disorganization, and consequences for occupational health: a review of recent research, *International Journal of Health Services*, **31**(2), 335–414.
Quinn, M. M., G. Sembajwe, A. M. Stoddard, D. Kriebel, N. Krieger, G. Sorensen, C. Hartman, D. Naishadham and E. M. Barbeau (2007), Social disparities in the burden of occupational exposures: results of a cross-sectional study, *American Journal of Industrial Medicine*, **50**(12), 861–875.
Raijman, R., S. Schammah-Gesser and A. Kemp (2003), International migration, domestic work, and care work undocumented Latina migrants in Israel, *Gender & Society*, **17**(5), 727–749.
Reid, A. (2012), Under-use of migrants' employment skills linked to poorer mental health, *Australian and New Zealand Journal of Public Health*, **36**(2), 120–125.
Reid, A., E. Lenguerrand, I. Santos, U. Read, A. D. LaMontagne, L. Fritschi and S. Harding (2014), Taking risks and survival jobs: foreign-born workers and work-related injuries in Australia, *Safety Science*, **70**, 378–386.
Reid, A., S. Peters, N. Felipe, E. Lenguerrand and S. Harding (2015), The impact of migration on deaths and hospital admissions from work-related injuries in Australia, *Australian and New Zealand Journal of Public Health*.
Ronda, E., A. A. Agudelo-Suárez, A. M. García, M. J. López-Jacob, C. Ruiz-Frutos and F. G. Benavides (2013), Differences in exposure to occupational health risks in Spanish and foreign-born workers in Spain (Itsal Project), *Journal of Immigrant and Minority Health*, **15**(1), 164–171.
Ronda Pérez, E., F. G. Benavides, K. Levecque, J. G. Love, E. Felt and R. Van Rossem (2012), Differences in working conditions and employment arrangements among migrant and non-migrant workers in Europe, *Ethnicity & Health*, **17**(6), 563–577.
Rugulies, R. and N. Krause (2008), Effort–reward imbalance and incidence of low back and neck injuries in San Francisco transit operators, *Occupational and Environmental Medicine*, **65**(8), 525–533.

Safe Work Australia (2014), *Work-Related Traumatic Injury Fatalities Australia 2013*, Canberra: Safe Work Australia.
Salvatore, M. A., G. Baglio, L. Cacciani, A. Spagnolo and A. Rosano (2013), Work-related injuries among immigrant workers in Italy, *Journal of Immigrant and Minority Health*, **15**(1), 182–187.
Sargeant, M. and E. Tucker (2009), Layers of Vulnerability in occupational safety and health for migrant workers: case studies from Canada and the UK, *Policy and Practice in Health and Safety*, **7**(2), 51–73.
Sauter, S., L. Murphy, M. Colligan, N. Swanson, F. Scharf, R. Sinclair, P. Grubb, L. Goldenhar, T. Alterman, J. Johnston, A. Hamilton and J. Tisdale (1999), *Stress at Work*, DHHS (NIOSH) Publication Number 99–101.
Schenker, M. (2008), Work-related injuries among immigrants: a growing global health disparity, *Occupational and Environmental Medicine*, **65**(11), 717–718.
Schenker, M. (2010), A global perspective of migration and occupational health, *American Journal of Industrial Medicine*, **53**(4), 329–337.
Shetterly, S. M., J. Baxter, L. D. Mason and R. F. Hamman (1996), Self-rated health among Hispanic vs non-Hispanic white adults: the San Luis Valley Health and Aging Study, *American Journal of Public Health*, **86**(12), 1798–1801.
Siegrist, J. (1996), Adverse health effects of high-effort/low-reward conditions, *Journal of Occupational Health Psychology*, **1**(1), 27–41.
Sincavage, J. R. (2005), Fatal occupational injuries among Asian workers, *Monthly Labor Review*, **128**(10), 49–55.
Smith, P. M. and C. A. Mustard (2009), Comparing the risk of work-related injuries between immigrants to Canada and Canadian-born labour market participants, *Occupational and Environmental Medicine*, **66**(6), 361–367.
Smith, P. M. and C. A. Mustard (2010), The unequal distribution of occupational health and safety risks among immigrants to Canada compared to Canadian-born labour market participants: 1993–2005, *Safety Science*, **48**(10), 1296–1303.
Smith, P. M., C. Chen and C. Mustard (2009a), Differential risk of employment in more physically demanding jobs among a recent cohort of immigrants to Canada, *Injury Prevention*, **15**(4), 252–258.
Smith, P. M., A. A. Kosny and C. A. Mustard (2009b), Differences in access to wage replacement benefits for absences due to work-related injury or illness in Canada, *American Journal of Industrial Medicine*, **52**(4), 341–349.
Somervell, P. D. and G. A. Conway (2011), Does the small farm exemption cost lives? *American Journal of Industrial Medicine*, **54**(6), 461–466.
Sørensen, O. H., P. Hasle and E. Bach (2007), Working in small enterprises: is there a special risk? *Safety Science*, **45**(10), 1044–1059.
Tiagi, R. (2015), Are immigrants in Canada over-represented in riskier jobs relative to Canadian-born labor market participants? *American Journal of Industrial Medicine*, **58**(9), 933–942.
Underhill, E. and M. Rimmer (2015), Layered vulnerability: temporary migrants in Australian horticulture, *Journal of Industrial Relations*, **0**(0), 1–19.
Vaughan, E. and B. Nordenstam (1991), The perception of environmental risks among ethnically diverse groups, *Journal of Cross-Cultural Psychology*, **22**(1), 29–60.
Villarejo, D., S. A. McCurdy, B. Bade, S. Samuels, D. Lighthall and D. Williams (2010), The health of California's immigrant hired farmworkers, *American Journal of Industrial Medicine*, **53**(4), 387–397.
Virtanen, M., M. Kivimäki, M. Joensuu, P. Virtanen, M. Elovainio and J. Vahtera (2005), Temporary employment and health: a review, *International Journal of Epidemiology*, **34**(3), 610–622.
Vives, A., C. Vanroelen, M. Amable, M. Ferrer, S. Moncada, C. Llorens, C. Muntaner, F. G. Benavides and J. Benach (2011), Employment precariousness in Spain: prevalence, social distribution, and population-attributable risk per cent of poor mental health, *International Journal of Health Services*, **41**(4), 625–646.

Wilkinson, M. (2014), Demonising 'the other': British government complicity in the exploitation, social exclusion and vilification of new migrant workers, *Citizenship Studies*, **18**(5), 499–515.
Woolfson, C. and B. Likic-Brboric (2008), Migrants and the unequal burdening of 'toxic' risk: towards a new global governance regime, *Debatte*, **16**(3), 291–308.
Zahm, S. H. and A. Blair (1993), Cancer among migrant and seasonal farmworkers: an epidemiologic review and research agenda, *American Journal of Industrial Medicine*, **24**(6), 753–766.
Zhang, X., S. Yu, K. Wheeler, K. Kelleher, L. Stallones and H. Xiang (2009), Work-related non-fatal injuries among foreign-born and US-born workers: findings from the US National Health Interview Survey, 1997–2005, *American Journal of Industrial Medicine*, **52**(1), 25–36.

15 Winds of change: climate change, migration and health

Celia McMichael

INTRODUCTION: CLIMATE CHANGE AND MIGRATION

Earth's climate has been relatively stable for thousands of years. For more than a century, however, industrialization has led to increased emissions of CO_2 and other greenhouse gases; there is now near-unanimous consensus among climate scientists that anthropogenic climate change is occurring. The atmosphere and ocean have warmed, the amounts of snow and ice have diminished, and the sea level has risen (IPCC 2014). Models predict that by the year 2100, Earth's mean surface temperature (relative to 1986– 2005) is likely to rise 0.3–1.7°C (low emissions scenario) to 2.6–4.8°C (high emissions scenario), sea levels (relative to 1986–2005) will rise 0.26–0.82m, increasing CO_2 concentrations will lead to further ocean acidification, and weather variability will increase significantly (IPCC 2014). The magnitude of the projected climatic changes is affected substantially by the choice of future emissions scenarios. These climatic changes will have significant impacts on humans, including patterns of migration, displacement and planned relocation (Foresight 2011; Warner et al. 2013). First, this chapter provides a broad overview of the relationship between climate change and migration; it then discusses the implications of climate-related migration for human health and wellbeing.

Currently, there are an estimated 232 million international migrants, approximately 740 million people migrating within their own country, and an unknown number of migrants in 'irregular' situations (IOM 2014). Drivers of contemporary migration include globalization, socioeconomic disparities, demographic change, skills shortages, political crises and shifting capital and opportunities. Climate change will further shape patterns of human migration in coming years and decades, as it amplifies and creates pressures that contribute to the displacement and migration of individuals, families and communities (ADB 2012; Black et al. 2011; McMichael et al. 2012).

The relationship between climate change and human migration is complex (Barnett and Webber 2009; Bardsley and Hugo 2010). Climate change produces environmental effects that can act as contributory and proximate causes of human migration and mobility, including both slow-onset change (e.g., sea-level rise, drought, food insecurity) and fast-onset changes (e.g., extremes of flooding, cyclones) (Birk and Rasmussen 2014). The relationship between slow-onset environmental change and migration is poorly understood; for example, there has been substantial discussion and debate regarding the impact on migration of drought in sub-Saharan Africa or sea-level rise in low-lying Small Island States, deltaic regions and coastal regions (IOM 2014). Approximately 10 per cent of the global population live in coastal communities that have an elevation of 10m or less above current sea levels, placing populations at risk of displacement with rising sea levels (Nicholls and Cazenave 2010). Fast-onset changes, particularly natural disasters, are often associated with shorter-term and short-distance displacement. While no single disaster can be attributed solely to climate change, scientific assessment indicates that – when viewed in aggregate – climate change is contributing to increasing frequency and intensity of extreme weather events in many regions of the world (Coumou et al. 2013). In 2013, 21.9 million people were newly displaced by environmental disasters. The great majority were displaced by weather-related disasters, with only a small minority by geophysical hazards (IDMC 2014). There is also substantial debate as to whether competition over diminishing resources (e.g., water, land) may contribute to conflict, which in turn precipitates forced displacement (Gemenne et al. 2014).[1]

Since 1990, when the Intergovernmental Panel on Climate Change (IPCC) noted that climate change could have significant impact on human migration, there have been many attempts to estimate future numbers of climate-related migrants. The complex interplay, however, between climatic changes and non-climate factors that contribute to migration, and the potential for local adaptive responses among at-risk populations, present serious challenges for the accuracy of projections of climate-related migration (Bardsley and Hugo 2010; Barnett and Webber 2009; Tacoli 2009). Furthermore, broad global estimates of climate-related migrants form an inadequate basis for formulating policies, including because they obscure the diversity of potential responses that will range across a spectrum of forced to voluntary, short- to long-distance, internal and cross-border, and permanent, circular, seasonal and short-term movement.

Environmental change rarely acts on its own to cause migration. Migration decisions are also shaped by social, economic, political, economic, demographic and other 'push' and 'pull' factors (see Figure 15.1). These include livelihood opportunities, economic resources, capacity to adapt to environmental changes, social networks, availability of services,

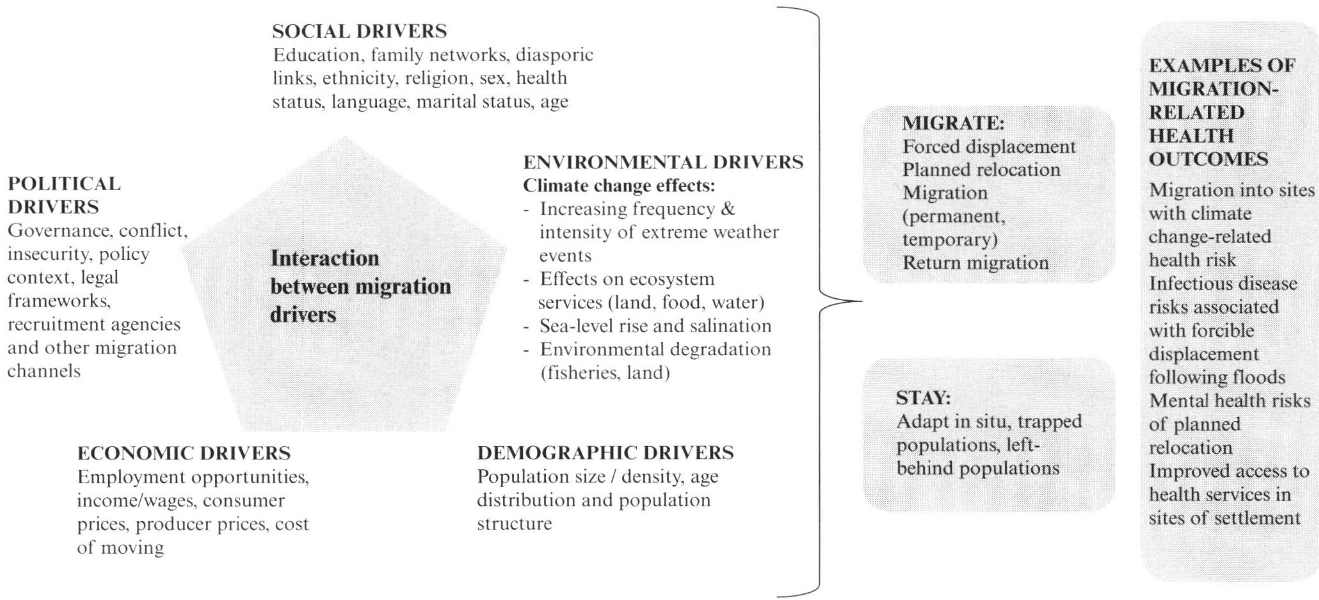

Figure 15.1 Climate change as a driver of migration and associated health outcomes

political/legal frameworks, perceived benefits of staying versus leaving, the significant barriers to migration for many people (particularly the poor and vulnerable), and civil conflict (Birk and Rasmussen 2014; Black 2001; Black et al. 2012; Foresight 2011; Morrisey 2009; Tacoli 2009; Warner et al. 2008). Bangladesh, for example, is situated on the Ganges-Brahmaputra river delta and is often cited as one of the most vulnerable countries to environmental change with threats of flooding, river bank erosion, storm surges, cyclones and droughts. While the migration of people both within and from Bangladesh can be partly attributed to environmental changes, migration is also shaped by other socioeconomic drivers including employment opportunities, economic expansion, industrialization, quality of public services, educational status, gender and age (Hugo and Bardsley 2014). The characteristics, composition and volume of migrants are linked to multiple dimensions of social systems as well as environmental and climatic changes.

Migration is increasingly presented as a strategic and adaptive response to climate variability and environmental change (Sow et al. 2016; Foresight 2011). It generates remittances, diversifies incomes, reduces pressure on homeland environments and resources, and contributes to the transfer of knowledge and skills. Recent research has demonstrated, for example, that environmental change affects human mobility most directly through livelihoods, with migration representing a means of livelihood diversification (Warner et al. 2013).

Climate-related migration, however, affects the health of people and populations as it presents both opportunities and threats for the well-being of migrants and host and home communities (Bowles et al. 2014; Carballo 2008; McMichael 2014; McMichael et al. 2012). Population health is not merely a collateral consequence, but rather a critical indicator of whether migration is a successful and sustainable adaptive response to climate change impacts. The following section explores how diverse migratory responses to climate change may affect population health.

CLIMATE-RELATED MIGRATION AND HEALTH OUTCOMES

Migration does not always present a risk to health. Health benefits can accrue via increased economic and educational opportunities, better nutrition, and better access to health services in destination sites. Further, many migrants are (initially) healthier than host populations because those who migrate generally have resources, good health and capacity that enable their movement (i.e., the 'healthy migrant effect'). The conditions surrounding migration processes, however, can increase health vulnerabilities for some, particularly those migrating within and between low-income countries, forcibly displaced populations and irregular migrants (Davies et al. 2011). With the prospect of increasing human migration and mobility in response to climate change impacts, it is important to understand the health risks and opportunities of those who migrate. The subsections below focus on potential health outcomes for migrants across different stages of the migration process, and with reference to different 'migrant types' (e.g., labour migrants, those involved in planned resettlement schemes). They consider the following stages of migration: pre-departure, transit, displacement, planned relocation, resettlement and return as they relate to climate change.

Because it is difficult to forecast the extent and nature of future climate-related migration and health outcomes, and given the limited level of contemporary migration that is clearly attributable to global environmental change, and the heterogeneity of migratory responses in response to environmental change, the case studies cited serve as an analogue for exploring potential future health outcomes of climate change-related migration.

PRE-DEPARTURE

In situ adaptation will prevail in the early stages of climatic change; people are strongly tied to place and will attempt to adjust and adapt their local socioeconomic systems rather than seek out opportunities elsewhere (Adger et al. 2005; Hugo and Bardsley 2014). Adaptation to climate change will occur across multiple scales and will include preventative, anticipatory and responsive actions – from rapid reactions following extreme weather events to long-term planning to reduce vulnerability (Marino 2012). An analysis of households affected by the 1994/1995 drought in north-western Bangladesh, for example, found that people adopted various *in situ* activities to cope including: borrowing money and selling land, household goods and livestock in order to buy food; consuming wild plants and tubers that are not normally eaten; agricultural adjustments to compensate for crop loss; and seeking resources and support from more affluent community members, local government and NGOs. There was extremely limited out-migration (Paul 1998).

Even as individuals, households, communities and countries seek to adapt *in situ* to critical impacts of climate change, the health of local populations may be affected. Epidemiological studies have identified climate change-related health risks with principal concerns including injury and fatalities related to severe weather events and heatwaves, food and water insecurity, food contamination, illness and fatality related to natural disaster, respiratory and cardiovascular disease related to air pollution, changing infectious disease patterns, and mental health consequences (McMichael 2013). Whether, and to what extent, these health threats will influence or drive migratory decisions is uncertain. For example, it is highly unlikely that changing distribution of dengue will drive migration, whereas drought and food insecurity can be precursors to migration. Nonetheless, these (pre-departure) health risks may shape the baseline health status of migrating populations when local responses to cope with climate change threats become inadequate (Hugo and Bardsley 2014).

CASE STUDY 1 THE NORTHWEST ARCTIC REGION, CLIMATE IMPACTS ON HEALTH AND RELOCATION

In the Northwest Arctic region, between 1949 and 2006, the average annual temperature increased by 1.8°C. In Northwest Alaska, climate change is resulting in delayed freeze-up, decreasing sea-ice, earlier breakup, storm surges, coastal erosion, and thawing permafrost. There are 12 communities in the region, the largest of which is Kotzebue (pop. 8,000), and the majority of residents are Inupiat Eskimos. There are no connecting roads between communities or with the rest of the state. Community members harvest caribou, seal, fish, whale, moose, berries, birds and edible plants. Employment opportunities relate to education, health, government, mining, transportation, fishing and construction; unemployment is about 16 per cent. The health of Indigenous people in the Arctic region has improved in the past 50 years. Due to their close relationship with nature, however, many Indigenous Alaskan people are vulnerable to emerging climate change-related health threats. Adverse health threats of climate change in the region include injury related to weather and ice conditions, respiratory infection, decline in the availability of traditional foods (e.g., caribou, moose) and an increasingly Western diet associated with (for example) cardiovascular disease and diabetes, and mental health issues linked with altered social, cultural and environmental conditions (Parkinson and Evengård 2015). Local *in situ* adaptive responses to climate change include adaptive engineering strategies to control erosion, public education, extreme weather early warning systems, health work force training, disaster preparedness and public policy developments (Brubaker et al. 2011). Yet Alaskan communities are among the first to be displaced by anthropogenic climate change, as coastal erosion and flooding events are compelling residents to relocate (Marino 2012). The state of Alaska and federal government agencies are working with some communities (i.e. Kivalina, Newtok and Shishmaref) to plan organized relocation. The health profile of those who relocate will be shaped in part by persistent climate change-related health concerns.

TRANSIT MIGRATION

Transit migration occurs as people move between places of origin and their planned destination, stopping for short periods or longer periods of up to several years or more (Zimmerman et al. 2011). The (contested) term 'transit migration' is most widely applied to irregular migrants. The vast majority of contemporary transit migration is politically and economically driven, rather than environmental. The threat that climate change will drive increases in cross-border transit migration is a preoccupation for many countries, such as European and North African states, yet the likelihood and magnitude of such migration remains unclear.

Transit migrants typically experience substantial risks to health and poor access to services (WHO 2010). Health risks emerge associated with the conditions and duration of transit migration – including overland flight on foot or via boats – which can lead to physical danger, trauma, hunger and exposure to violence (IOM 2013). During transit, migrants can be exposed to health risks in new locations or carry pathogens to new sites (McMichael et al. 2012; Zimmerman et al. 2011). For example, the resurgence of malaria in border regions of Asia, including drug-resistant falciparum malaria, has been attributed in part to cross-border and transit migration (Hugo 2013). Living and working conditions in sites of transit and temporary settlement are also key determinants of health. Health risks associated with transit migration have received limited research focus, but could become a concern where climate change contributes to and amplifies migration push factors, such as livelihood insecurity, leading to transit migration.

CASE STUDY 2 TRANSIT MIGRATION AND HEALTH IN MOROCCO

A recent study explored transit migration of West African fisher people in Morocco in the context of climate change (Sow et al. 2016). Globally, fishery productivity will be challenged by marine species redistribution and marine biodiversity reduction (IPCC 2014). In West Africa, climate change is having adverse impacts on marine and inland fisheries: on the West Atlantic African coast, climate variability and changing upwelling patterns have led to changes in the quantity and distribution of fish species. Increasingly warm and acidified water will affect the coral ecosystem, which further contributes to declining fish stocks. West African fishers have a long history of movement and migration, associated with seasonal changes and economic drivers. The negative affect of climate change and overfishing on fisheries in West Africa is now also contributing to decisions to emigrate among those who fish for a living (Sow et al. 2016). Many migrants from West Africa regard Morocco as a transit country before reaching the final destination; Europe, Persian Gulf countries and Asia. This is the case particularly for migrants from Senegal, Niger, Mali, Libya, Ivory Coast and Guinea who are exempted from visas to Morocco. Migration may offer opportunities to build economic and social capital among migrants and to transfer knowledge, technology, remittances and other resources to sites of origin. However, illegal migrants (in sites of transit) experience much hardship. Most West Africans living in Morocco do not have legal status, institutional support or social protection, they live in precarious conditions, are at risk of being expelled, suffer from exploitation and racism, have limited employment opportunities and live in poor-quality housing (Keygnaert et al. 2014). As numerous reports highlight, these socioeconomic conditions contribute to substantial health threats for transit migrants, including violence, poor mental health and infectious disease risks (Hugo 2013).

DISPLACEMENT

Climate change will contribute to temporary population displacement, particularly in response to extreme weather events (e.g., floods, cyclones). Extreme weather events can lead to adverse health outcomes and infectious disease outbreaks, particularly when they result in large-scale population displacement. The communicable disease profile of displaced populations after natural disasters is determined largely by the availability and accessibility of safe water and latrines, nutritional status, living conditions, presence of vector breeding sites, exposure to disease vectors and reservoir animal hosts (e.g., mosquitoes, rodents), levels of immunity to vaccine-preventable diseases, and access to healthcare services (Watson et al. 2007). Common infectious diseases in post-disaster contexts include diarrhoeal disease, measles, meningitis, acute respiratory infection, vector-borne diseases (malaria, dengue), tuberculosis and malaria (IFRC 2007; Toole 2006; Watson et al. 2007). Prolonged health impacts of natural disaster for displaced populations may include disruption of disease surveillance and health programmes (e.g., immunization), food insecurity and food scarcity due to limitation of agricultural and farming activities, and interruption of treatment regimens (Kouadio et al. 2012). The risk of water-borne infectious disease outbreaks among displaced populations can be reduced through provision of clean water in the disaster-response (Cairncross and Alvarinho 2006; Kondo et al. 2002).

Caution is required in drawing lessons from a global literature on disaster, displacement and health outcomes. Floods and other environmental disasters vary greatly in their nature, size and the vulnerability of the populations they affect. In low-income settings, however, there are typically limited emergency and support services, limited infrastructure and people have little capacity to protect themselves (Kondo et al. 2002).

CASE STUDY 3 DISASTER, DISPLACEMENT AND DIARRHOEA

In recent years, floods in Thailand, Pakistan, Vietnam and Nepal have inundated vast areas, forcibly displacing many thousands of people (Hugo and Bardsley 2014). Flooding is often associated with an increase in cases or outbreaks of infectious diseases including diarrhoea, malaria and leptospirosis. Diarrheal disease epidemics have been attributed to faecal contamination of water (at source and during transportation and storage), shared cooking pots, shortage of food, scarcity of soap and contaminated food. In 2000, flooding in Mozambique resulted in large-scale population displacement and a significant increase in the incidence of diarrheal diseases. In the months following the floods there were an estimated 8,000 additional cases and 447 deaths from diarrhoeal disease (Cairncross and Alvarinho 2006). The Mozambique floods also increased the number of malaria cases by a factor of 1.5–2 as compared with 1999 and 2001 rates (Kondo et al. 2002).

PLANNED RELOCATION

Climate change is expected to lead to planned relocation of communities. Planned relocation may be necessary where areas become prone to increasingly severe and frequent sudden-onset natural disasters (e.g., flood areas), where livelihoods are undermined by slow-onset effects (e.g., increasing drought frequency), where lands are required for mitigation and adaptation projects (e.g., water reservoirs), or where land becomes unsuitable or unavailable for habitation (e.g., due to sea-level rise). Planned relocation should be considered a last resort, when other adaptive strategies have failed (Adger et al. 2005; Tacoli 2009; Bardsley and Hugo 2010). It requires the regeneration of livelihoods and construction of new homes and public infrastructure. Most experiences of planned relocation have occurred in the context of development forced displacement and resettlement (DFDR) projects.

Health indicators are not typically included in DFDR monitoring and evaluation, but there is some evidence that well-designed, financed and implemented relocation processes can improve outcomes for affected populations (Weerasinghe 2014). For example, the Koto Panjang dam construction project was initiated to meet increasing demand for electricity in central Sumatra, Indonesia. Between 1991 and 2000, approximately 5,000 households were relocated in order to allow inundation of ten villages during the construction of the dam. A survey conducted in 2010, more than a decade post-resettlement, found that resettled households had significantly improved access to electricity, living conditions, clean drinking water and health services (Karimi and Taifur 2013). Existing studies indicate overwhelmingly, however, that resettled communities are worse-off following DFDR, particularly where relocation is poorly planned and implemented. For example, the Three Gorges Dam in China is estimated to have led to the forced displacement and resettlement of 1 million people, with as many as 4 million anticipated to be relocated. For populations relocated for the Three Gorges Dam, health concerns have emerged associated with livelihood and food security, psychosocial impacts of relocation, toxicological impacts of the dam, shifting disease dynamics and erosion of social support systems (Kittinger et al. 2010; McMichael 2015).

CASE STUDY 4 PLANNED RELOCATION IN SRI LANKA

Planned relocation, where necessary, should seek to provide opportunity for human development and progressive social change. In Sri Lanka, the Lunawa Environmental Improvement and Community Development Project aimed to improve the storm water drainage system and rehabilitating existing canals and streams. A total of 18,000 households consisting of low-income slum-dwellers were directly and indirectly affected by the project and 883 families were entitled for resettlement. The resettlement process was founded on extensive consultation with affected community members and strategic partnerships between the government of Sri Lanka, UNHABITAT, municipal councils, local NGOs and the Japan Bank for International Cooperation. Project benefits included security of tenure, livelihood development, access to banking services and improved infrastructure and services (i.e., solid waste management, wastewater disposal, sewage disposal and renovation of internal roads) (UNHABITAT 2009). The challenge is for climate-related planned relocation to occur, where necessary, via participatory and careful approaches to planning and relocation in order to restore the standards of living of relocated populations and ensure good health of people and communities.

RESETTLEMENT IN DESTINATION SITES

Migration can be understood as a risk management and adaptation response that reduces vulnerability to climate change. Current migration in Pacific Island nations, for example, is widespread and often leads to positive outcomes for migrants and their families and home communities; it can improve access to social and financial capital, reduce pressure on natural resources, and allow flexible responses to socioeconomic and environmental pressures and change. Policies that support migration allow adaptation to be *done by* rather than *done to* people, as they give people increased control over the decisions they make about climate change adaptation (Barnett et al. 2013).

It is likely that voluntary migration and resettlement will follow existing migration pathways, and will predominantly comprise internal migration. In many low-income agricultural-based economies, such as many African nations, rural–rural migration is prevalent, urban–urban movement occurs in regions with high levels of urbanization, and rural–urban migration is higher in areas with high economic growth and growing industry and services sectors (Tacoli 2009). The health impacts of climate change for resettling populations will depend substantially on the nature, location and context of the migration process: health consequences will be shaped by policy and legal contexts, health services and conditions in sites of settlement, and resources and capacity of migrants. There are some scenarios where the health of resettled populations may improve. Migration to many urban-poor areas, however, is associated with substantial risks to health due to overcrowding, inadequate water and sanitation facilities, poor working conditions and underemployment, income instability and increased pressure on infrastructure and services (McMichael et al. 2012).

CASE STUDY 5 URBAN MIGRATION AND SETTLEMENT IN THE PACIFIC

In Pacific Island towns and cities, there is likely to be a substantial climate change-related increase in migrants. Rates of urbanization are expected to increase throughout the region, and this is likely to be increased by climate change impacts as sea-levels rise and as livelihoods in rural areas and outer islands become more difficult to sustain. Fiji's National Climate Change Policy states that 'land loss and reduction of arable land could lead to migration to urban centres, resulting in overcrowding' (Republic of Fiji 2012: 64). Urban atolls (e.g., South Tarawa, Kiribati; Funafuti, Tuvalu) already have high population densities and related problems of fresh water supply and quality, waste disposal and inadequate housing supply. Suva, the capital of Fiji, is the main destination for internal migration in Fiji, and in informal urban settlements – such as the Suva-Nausori corridor – there is a high level of poverty, inadequate sanitation and water supply, and elevated exposure to infectious disease (Narsey 2008). In the Pacific Islands, resettling migrants in urban-poor areas are likely to be exposed to health threats in sites of settlement (Campbell and Warrick 2014).

Further, in a contemporary era of widespread migration, existing population movement will occur in the context of changing climatic conditions. People will migrate to areas that are exposed to adverse environmental risks such as storm surges, floods, droughts and extreme weather events and, consequently, may face elevated health threats (Foresight 2011; Sward 2008; Wirawan 2010). Accordingly, the broader migrant population may experience climate-related health risks. In India, recent census data shows that for the first time, India's urban population has increased more rapidly than its rural population, mostly due to rural–urban migration (IOM 2014). Yet climate change is associated with particular threats to the health of urban populations. Epidemiological studies indicate that during heatwaves, heat stress and mortality rates are higher in dense urban areas compared to rural areas due to the urban heat island effect (largely due to heat storage in buildings and sealed roads), and the lack of surface moisture and lower wind speeds in urban areas (Azhar 2014). While there are many benefits of city living, migrants in urban-poor areas may be particularly vulnerable to climate change-related health risks. The death toll from the May 2015 heatwave in India, for example, exceeded 2,500 people, and many of those who died were construction workers in urban areas who were unable to heed official advice to stay indoors (ABC News 2015; *Telegraph* 2015). Similarly, the 2015 heatwave in Pakistan resulted in more than 1,000 deaths in Karachi, and migrant workers with little access to shelter from the sun were identified as being at risk of heat stroke and heat-related mortality (Dearden 2015). As Kjellstrom et al. (2013: 64) state, climate change will increase heat-related risks to occupational health hazards and potentially death if people work beyond physiological limits, as was the case in 2015 for urban-based migrant workers in India and Pakistan.

RETURN

Research suggests that 'environmental migration' predominantly occurs within countries and that people typically return to their sites of origin when conditions allow (Tacoli 2009; McLeman and Hunter 2010; Oliver-Smith 2012). The health of returning migrants is determined by cumulative exposure to health risks prior to migration, during migration processes and following return. Migrants who receive low wages, live in inadequate housing, have poor nutrition and face barriers to accessing health service often return home less healthy than when they left. They may need health-care that is not available upon return, particularly in low-resource settings, or which they cannot afford (Davies et al. 2011). Returning migrants may be responsible for introducing new pathogens to the local population (Zimmerman et al. 2011). For many labour migrants, however, saved income and remittances can support a healthier lifestyle and improved healthcare options for themselves and their family (Zimmerman et al. 2011).

CASE STUDY 6 HURRICANE KATRINA AND RETURN MIGRATION

Hurricane Katrina struck New Orleans, Louisiana on 29 August 2005; the protective levees failed, producing a catastrophic flood. In the days following, all residents were evacuated, except police, fire fighters and search and rescue teams. A month later neighbourhoods were deemed safe following the removal of flood water, and were reopened for occupancy. A study of 569 poor, predominantly African-American Hurricane Katrina survivors – all of whom returned to New Orleans – examined the extent to which pre-disaster health problems (i.e., asthma, high blood pressure, diabetes, high cholesterol, heart problems, other physical health problems, migraines, back pain, digestive problems) predicted subsequent neighbourhood poverty following their return. Although health problems were not associated with neighbourhood poverty at baseline, baseline health problems were predictive of living in higher poverty areas by 2009–2010. People with diagnosed health conditions experienced larger and stronger effects even after adjusting for insurance status. Results indicate the potential for an environmental disaster to spur selective mobility into neighbourhoods following return, based on pre-disaster health status. Better health conferred an advantage in this highly mobile sample, providing opportunity to 'leverage the tragedy of Hurricane Katrina into an opportunity' (Arcaya et al. 2014). This suggests that among returning populations, those with poor health status may experience particular vulnerabilities.

LEFT-BEHIND AND 'TRAPPED' POPULATIONS

Migration also has an impact on the lives and wellbeing of left-behind populations. The UK government's Foresight report (2011) focusing on migration and global environmental change contends that the greatest risks will be borne by those who are unable or unwilling to migrate. In their analysis of households in rural Bangladesh, Gray and Mueller (2012), illustrate that direct exposure to climate change threats (i.e., crop failure due to rainfall deficits) can limit migration and mobility among poor and food-insecure households through resource constraints, while higher-income households are more likely to use migration as an adaptive response. These findings challenge the widely accepted narrative advanced in public dialogue that the poor and vulnerable are most likely to migrate in the face of climate change threats. Left-behind and 'trapped' populations, who do not have the social and economic capital required to migrate, may be among the most vulnerable and at greatest risk of adverse health consequences such as undernutrition and malnutrition. They may be left behind in sites with environmental threat and decreasing levels of capital investment as the more mobile and wealthy move out (temporarily or permanently).

CONCLUDING DISCUSSION

Globally, the impacts of climate change will amplify migration and migration complexity. It is widely argued that migration will be an effective way in which people adapt and build resilience in the face of climate change threats (Hugo and Bardsley 2014). As Tacoli (2009: 514) writes, 'what is needed urgently is a radical change in perceptions of migration and a better understanding of the role that local and national institutions need to play in making mobility be seen as part of the solution rather than the problem'. The 2010 Cancun Adaptation Framework calls upon parties to undertake 'measures to enhance understanding, coordination and cooperation with regard to climate change-induced displacement, migration and planned relocation, where appropriate, at national, regional and international levels' (UNFCCC 2010). In the UK's Foresight report (2011), migration is presented as building long-term resilience to environmental change among individuals, households and communities, and policymakers are encouraged to promote migration for those suffering adverse environmental changes.

There are good social, geopolitical and policy-related reasons for understanding migration as an adaptive response, rather than a crisis to be managed and stemmed. Yet it is contrary to values of equality and social justice that the 'haves' of the world should produce vast quantities of greenhouse gas emissions while the 'have-nots' suffer the detrimental effects of climatic changes – whether that be loss of habitable land with rising seas, or erosion of livelihood with depleted fisheries – and must migrate in order to seek, for example, opportunities for income diversification. This provides a reminder that climate change mitigation remains the foremost priority, requiring significantly enhanced international cooperation and urgent and deep cuts in greenhouse gas emissions.

And yet, given that past emissions have committed the world to a certain amount of accelerated warming, programme and policy responses are required to address and support climate change-related migration. The heterogeneity of migration, displacement and planned relocation scenarios means that policy responses to climate-related migration cannot be discussed in generic terms (McAdam 2010). This is true of efforts to address the health risks and opportunities in relation to climate-related migration. Following extreme weather events, tailored public health measures for forcibly displaced populations should include: surveillance systems for early case detection and treatment; adequate site planning; appropriate management of water and sanitation systems; adequate food supplies and storage; and strong vector control and vaccination programmes (Kouadio et al. 2012). Lessons from DFDR suggest that when planned relocation is unavoidable, the scale of displacement should be minimized, planning processes should have sufficient lead time and directly involve affected communities, relocation should provide for appropriate land acquisition and sufficient financing, and there should be long-term attention to restoring and improving lives and livelihoods (Ferris 2012; Warner et al. 2013). However, in many situations climate-related migrants will not represent a distinct group that can be the target of policy responses. While climate change may contribute to rural–urban migration, for example, rural–urban migrants do not comprise the majority of the urban poor, nor is climate change (currently) the primary driver of rural–urban migration. Accordingly, the health of climate-related migrants in urban settings will need to be addressed through broader urban health policies and programmes.

Assessment of the associations between climate change, migration and health outcomes involve multiple uncertainties in relation to the exposure–response relationships (e.g., drought and forced displacement), geographical and temporal variability, climate scenarios, limited available empirical data, questions regarding the applicability of analogous examples to long-term projections, and multifactorial causal webs. These uncertainties do not mean, however, that appropriate climate change adaptation cannot occur. Approaches that focus on enhancing the capacity of society, health systems and migration frameworks and policies to deal with changes and uncertainties are important, as are 'no-regret' options that make sense due to co-benefits of climate change adaptation policies for other policy issues (Wardekker et al. 2012).

Good health is an essential asset of any population; in the face of climate threats, the adaptive potential of migration will be defined in part by health outcomes for source community, host community and migrant populations. There will need to be nuanced and significant policy improvements in many areas: climate-sensitive policies that build resilience and reduce the need to migrate away from adversely affected areas; effective migration management that protects the rights and wellbeing of migrants; stronger governance; more appropriate funding mechanisms to facilitate climate change adaptation; and expanded and improved development assistance mechanisms (Hugo and Bardsley 2014). Substantial institutional and sociocultural change at a local, national and global level is required in order to respond to climate-related migration, and this will take time to achieve (Bardsley and Hugo 2010). And yet some impacts of climate change on migration are already in evidence. In order to support migration as an adaptive response to climate change, it is important to better understand and respond to health impacts for diverse migrant populations.

NOTE

1. Darfur is often cited as an example of a conflict emerging from dwindling resources due to climate change impacts, yet others have highlighted the significant impacts of inequitable wealth and power distributions, government agricultural policies that favoured industrialized farms over small-scale farmers, and the nationalization of land in 1970 that led to the marginalization of pastoralists.

REFERENCES

ABC News (2015), India heatwave death toll tops 1,100 as New Delhi roads melt in near-50-degree temperatures, available online at www.abc.net.au/news/2015-05-26/india-heatwave-kills-1100-as-capitals-roads-melt/6499264.

ADB (2012), *Climate Change and Migration in Asia and the Pacific: Draft Edition*, Manila: Asian Development Bank.

Adger, W. N., N. W. Arnell and E. L. Tompkins (2005), Successful adaptation to climate change across scales, *Global Environmental Change*, **15**, 77–86.

Arcaya, M., S. V. Subramanian, J. E. Rhodes and M. C. Waters (2014), Role of health in predicting moves to poor neighbourhoods among Hurricane Katrina survivors, *PNAS*, **111**(46), 16246–16253.

Azhar, G., D. Mavalankar, A. Nori-Sarma, A. Rajiva, P. Dutta, A. Jaiswal, A., P. Sheffield, K. Knowlton and J. Hess (2014), Heat-related mortality in India: excess all-cause mortality associated with the 2010 Ahmedabad Heat Wave, *PLOS One*, **9**(3), e91831.

Bardsley, D. and G. Hugo (2010), Migration and climate change: examining thresholds of change to guide effective adaptation decision-making, *Population and Environment*, **32**(2), 238–262.

Barnett, J. and M. Webber (2009), *Accommodating Migration to Promote Adaptation to Climate Change: A Policy Brief Prepared for the Secretariat of the Swedish Commission on Climate Change and Development and the World Bank Development Report 2010 Team*, Stockholm: Commission on Climate Change and Development.

Barnett J., S. O'Neill, S. Waller and S. Rogers (2013), Reducing the risk of maladaptation in response to sea-level rise and urban water scarcity, in S. Moser and M. Boykoff (eds.), *Successful Adaptation to Climate Change: Linking Science and Policy in a Rapidly Changing World*, London: Routledge, pp. 37–49.

Birk, T. and K. Rasmussen (2014), Migration from atolls as climate change adaptation: current practices, barriers and options in Solomon Islands, *Natural Resources Forum, Special Issue: Small Island Developing States*, **38**(1), 1–13.

Black, R. (2001), *Environmental Refugees: Myth or Reality?* Brighton: UNHCR, University of Sussex.

Black, R., R. Stephen, G. Bennet, S. Thomas and J. Beddington (2011), Migration as adaptation, *Nature*, **478**, 447–449.

Black, R., N. W. Arnell, W. N. Adger, D. Thomas and A. Geddes (2012), Migration, immobility and displacement outcomes following extreme events, *Environmental Science and Policy*, **27**(S1), S32–S43.

Bowles, D. C., R. Reuveny and C. D. Butler (2014), Moving to a better life? Climate, migration and population health, in C. D. Butler (ed.), *Climate Change and Global Health*, Wallingford: CAB International, pp. 135–143.

Brubaker, M. J. Berner, R. Chavan and J. Warren (2011), Climate change and health effects in Northwest Alaska, *Global Health Action*, **4**.

Cairncross, S. and M. Alvarinho (2006), The Mozambique floods of 2000: health impact and response, in R. Few and F. Matthies (eds.), *Flood Hazards and Health: Responding to Present and Future Risks*, London: Earthscan, pp. 111–127.

Campbell, J. and O. Warrick (2014), *Climate Change and Migration Issues in the Pacific*, Fiji: UNESCAP.
Carballo, M., C. Smith and K. Pettersson (2008), Climate change and displacement: health challenges, *Forced Migration*, **31**, 32–33.
Coumou, D., A. Robinson and S. Rahmstorf (2013), Global increase in record-breaking monthly-mean temperatures, *Climate Change*, **118**, 771–782.
Davies, A., R. Borland, C. Blake and H. West (2011), The dynamics of health and return migration, *PLOS Medicine*, **8**(6), e1001046.
Dearden, L. (2015), Pakistan heatwave: death toll tops 400 I Karachi as morgues overflow and power cuts worsen crisis, available online at www.independent.co.uk/news/world/asia/pakistan-heatwave-death-toll-tops-400-in-karachi-as-morgues-overflow-and-power-cuts-worsen-crisis-10339798.html.
Ferris, E. (2012), *Protection and Planned Relocations in the Context of Climate Change, UNHCR, Legal and Protection Policy Research Services*, available online at www.unhcr.org/5024d5169.pdf.
Foresight (2011), *Migration and Global Environmental Change: Future Challenges and Opportunities* London: Government Office for Science.
Gemenne, F., J. Barnett, W. N. Adger and G. D. Dabelko (2014), Climate and security: evidence, emerging risks, and a new agenda, *Climatic Change*, **123**(1), 1–9.
Gray, C. L. and V. Mueller (2012), Natural disasters and population mobility in Bangladesh, *PNAS*, **109**(16), 6000–6005.
Hugo, G. (2013), Migration and health, in *Situation Report on International Migration in South and South-West Asia: Asia-Pacific RCM Thematic Working Group on International Migration including Human Trafficking*, Bangkok: UNESCAP.
Hugo, G. and D. Bardsley (2014), Migration and environmental change in Asia, in E. Piguet and F. Lazko (eds.), *People on the Move in a Changing Climate: Global Migration Issues*, Dordrecht: Springer.
IDMC (2014), *Global Estimates 2014: People Displaced by Disasters*, Geneva: Internal Displacement Monitoring Centre, available online at www.internal-displacement.org/assets/publications/2014/201409-global-estimates2.pdf.
IFRC (2007), *The John Hopkins and Red Cross and Red Crescent Public Health Guide in Emergencies*, Geneva: International Federation of Red Cross and Red Crescent Societies.
IOM (2013), *International Migration, Health and Human Rights*, Geneva: International Organization for Migration.
IOM (2014), *Global Migration Trends: An Overview*, Geneva: Migration Research Division, International Organization for Migration.
IPCC (2014), *Climate Change 2014 Synthesis Report Summary for Policymakers*, available online at www.ipcc.ch/pdf/assessment-report/ar5/syr/AR5_SYR_FINAL_SPM.pdf.
Karimi, S. and W. Taifur (2013), Resettlement and development: a survey of two of Indonesia's Koto Panjang resettlement villages, *International Journal of Water Resources Development*, **29**(1), 35–49.
Keygnaert, I., A. Dialmy, A. Manço, A., J. Keygnaert, N. Vettenburg, K. Roelens and M. Temmerman (2014), Sexual violence and sub-Saharan migrants in Morocco: a community-based participatory assessment using respondent driven sampling, *Globalization and Health*, **10**, 32.
Kittinger, J., K. Coontz, Z. Yuan, Y. Han, X. Zhao and B. Wilcox (2010), Toward holistic evaluation and assessment: linking ecosystems and human well-being for the Three Gorges Dam, *EcoHealth*, **6**(4), 601–13.
Kjellstrom, T., B. Lemke and M. Otto (2013), Mapping occupational heat exposure and effects in South-East Asia: ongoing time trends 1980–2011 and future estimates to 2050, *Industrial Health*, **51**, 56–67.
Kondo H, N. Seo, T. Yasuda, M. Hasizume, Y. Koido, N. Ninomiya and Y. Yamamoto (2002), Post-flood-infectious diseases in Mozambique, *Prehospital Disaster Medicine*, **17**, 126–133.
Kouadio, I., S. Aljunid, T. Kamigaki, K. Hammad and H. Oshitani (2012), Infectious

diseases following natural disasters: prevention and control measures, *Expert Review of Anti-infective Therapy*, **10**(1), 95–104.
Marino, E. (2012), The long history of environmental migration: Assessing vulnerability construction and obstacles to successful relocation in Shishmaref, Alaska, *Global Environmental Change*, **22**, 374–381.
McAdam, J. (2010), 'Disappearing states', statelessness and the boundaries of international law, in J. McAdam (ed.), *Climate Change and Displacement: Multidisciplinary Perspectives*, Oxford/Portland: Hart Publishing, pp. 105–130.
McLeman, R. A. and L. M. Hunter (2010), Migration in the context of vulnerability and adaptation to climate change: insights from analogues, *Wiley Interdisciplinary Reviews–Climate Change*, **1**(3), 450–461.
McMichael, A. J. (2013), Globalization, climate change and human health, *NEJM*, **368**, 1335–1343.
McMichael, C. (2014), Climate change and migration: food insecurity as a driver and outcome of climate change-related migration, in A Malik, E. Grohmann and R. Akhtar (eds.), *Environmental Deterioration and Human Health: Natural and Anthropogenic Determinants*, Dordrecht, Heidelberg, London and New York: Springer.
McMichael, C. (2015), Climate change-related migration and infectious disease, *Virulence*, **6**(6), 1–6.
McMichael, C., J. Barnett and A. J. McMichael (2012), An ill wind? Climate change, migration and health, *Environmental Health Perspectives*, **120**(5), 646–654.
Morrisey, J. (2009), *Environmental Change and Forced Migration: A State of the Art Review*, Oxford: University of Oxford, Refugee Studies Centre.
Narsey, W. (2008), *The Quantitative Analysis of Poverty in Fiji*, Suva: Vanuavou Publications.
Nicholls, R. J. and A. Cazenave (2010), Sea-level rise and its impact on coastal zones, *Science*, **328**(5985), 1517–1520.
Oliver-Smith, A. (2012), Debating environmental migration: society, nature and population displacement in climate change, *Journal of International Development*, **24**(8), 1058–1070.
Paul, B. (1998), Coping mechanisms practised by drought victims (1994/5) in North Bengal, Bangladesh, *Applied Geography*, **18**(4), 355–373.
Parkinson, A. and B. Evengård (2015), Climate change and health in the Arctic, in C. D. Butler (ed.), *Climate Change and Global Health*, Wallingford: CABI Publishing, pp. 206–216.
Republic of Fiji (2012), *National Climate Change Policy*, Suva: Secretariat of the Pacific Community.
Sow, P., E. Marmer and J. Scheffran (2016), Between the heat and the hardships: climate change and mixed migration flows in Morocco, *Migration and Development*, **5**(2).
Sward J. (2008), *Migration and Climate Change: How Will Climate Shifts Affect Migration Trends?* Briefing Paper No. 12, Brighton: Development Research Centre on Migration, Globalisation and Poverty.
Tacoli, C. (2009), Crisis or adaptation? Migration and climate change in a context of high mobility, *Environment and Urbanization*, **21**(2), 513–525.
Telegraph (2015), India heatwave: death toll passes 2,500 as victim families fight for compensation, *The Telegraph*, available online at www.telegraph.co.uk/news/worldnews/asia/india/11645731/India-heatwave-death-toll-passes-2500-as-victim-families-fight-for-compensation.html.
Toole, M. J. (2006), 'Forced migrants: refugees and internally displaced persons', in B. Levy and V. Sidel (eds.), *Social Injustice and Public Health*, Oxford: Oxford University Press, pp. 190–204.
UNFCCC (2010), *Advance Unedited Version, Draft Decision -/CP.16. Outcome of the Work of the Ad Hoc Working Group on Long-Term Cooperative Action under the Convention*, United Nations Framework Convention on Climate Change, available online at http://unfccc.int/files/meetings/cop_16/application/pdf/cop16_lca.pdf.
UNHABITAT (2009), *Innovative Approaches for Involuntary Resettlement: Lunawa*

Environmental Improvement & Community Development Project. Nairobi, Kenya, available online at www.preventionweb.net/files/13586_2870alt.pdf.
Wardekker, J., A. de Jong, L. van Bree, W. Turkenburg, J. van der Sluijs (2012), Health risks of climate change: an assessment of uncertainties and its implications for adaptation policies, *Environmental Health*, **11**, 67.
Warner, K., T. Afifi, O. Dun, M. Stal and S. Schmidl (2008), *Human Security, Climate Change and Environmentally Induced Migration*, Bonn: United Nations University.
Warner, K. T. Afifi, W. Kälin, S. Leckie, B. Ferris, S.F. Martin and D. Wrathall (2013), *Changing Climates, Moving People: Framing Migration, Displacement and Planned Relocation*, Policy Brief No. 8, Bonn: United Nations University Institute for Environment and Human Security.
Watson J, M. Gayer and M. Connolly (2007), Epidemics after natural disasters, *Emerging Infectious Disease*, **13**(1), 1–5.
Weerasinghe, S. (2014), *Planned Relocation, Disasters and Climate Change: Consolidating Good Practices and Preparing for the Future*, Geneva: UNHCR.
Wirawan, M. (2010), Public health responses to climate change impacts in Indonesia, *Asia-Pacific Journal of Public Health*, **22**(1), 25–31.
WHO (2010), *Health of Migrants: The Way Forward: Report of Global Consultation*, Geneva: World Health Organization.
Zimmerman, C., L. Kiss and M. Hossain (2011), Migration and health: a framework for 21st century policy-making, *PLOS Medicine* **8**(5): e1001034.

PART V

SPECIFIC HEALTHCARE NEEDS AND PRIORITIES

16 Disability and chronic illness

Gudbjorg Ottosdottir and Ruth Evans

INTRODUCTION

The World Health Organization (WHO) estimates that 15 per cent of the global population are disabled people (WHO and World Bank, 2011). The majority of disabled people live in the Global South and the incidence of poverty among disabled people is higher than in the general population in this region of the world (Mitra et al. 2013). This is due to limited rights to public welfare support, greater health-related expenditure and barriers to participation in employment and education (Groce et al. 2011), which are influenced by wider national and global processes and inequalities that constrain government spending and public welfare systems. In much of the Global North, disabled people's rights to participate in social life and to receive support are recognised in policy and designated support may be provided. Yet despite considerable advances in international and national policies, and the greater involvement of diverse groups of disabled people in decision-making processes, disabled people globally continue to experience multidimensional inequalities and disadvantages in their life chances and opportunities (Mitra et al. 2013; Groce et al. 2011).

Disabled people may become displaced as a result of extreme poverty and lack of social protection, environmental disasters or war. Approximately 2.3 million to 3.3 million internally displaced persons are estimated to be disabled people (UNHCR 2014). However, disabled people may be left behind during displacement, because they lack social protection, support and the power or resources needed to negotiate migration routes (Straimer 2010). To date, there are no official statistics about the numbers of disabled people involved in migration across international borders (Shivji 2010; Simmons 2010). The vast majority of disabled people face significant structural barriers, as well as barriers to migration (Grech and Pisani 2015; WHO and World Bank 2011). This is because of negative connotations associated with disability and assumptions in national immigration policies that disabled people are 'unproductive' and will not contribute economically or socially to their country of settlement (El-Lahib and Wehbi 2012). Disabled people tend to be ignored in migration policy and interventions and have restricted rights to employment and welfare support because of their status as migrants in receiving countries; they are often unable to access the same level of health and social care support that other disabled citizens in receiving countries are entitled to, which further compounds negative experiences of disability and social exclusion. This applies particularly in European countries where migrants from countries outside the EU, asylum-seekers and undocumented migrants have unequal entitlements to support (see Harris and Roberts 2004; European Migration Network 2014).

The links between disability and migration have been generally neglected in the literature to date; often disability is only referred to as a potential outcome of migration because of the association between poverty, poor health, housing and employment conditions among migrants (Rechel et al. 2013; Ryan et al. 2009). Migrants are considered at higher risk of becoming chronically ill or disabled than the general population because of poorer living conditions and limited entitlements to welfare support (Sole-Auro and Crimmins 2008; Sundquist 1995). Migrants with a marginalised legal status, such as asylum-seekers or those with insecure or no legal status, may be more likely to experience disability, chronic illness or other physical or mental health problems (Allsopp et al. 2014; Jayaweera 2014; Raphaely and O'Moore 2010). The few available studies of disabled migrants' experiences offer important insights into how disability intersects with cultural, social, economic and global processes to constrain participation and shape the agency of disabled people involved in migration (Grech and Pisani 2015). At the international scale, the situation of disabled migrants has only recently been acknowledged, following the establishment of the United Nations Convention on the Rights of Persons with Disabilities (UNCRPD) in 2008. Given the lack of statistical evidence, knowledge about disabled migrants' experiences and the lack of policy engagement with such critical issues, the picture of disability and migration that we discuss is rather complex.

In this chapter, we first provide insight into key conceptual understandings of disability and chronic illness. We then discuss the policy context of migration, disability and chronic illness. We focus on the specific situation of asylum-seekers with disability or chronic illness and provide a case study of the UK context, drawing on literature, policy and our own empirical research on disability, HIV and caring relations among asylum-seeking and refugee families.

UNDERSTANDING DISABILITY AND CHRONIC ILLNESS

A 'medical model' of disability dominated approaches to disability in the Global North until relatively recently and continues to exercise a significant hold over attitudes and responses to disability globally. The 'medical model' regarded disability as largely an 'individual misfortune' or private 'tragedy' or 'abnormality' that needed to be treated, cured or prevented by medical intervention alone (Oliver 1990; Gleeson 1999). The disability movement, led primarily by activists and allies in the UK and the USA from the 1970s onwards, rejected such medical, rehabilitative models of disability and developed instead a 'social model' of disability to highlight the sociocultural, economic, political and environmental barriers that prevented disabled people's participation in society.

The 'social model' focused on changing society to facilitate the participation and inclusion of disabled people, rather than on efforts to 'rehabilitate' individuals and overcome biological constraints of the body. Political lobbying and campaigning underpinned by a social model approach to disability have led to significant changes in disabled people's access to education, employment, health and social care and welfare provision (Priestley 2003). Disability activists and allies demanded disabled people's rights to participate in all aspects of society on an equal basis with non-disabled people, under the often cited slogan, 'Nothing about us without us'.

The social model has, however, come under increasing criticism in recent decades for being gender-, race- and class-blind, speaking mainly of the experiences of white middle-class men with physical impairments in the Global North. It paid little attention to the experiences of women and others from socially disadvantaged backgrounds with diverse impairments and the majority of the global population of disabled people who live in the Global South (Imrie and Edwards 2007). Feminist disability scholars highlighted the failure of the social model to recognise personal, embodied experiences of impairment and chronic illness as part of people's diverse experiences of disability (Butler and Parr 1999; Dyck 2010; Morris 1991). Wendell (2001) argues that social model proponents' resistance to the idea of identifying disability with 'illness' (due to its association with the medical model) in fact served to prioritise the experiences of 'healthy' disabled people and neglect the diverse experiences of people living with pain or other physical (or mental health) complications linked to impairments that affect their health. The call of some disability scholars to 'bring the body back' into disability studies is not merely for theoretical reasons but also to respond to the real support needs of disabled people (Loja et al. 2012; Kröger 2009).

Indeed, conceptualising chronic illness as 'disability' poses a fundamental challenge to the social model of disability, which seeks to distance itself from medical discourses. Those living with chronic illness may choose to identify according to their biomedical diagnosis rather than according to a more generalised notion of 'disability'. Hughes (2009) notes that the interests and concerns of such 'biosocial' groups and the disability movement diverge in a number of ways: biomedical diagnosis and impairment are central to the identification of 'biological citizens'; biosocial groups are likely to 'gather and embrace the specialised medical and scientific knowledge associated with their condition' and medicine is perceived as a 'potential ally' in contrast to the rejection of medical approaches by the disability movement (Hughes 2009: 678). Identification as a biosocial group, however, may limit access to entitlements under disability legislation and potentially perpetuate the stigma surrounding both disability and some chronic (often life-limiting) illnesses (Evans et al. 2016).

People living with HIV can be regarded as such a biosocial group, who do not identify as 'disabled people' and are often not defined as such in law or social policy unless they have specific long-term impairments, although the UK and Australia are notable exceptions, according protection to people living with HIV under national disability legislation (Evans and Atim, 2011). The activism and advocacy of networks of people living with HIV in the Global South have been crucial to securing free access to life-prolonging antiretroviral medical treatment in many resource-constrained contexts. Nevertheless, the continuing stigma surrounding HIV, which is often gendered, combined with a lack of entitlements to support, may lead to significant experiences of discrimination, destitution and insecurity among migrant women living with HIV and their children in the UK (Evans and Becker 2009).

An increasing body of literature has shown that sociocultural constructions of disability and 'healthy/ill' bodies and the ways that people are treated vary cross-culturally and are shaped by personal, embodied and collective experiences, as well as by social differences (such as gender, class, race, ethnicity, socioeconomic status), and wider structural processes such as national and international policies and welfare provision in different geographical and historical contexts.

Recent international policy acknowledges the interaction between biological, psychosocial and environmental dimensions of disability. The UNCRPD, rapidly ratified by many countries after it was introduced in 2008, demonstrates a renewed global commitment to recognise disability as not merely a personal matter but as a bio-psychosocial and human rights concern. The bio-psychosocial model endorsed by the UN and WHO arose from a growing concern about the seeming lack of attention to 'impairment' and global differences in the experiences of disabled people within social model approaches. The bio-psychosocial model endorses a human rights approach to disability, while recognising that disability is a medical, personal and a social matter. The Convention aims to 'ensure and promote the full realization of all human rights and fundamental freedoms for all persons with disabilities without discrimination of any kind on the basis of disability' (UN 2008).

DISABILITY, CHRONIC ILLNESS AND THE UN'S POSITION

The UNCRPD and UN Refugee Agency (UNHCR) have sought to address the situation of disabled people in migration processes. The UNCRPD refers to migrants in Article 18 on the liberty of movement and nationality:

> 1. States Parties shall recognize the rights of persons with disabilities to liberty of movement, to freedom to choose their residence and to a nationality, on an equal basis with others, including by ensuring that persons with disabilities:
>   (a) Have the right to acquire and change a nationality and are not deprived of their nationality arbitrarily or on the basis of disability;
>   (b) Are not deprived, on the basis of disability, of their ability to obtain, possess and utilize documentation of their nationality or other documentation of identification, or to utilize relevant processes such as immigration proceedings, that may be needed to facilitate exercise of the right to liberty of movement;
>   (c) Are free to leave any country, including their own;
>   (d) Are not deprived, arbitrarily or on the basis of disability, of the right to enter their own country.
>
> (UN 2008)

Nation-states that have ratified the UNCRPD are obliged to promote and develop policies on disability that provide equal access to opportunities for welfare, health and social care, and any other support required in order for all disabled people (including migrants) to participate fully in society. Yet despite ratifying the Convention, the UK, Malaysia and Thailand have maintained a reservation on Article 18, excluding immigration policies from the Convention's obligations. Australia recently lifted the reservation it had on Article 18 (UN 2015).

Furthermore, the UNHCR launched its *Conclusion on Refugees Living with Disabilities and Other Persons Living with Disabilities Protected and Assisted by UNHCR* in 2010 in order to demonstrate the UN's commitment to specifically address the situation of disabled asylum-seekers, refugees and other migrants who have been displaced (UN 2008; UNHCR 2010). The *Conclusion* focuses exclusively on disabled people in need of humanitarian protection following displacement and includes men, women and children who have become displaced internally and across nation-states because of a variety of environmental, political and social reasons endangering their lives. Yet it has been criticised for lacking any further guidelines concerning how to respond to disabled asylum-seekers in receiving countries (Straimer 2011). Disabled asylum-seekers, as well as migrants who hold limited entitlements to support, may be denied status as a disabled person in receiving countries if, for example, their disability is not visible or they do not qualify for a care assessment on the basis of having visible 'care needs', which further marginalises those with 'invisible' chronic illnesses, mental health problems or other disability (Harris and Roberts 2004).

In reality, the ratification of the UNCRPD and UNHCR's *Conclusion* have not necessarily translated into actual rights for disabled people. In many countries, disabled people continue to be devalued and stigmatised due to sociocultural constructions of the problematic, 'abnormal' nature of disability, and because of legislation, public policy and service provision that are based primarily on medical model approaches to disability (Groce et al. 2011). Furthermore, despite significant improvements to legislation and service provision in many countries, including the UK, disabled people continue to experience inequality and marginalisation in the labour market, education and other aspects of society (Hughes 2015). Disabled migrants with limited entitlements to welfare, health and social care are even more likely to face poverty, inequality and destitution than other migrants (Ward et al. 2008). Their situation has been exacerbated in recent years by increasingly restrictive immigration policies, austerity and cuts to public welfare services following the global financial crisis in 2008, despite the adoption of laws and policies underpinned by a social model and/or human rights approach to disability in many receiving countries in Europe and elsewhere in the Global North.

THE POLICY CONTEXT OF MIGRATION, DISABILITY AND CHRONIC ILLNESS IN SETTLEMENT COUNTRIES

The introduction of the UNCRPD has been broadly welcomed among disability organisations and, in theory at least, appears to have positive implications for the human rights of disabled migrants. In reality, migrants with disability or chronic illness face challenges in gaining acceptance of their status as disabled people and in gaining entry because of increasingly restrictive immigration policies in many receiving countries (Straimer 2011). Disabled migrants face significant structural barriers in accessing health and social care support because of ever-tightening criteria used to determine eligibility and definitions of disability and 'care needs'. Coupled with language and sociocultural barriers and limited resources to address diverse needs within migrant and black and minority ethnic (BME) communities, disabled migrants often experience multiple barriers to support that prevent their participation in society on an equal basis with non-disabled people (Trotter 2012; Cole and Burke 2012).

As noted earlier, knowledge about the needs of migrants with disability or chronic illness is very limited. In migrant studies, disability is usually only referred to as a medical condition that a migrant may have been born with, or that may have developed during settlement. Many disabled migrants come from low-income countries where disability and poverty are intrinsically linked; while some individuals may have been born with impairments, many impairments are caused by poor living conditions in the country of origin and difficult experiences associated with migration and settlement (Straimer 2011; Harris 2003). Poverty, insecure housing and hazardous employment environments negatively impact on the physical and social health of individuals, which can result in disability (Zimmer 2008). Further barriers to accessing support in receiving countries include sociocultural barriers related to negative personal and social experiences of disability and inexperience in receiving welfare support in the Global South, combined with a failure of services and policy to address migrants' diverse support needs (Groce et al. 2011; Lamichhane et al. 2014). Due to these structural inequalities, comparative research between European countries suggests that migrants that are relatively 'healthy' on arrival are at a much higher risk of developing chronic impairments and poorer health outcomes than other groups in receiving countries where they have settled (Rechel et al. 2013; Sole-Auro and Crimmins 2008; Sundquist 1995). Sole-Auro and Crimmins (2008: 861) conclude that, 'there is little evidence of the "healthy migrant" in European populations'.

Statistical evidence about chronic illness among migrants has several shortcomings. No reliable figures currently exist about the prevalence of chronic ill-health among the migrant population in the UK, for example, although 'non-UK born' migrants, particularly those from South Asia (especially Pakistan and India) and sub-Saharan Africa, are disproportionately affected by infectious diseases, such as TB, Hepatitis B and C and HIV, than 'UK-born' people, which may be due in part to the higher prevalence of these infections in their countries of origin (Health Protection Agency 2006; Health Protection Services 2011; Jayaweera 2014). The majority of cases of TB, HIV in heterosexuals, malaria and enteric fever reported in the UK were found among migrants (Wagner et al. 2013). Unlike for infectious diseases, however, evidence by country of birth for non-communicable diseases is limited. Jayaweera (2014) concludes that a comprehensive overview of the health of migrants in the UK is hindered by the fact that much existing evidence on health includes ethnic group but not migration variables, such as country of birth, length of residence in the UK or immigration status, which often reveal significant differences.

While BME communities are likely to face a multitude of structural barriers to health and social support that they may share with migrants, studies in the UK often pay little attention to migrants' differential position and specific needs in accessing welfare services. Moreover, disabled migrants tend to be overlooked in policy and research on BME disabled people and those who care for them (Carers UK 2014; Children's Society et al. 2012).

Migrants in many receiving countries also face increasing public hostility and stigmatisation due to unfounded media portrayals of migrants as 'health tourists' (Jayaweera 2014). This notion is often used to question migrants' access to healthcare and the welfare system, with the claim that migrants are a 'burden' to national economies. The UK Department of Health's (2013) recent public consultation, for example, emphasises the need to regulate migrants' access to National Health Service healthcare by introducing fees for migrants from states outside of the European Economic Area (EEA). Research suggests, however, that migrants from within (rather than outside) the EEA entering the UK for medical purposes and health tourism produces financial gains rather than a drain on the NHS (Hanefield et al. 2013). The Department of Health's emphasis on the role of front-line health services in identifying chargeable migrants means that healthcare professionals, such as general practitioners (GPs), are under pressure to not only deliver clinical practice, but also to control entitlements to health services (Ottosdottir and Evans 2014: i59). Indeed, Pussetti and Barros (2012) highlight the racialised nature of European countries' public health and social care policy, which often constitute migrant populations as 'unsanitary citizens'. Following this overview of the policy context of migration, disability and chronic illness, we now discuss the specific situation of asylum-seekers with disability or chronic illness in receiving countries.

ASYLUM-SEEKERS WITH DISABILITY OR CHRONIC ILLNESS

An estimated 3.5 million to 5 million of the global population of displaced people are disabled people (Pisani and Grech 2015). Research with asylum-seekers has focused on the physical and mental effects of conflict and war in countries of origin; material and social disadvantage associated with migration and settlement processes, including isolation, loss of social status, poverty and insecure legal immigration status; and the impact of government policies such as detention and dispersal in the receiving society (Roberts and Harris 2002; Ward et al. 2008; Jayaweera 2014). Asylum-seekers and refugees are likely to have higher health needs than other migrant groups. Studies in the UK and systematic reviews of studies across European countries point to higher rates of depression and anxiety among asylum-seekers and refugees compared to the national population or other migrant categories (Raphaely and O'Moore 2010; Jayaweera 2014). Children and women who have suffered sexual and physical abuse are regarded as particularly vulnerable groups (Women's Refugee Commission 2014).

The majority of research on disabled asylum-seekers is based on health studies informed by the medical model of disability. Research examines the impact of forced migration on an individual's physical and psychological health and 'functioning', painting a general picture of complex impairments in forced migrant populations, with a high prevalence of mental health problems (Mollica et al. 1999; Silove et al. 1998). In their study of Bosnian refugees in Australia for example, Momartin et al. (2003) found that a high proportion of participants suffered from mental health problems, showing clinical symptoms of post-traumatic stress disorder.

Only a few studies have examined the situation of disabled asylum-seekers and refugees from a social or bio-psycho-social model of disability perspective, highlighting the detrimental material and social conditions generally found in settlement countries (Ruiz-Casares et al. 2010; Steel et al. 2006; Roberts and Harris 2002). Asylum-seekers in many countries in Europe experience prolonged periods of insecure immigration status and limited levels of subsistence support; they may be subject to deportation or detention processes; and are highly vulnerable to poverty and destitution, which significantly impacts on their health and wellbeing (Ryan et al. 2009). While the focus is often on barriers to care support, research is usually conducted with non-disabled people and disability is viewed as a mere outcome of the migration and settlement process (ICAR 2006; Crawley et al. 2011; Children's Society 2012). Straimer (2010, 2011) comments that European national policies on asylum and disabled asylum-seekers tend to be based on the medical model and do not seem to take on-board the recommendations made by the UNHCR on the situation of disabled people in forced migration contexts. Disabled women and children in particular, face significant barriers to social support and fulfilment of their rights to equal participation in settlement countries (Women's Refugee Commission 2014).

The little available literature reveals multiple legal, cultural, policy, language and information barriers to accessing formal care facing disabled asylum-seekers (see Harris and Roberts 2004; Sales and Hek 2004; Roberts and Harris 2002; Guhan and Liebling-Kalifani 2011; Humpries 2004). In comparison to other disabled people, disabled asylum-seekers appear to have heightened vulnerability to poverty and social exclusion because of their legal status, restricted entitlements to health, social care and welfare support, raised thresholds in care assessments and the failure of refugee organisations, disability organisations and local authorities to adequately address their needs (Roberts and Harris 2002).

CASE STUDY: ASYLUM-SEEKERS WITH DISABILITY AND CHRONIC ILLNESS AND INFORMAL CARERS IN THE UK

Given the limited evidence about the situation of disabled asylum-seekers in receiving countries, in the remainder of this chapter, we draw on available literature and our own empirical studies to provide a case study of disabled asylum-seekers and carers' access to welfare support, health and social care in the UK.

Asylum-seekers in the UK have a recognised legal status (unlike 'undocumented migrants') and are granted limited entitlements to public welfare support, although this is only approximately 70 per cent of the public benefits (such as Income Support Allowance) that are available to British citizens or those who have been granted refugee status (Home Office 2014; UK Government 2014). Asylum-seekers and 'undocumented' migrants face additional structural barriers to accessing employment, education and health and social care support in the UK because of their limited or lack of entitlements and lack of, or illegal, access to the labour market (ICAR 2006; Harris 2003). Furthermore 'irregular' or 'undocumented' migrants have very limited entitlement to healthcare within the NHS and often lack the resources to fund alternative treatment (Medical Protection Society 2015). Both of these categories of migrants (asylum-seekers and undocumented migrants) continue to be relatively hidden within research and policy on disability, care and migration, despite their often acute experiences of destitution and marginalisation (Harris 2003; Roberts and Harris 2002; Ward et al. 2008). Furthermore, although refugees whose asylum claims have been upheld and who have been granted indefinite leave to remain in the UK have the same legal entitlements to welfare support as British citizens, they may continue to experience structural inequalities (such as in entering the labour market), ongoing chronic illness or disability that may have resulted from extended periods living in poverty and destitution as an asylum-seeker and sociocultural barriers to accessing health and social care support (Fell and Fell 2013; Harris and Roberts 2004; Yeo 2015).

In UK asylum support policy, no reference is made to the needs and rights of disabled migrants other than the use of the term 'care needs', which is used to determine eligibility for care support for all disabled people (UK Government 1990, 1999). In order to qualify for care support, disabled asylum-seekers and people with 'no recourse to public funds' must have 'critical needs' that result from impairment or age and not merely from their living conditions (SCIE 2010, 2013). Furthermore, disabled people are regarded as 'vulnerable' rather than being considered as social actors with capabilities (Katsapaou 2013). Hence, social care and housing may be granted only to disabled asylum-seekers with significant impairments who are deemed to be in need of assistance with activities of daily living (SCIE 2010, 2013).

Ottosdottir's (2015) study of asylum-seekers and refugees with disability and chronic illness in the south-east of England confirmed these findings. Despite the option to use human rights assessments to provide social care for asylum-seekers with limited entitlements, social workers explained that local authorities usually sought identification of 'critical needs', rather than their assessments being informed by human rights principles:

> You need to have care needs first, yeah! [. . .] You have to have an eligible care need for us to provide a service [to asylum-seekers whose claims or appeals have been rejected]. The care need is the gateway into the service with us.
>
> (Ronalda,[1] social worker in a local authority).

Professionals in statutory and third sectors that provided health and social care support struggled to respond to the care needs of disabled asylum-seekers because of the strict eligibility criteria required for care assessments, and the conflictual nature of social policies designed to meet the needs of 'vulnerable adults and children' and immigration policies that applied to those in the asylum system (Grady 2004; Sales and Hek 2004; Robinson 2013; Ottosdottir and Evans 2014). Statutory sector professionals, such as social workers, experienced tensions between the legal framework governing the situation of asylum-seekers and their efforts to address their human rights and care needs (Ward et al. 2008; Newbigging and Thomas 2011; Ottosdottir and Evans 2014). In Ottosdottir's (2015) research, social workers expressed frustrations about the ethical dilemmas they faced when they were under pressure from the local authority to withhold support to asylum-seekers with limited entitlements because of funding constraints. Support must be negotiated between local authorities, the Home Office and even the NHS, and social workers felt that they were at risk of losing sight of fundamental human rights principles and their professional ethics of care (underpinned by a holistic approach to the person's needs) when they became involved in such negotiations (Ottosdottir 2015; Ottosdottir and Evans 2014).

In the light of multiple barriers to formal support, disabled asylum-seekers in the UK often rely on informal sources of support, such as children, relatives, friends and others, to provide – sometimes substantial – regular care to meet their needs. Ottosdottir's (2015) study revealed that most family and friends interviewed who were caring for disabled asylum-seekers had not received a carers' assessment or support as carers from the local authority, the third sector or from the NHS. Carers may also keep their caring role hidden due to a fear of deportation and discovery of their family's insecure immigration status. As Charlotte (aged 21) from Uganda, who cared for her mother with HIV, explained:

> My mum always used to tell me stories about her friends that had been . . . sleeping at their house and immigration came and just took them, you know because they did not have leave to remain. Not that they were illegal but they did not have the confirmed status. So she always used to worry about that they would suddenly appear . . . My mum used to say, 'Listen you are not like any of these children. If your friends are going wherever and start to have fun, you should think that for you that is not normal because for one, you don't have leave to remain and you don't have the money', so always those two things.

Disabled migrants and carers may therefore 'remain hidden' from services or be considered 'hard to reach' by professionals due to such fears, which may prevent them from seeking support (Harris and Roberts 2004). Other reasons cited for the invisibility of disabled migrants and carers within statutory and third-sector social care and support services included a lack of policy implementation, limited professional efforts to engage with the specific needs of migrants with disability or chronic illness and the fact that migrants assume caring roles on the basis of expected sociocultural norms of family roles and relationships (Ottosdottir 2015). The scarcity of research and knowledge about families' experiences of disability and care further hinders the development of appropriate support (Roberts and Harris 2002; Harris and Roberts 2004; Trotter 2012; Yeo 2015).

In the UK, third-sector organisations are beginning to recognise the potentially high levels of caring that young people in asylum seeking families and in families' without recourse to public funds' take on (Children's Society 2013). Young carers in asylum-seeking families may be more likely to experience higher levels of caring responsibilities than 'young carers' in non-migrant families because of the unmet needs of their disabled parents/relatives, in addition to the often lengthy periods of insecure legal status and limited entitlements to health, social care and welfare support.

Evans' (2011) research with African migrant mothers living with HIV and children caring for them who were seeking asylum or who had been granted refugee status or British citizenship, suggested that young people's regular responsibilities for household chores, childcare and provision of emotional support were interspersed with periods of more intensive care for their parent during episodes of ill health or hospitalisation. Many mothers living with HIV expressed feelings of frustration, sadness and guilt that they had to rely on their children to care for them when they were ill.

For young people from asylum-seeking families, the emotional impacts of supporting a parent/relative with a life-limiting illness were exacerbated by pressures associated with their insecure immigration status and a sense of isolation and lack of alternative support (Evans 2011). Crystal (aged 15), who cared for her mother and brother with HIV in an asylum-seeking family from Uganda, emphasised the need for security for her and her family's future:

> To know that we can settle down because the Home Office is not replying to us and mum can't work and I can't get a part time job and no one, it's just we need to have that assurance that yes we are going to stay in this country, that we don't need to be worrying about every time they're sending people to their country that it's going to be us next or something. We just need security.
>
> (Evans 2011: 354)

The profound sense of insecurity mothers and young people felt about whether they would be allowed to remain in the UK was linked to a fear of deportation and potential loss of access to life-prolonging anti-retroviral therapy that returning to their country of origin would entail (Evans 2011: 348). Caring relationships and young people's and mothers' mobility and access to support at the local level were thus influenced by wider structural processes such as global inequalities in access to HIV treatment and restrictive immigration policies (Evans 2011).

Young adults carers (aged 18–24) in asylum-seeking families also face significant challenges in their transitions to adulthood because of their caring responsibilities, as well as their legal status and sustained periods without entitlements to employment and education (Children's Society 2013; Becker and Becker 2008). Ottosdottir's (2015) research suggests that young adult carers in asylum-seeking families faced major barriers in making the transition into university education. Young adult carers with different legal status than the rest of their families faced great difficulties.

Susan (aged 21) from Zimbabwe who had a different legal status from the rest of her family and who cared for her mother with HIV, explained that she would not qualify for reduced university fees until she had gained 'indefinite leave to remain', despite having lived in the UK for ten years on consecutive limited 'leave to remain' permits:

> I will probably be near 30 years old then you know. I mean I want to do my education now! Unfortunately it is not going to work for me so I am hoping to get a good job that pays me well so that I can put myself through school.

Migrant young people from non-EU countries struggled to pay the much higher university fees than home/EU students and may postpone higher education, further compounding structural inequalities and discrimination they may face in the labour market and in their future life chances.

In addition to these barriers, a lack of cooperation between refugee and mainstream disability organisations in supporting disabled asylum-seekers has been noted in the UK (Ward et al., 2008). Refugee organisations often carry the burden of support, and disability support organisations do not appear to be involved in supporting disabled people from forced migrant backgrounds. In addition, carers organisations, including those providing young carer support services, are often not in contact with young people or other family members providing informal care in asylum-seeking and refugee families (Evans and Becker 2009; Greenwood et al. 2015).

While many local authorities emphasise diversity and family-focused approaches, a recent UN report suggests that many strategies have failed to reach families or meet the diverse support needs of children and adults in the UK asylum system (UNHCR 2013). Limited evidence was found of 'good practice' in social care with forced migrant families; professionals and agencies struggled to identify care needs, including those of disabled people, young carers and adult carers (SCIE 2010). The 'complexity' of care needs among asylum-seekers with disability or chronic illness; professionals' lack of awareness of entitlements; difficult interagency partnerships between organisations who work with asylum-seekers and those 'without recourse to public funds' were cited as key issues that had a negative impact on professional interactions with forced migrant families with care needs (SCIE 2010).

CONCLUSION

In this chapter we have analysed the complex linkages between migration, disability, chronic illness and care support. We provided an overview of key conceptual approaches to disability and chronic illness. We then discussed the policy context of migration, disability and chronic illness, highlighting the shortfalls of existing knowledge and the lack of engagement with asylum-seekers and refugees, despite their often high care needs. The specific situation of asylum-seekers with disability or chronic illness was discussed through a case study of the UK context, drawing on available literature, policy and our own empirical research on disability, HIV and caring relations among asylum-seeking and refugee families. Our analysis of the situation of asylum-seekers with disability and chronic illness revealed that this group faces major barriers in accessing appropriate health, social care and welfare support. The unmet care needs of disabled asylum-seekers also impact on informal family carers, including children and young adults, whose substantial caring responsibilities and their legal status and limited entitlements to support affects their wellbeing, education and transitions into adulthood.

NOTE

1. Pseudonyms have been used throughout the case study section to protect research participants' identities.

REFERENCES

Allsopp, J., N. Sigona and J. Phillimore (2014), *Poverty among Refugees and Asylum Seekers in the UK: An Evidence and Policy Review*, available online at www.birmingham.ac.uk/Documents/college-social-sciences/social-policy/iris/2014/working-paper-series/IRIS-WP-1-2014.pdf.

Becker, F. and S. Becker (2008), *Young Adult Carers in the UK: Experiences, Needs and Services for Carers Aged 16–24*, London: Princess Royal Trust for Carers.

Butler, R. and H. Parr (eds.) (1999), *Mind and Body Spaces: Geographies of Illness, Impairment and Disability*, London and New York: Routledge.

Carers UK (2014), *Facts About Carers*, available online at www.carersuk.org/for-professionals/policy/policy-library/facts-about-carers-2014.

Children's Society (2012) *I Don't Feel Human: The Experiences of Destitution among Young Refugees and Migrants*, London: The Children's Society, available online at www.childrenssociety.org.uk/news-views/press-release/report-shocking-destitution-among-asylum-seeking-and-migrant-children.

Children's Society (2013), *Hidden from View: The Experiences of Young Carers in England*, London: The Children's Society, available online at www.childrenssociety.org.uk/sites/default/files/tcs/report_hidden-from-view_young-carers_final.pdf.

Children's Society, ADASS and ADCS (2012), *Working Together to Support Young Carers and Their Families*, available online at www.youngcarer.com/sites/default/files/imce_user_files/PTP/mou_young_carers_2012.pdf.

Cole, A. and C. Burke (2012), *Reaching Out to People with Learning Disabilities and Their Families from Black and Minority Ethnic Communities*, Foundation for People with

Learning Disabilities, available online at www.learningdisabilities.org.uk/content/assets/pdf/publications/reaching-out-report1.pdf?view=Standard.
Crawley, H., J. Hemmings and N. Price (2011), *Coping with Destitution*, Oxford: Oxfam, available online at http://policy-practice.oxfam.org.uk/publications/coping-with-destitution-survival-and-livelihood-strategies-of-refused-asylum-se-121667.
Department of Health (2013), *Sustaining Services, Sustaining Fairness*, available online at www.gov.uk/government/uploads/attachment_data/file/210438.
Dyck, I. (2010). Geographies of disability: reflections on new body knowledges, in V. Chouinard, E. Hall and R. Wilton (eds.), *Towards Enabling Geographies: 'Disabled' Bodies and Minds in Society and Space*, Farnham: Ashgate Publishing Limited, pp. 253–264.
El-Lahib, Y. and S. Wehbi (2012), Immigration and disability: ableism in the policies of the Canadian state, *International Social Work*, **55**(1), pp. 95–108.
European Migration Network (2014), *Migrant Access to Social Security and Healthcare: Policies and Practice*, available online at http://ec.europa.eu/dgs/home-affairs/what-we-do/networks/european_migration_network/reports/docs/emn-studies/final_synthesis_report_migrant_access_to_social_security_final_3july2014_en.pdf.
Evans, R. (2011), Young caregiving and HIV in the UK: caring relationships and mobilities in African migrant families, *Population, Space and Place*, **17**(4), 338–360.
Evans, R. and A. Atim (2011), Care, disability and HIV in Africa: diverging or interconnected concepts and practices, *Third World Quarterly*, **32**(8), 1437–1454.
Evans, R. and S. Becker (2009), *Children Caring for Parents with HIV and AIDS: Global Issues and Policy Responses*, Bristol: Policy Press.
Evans, R., Y. Adjei-Amoako and A. Atim (2016), Disability and HIV: critical intersections, in S. Grech and K. Soldatic (eds.), *Disability in the Global South: The Critical Handbook*, Berlin: Springer.
Fell, B. and P. Fell (2013), Welfare across borders: a social work process with adult asylum seekers, *British Journal of Social Work*, **44**(5), 1322–1339.
Gleeson, B. (1999), *Geographies of Disability*, London: Routledge.
Grady, P. (2004), Social work responses to accompanied asylum-seeking children, in D. Hayes and B. Humpries (eds.), *Social Work, Immigration and Asylum: Debates, Dilemmas and Ethical Issues for Social Work and Socia Care Practice*, London: Jessica Kingsley Publishers, pp. 132–150.
Grech, S. and M. Pisani (2015), Editorial: towards a critical understanding of the disability/forced migration nexus, *Disability and the Global South*, **2**(1), pp. 416–420.
Greenwood, N., R. Habibi, R. Smith and J. Manthorpe (2015), Barriers to access and minority ethnic carers' satisfaction with social care services in the community: a systematic review of qualitative and quantitative literature, *Health & Social Care in the Community*, **23**(1), 64–78.
Groce, N., G. Kembhavi, S. Wirz, R. Lang and J-F. Trani (2011), *Poverty and Disability*, London: Leonard Cheshire Disability and Inclusive Development Centre University of London.
Guhan, R. and H. Liebling-Kalifani (2011), The experience of staff working with refugees and asylum seekers in the United Kingdom: a grounded theory exploration, *Journal of Immigrant and Refugee Studies*, **9**, 205–228.
Hanefield, J., N. Lunt and R. Smith (2013), Health tourism and the NHS: facts or fiction? *Lancet*, **382**(9890), e2.
Harris, J. (2003), All doors are closed to us: a social model analysis of the experiences of disabled refugees and asylum seekers in Britain, *Disability & Society*, **18**(4), 395–410.
Harris, J. and K. Roberts (2004), Not our problem: the provision of services to disabled refugees and asylum-seekers, in D. Hayes and B. Humpries (eds.), *Social Work, Immigration and Asylum*, London: Jessica Kingsley Publishers, pp. 151–161.
Health Protection Agency (2006), *Migrant Health: Infectious Diseases in Non-UK Born Populations in England, Wales and Northern Ireland: A Baseline Report*, London: HPA Centre for Infections.
Health Protection Services (2011), *Migrant Health: Infectious Diseases in Non-UK Born*

Populations in the United Kingdom: An Update to the Baseline Report, 2011, London: Health Protection Agency.
Home Office (2014), *Public Funds*, available online at www.ukba.homeoffice.gov.uk/visas-immigration/while-in-uk/rightsandresponsibilities/publicfunds.
Hughes, B. (2009), Disability activisms: social model stalwarts and biological citizens, *Disability & Society*, **24**(6), 677–688.
Hughes, B. (2015), Disabled people as counterfeit citizens: the politics of resentment past and present, *Disability & Society*, **30**(7), 991–1004.
Humpries, B. (2004), Refugees, asylum seekers, welfare and social work, in D. Hayes and B. Humpries (eds.), *Social Work, Immigration and Asylum: Debates, Dilemmas and Ethical Issues for Social Work and Social Care Practice*, London: Jessica Kingsley Publishers, pp. 42–58.
ICAR (2006). *Destitution Amongst Refugees and Asylum Seekers in the UK*, available online at www.icar.org.uk/Destitution%20briefing.pdf.
Imrie, R. and C. Edwards (2007), The geographies of disability: reflections on the development of a sub-discipline, *Geography Compass*, **1**(3), 1659–1680.
Jayaweera, H. (2014), *Health of Migrants in the UK: What Do We Know?* Oxford: The Migration Observatory, University of Oxford.
Katsapaou, C. (2013), *Response to Vulnerability in Asylum*, Budapest: UNHCR, available online at www.unhcr-centraleurope.org/en/what-we-do/caring-for-the-vulnerable/caring-for-the-vulnerable-in-asylum.html.
Kröger, T. (2009), Care research and disability studies: nothing in common? *Critical Social Policy*, **29**(3), 398–420.
Lamichhane, K., D. B. Paudel and D. Kartika (2014), *Analysis of Poverty between People with and without Disabilities in Nepal*, Tokyo: JICA Research Institute, available online at https://jica-ri.jica.go.jp/publication/assets/jica_ri_wp_no.77_2014_2.pdf.
Loja, E., M. E. Costa, B. Hughes and I. Menezes (2012), Disability, embodiment and ableism: stories of resistance, *Disability & Society*, **28**(2), 190–203.
Medical Protection Society (2015), *Health Care for All?* Available online at www.medicalprotection.org/uk/casebook/casebook-september-2014/healthcare-for-all.
Mitra, S., A. Posarac and B. Vick (2013), Disability and poverty in developing countries: a multidimensional study, *World Development*, **41**, 1–18.
Mollica, R. F., K. McInnes, N. Sarajlic, J. Lavelle, I. Sarajlic and M. Massagli (1999), Disability associated with psychiatric comorbidity and health status in Bosnian refugees living in Croatia, *Journal of American Medical Association*, **282**(5), 433–439.
Momartin, S., V. Silove, Z. Manicavasagar and Z. Steel (2003), Dimensions of trauma associated with posttraumatic stress disorder (ptsd) caseness, severity and functional impairment: a study of Bosnian refugees resettled in Australia, *Social Science & Medicine*, **57**(5), 775–781.
Morris, J. (1991), *Pride against Prejudice: Transforming Attitudes to Disability*, London: Women's Press.
Newbigging, K. and N. Thomas (2011), Good practice in social care for refugee and asylum-seeking children, *Child Abuse Review*, **20**(5), 374–390.
Oliver, M. (1990), *The Politics of Disablement*, London: Macmillan.
Ottosdottir, G. (2015), *Everyday Geographies of Disability, Care and Forced Migration in the South-East of England*, PhD Dissertation, University of Reading.
Ottosdottir, G. and R. Evans (2014), Ethics of care in supporting disabled forced migrants: interactions with professionals and ethical dilemmas in health and social care in the south-east of England, *British Journal of Social Work*, **44**(1), 53–69.
Pisani, M. and S. Grech (2015), Disability and forced migration: critical intersectionalities, *Disability and the Global South*, **2**(1), 421–441.
Priestley, M. (2003), *Disability: A Life Course Approach*, Cambridge: Polity Press.
Pussetti, C. and V. Barros (2012), The care of the immigrant self: technologies of citizenship and the healthcare sector, *International Journal of Migration, Health and Social Care*, **8**(1), 42–50.

Raphaely, N. and E. O'Moore (2010), *Understanding the Health Needs of Migrants in the South East Region*, London: Health.
Rechel, B., P. Mladovsky, D. Ingleby, J. P. Mackenbach and M. McKee (2013), Migration and health in an increasingly diverse Europe, *The Lancet*, **381**(9873), 1235–1245.
Roberts, K. and J. Harris (2002), *Disabled People in Refugee and Asylum Seeking Communities*, Bristol: Joseph Rowntree Foundation/Policy Press.
Robinson, K. (2013), Supervision found wanting: experiences of health and social workers in non-government organisations working with refugees and asylum seekers, *Practice: Social Work in Action*, **25**(2), 87–103.
Ruiz-Casares, M., C. Rousseau, I Derluyn, C Watters and F. Crépeau (2010), Right and access to healthcare for undocumented children: addressing the gap between international conventions and disparate implementations in North America and Europe, *Social Science & Medicine*, **70**(2), 329–336.
Ryan, D. A., F. E. Kelly and B. D. Kelly (2009), Mental health among persons awaiting an asylum outcome in Western countries: a literature review, *International Journal of Mental Health*, **38**(3), 88–111.
Sales, R. and R. Hek (2004), Dilemmas of care and control: the work of an asylum team in a London borough, in D. Hayes and B. Humpries (eds.), *Social Work, Immigration and Asylum: Debates, Dilemmas and Ethical Issues for Social Work and Social Care Practice*, London: Jessica Kingsley Publishers, pp. 59–76.
SCIE (2010), *Good Practice in Social Care with Refugees and Asylum Seekers*, London: Social Care Institute for Excellence, available online at www.scie.org.uk/publications/guides/guide37/files/guide37.pdf.
SCIE (2013), *Fair Access to Care Services (FACS): Prioritising Eligibility for Care and Support*, London: Social Care Institute for Excellence, available online at www.scie.org.uk/publications/guides/guide33/files/guide33.pdf.
Shivji, A. (2010), Disability in displacement, *Forced Migration Review*, **35**, 4–7.
Silove, D., Z. Steel, P. McGorry and P. Mohan (1998), Trauma exposure, postmigration stressors, and symptoms of anxiety, depression and posttraumatic stress in Tamil asylum seekers: comparison with refugees and immigrants, *Acta Pscychiatrica Scandinavia*, **97**(1), 175–181.
Simmons, K. (2010), Addressing the data challenge, *Forced Migration Review*, **35**, 10–12.
Sole-Auro, A. and E. M. Crimmins (2008), Health of immigrants in European countries, *International Migration Review*, **42**(4), 861–876.
Steel, Z., S. Momartin, D. Silove, M. Coello, J. Aroche and K. W. Tay (2006), Two-year psychosocial and mental health outcomes for refugees subjected to restrictive or supportive immigration policies, *Social Science & Medicine*, **72**(7), 1149–1156.
Straimer, C. (2010), *Vulnerable or Invisible? Asylum Seekers with Disabilities in Europe*, available online at www.unhcr.org/4cd9765b9.html.
Straimer, C. (2011), Between protection and assistance: is there refuge for asylum seekers with disabilities in Europe? *Disability & Society*, **26**(5), 537–551.
Sundquist, J. (1995), Ethnicity, social class and health: a population-based study on the influence of social factors on self-reported illness in 223 Latin American refugees, 333 Finnish and 126 South European labour migrants and 841 Swedish controls, *Social Science & Medicine*, **40**(6), 777–787.
Trotter, R. (2012), *Over-Looked Communities, Over-Due Change: How Services Can Better Support BME Disabled People*, London: Scope, available online at www.scope.org.uk/Scope/media/Images/Publication%20Directory/Over-looked-communities-over-due-change.pdf?ext=.pdf.
UK Government (1990), *National Health Service and Community Care Act 1990*, London: HMSO, available online at www.legislation.gov.uk/ukpga/1990/19/contents.
UK Government (1999), *Immigration and Asylum Act 1999*, London: HMSO, available at: http://www.legislation.gov.uk/ukpga/Geo6/11-12/29/section/21 [Accessed 20 January 2014].
UK Government (2014), *Income Support*, London: HMSO, available online at www.gov.uk/income-support/what-youll-get.

UN (2008), *Convention on the Rights of Persons with Disabilities*, available at www.un.org/disabilities/default.asp?navid=12&pid=150.

UN (2015), *UN Treaty Collection*, available online at https://treaties.un.org/Pages/ViewDetails.aspx?src=TREATY&mtdsg_no=iv-15&chapter=4&lang=en.

UNHCR (2010), *Conclusion on Refugees with Disabilities and Other Persons with Disabilities Protected and Assisted by UNHCR*, available online at www.unhcr.org/4cbeb1a99.html.

UNHCR (2013), *Considering the Best Interests of the Child within a Family Seeking Asylum*, London: UNHCR, available online at www.unhcr.org.uk/fileadmin/user_upload/docs/UNHCR-Best_Interest-screen.pdf.

UNHCR (2014), *People with Disabilities*, available online at www.unhcr.org/pages/4a0c310c6.html.

Wagner, K. S., J. Lawrence, L. Anderson, Z. Yin, V. Delpech, P. L. Chiodini, C. Redman and J. Jones (2013), Migrant health and infectious diseases in the UK: findings from the last 10 years of surveillance, *Journal of Public Health*, **35**(1), 28–35.

Ward, K., N. Amas and J. Lagnado (2008), *Supporting Disabled Refugees and Asylum Seekers: Opportunities for New Approaches*, London: London Metropolitan Support Trust, available online at www.metropolitan.org.uk/images/Disability-Report.pdf.

Wendell, S. (2001), Unhealthy disabled: treating chronic illnesses as disabilities, *Hypatia*, **16**(4), 17.

WHO and World Bank (2011), *World Report on Disability*, available online at www.who.int/disabilities/world_report/2011/report/en.

Women's Refugee Commission (2014), *Disability Inclusion: Translating Policy into Practice in Humanitarian Action*, available online at http://womensrefugeecommission.org/programs/disabilities/disability-inclusion.

Yeo, R. (2015), Disabled asylum seekers? They don't really exist': the marginalisation of disabled asylum seekers in the UK and why it matters, *Disability and the Global South*, **2**(1), 523–550.

Zimmer, Z. (2008), Poverty, wealth inequality and health among older adults in rural Cambodia, *Social Science & Medicine*, **66**(1), 57–71.

17 Mental health and forced migration: the case of Chilean exiles in the UK

Jasmine Gideon

INTRODUCTION

As the number of refugees fleeing from conflict continues to grow, there has been increased recognition of the mental health issues many refugees and asylum-seekers[1] experience. Yet, much of this work has applied bio-medical approaches, most notably Western models of post-traumatic stress disorder (PTSD) and depression, to 'measure' the impact of trauma experienced by refugees and those now living in exile. Moreover, there is still a tendency to conceptualise refugees and exiles as 'passive victims' and see them as a homogenous group with discussion of axis of difference such as gender, race, class and sexuality notably absent (Hyndman 2010; Bermudez 2013). While the health needs of women have been considered by some authors in refugee health debates, the focus has tended to be on health needs in the early years in host countries or the impact of sexual violence on women with very little analysis of the gendered experiences of long-term exile. Understanding how gendered norms, roles and relationships shape experiences of exile is critical if we are to also understand how these differences impact on health and wellbeing (Gideon 2016).

The chapter starts with a review of two contending approaches to the mental health of refugees that dominate the academic literature. The analysis then considers the case of long-term Chilean exiles in the UK to explore how people live with the long-term impacts of trauma and how the experiences of exile shape individuals' lives. Drawing on material from narrative interviews (conducted between September 2014 and November 2015) with 40 Chilean exiles living in Cambridge, London and Sheffield, the chapter reflects on how far the Chilean experience 'fits' into these wider debates and contemplates the coping strategies adopted following their expulsion from Chile during the military dictatorship of General Pinochet (1973–1990).

APPROACHES TO REFUGEE MENTAL HEALTH

To date, much of the analysis of the mental health of migrants has focused on the experiences of those recognised as refugees, and has predominantly focused on a Western biomedical model of trauma that concentrates on the psychological sequelae to trauma. Yet as Watters (2001) argues, such methods fail to acknowledge the social, political and economic factors that shape refugees' lives, as well as acknowledging their responses to these processes; moreover, within biomedical paradigms, limited space is offered for refugees to define their own needs and priorities. Others have suggested that there has also been a tendency to focus on the impact of refugees' exposure to violence in their home country, rather than taking into account the stressors encountered by refugees once they leave; that is, post-migration or exile-related stressors (Miller et al. 2002: 341).

Brough and colleagues argue that in the context of the 'medicalisation of distress', macro political events are transferred 'into a series of micro, medicalised experiences inappropriately divorced from both the wider contexts of their creation and the political commitments required for their solutions' (Brough et al. 2012: 210). In seeking to understand how this approach to refugee health has come to dominate practice, Summerfield (1999: 1449) reflects how in the latter half of the twentieth century, medicine and psychology 'have displaced religion as the source of explanations for the vicissitudes of life, and of the vocabulary of distress'. Yet, according to Summerfield, it was the recognition of PTSD in 1980 that marks the start of increasingly medicalised approaches to mental health and introduced the term 'trauma' into the 'refugee health' discourse. Ideas around PTSD emerged from the work of the anti-war movement in the United States, which argued that Vietnam War veterans were not just perpetrators of violence, but were also victims, traumatised by roles thrust on them by the US military establishment. They lobbied for veterans to receive a distinctive and specialised medical care organised around a diagnosis of PTSD – the successor to older formulations like shell shock or war neurosis (Summerfield 1999: 1450). As critics have argued, this has led to the development of a whole industry oriented at sustaining the wide-scale medical intervention required in both humanitarian and everyday contexts of mental trauma (Pupavac 2002; Theidon 2013; Watters 2001; Westoby and Ingamells 2010).

However, there has been a questioning of the construction of trauma as an individual pathology that can be addressed through a narrow application of mental health technologies. Indeed as Summerfield argues:

> Health and illness have social and political roots: post-traumatic reactions are not just a private problem, with the onus on the individual to recover, but an indictment of the socio-political forces that produced them.
>
> (Summerfield 2000: 234)

Research has found inconsistencies in rates of PTSD and depression and has shown general unpredictability in terms of reactions to trauma across cultural groups. As Pupavac (2002) argues, distressing experiences do not automatically translate into post-traumatic stress disorder, and there is a clear need to distinguish between the two and avoid classifying all refugees as traumatised, despite growing pressures to do so; for example, in the context of humanitarian crises. This has led to the questioning of the suitability of Western trauma models as a framework for addressing refugee experiences (Borwick et al. 2013).

Nevertheless, an alternative perspective can be found in the literature – one that moves towards more salutogenic understandings of 'resilience' among refugees. Commentators have argued that there is much value in applying a resilience 'lens' to understand the refugee experience, since it affords the opportunity to de-medicalise the 'needy victim' status often attached to the refugee label (Sherwood and Liebling-Kalifani 2012; Schweitzer et al. 2007). As Marlowe (2010) comments, *a priori* assumptions of refugees as traumatised or damaged can limit potential opportunities that can help people 'move on' and contribute to the healing process. Sudanese participants in his research in Australia, for example, expressed concerns about being labelled as 'traumatised' as this could jeopardise future job prospects.

Critics have also pointed to the limitations of an overemphasis on purely quantitative methods to understand mental health. As Ghorashi (2008: 117, cited in Marlowe 2010: 12) argues, 'in order to capture refugees' experiences and narratives it is necessary to create space within research to be able to notice the untold within the interviews'. Miller and colleagues (2002) advocate the importance of recognising concerns such as a loss of identity and crises of existential meaning that are largely overlooked within quantitative analyses. Moreover, other studies point to the importance of the 'ordinary' nature of responses to trauma and suggest that it is essential we differentiate between the 'extra-ordinariness' of the trauma and the often very 'ordinary' responses to traumatic events (Marlowe 2010) that can be shaped by factors including religious or political views (Gorman et al. 2003; Marlowe 2010). Drawing on the experiences of Somali and Zimbabwean refugee women in the UK, Sherwood and Liebling-Kalifani (2012) argue that 'everydayness' is itself an achievement and a potential aspect of resilience. Within their study, notions of resilience were not predefined, but instead conceptualised as the dynamic progression of mundane activities and the ordinary process of moving through daily life challenges and opportunities. Resilience means more than overcoming past experiences and involves 'a dynamic process of shifting, changing, building, learning and moving on' (Pulvirenti and Mason 2011: 46).

Other forms of resilience and methods of coping lie in cognitive processes in the form of interpretations and perceptions of themselves and their situation (Khawaja et al. 2008). Such 'inner resources' include taking a positive approach, identifying strengths, reinforcing the determination to cope and self-perception as a survivor rather than a victim (Gorman et al. 2003). As interviews with Chilean respondents highlight later in this chapter, this has been a critical strategy for many exiles.

Some attention has been given to the gender dimensions of 'coping', with some commentators suggesting that women are often better able to cope with the challenges of exile precisely because of their gender roles and responsibilities (Jansen 2008; Holm Pedersen 2012). Research has shown how, in the context of refugee camps, women's caring role means that they are able to maintain some semblance of normalcy in their daily activities – something that is reinforced once again after resettlement (Jansen 2008). In contrast, male exiles can struggle with the challenges of downward social mobility and the loss of traditional masculine roles, particularly as the household breadwinner (Kabachnik et al. 2013; Marlowe 2011; Szczepanikova 2015). However, two studies of the Chilean case (Kay, 1988; López, 1998) show how the needs of female refugees were often overlooked. Since it was predominantly men who had been imprisoned, their needs were prioritised while the indirect repression women endured was ignored (López 1998: 191). Yet these women faced particular challenges that were exacerbated by their position as 'heroes' wives' and the expectations this placed upon them (López 1998: 190).

Critics have also pointed to the need to avoid arbitrary assumptions about what constitutes a resilient or a non-resilient response to a particular life event (Sherwood and Liebling-Kalifani 2012; Ungar 2003: 88). Rather than focusing on specific traits of resilience, it is more useful to understand resilience as a dynamic process while at the same time acknowledging its 'everydayness'. Yet there is a need to acknowledge that exile-related stressors such as social isolation, unemployment and discrimination can be strongly associated with levels of depression and anxiety and may exacerbate symptoms of war-related trauma (Miller et al. 2002: 342). Focusing on resilience as a process can therefore also shed some light on the ways in which the experience of exile changes over time and exiles may overcome these initial stressors. Moreover, understanding resilience in this way can help shift away from an overemphasis on individualised responses and instead allow a broader focus on the ways in which exiled communities have responded to traumatic events, thus acknowledging the importance of recognising the sociopolitical context of situations. As the Chilean case demonstrates, shifts in the sociopolitical situation can also impact on resilience.

REFUGEES, EXILES AND THE CHILEAN EXPERIENCE

The term 'exile' can be used in many different ways and, as commentators have noted, it can be 'voluntary or involuntary, self-imposed or other-imposed, and may be near or far, short-term or long-term or permanent' (Lumsden 1999: 32). In the Chilean case, the term has been used to refer to those individuals and their families who were exiled from the country following the brutal military coup led by Augusto Pinochet on 11 September 1973. It has been suggested that around 200,000 Chileans were exiled internationally, 3,000 of whom came to the UK (Hirsch 2016: 2). Yet since the return to more democratic forms of government in 1990, some authors have suggested that the Chilean exiles should now be considered as 'post-exile' because despite the (theoretical[2]) possibility of returning to Chile, many exiles continued to live in their adopted countries (Olsson 2009; Roniger 2015).

The context of exit and arrival into exile is clearly important (Bermudez 2013) and has the potential to shape the long-term health and wellbeing of refugees (Correa-Velez et al. 2015; McMichael et al. 2015). In order to better capture these differences, commentators have suggested three distinct categories of refugees, which allow for a more nuanced analysis: activist, accidental or security and dependent refugees (Landolt and Goldring 2006; Bermudez 2013). Landolt and Goldring (2006) developed their typology as a response to the experiences of Chileans and Colombians in Canada. Activist refugees were those who had a history of left-wing political participation and had consequently received threats, been detained and imprisoned and suffered kidnapping or assassination attempts. 'Security' or 'accidental' refugees referred to those 'leaving because of the generalised violence and insecurity' and those 'who are unwittingly drawn into politics and become targets of political violence' respectively (Landolt and Goldring 2006: 16). In the Chilean case, many of these 'security' refugees were women who were the wives and partners of activist refugees and although not necessarily politically active themselves, did not support the Pinochet regime and held left-wing views. This contrasts with the case of dependent refugees, also frequently women, who move abroad primarily to accompany their male relatives and so may find it harder to adapt to a new society (Bermudez 2013). This typology is helpful for examining the case of Chilean exiles in the UK where the majority who arrived in the 1970s and early 1980s were either activist or accidental/security refugees.

The Chilean case is an important one given the longevity of the exile community in the UK and offers important insights into how the context of arrival can shape health and wellbeing. Salvador Allende's socialist government in Chile had generated considerable attention across the world, and following the military coup there was overwhelming support throughout the UK for the plight of the Chileans. Given the severity of the coup and the extensive arrests, imprisonment and torture of anyone suspected of opposing the military government, a strong solidarity network emerged within the UK to try and support refugees coming from Chile and to push for the release of political prisoners (Angell 2010).

International efforts directed through the Intergovernmental Committee on European Migration (ICEM)[3] were also made to offer assistance to those who were either at risk of detention or re-arrest as well as those in prison and concentration camps across Chile. The ICEM were active in negotiating an agreement in Chile that allowed some political prisoners to have their sentence commuted to exile. Once visas were negotiated for prisoners, ICEM handled their travel arrangements and in total assisted around 3,000 prisoners to leave under this programme (Angell and Carstairs 1987: 151).

Within the UK, several organisations were also established – these included the Joint Working Group for the Resettlement of Refugees (Joint Working Group), Academics for Chile and the World University Service (WUS). The WUS played a central role in offering scholarships for Chilean refugee students to continue their studies in the UK but the majority of the refugees arrived via the Joint Working Group. In the interviews conducted for this study, the majority of respondents reflected positively on the way in which they had been welcomed to the UK and the importance of this for them. As one woman reflected

> It was so emotional, because English people were so nice, so kind to us. They received us with love. [Laugh]. We, we felt love from them. And helping in any way . . . bringing us things, clothes, furniture, every day, it was so nice. And the Chilean people who were there already . . . although we didn't know any of them, we were like a big family. It was so nice.

The Joint Working Group and WUS played a critical role in supporting the Chilean exiles with practical issues, and for many exiles the input from these groups has had a lifelong impact in terms of making them feel welcome and offering them essential support in accessing housing, education and UK bureaucracy. However, since the main focus was on getting people safely out of Chile and in meeting their immediate resettlement needs, little attention was given to the mental health needs of these refugees, a situation exacerbated by the ad hoc nature of the solidarity work and the fact that few of those running the organisations were experienced in working with refugees.

RESPONSES TO EXILE AMONG THE UK-BASED CHILEAN COMMUNITY

The majority of respondents in the research did feel that overall they were in good health despite age-related difficulties for some and the ongoing psychological impact of their experiences. This is illustrated in the following quote from Claudia, an ex-political prisoner. She had worked in the NHS in the UK and so reflects on her own situation compared to many of those people she encountered through her job.

> I had read so many reports . . . about people younger than me, you know, a stroke, MS, cancer, you name it. And sometimes I tried to benchmark with some of those people. So I think that I'm extremely lucky, I'm really lucky, I'm 63 I haven't had any strokes, but I have thyroid problems but that is all . . . I have never been diagnosed by anybody but I think that I probably have got PTSD . . . but I have never had clinical depression . . . But I feel that is post-traumatic stress disorder, and the main thing is how mental health is approached in this country, and [it is about whether or not] are you able to function? I have been able to function, my fitness level is very good . . . so if that is the benchmark, I feel very well.
>
> (Claudia, ex-political prisoner, aged 63)

While it is important to acknowledge that the research sample only included those who were willing to talk and therefore was unlikely to have captured those people who felt that they were not able to cope, the interviews do offer important insights into how people make sense of traumatic events in their lives and are able to move forward with the healing process or at least cope with life. As the quote above illustrates, this is, of course, not to suggest that people did not continue to suffer some of the long-term consequences of their experiences in Chile. Many spoke of suffering flashbacks, having nightmares and other possible symptoms of PTSD. Indeed in one interview, the respondent explained how a recent holiday to a mountainous place set off a series of flashbacks for her

> There was something about the scenery . . . when we arrived at [the concentration camp] and they took off the blindfold I saw mountains and the scene [in the holiday destination] was the same . . . I just collapsed, it was terrible.
>
> (Marta, activist refugee).

It is worth noting that in the case of Chilean refugees, the majority arrived in the early to mid-1970s and so their arrival predated the 'discovery' of PTSD. This may also explain why more emphasis was placed on offering practical support, i.e., attempting to address the 'stressors of exile', rather than focusing on the potential mental health needs of refugees – moreover, few of the refugees themselves even thought about the long-term impacts of the trauma on their mental wellbeing, as one respondent explained:

> You felt that you have to cope on your own. You needed to be able to cope with things so it never occurred to me to ask for any support either.
>
> (Silvia, activist refugee)

Recognising the sociopolitical context in which trauma occurs is also critical in our understanding of the subsequent responses of individuals (Summerfield 2000). This is reflected in the words of one female activist refugee who explained how the realisation that she was not responsible for the torture she endured was critical in helping her move on in life. She had been a university student at the time of the coup and was subsequently imprisoned.

> I didn't choose the torture or being treated like that. They did that to me so why on earth should I feel unhappy inside for what they did? And I thought, well, I'm not going to carry their guilt because they should be the ones feeling bad for what they did. . . . And I thought, well, this is something that I don't want to do – feeling for what Pinochet did because . . . it wasn't my fault; I didn't do anything that really merited what they did to me, so why on earth I'm going to feel unhappy . . . carrying this thing for the rest of my life. And I thought, no, I'm not going to do that so I enjoy what I do [laughs]. It's not a lot but I go and I attend anything that is going on that I can take something from, learn something or see something and be in touch with people.
>
> (Silvia, activist refugee)

Similar views were expressed by other respondents. Yet for a number of people it was Pinochet's arrest in 1998 that changed how they made sense of their imprisonment and torture. One respondent reflected:

> The Pinochet detention marked a landmark . . . [it became clear that] we were the victims – the sense of guilt that they instil in you – that you are the reason you are here – it's your own fault, you did something wrong – the guilt is something they instil in you . . . [But] with Pinochet's detention it was clear that we were not guilty, we were pushed, we were forced into a situation, but we didn't

> have any control – so at that point there is a retaliation and a realisation that we were victims of a clear state repression.
>
> (Clara, activist refugee)

She also explained how this realisation enabled her to start to make sense of everything that happened and this was an important step in helping her to move on with her life and her relationships, particularly with family in Chile who had suffered considerably – both economically and emotionally – following her arrest and detention. She concluded 'the reason I felt better was that I started to rationalise my sense of guilt'.

RELATIONSHIP WITH FORMAL HEALTH SERVICES

One theme that emerged very clearly from the majority of interviews was a reluctance to discuss mental health issues with GPs or other health professionals. While a significant number of respondents revealed that they did still experience repercussions stemming from their imprisonment and/or torture – and, in the case of the security refugees, their experiences of searching for their husbands and other family members who were 'disappeared' – very few sought help from the NHS. The constraints to accessing formal health services encountered by migrants and refugees have been widely discussed in the literature (Thomas and Gideon 2013). A number of formal and informal barriers have been identified which can include lack of knowledge of the system, language difficulties, prejudice and racism on the part of providers. Yet in contrast to some of the more recent Latin American migrant groups in the UK (Gideon 2013), the Chilean exile population actively engages with the NHS around broader health issues and in my interviews respondents did not identify any particular constraints to access. Some recounted occasions, particularly in the early years of their exile, where they had experienced racism and prejudice on using services but many also reported positive, or at least neutral, relationships with their GP. Nevertheless within the interviews, a large number of respondents expressed a clear reluctance to engage with GPs and other health professionals over mental health issues or to reveal their history to health staff. Watters (2001) points to the importance of trust as an essential prerequisite for the development of any therapeutic mental health work with refugees, yet as respondents reveal in the interviews, many did not have much confidence in the ability of GPs to help them or direct them to appropriate services. This lack of trust was clearly expressed by one respondent, who recounted how medical staff had not believed her story. She had been detained and tortured by the military in Chile and as a result of her injuries she was hospitalised following her arrival in the UK in 1976. She was subsequently referred for counselling but had a very negative experience. She recalled how the therapist refused to believe that she had been detained in a concentration camp and told her that such camps had ceased to exist after World War II. She also then saw him gesticulate to a colleague that 'she was crazy' and so after that she decided to discontinue with the counselling. Ironically when in the 2000s she presented to a GP with serious physical pain, particularly stomach problems, he told her that she should see a psychiatrist because she had been a refugee and was clearly experiencing some degree of PTSD. Although she was referred to hospital for the pain, she was told it was nothing serious and again it was suggested that she seek psychiatric help. She was eventually diagnosed with stomach cancer when she insisted on being transferred to a different hospital (Teresa, activist refugee).

The lack of trust was also clearly articulated by another respondent who had recently tried to raise the issue of memory loss with her GP. She had been tortured by the military government and as a result now had several periods of her life that she had no recollection of whatsoever – similar symptoms were also reported by a small number of other respondents. As the respondent explained, she had not pursued her search for 'solutions' within the NHS because she lacked confidence in the response of healthcare professionals. She recounted her experiences of a visit to a GP

> Because sometimes you lack trust . . . I had mentioned the memory thing to my GP . . . and he said, oh no, [laughs] he said, oh, I've also got problem but I keep a notebook and . . . I keep this at work and I put everything that I need to do . . . And he said, oh no, don't worry then . . . I haven't told him that I was tortured. I said, no, because I really need something. He said, oh no, it's age; we all get that. Look here in my calendar. I put in there what I have to do because I always forget. So he really dismissed these memory things.

Yet as the following extract highlights, it is often about more than a lack of trust. She did subsequently see another doctor who suggested she challenge the doctor who had dismissed her.

> He said, oh, you have been having memory problem, I said, yes, and what did he say. He said, oh, he said that yes and he was really upset. He said . . . you should go back to him and say that he should send you . . . There are some memory clinics, I think. And I haven't done that actually, because I think that I need something more than a memory clinic. It's not because . . . I keep really active; I read and study and do things like that, so I don't think it's just the normal age-related memory loss. Mine is something else because there are too many gaps, too important things for my life actually. I think that, yeah. So, yeah, I, uh, probably need to do something about that. I don't know if my GP, has that same attitude. How do you get him to understand that role? Yeah, if he thinks that there is nothing you can do because it's your age?

> Interviewer: And you wouldn't tell him you'd been tortured and that's. . .
> I'm not sure if that would make any difference. Maybe, I don't know actually. I haven't, I haven't tried that one with him. He might be more sympathetic or maybe not; I don't know. I could try actually, I should.
>
> (Silvia, activist refugee)

Many respondents also felt that the structure and remit of the NHS was not appropriate for providing the kind of mental health support that exiles might need. Critics have suggested that one limitation of the biomedical approach to looking at the mental health of refugees is that their experiences are 'condensed into that which is deemed "clinically significant"' Watters 2001: 1710). The refugee's story is therefore structured within a framework of a biomedical explanatory model and the telling of refugees' stories takes place within a clinical arena in which the process of narrating the story is, in itself, viewed as having a therapeutic effect (Watters 2001). Yet, refugees are rarely given a voice in policy debates around the most appropriate forms of treatment or prioritising their needs in terms of service provision. As Watters notes:

> Refugees may be the subject of institutional responses that are influenced by stereotypes and the homogenising of refugees into a single pathologised identity.
>
> (Watters 2001: 1710).

This resonates with my own findings where other respondents also clearly articulated that they did not feel that the NHS could help them. In the first excerpt, a male ex-political prisoner, recounted ongoing nightmares and panic attacks that he still suffered from, but said he had never discussed this with his GP or other medical professional. When asked if he had ever discussed his situation with the GP he replied: 'No never . . . No because they, I won't say, I won't say all of them but they, most of the GPs here they are prescribers' (Roberto, activist refugee).

He went on to talk about how GPs are just an entry point to the NHS and lack specialist knowledge so their response to problems is simply to prescribe medication. He then talked about how he considered himself to be very healthy and did not take medication but instead preferred to look after himself through eating well and maintaining a healthy lifestyle. He also explained how he dealt with any feelings of depression and isolation, particularly in the early years of exile

> You don't have access to things, so you become more and more isolated, and you have to feed yourself which for me is studying, reading, motivating meetings, so I never had time to think about myself in that way.

His comments also highlight the reluctance expressed by many respondents to see themselves as victims.

Another theme expressed by several respondents was that they felt that GPs were also not interested in their history because their focus was on the clinical aspects of a problem, even if the problem itself was a result of torture and therefore there was no point in telling doctors and making them feel uncomfortable

> And in the first place it may be because it's not relevant to, to the clinical aspect or something, but people probably are not comfortable with it, with the subject.
>
> (Ana, security refugee)

In another case, the respondent had a number of physical symptoms that she considered were the direct result of torture she had experienced – including being pushed down a flight of stone stairs. She explained that that she was also reluctant to discuss her situation with her GP, although she thought it was probably noted in her medical records that she had been the victim of torture.

> Because obviously, I don't know, in my records it said about the situation of the torture. But . . . but . . . people don't understand. They just can't . . . can't. They can't. . . . Look, if I'm very honest, the more I do, I feel a lot of solidarity with the people . . . with the Chileans that have been tortured. Yes? Because they're elderly now, like me, that have been tortured, yes? We are experiencing a lot of problems. A lot of problems. And they are not things that the NHS could solve for us.
>
> Interviewer: Why do you think that, though?
>
> [Pause]. We are damaged. I think that's the right word.
>
> (Diana, activist refugee)

In some cases, the feeling that there was nothing that could be done to help people in their suffering can have devastating consequences. One woman recounted how her husband had committed suicide as he could no longer cope with the pain and anguish that he continued to experience. She explained how difficult it had been to support her partner:

> It was very hard because he suffered from depression but he wouldn't get help . . . Not the help he needed . . . He was taking some antidepressants and I said, well, I cannot do any more . . . you need some kind of therapy. [He said] No, nobody would understand because I don't want to change . . . he thought that he would talk to someone, that it would change his soul; the way he was, because . . . I said, no, you can look at things in another way, you know . . . he's suffering, you know, because he suffered a lot, you know. He was . . . he was in prison nearly five years, and a lot of people survive somehow, but he couldn't. His music helped him; that was his food for his soul, but the last couple of few years he was becoming more . . . and we talked about him going back to

> [Chile] . . . because he said, I want to be first time on my own to sort it out . . . because he said that his trial started 40 years ago because his dreams were cut off, and the children and the life we had helped him but it was always on his mind that he had lost something that he could never recover and he couldn't get over it. I never thought that he could take his life.
>
> (Telma, security refugee)

COMMUNITY AND RESILIENCE

In line with wider debates around refugees' responses to trauma, many of the Chilean exiles had found their own ways of coping and developing resilience that did not necessarily involve engagement with formal health services. For many respondents, the theme of 'community' emerged very clearly from the interviews and reinforces wider debates around the importance of social networks in promoting better health (Kawachi et al. 1999). Many respondents stressed the importance of the Chilean community and Chile solidarity networks that offered critical support following their arrival in the UK, and also talked about the positive role the Chilean community continued to play in their life today.

In some cases, respondents' experiences reinforce the connections between resilience and the performance of ordinary, everyday activities in exile – many of which were gendered. Many middle-class women had previously employed domestic workers in Chile, so for these women many of the everyday tasks they had to take on when they arrived in the UK were new (Kay 1988). One woman, an ex-political prisoner, spoke of arriving in London alone with her three young children and the immediate challenges she faced. She explained how with the help of another Chilean family who were living in the same street as her she learnt to cook – they exchanged recipes and taught each other as the other family were also unused to cooking for themselves. At the same time, the children in the two families became friends and this all helped in coping with the situation they were all in. She talked about how critical the friendships were to the wellbeing of the children, especially as no other support was given to them at the time.

In another interview, the respondent had accompanied her husband into exile and talked of the sense of relief she felt when arriving in London and being accommodated in bed and breakfast accommodation with other Chileans until alternative housing became available.

> My, my big happiness was when, when, um, I saw the, this big Chilean family in the hotel, because it looked like, it was like a big family. Everybody was telling their stories and trying to help each other.
>
> (Alejandra, security refugee)

However, although they were appreciative of the accommodation, there were also challenges, particularly if they were there with children, as they were not allowed to stay in the B&B during the day, so spent much of the time roaming the streets, and in winter trying to keep warm. As Alejandra, who had worked as a teacher in Chile, explained:

> It was mad . . . We couldn't control the children, so we started to organise . . ., I asked one of [the women who was a] teacher . . . there were two other teachers, and with me, four teachers, and so with the social workers, we organised. We made a little school inside the, the hotel, to control the children, because it was mad. Children were running on the street, um, going to the shop, they were stealing. My children saying, mummy, that boy, he took a chocolate . . . [Laughter]. So, I was scared for our children. It was bad, a bad experience.

This subsequently became a more long-term fixture with Chileans in both London and Sheffield, where they organised Saturday schools for the children. Here too the gender dimensions of resilience can be seen – women's role as 'carers' and 'educators' shapes the ways in which they respond to the challenges of exile. Several women found the schools offered an opportunity to develop new support networks, replacing the family and kinship networks they had been forced to leave behind in Chile. For some, the schools also offered a means of protection for their children from potential psychological damage, as they felt it provided them with a sense of community and shared experience.

RESILIENCE, POLITICAL SOLIDARITY AND ACTIVISM

For many Chilean exiles, political activism has formed an integral part of their lives in exile. Respondents talked about the support and friendships they found in the Chilean community or through other forms of political activism, especially in the early years of exile. This is exemplified in the following quote:

> So it was very hectic at first here, I would say it was very hectic. There were meetings all the time, like the meetings with the student committees, things to do with the Chilean community, it was an eye-opener, I started making friends with some English people here in London, but I was happy.
>
> (Jaime, activist refugee)

In the early years, the intensity of solidarity work meant that there was little time to think about one's problems. However, at the same time, many saw this as a way of moving forward and making sense of what happened to them:

> Most of the Chileans they, they stopped their clock on the 11th of September and that's it, that's all, poor me, and I think my attitude wasn't that. My attitude is OK, I'm going to go somewhere else, I have to do something somewhere else, I will be useful, we all have the capacity, the potential to develop you know.
> (Roberto, security refugee)

Another respondent explained how his job, which involved working with other refugees who had experienced trauma, helped him to make sense of his own situation and feel positive about himself and the work he was doing.

> So I'm happy with what I did, in fact over the years I've discovered that if I could restart my life I would have studied law rather than journalism . . . you know law can be subversive, that I realise, you know it can be a good science and you can use it to do good.
> (Silvia, activist refugee, aged 63)

Similarly, Silvia also felt her political activism helped her to cope with life in exile. She talked at length about the different activities she took on in the aftermath of her arrival, including taking up a WUS grant to study at university while travelling the country to carry out solidarity work.

She reflected how her activism helped her to maintain a positive approach to life. She recalled: 'I don't remember ever having sat and thinking oh I went through all this and I'm so sad. No, I didn't have time. I didn't allow time for myself.' She also emphasised the importance of political activism and being resilient as a critical means of survival after her imprisonment:

> And also because during the time I was in prison, for me you know it's a survival tool . . . I thought oh no, Pinochet, what Pinochet wanted with all this is to defeat you, to make you unhappy and it would be a, a triumph . . . To Pinochet if I am sorry, if I'm ill, if I'm defeated and I will never, ever give them this success . . . they didn't win because I have done my life and I came here and I did as much work as I could, went back to Chile, worked underground. I was part of the whole movement again and I was really active and all that and I thought well, you know, this is my, this is what – my vengeance, if you want [laughs] to them.

Nevertheless, she does reflect that with the passing of time, she acknowledges that she may have had some mental health needs that were never addressed:

> Now actually, if you asked me, I probably should have paid more attention to myself because I feel I had a lot of . . . If I look that I think that a lot of things are because of that.

Many of the activist refugees – male and female – spoke about the ongoing importance of political activism and how it provided them a sense of purpose in exile and indeed post-exile. While some people still focused their attention on Chile – for example, raising money following the 2010 earthquake – others had turned their attention to British politics or other global justice issues. A male respondent explained the importance of his activism: he had been working in Santiago, after being dismissed from his job and threatened as a consequence of his political affiliations he fled to Argentina with his family. Following the coup and rising tensions in Buenos Aires he came to the UK with his family and the support of the Joint Working Group. After a number of years, he had ended up working in a refugee support organisation, which he suggested had been central to his 'moving on' in life. He talked about how exile had been a positive experience in many ways, particularly as he felt his work in the charity sector was very rewarding and gave him an opportunity to help others.

Limits of 'Community'

It is also important to recognise the limits of 'community' and recognise that while for some it can be a source of support, for others it may be a source of tension, particularly in relation to health and wellbeing (Menjívar 2002; Escandell and Tapias 2010; Gideon 2011). Indeed, at times, refugees may opt to isolate themselves as a means of protecting themselves and avoiding painful memories elicited during social interactions (Miller et al. 2002).

In the Chilean case, the vast majority of exiles were related to different political parties but they were also separated by strong ideological divisions (Angell and Carstairs 1987). For some this emphasis on 'the political' created a challenge of belonging, and as one observer noted, if you were not involved in politics then 'the community' were not interested in you.

> Political parties were the only institutions that counted in exile and were a means of social control replacing the extended family. As I had resigned from my political party, my private problems were of no concern to them. Consequently, I became isolated and had to rely on sporadic support.
>
> (López 1998: 192)

This was particularly significant for the female security refugees who were frequently reduced to their dependent role rather than being acknowledged as an exile in their own right (López 1998; Kay 1988).

Yet as respondents in my own interviews suggested, today these political divisions are no longer so divisive. The arrest of Pinochet in 1998 had done much to heal the rift between different sections of the community and bring people closer together. At the same time, Pinochet's arrest and the public acknowledgement of the nature and extent of the torture meted out to political prisoners also changed the dynamics of relationships among many Chilean exiles. As one woman explained:

> I have lots of women friends now, Chilean women friends, and we sort of seek each other out. What happened with the 40 years is that lots of people who had been political prisoners and perhaps have never said because it's very shameful for them because now we all know what happened to all of them. Yes but anyway it's horrible . . . but we enjoy each other's company . . . [and we meet] to talk. And that has opened up with the years.
>
> (Isabel, security refugee)

Other respondents expressed similar views and suggested that with age they had found themselves more drawn to the Chilean community, given their shared experience of living through the military coup and life in exile. Several stressed how they felt an affinity with other Chileans that they did not feel with British friends and emphasised that with other Chileans they felt that there was 'no need to explain ourselves' (Isabel, security refugee).

GENDER AND COPING

Interviews with female 'security' refugees offer a slightly different perspective on the importance of political activism. While many of the women were also very active in political solidarity work, here too roles were often gendered and they were frequently responsible for cooking food for events and fundraising rather than activities such as public speaking, which were the domain of the activist refugees. Critics have noted that despite women's political activism both during the Allende government and as part of the opposition movement under the military regime, women's maternal role was never questioned and continued to shape Chilean society (Thomas 2013; Hiner 2015). Indeed, Kay notes how questions of gender equality were not part of the Popular Unity project and the absence of a gender critique meant that 'male–female relations were carried into exile largely unexamined' (Kay 1988: 5). Several women interviewed for my study hinted at tensions they felt at times, mostly in relation to their gender roles where they were left at home to look after the children while their husbands spent time travelling round the UK giving talks about their experiences in Chile.

> You know when people come here they wanted to give something back in a way so they got quite involved with the Chile Solidarity campaign. And at that time it was a big campaign so sometimes you felt that rather than being with

> you they were doing all this kind of activity . . . but also that sometimes you were left . . . not often but sometimes you said, oh why does he keeps going to that? And . . . and stay with us or go out with us or, but, um, in general it wasn't really a big deal.
>
> (Elena, security refugee)

Other women – predominantly security refugees – spoke of the way in which the strongly patriarchal norms that continue to govern men's behaviour left them feeling alienated from the community. For some women, particularly single women, this was evident in the behaviour of some of the men towards them and they spoke of their patriarchal attitudes, frequently expressed in the form of lewd comments, which left them feeling uncomfortable.

> Sometimes when I go to Chilean parties and events the men make me feel uncomfortable. They always tell me that you only have all these problems because you don't have a man . . . I have to just laugh though so I can still be part of the group. But I don't like it.
>
> (Ximena, security refugee, 66)

Some women opted to distance themselves from the Chilean community, but this left them without a support network:

> The other Chileans don't really talk to me . . . They don't ever help me, they think I am a snob but the thing is I don't like what the men say to me.
>
> (Rosario, security refugee)

Other studies have considered the ways in which rigid gender norms have shaped health seeking behaviour among Chileans (Cianelli et al. 2008; Cárdenas et al. 2012). Interviews in my research also alluded to some of the ways in which the pressure of gender norms shaped their behaviour. In one case, echoing López's earlier argument about the importance of playing the 'hero's wife', one woman talked about the difficulties of having to attend solidarity events where she made and sold empanadas along with the other wives, and about the pressures she felt to behave as the 'perfect wife' of a man who had been a widely respected high-profile activist in Chile. Yet she explained how when they returned home after such events he would become extremely violent and aggressive, but she felt unable to talk to anyone else in the community about this because of the respect he had among Chileans (Ximena, security refugee). Other studies have also suggested that gendered norms continue to shape Chilean women's responses to abusive husbands and they are reluctant to confront the problem, especially since wider societal norms permit men to behave in this way (Cianelli et al. 2008; Vandello et al. 2009). While other respondents told me anecdotally about women they knew in the community who continued to suffer domestic abuse, no one spoke about this directly to me in the interviews. It is clearly an area that needs careful examination in the future.

CONCLUSIONS

The experience of Chilean exiles in the UK points to the complexities of lifelong exile and how the impacts of trauma are incorporated into daily life in multifarious ways. Many of those exiled were tortured and imprisoned while others coped with the effect of having friends and family 'disappeared' and had to endure daily life under one of the most repressive regimes of the twentieth century. Yet as the discussion has highlighted, while more than 40 years have passed since the military coup of 11 September 1973, the repercussions of the era continue to shape – to varying degrees – the health and wellbeing of the exiled community. While many people are able to develop resilience, this does not detract from the fact that they may be 'damaged'. However, the Chilean experience also highlights how inextricably linked trauma and survival are to wider socio-political questions – many respondents in this study for example, saw the arrest of Pinochet as a significant landmark in their ability to 'move on' in life.

Yet for the majority of Chileans, their arrival in the UK predated the 'discovery' of PTSD, mental illness was heavily stigmatised and treatment options were scarce. Specialist organisations such as the Medical Foundation for the Care of Victims of Torture[4] did not emerge until the mid-1980s and as many respondents articulated, few felt that they either needed or wanted any form of mental health intervention. In some cases, where people did receive mental health interventions, their experiences reinforce some of the concerns raised in the wider literature. As a consequence of being seen primarily as 'passive victims', this meant that subsequent health complaints were not necessarily fully explored and on occasion physical ailments were seen by doctors as being psychosomatic. Such reductionist categories mean that little – if any – attention is given to the causes of health complaints nor is any attempt made to understand the ongoing social context in which the health issue is experienced; for example, via gendered and cultural norms. Given the limited resources currently assigned to the mental health needs of migrants (Lamb et al. 2011), 'long-term' migrant populations are unlikely to be considered as a priority group and so few opportunities exist to revisit their needs. As a consequence, people will continue to live with the long-term impacts of trauma, which could potentially be alleviated with more nuanced approaches to mental health that recognise the diverse ways in which people cope with varying degrees of success.

NOTES

1. While it is important to acknowledge the mental health needs of asylum-seekers, in this chapter I will use the term 'refugee' to refer to all those fleeing violence, persecution and conflict, not just those who have officially been recognised as refugees.
2. Several studies highlight the challenges of return migration for those who were exiled under Pinochet (Hirsch 2016; Roniger 2015).
3. This was a precursor to the International Organization for Migration.
4. This is now known as Freedom from Torture.

REFERENCES

Angell, A. (2010), Academics for Chile, available online at www2.warwick.ac.uk/fac/arts/history/research/projects/chileanexileinuk/testimonies/documents/alan_angell.pdf.

Angell, A. and Carstairs, S. (1987), The exile question in Chilean politics, *Third World Quarterly*, **9**(1), 148–167.

Bermudez, A. (2013), A gendered perspective on the arrival and settlement of Colombian refugees in the United Kingdom, *Journal of Ethnic and Migration Studies*, **39**(7), 1159–1175.

Borwick, S., R. D. Schweitzer, M. Brough, L. Vromans and J. Shakespeare-Finch (2013), Well-being of refugees from Burma: a salutogenic perspective, *International Migration*, **51**(5), 91–105.

Brough, M., R. Schweitzer, J. Shakespeare-Finch, L. Vromans and J. King (2012), Unpacking the micro–macro nexus: narratives of suffering and hope among refugees from Burma recently settled in Australia, *Journal of Refugee Studies*, **26**(2), 207–225.

Cárdenas, M., J. Barrientos, F. Gómez and D. Frías-Navarro (2012), Attitudes toward gay men and lesbians and their relationship with gender role beliefs in a sample of Chilean university students, *International Journal of Sexual Health*, **24**(3), 226–236.

Cianelli, R., L. Ferrer and B. J. McElmurry (2008), HIV prevention and low-income Chilean women: machismo, marianismo and HIV misconceptions, *Culture, Health and Sexuality*, **10**(3), 297–230.

Correa-Velez, I., S. Gifford and C. McMichael (2015), The persistence of predictors of well-being among refugee youth eight years after resettlement in Melbourne, Australia, *Social Science and Medicine*, **142**, 163–168.

Escandell, X. and M. Tapias (2010), Transnational lives, travelling emotions and idioms of distress among Bolivian migrants in Spain, *Journal of Ethnic and Migration Studies*, **36**(3), 407–423.

Gideon, J. (2011), Exploring migrants' health seeking strategies: the case of Latin American migrants in London, *International Journal of Migration, Health and Social Care*, **7**(4), 197–208.

Gideon, J. (2013), Access versus entitlements: the health seeking behaviour of Latin American migrants in London, in F. Thomas and J. Gideon (eds.), *Migration, Health and Inequality*, London: Zed Books.

Gideon, J. (ed.) (2016), *Handbook on Gender and Health*, Cheltenham: Edward Elgar Publishing.

Ghorashi, H. (2008), Giving silence a chance: the importance of life stories for research on refugees, *Journal of Refugee Studies*, **21**(1), 117–132.

Gorman, D., M. Brough and E. Ramirez (2003), How young people from culturally and linguistically diverse background experience mental health: some insights for mental health nurses, *International Journal of Mental Health Nursing*, **12**, 194–202.

Hiner, H. (2015), 'Memory speaks from today': analyzing oral histories of female members of the MIR in Chile through the work of Luisa Passerini, *Women's History Review*, **25**(3), 382–407.

Hirsch, S. (2016), Chilean exiles, reconciliation and return: an alternative view from below, *Journal of Refugee Studies*, **29**(1), 82–97.

Holm Pedersen, M. (2012). Going on a Class journey: the inclusion and exclusion of Iraqi refugees in Denmark, *Journal of Ethnic and Migration Studies*, **38**(7), 1101–1117.

Hyndman, J. (2010) 'Introduction: the feminist politics of refugee migration', *Gender, Place & Culture*, **17**(4), 453–459.

Jansen, S. (2008), Misplaced masculinities: status loss and the location of gendered subjectivities amongst 'non-transnational' Bosnian refugees' anthropological theory, **8**(2), 181–200.

Kabachnik, P., M. Grabowska, J. Regulska, B. Mitchneck and O. Mayorova (2013), Traumatic masculinities: the gendered geographies of Georgian IDPs from Abkhazia, *Gender, Place & Culture: A Journal of Feminist Geography*, **20**(6): 773–793.

Kawachi, I., B. P. Kennedy and R. Glass (1999), Social capital and self-rated health: a contextual analysis, *American Journal of Public Health*, **89**(8), 1187–1193.

Kay, D. (1988), The politics of gender in exile, *Sociology*, **22**(1), 1–21.

Khawaja, N. G., K. M. White, R. Schweitzer and J. H. Greenslade (2008), Difficulties and coping strategies of Sudanese refugees: a qualitative approach, *Transcultural Psychiatry*, **45**(3), 489–512.

Lamb, J., P. Bower, A. Rogers, C. Dowrick and L. Gask (2011), Access to mental health in primary care: a qualitative meta-synthesis of evidence from the experience of people from 'hard to reach' groups, *Health*, **16**(1), 76–104.

Landolt, P. and L. Goldring (2006), Activist dialogues and the production of refugee political transnationalism: Chileans, Colombians and non-migrant civil society in Canada, available online at www.researchgate.net/profile/Luin_Goldring/publication/242152457_Activist_dialogues_and_the_production_of_refugee_political_transnationalism_Chileans_Colombians_and_non-migrant_civil_society_in_Canada/links/00b7d53347f3d9078e000000.pdf.

López, H. (1998), Internal exile, exile and return: a gendered view, *Journal of Refugee Studies*, **11**(2), 189–198.

Lumsden, D. P. (1999), Broken lives? Reflections on the anthropology of exile and repair, *Refuge*, **18**(4), 30–40.

Marlowe, J. M. (2010), Beyond the discourse of trauma: shifting the focus on Sudanese refugees, *Journal of Refugee Studies*, **23**(2), 183–198.

Marlowe, J. M. (2011), 'Walking the line': southern Sudanese masculinities and reconciling one's past with the present, *Ethnicities*, **12**(1), 50–66.

McMichael, C., C. Nunn, S. M. Gifford and I. Correa-Velez (2015), Studying refugee settlement through longitudinal research: methodological and ethical insights from the good starts study, *Journal of Refugee Studies*, **28**, 238–257.

Menjívar, C. (2002), The ties that heal: Guatemalan immigrant women's networks and medical treatment, *International Migration Review*, **36**(2), 437–466.

Miller, K. E., G. J. Worthington, J. Muzurovic, S. Tipping and A. Goldman (2002), Bosnian refugees and the stressors of exile: a narrative study, *American Journal of Orthopsychiatry*, **72**(3), 341–354.

Olsson, E. (2009), From exile to post-exile: the diasporisation of Swedish Chileans in historical contexts, *Social Identities*, **15**(5), 659–676.

Pulvirenti, M. and G. Mason (2011), Resilience and survival: refugee women and violence, *Current Issues in Criminal Justice*, **23**(1), 37–52.

Pupavac, V. (2002), Pathologizing populations and colonizing minds: international psychosocial programs in Kosovo, *Alternatives*, **27**, 489–511.
Roniger, L. (2015), Displacement and testimony: recent history and the study of exile and post-exile, *International Journal of Politics, Culture & Society*, **28**(1).
Schweitzer, R. and J. H. Greenslade and A. Kagee (2007), Coping and resilience in refugees from the Sudan: a narrative account, *Australian and New Zealand Journal of Psychiatry*, **41**(3), 282–288.
Sherwood, K. and H. Liebling-Kalifani (2012), A grounded theory investigation into the experiences of African women refugees: effects on resilience and identity and implications for service provision, *Journal of International Women's Studies*, **13**(1), 86–108.
Summerfield, D. (1999), A critique of seven assumptions behind psychological trauma programmes in war-affected areas, *Social Science and Medicine*, **48**, 1449–1462.
Summerfield, D. (2000), War and mental health: a brief overview, *BMJ*, **321**, 232–235.
Szczepanikova, A. (2015), Chechen women in war and exile: changing gender roles in the context of violence, *Nationalities Papers: The Journal of Nationalism and Ethnicity*, **43**(5), 753–770.
Theidon, K. (2013), *Intimate Enemies: Violence and Reconciliation in Peru*, Philadelphia: University of Pennsylvania Press.
Thomas, F. and J. Gideon (2013), *Migration, Health and Inequality*, London: Zed Books.
Thomas, G. (2013), *Contesting Legitimacy in Chile: Familial Ideals, Citizenship, and Political*, University Park: Pennsylvania State University Press.
Ungar, M. (2003), Qualitative contributions to resilience research, *Qualitative Social Work*, **2**(1), 85–102.
Vandello, J., D. Cohen, R. Grandon and R. Franiuk (2009), Stand by your man: indirect prescriptions for honorable violence and feminine loyalty in Canada, Chile, and the United States, *Journal of Cross-Cultural Psychology*, **40**(1), 81–104.
Watters, C. (2001), Emerging paradigms in the mental health care of refugees, *Social Science and Medicine*, **52**, 1709–1718.
Westoby, P. and A. Ingamells (2010), A critically informed perspective of working with resettling refugee groups in Australia, *British Journal of Social Work*, **40**, 1759–1776.

18 Mobility, migration and generalised HIV epidemics: a focus on sub-Saharan Africa

Jo Vearey

BACKGROUND

Globally, and within the sub-Saharan African (SSA) region, there is an increasing recognition of the need to better understand and respond to migration – including movement across national borders and within countries – when planning health and, specifically, HIV programmes (for example, see Desmond Tutu Foundation 2011; Núñez Carrasco et al. 2011; Richter et al. 2014; SADC Directorate for Social and Human Development and Special Programs 2009, 2012; UNAIDS 2014a; Vearey 2011b, 2014; World Health Assembly 2008). Migration and mobility have been shown to affect the acquisition, transmission and management of HIV at an individual level in multiple ways (for example, see Camlin et al. 2010; Collinson 2010; Deane et al. 2010; McGrath et al. 2015), yet most responses to HIV – including renewed efforts at addressing structural determinants of HIV – fail to engage with the movement of people (Vearey 2014; Vearey et al. 2011). If considered within programmatic or policy responses, such as in the development of regional responses or National Strategic Plans (NSPs) for HIV, migration is exceptionalised – even within contexts where mobility is a prevalent norm – and migrants are considered a high-risk, 'key population' (Aggleton et al. 2014; UNAIDS 2014a). In such cases, migration refers to movements across national borders, and the more prevalent movements of people within countries are not considered (Vearey 2014). Such responses fail to engage with the complexity and heterogeneity of diverse population movements, rather targeting 'problematic', individual migrants who are (unfairly) blamed for the (continued) spread of HIV with no consideration of the broader contextual factors that are likely to be affecting aspects of the management of HIV associated with mobility – including treatment continuity and combination prevention approaches (for example, see Aggleton et al. 2014; Camlin et al. 2010; Colebunders and Kenyon 2015; Hirsch 2014; Kenyon et al. 2014; Todrys and Amon 2009). Importantly, such responses fail to incorporate consideration of migration-aware responses: a whole-system response whereby population movement is embedded as a central concern in the design of interventions, policy and research (Vearey 2014). While the body of evidence exploring associations between the global HIV pandemic, localised epidemics and the movement of people is increasing, challenges to improving our understanding and capacity to respond effectively remain. These challenges will be discussed in the chapter, including: limited consideration of the complexity and diversity of population movements that, in turn, limits research, evidence and practice; non-standardised ways in which migration and mobility are defined and measured, leading to an inability to compare findings between different contexts; and, ongoing – and in some contexts, increasing – anti-(im)migrant rhetoric that overshadows evidence-informed, rational public health discussions and decision-making.

Human mobility shaped early HIV epidemics by providing opportunities for the connection of high and low prevalence and incidence settings (for example, see Deane et al. 2010; Docquier et al. 2014; Lurie and Williams 2014); this is particularly true in the southern African region, one associated with a long history of restricted (im)migration and controlled male labour migration for work in the gold mines of South Africa (Lurie and Williams 2014). Today, the SSA region is home to a generalised HIV epidemic (GHE) that makes up the largest population of people living with HIV globally (UNAIDS 2015), and high levels of diverse population movements. New evidence, that makes use of 'peak HIV prevalence', indicates that the contemporary movements of people within the region – including people moving in search of improved livelihood opportunities, for work and study, to join family members, and to escape political persecution – are not associated at a population level with the spread of HIV within SSA; there is no association between national migration levels and national HIV prevalence (Kenyon et al. 2014). However, evidence exists to support individual-level associations between migration and the spread of HIV (for example, Baltazar et al. 2015; Camlin et al. 2010; Corno and de Walque 2012; Deane et al. 2010; Lurie 2006; McGrath et al. 2015), and the high prevalence of population mobility associated with the region today is likely to impact other aspects of a GHE – particularly combination prevention approaches; '[m]obility might have a greater effect on antiretroviral adherence than on HIV transmission' (Colebunders and Kenyon 2015: e223).

In 2015, the SSA region remains home to the largest number of people living with HIV – and while some successes have been reported, such as increased numbers of people on treatment, fewer deaths and a reduction in new cases of HIV per year (UNAIDS 2015) – challenges remain to the development and implementation of effective interventions to address the structural drivers of HIV, including the current drive to developing combination prevention interventions (see Parkhurst and Hunsmann 2015). For responses to HIV to be more successful in the SSA region, they must become migration-aware: population mobility, and the diversity of such movements, must be embedded as a core component of any research or response that aims to address HIV in SSA. Drawing on literature and evidence relating to contemporary population movements within the region, and their associated developmental challenges, the chapter shows that there is an urgent need for health and HIV programmers working in SSA to consider five key contextual issues. These are summarised below and discussed in more detail later on:

1 The prevalent movement of people in search of improved livelihood opportunities within the region, including those moving for work and study opportunities, within a country and across borders, including those who move irregularly or becoming irregular (i.e., overstaying the time allowed on a visitor's visa), working informally (and possibly illegally) and working in the sex industry, which is currently criminalised throughout the region (e.g., Richter et al. 2014; Vearey et al. 2011).
2 The role of mobility in urbanisation and urban HIV epidemics – specifically urban informal spaces where many migrants enter the city and where HIV prevalence is found to be double that of urban formal areas (e.g., Bocquier 2008; Kamndaya et al. 2014, 2015; Vearey et al. 2010; Vearey 2013a).
3 Movement to access HIV treatment and care (e.g., Clark et al. 2007; Collinson 2010; Lurie and Williams 2014; Nunez et al. 2010).
4 The limited governance and health systems capacity to respond to both HIV and migration (e.g., Misago et al. 2010; Landau et al. 2011a, 2011b; Landau and Amit 2014; Landau and Wa Kabwe Segatti 2009; Segatti and Landau 2011; Vearey 2011b).
5 The movements associated with conflict and post-conflict situations (e.g., de Waal 2010; Mills et al. 2006; Mock et al. 2004; Roberts and Patel 2010; Vearey 2013b).

Responding effectively to these five contextual issues is particularly important in the era of antiretroviral therapy (ART-era), and at a time where calls are being made for a (renewed) focus on addressing structural drivers of HIV, engaging with the complexity of GHEs, and developing combination prevention approaches – where responses attempt to bring biomedical, behavioural and structural aspects of HIV together (see Kurth et al. 2011; Parkhurst and Hunsmann 2015). As Parkhurst and Hunsmann (2015) rightly point out, this is a critical time – a strategic opportunity – for (re)focusing on structural drivers of HIV; in this chapter, it is argued that population mobility is one such prevalent structural reality affecting HIV policy and programming in multiple ways.

UNDERSTANDING MIGRATION AS A STRUCTURAL DRIVER OF HIV: INDIVIDUAL AND POPULATION-LEVEL IMPLICATIONS

> Migration is not only the geographical movement of persons from one country or locality to another, but movement within and between social and sexual networks.
>
> (Cassels et al. 2014: 8)

The published literature indicates that a complex – and contested – relationship exists between population mobility and HIV transmission (for example, see Bennett and Williams 2013; Brockerhoff and Biddlecom 1999; Camlin et al. 2010; Cassels et al. 2014; Clark et al. 2007; Coffee et al. 2007; Colebunders and Kenyon 2015; Collinson et al. 2014; Crush et al. 2005: 200; Crush 2002; Deane et al. 2010; Decosas et al. 1995; Docquier et al. 2014; Gerritsen et al. 2013; Kenyon et al. 2014; Lurie and Williams 2014; Vearey 2012; Weine and Kashuba 2012; Welaga et al. 2009). Critical to unpacking this complexity is the need to better engage with associations demonstrated at the individual level, and those at the population level: individual-level associations between HIV and migration are not found to be relevant at a population level (Kenyon et al. 2014).

> A number of papers have made the 'atomistic fallacy' of inferring that migration is a driver of HIV prevalence based on individual-level studies showing a correlation between migration and HIV prevalence. This inference fallacy has then led some authors to conclude that migration is central to the genesis of GHEs. Some researchers, for example, deduce from an individual-level study showing an association between migration and HIV incidence that young women engaging in sex with migrant men is the key driver in the spread of HIV infection (in Southern Africa).
>
> (Kenyon et al. 2014: 2)

The implication is that the movement of people does not explain current HIV epidemiology; historically, migration impacted the spread of HIV in SAA but as epidemics have become generalised, evidence suggests that mobility is no longer important (Coffee et al. 2007; Kenyon et al. 2014; Mundandi et al. n.d.). With that said, migration does impact (drive) other aspects of the HIV epidemic, including mediating HIV treatment seeking and adherence. This has important implications for the development of appropriate combination prevention programmes; as HIV becomes an increasingly chronic condition, questions are raised about its management in a context of high mobility (Lurie and Williams 2014). For example, there is a need to ensure that people living with HIV are able to access continued treatment regardless of their mobility trajectory (Vearey 2014). As indicated earlier, a particular challenge is related to the ways in which population mobility – a norm within the SSA region – is exceptionalised and vilified in the context of HIV:

> Sad to say, recognition of the positive aspects of mobility is rarely present in the HIV literature, which more often than not focuses on difficulties, problems and risks as we will see below. Moreover, the term treats mobility as if it is a new phenomenon and, therefore, a form of 'risk to be contained', rather than as a long-term characteristic of particular communities and countries.
>
> (Aggleton et al. 2014: 262)

Improved evidence and understanding is required to assist in challenging such negative rhetoric and supporting the development of informed, rational public health responses to HIV in a context associated with the prevalent social norm of population movement. This includes working to better position migration as a key structural determinant of HIV: one that while not associated with the propagation of HIV at a population level (Kenyon et al. 2014), is associated with HIV risk profiles at an individual level (for example, Deane et al. 2010) and affects key aspects of the management of the current GHE in SSA. Strengthening the understanding of the role of migration will assist in the development of migration-aware responses that are needed to support a more successful response to HIV in the SSA region.

MIGRATION AS A KEY STRUCTURAL DETERMINANT OF HIV

In line with the evidence indicating that associations between migration status and HIV at an individual level do not bear out at a population level (Kenyon et al. 2014), there is an increasing recognition that HIV risk is not an individual behaviour, but something mediated and influenced by a range of structural determinants or drivers, including social, economic and political factors (for example, Auerbach et al. 2011; Kippax et al. 2013; Parker et al. 2000; Parkhurst and Hunsmann 2015; Seeley et al. 2012). With this in mind, a social determinants of health framework (WHO 2008) is used to explore migration and HIV in SSA, whereby population movements are considered key structural determinants of HIV (for example, see Hirsch 2014; Vearey 2013a). Hirsch calls for a focus on the meso-level social processes that mediate HIV risks in order to move beyond the proximate drivers of HIV (such as individual behaviour) to the role of policy (Hirsch 2014). Awareness of the roles that migration plays at individual and population levels

> points to the need to recognise the multiple reasons for migration, the differing migration flows that result and finally the diverse behavioural practices that arise in given settings. It also requires the knowledge of local epidemiological context to see how these may play out with regard to more proximal determinants of HIV infection.
>
> (Deane et al. 2010: 1459).

Ultimately, there is a need to improve our ways of defining and measuring migration that engage with the heterogeneity of population movements and allow for comparisons across time and place. Importantly, there is a need to determine whether existing measures of migration are appropriate in the ART-era – i.e., are our measures sufficiently sensitive and specific to capture the nuances of population movements (McGrath et al. 2015).

DEFINING AND MEASURING MIGRATION

> Migration and HIV studies are subject to many methodological and measurement challenges in part because there are many forms of migration, from short-term circular labor migration to lifetime rural to urban migratory patterns. Consequently, our understanding of the etiologic impact of migration on HIV risk is mixed, has evolved with the changing epidemic stage, and depends on social context and measurement methods across studies.
>
> (Cassels et al. 2014: 2)

As highlighted by Cassels et al. (2014) above, migration is a heterogeneous process; the SSA region is associated with various forms of population movement that connect various places and spaces, including households and communities of origin, transit and destination. These movements – that include movement within countries and across national borders – are driven by various processes, including: job-seeking; formal, organised labour migration; forced migration due to political conflict or a natural disaster; health- and help-seeking, including care-seeking – particularly when an individual is too sick to work and returns to be cared for 'back home' (for example, see Clark et al. 2007; Collinson 2010; Nunez et al. 2010); and diverse movements associated with post-conflict settings (for example, see Vearey 2013b). These drivers can create different movement trajectories, some are well-planned, others are in response to more immediate danger or difficulty. Movement can be circular, or oscillating, involving regular movement between the household of origin and a place/s of work (such as seasonal agricultural work), job-seeking or staying with family members located elsewhere. Other migrations are more permanent, but connections to the household of origin may remain through, for example, the remittance of money, food or goods. Processes of return migration take place as part of circular migration, or in a post-conflict setting. It is this heterogeneity that makes measuring and understanding linkages between migration and HIV challenging.

In spite of a recognition that the movement of people is a dynamic and non-linear process (as briefly outlined above) (Cassels et al. 2014), ways of defining and measuring migration within HIV research studies are limited and much of the epidemiological literature has made use of 'abstract definitions of mobility' (Deane et al. 2010). Frustratingly, 'insights from the broader field of migration studies are rarely invoked to explain the relationship between HIV/AIDS and migration' (Deane et al. 2010). The result is that studies are unable to engage with the complexity of the migration experience, erase difference and rely on simplified – and differing – single measures of movement that result in contradictory and non-comparable research findings (Aggleton et al. 2014; for example, see Cassels et al. 2014; Deane et al. 2010; McGrath et al. 2015; Weine and Kashuba 2012). A key implication moving forward is the need for HIV and migration scholars to engage each other more effectively in the design and interpretation of research exploring mobility and HIV within SSA, and – ultimately – in the design and implementation of improved interventions. Methodological innovation is required, including making use of expanded definitions of a household to allow for the migratory composition of households to be considered, and more nuanced measures of mobility and migration that ensure the heterogeneity of movement are captured (McGrath et al. 2015). Cassels et al. (2014) suggest the development of a 'network-dyadic conceptual model' for exploring the relationships between migration, mobility and HIV. This is in recognition of the fact that 'migration is a dynamic process, and the role of migration in HIV transmission is a non-linear function of individual, dyadic, and network features regardless of context. Network-based epidemic models and other mathematical models are becoming more common in the field, and will be useful to test complex pathways between migration and HIV transmission at multiple scales' (Cassels et al. 2014: 9). While there is clearly a need to develop improved models for exploring the complexity of migration and HIV dynamics, it is also necessary to work with existing evidence and understandings to improve current programmatic responses; this includes working to improve local responses to local HIV and migration contexts.

CONTEXT SPECIFIC UNDERSTANDING: LOCAL EPIDEMICS, LOCAL RESPONSES

> [D]evelopment of research and intervention strategies should proceed with caution unless the local context of migration and mobility is understood and can be incorporated.
>
> (McGrath et al. 2015: 7)

As outlined earlier, there is a need to understand the ways in which mobility and migration interact with HIV in a range of different contexts – both spatially and temporally (Deane et al., 2010). This includes recognising that people who move are exposed to multiple environments at different times during their migratory journeys (Deane et al., 2010; McGrath et al., 2015), including different epidemiological profiles; the ways in which different contexts are linked to each other through migration have implications for HIV programming in SSA. While understanding the challenges outlined above regarding the difficulties faced in developing standardised and comparative measures of migration, we do urgently require 'more nuanced understandings of both the manifestations of migration and the resulting changes in proximate determinants of HIV infection in different settings and at different times' (Deane et al. 2010). This includes improving understandings of local epidemics in order to develop appropriate responses (McGrath et al. 2015; UNAIDS 2014b): local migration profiles should be incorporated as a key component of such localised assessments. Importantly, where individual-level associations with migration and HIV exist, it is the context of migration that affects HIV-risk profiles, not being a migrant per se (Camlin et al. 2010). With this in mind, five key contextual issues have been identified as potential focus areas for future research and intervention: (1) movement in search of improved livelihood opportunities; (2) the role of mobility in urbanisation and urban HIV epidemics; (3) movement to access treatment and care; (4) limited governance and capacity of health systems to respond to both HIV and migration; and (5) movement associated with conflict and post-conflict situations. These five issues present evidence challenging some prevailing assumptions relating to population mobility and HIV; the hope is that (re)thinking about these issues will positively influence policy and programmatic decision-making in the SSA region.

MOVEMENT IN SEARCH OF IMPROVED LIVELIHOOD OPPORTUNITIES

The most prevalent form of movement within the SSA region – both within and between countries – involves the search for improved livelihood opportunities. This includes people moving for work and study opportunities, and job-seekers. A systematic review of literature exploring determinants of HIV risk in relation to migration and labour explored four determinants – namely policy, sociocultural context, health and mental health, and sexual practices – and concluded that

> [t]he policy determinants most often associated with HIV risk were: prolonged and/or frequent absence, financial status, and difficult working and housing conditions. The sociocultural context determinants most often associated with HIV risk were: cultural norms, family separation, and low social support. The health and mental health factors most often associated with HIV risk were: substance use, other STIs, mental health problems, no HIV testing, and needle use. The sexual practices most often associated with increased HIV risk were: limited condom use, multiple partnering, clients of sex workers, low HIV knowledge, and low perceived HIV risk. Magnitude of effects through multivariate statistics were demonstrated more for health and mental health and sexual practices, than for policy or sociocultural context.
>
> (Weine and Kashuba 2012: 1, emphasis added)

In South Africa, the country receiving the greatest number of migrants from the southern African region, an increasingly restrictive Immigration Act presents challenges for job-seekers and lower-skilled migrants who may be forced to cross a border in an irregular way, or who become irregular during their stay in the country, through overstaying the time allowed on a visitor's visa, for example. This can include challenges in accessing public healthcare for HIV testing or continued access to ART; difficulties in accessing the formal job market and, as a result, engaging in informal livelihood activities that may increase risk of acquisition of HIV and are omitted from national HIV workplace responses. Currently, there are no regional job-seeker permits and informal employment does not qualify for a work permit. Many migrants – both from within the country and from elsewhere – engage in informal (and possibly illegal) work, and some find work within the sex industry, which is currently criminalised throughout the region (e.g., Richter et al. 2014; Vearey et al. 2011).

Increasing numbers of women are moving independently in search of work and, while there is some evidence that women are more likely to migrate shorter distances compared to men, research conducted in rural KZN (South Africa) has shown that female migrants bear an increased HIV risk profile compared to their male migrant counterparts (Camlin et al. 2010). The exact reasons for this require further in-depth research, including the need to improve our understandings of the destinations of rural female migrants: for example, are they more likely to be resident in urban areas associated with a higher HIV prevalence and incidence than their male counterparts, such as within urban informal areas where HIV prevalence is known to be double that of urban formal areas (Camlin et al. 2010).

THE ROLE OF MOBILITY IN URBANISATION AND URBAN HIV EPIDEMICS

Linked to the challenges raised above, the majority who move in search of improved livelihoods travel to urban centres, often entering the city through peripheral, informal areas where HIV prevalence is found to be double that of urban formal areas (e.g., Bocquier 2008; Greif et al. 2010; Greif and Nii-Amoo Dodoo 2011; Kamndaya et al. 2014, 2015; Vearey et al. 2010; Vearey 2013a). This requires careful consideration when exploring linkages between migration and HIV; an urban health or social determinants of urban health (SDUH) lens will assist in unpacking the complexities associated with the interlinked challenges of migration, HIV and informal settlements (Vearey 2011a, 2013a).

MOVEMENT TO ACCESS TREATMENT AND CARE

Historically, the focus on the associations between migration and HIV have focused on the ways that population mobility affects the HIV risk-profile of individuals but there is a need to better understand the ways that HIV may affect migratory decisions and patterns.

> How do migrants negotiate access to care, for example, after they leave urban employment? How do people who migrate frequently negotiate daily pill regimens, and how and where do they decide to get treated. Do migrants prefer to access treatment for some diseases in rural areas, while for other diseases in urban areas? These and other related questions about the role of migration in accessing and negotiating treatment are among the new important questions raised by migration and health today.
>
> (Lurie and Williams 2014: 39)

Literature from South Africa – exploring both internal and cross-border mobilities – clearly demonstrates the ways in which the health status – mediated by HIV – of migrants influences decisions to migrate, namely to return to a rural home when an individual is too sick to work (Clark et al. 2007; Collinson 2010; Lurie and Williams 2014; Nunez et al. 2010). This clearly highlights the complexity of exploring health-determined migration: it is often assumed that individuals travel to other countries or into urban areas in order to seek healthcare (including HIV treatment) but evidence indicates the importance of returning home, and to receiving care and support from family members. This, ultimately, places a higher HIV burden of care on rural areas from where many urban migrants originate – at the level of the household and healthcare system (for example, see Nunez et al. 2010). In terms of decision-making related to accessing HIV treatment, individuals may choose to access facilities that are not close to their place of residence and, for non-national migrants, they may choose to return to their country of origin at regular intervals to access treatment. Such complex dynamics relating to help- and healthcare-seeking behaviour of different migrant groups need to be better understood to assist in developing and implementing effective systems for ensuring treatment continuity, for example through the use of standardised patient-held records (health passports) and referral letters (Vearey 2014).

LIMITED GOVERNANCE AND HEALTH SYSTEMS CAPACITY TO RESPOND TO BOTH HIV AND MIGRATION

Understanding of population mobility as a governance issue is generally poor within the SSA region. Migration scholars have previously highlighted the limited governance structures to adequately deal with population mobility at various levels, including at the local level; immigration management, through national immigration and refugee acts, is often the sole, national response to migration – one that works to further securitise national borders and restrict population movement (e.g. Landau and Amit, 2014; Landau and Wa Kabwe Segatti, 2009; Segatti and Landau, 2011; Vearey, J., 2011). As a result, governance responses to migration are limited and do not engage with internal movements; combined with an overburdened and struggling public healthcare system, opportunities for developing migration-aware HIV programmes are limited. Opportunities exist for creating partnerships with scholars and practitioners working on migration and mobility in the region in order to collectively develop improved migration-aware responses to HIV.

MOVEMENT ASSOCIATED WITH CONFLICT AND POST-CONFLICT SITUATIONS

> As with many issues associated with the movement of people, linkages between mobility, HIV, conflict and post-conflict settings have often been based on conjecture rather than fact. Conflict was assumed to increase transmission of HIV, and displaced populations, refugees and armed forces were presumed to have higher HIV prevalence than host communities. However, recent evidence challenges these assumptions.
>
> (Vearey 2013b: 439)

It was previously assumed that conflict and post-conflict situations were associated with an increased incidence of HIV; however, as with much of the literature exploring mobility and HIV, conflicting evidence exists, suggesting that the relationship between these contexts and HIV is more complex than previously assumed (e.g., de Waal et al. 2010; Lowicki-Zucca et al. 2008; Mills et al. 2006; Mock et al. 2004; Roberts and Patel 2010; Spiegel et al. 2007; Vearey 2013b). The SSA region is home to a range of conflict and post-conflict settings, associated with varying migration dynamics. In the move towards developing migration-aware HIV programmes, the specific – and complex – contexts of conflict and post-conflict settings must be considered.

CONCLUSION

> While we must still be interested in migration induced disease – and in finding ways to mitigate the additional health risks of migration, we must increasingly turn our attention to disease-induced migration, where sick people may change their patterns of migration in order to access quality care.
>
> (Lurie and Williams 2014: 39)

In 2015, HIV is associated with different contextual realities, opportunities and challenges than those of the early days of the epidemic. A central success is the availability of treatment – turning HIV into a chronic, rather than life-threatening, condition – and possibilities for using 'treatment as prevention' now exist. Such new opportunities, however, come with new challenges: addressing the HIV epidemic in SSA in 2015 requires a response to structural drivers and effective combination prevention. A key structural driver – the movement of people – presents different challenges today than during the early stages of the epidemic. While migration was implicated in the early spread of HIV and individual-level associations between migrant status and HIV risk still exist, contemporary movements of people in the SSA region present challenges to the successful implementation of treatment programmes and must be considered in order to develop migration-aware HIV interventions.

While the body of evidence exploring associations between the global HIV pandemic, localised epidemics and the movement of people is increasing, challenges to improving our understanding and translating new knowledge into effective interventions remain. A central challenge relates to the limited consideration of the complexity of population movements that – in turn – limits research, evidence and practice. Improved – non-standardised – ways in which migration and mobility are defined and measured in relation to the GHE in SSA are needed, requiring migration, public health, epidemiology and HIV prevention scholars to collaborate. Additionally, ongoing – and in some contexts, increasing – anti-(im) migrant rhetoric overshadows attempts at evidence-informed, rational public health discussions and decision-making. The politics of migration and health remain central barriers to improving responses at regional, national and local levels, and concerns are raised as to whether government responses meet the (diverse) needs of (diverse) migrant populations (for example, see McGrath et al. 2015; Vearey 2014). While more research is needed, particularly in order to generate better understandings of the different experiences of diverse migrant groups in relation to HIV within the SSA region, it is an opportune time to take advantage of the (renewed) focus on structural interventions and combination prevention programmes (Parkhurst and Hunsmann 2015).

RECOMMENDATIONS

In order to support the development of migration-aware HIV programmes, the following recommendations are made:

- Public health, epidemiology, HIV prevention and migration scholars and practitioners need to engage in order to share insights relating to migration and mobility in the SSA region.
- Different spheres of governance need support in improving understandings of and responses to mobility and HIV.
- Improved measures of migration and HIV are needed, including expanded definitions of a household to capture non-resident migrant household members (McGrath et al. 2015; UNAIDS 2014a).
- Population-level associations cannot automatically be inferred between migration and HIV if found at an individual level (Kenyon et al. 2014).
- The role of the private sector in supporting migration-aware HIV

responses – particularly in relation to formalised migrant labour (Hirsch 2014) – needs to be explored.

- Exploration of a (potential) shift 'from migration-induced disease to disease-induced migration' (Lurie and Williams 2014: 39) where the (potential) role of HIV-treatment-induced movement needs to be understood and responded to.

REFERENCES

Aggleton, P., S. A. Bell and A. Kelly-Hanku (2014), 'Mobile men with money': HIV prevention and the erasure of difference, *Global Public Health*, **9**, 257–270.

Auerbach, J. D., J. O. Parkhurst and C. F. Cáceres (2011), Addressing social drivers of HIV/AIDS for the long-term response: conceptual and methodological considerations, *Global Public Health*, **6**, S293–S309.

Baltazar, C. S., R. Horth, C. Inguane, I. Sathane, F. César, H. Ricardo, C. Botão, Â. Augusto, L. Cooley, B. Cummings, H. F. Raymond and P. W. Young (2015), HIV prevalence and risk behaviors among Mozambicans working in South African mines, *AIDS and Behavior*, **19**, 59–67.

Bennett, R. and B. Williams (2013), Oscillating migration driving HIV and TB in sub-Saharan Africa, *SACEMA Quarterly*, March 2013.

Bocquier, P. (2008), Urbanisation in developing countries: is the 'Cities Without Slums' target attainable? *International Development Planning Review*, **30**.

Brockerhoff, M. and A. E. Biddlecom (1999), Migration, sexual behavior and the risk of HIV in Kenya, *International Migration Review*, **33**, 833–856.

Camlin, C. S., V. Hosegood, M-L. Newell, N. McGrath, T. Bärnighausen and R. C. Snow (2010), Gender, migration and HIV in Rural KwaZulu-Natal, South Africa. *PLOS One*, **5**, e11539.

Cassels, S., S. M. Jenness and A. S. Khanna (2014), Conceptual framework and research methods for migration and HIV transmission dynamics, *AIDS and Behavior*, **18**, 2302–2313.

Clark, S. J., M. A. Collinson, K. Kahn and S. M. Tollman (2007), Returning home to die: circular labour migration and mortality in rural South Africa, *Scandinavian Journal of Public Health*, **35**, 35–44.

Coffee, M., M. N. Lurie and G. P. Garnett (2007), Modelling the impact of migration on the HIV epidemic in South Africa, *Aids*, **21**, 343–350.

Colebunders, R. and C. Kenyon (2015), Behaviour, not mobility, is a risk factor for HIV, *The Lancet*, **HIV 2**, e223–e224.

Collinson, M. A. (2010), *Striving Against Adversity: The Dynamics of Migration, Health and Poverty in Rural South Africa*, Global Health Action 3.

Collinson, M. A., M. J. White, P. Bocquier, S. T. McGarvey, S. A. Afolabi, S. J. Clark, K. Kahn and S. M. Tollman (2014), *Migration and the Epidemiological Transition: Insights from the Agincourt Sub-District of Northeast South Africa*, Global Health Action 7.

Corno, L. and D. de Walque (2012), Mines, migration and HIV/AIDS in Southern Africa, *Journal of African Economies*, **21**, 465–498.

Crush, J. (ed.) (2002), *Spaces of Vulnerability: Migration and HIV/AIDS in South Africa*, Migration Policy Series No. 24.

Crush, J., B. Williams, E. Gouws and M. Lurie (2005), Migration and HIV/AIDS in South Africa, *Development Southern Africa*, **22**, 293–318.

Deane, K. D., J. O. Parkhurst and D. Johnston (2010), Linking migration, mobility and HIV: linking migration, mobility and HIV, *Tropical Medicine & International Health*, **15**, 1458–1463.

Decosas, J., F. Kane, J. K. Anafi, K. D. R. Sodji and H. U. Wagner (1995), Migration and AIDS, *Lancet*, **346**, 826–828.
Desmond Tutu Foundation (2011), *Key Populations Key Solutions: A Gap Analysis and Recommendations for Key Populations and HIV in South Africa*, Policy Brief.
de Waal, A., J. Klot, M. Mahajan, D. Huber, G. Frerks and S, M'Boup (2010), HIV/AIDS, security and conflict: new realities, new responses, *Forced Migration Review*, October, 6–8.
Docquier, F., C. Vasilakis and D. Tamfutu Munsi (2014), International migration and the propagation of HIV in sub-Saharan Africa, *Journal of Health Economics*, **35**, 20–33.
Gerritsen, A., P. Bocquier, M. White, C. Mbacké, N. Alam, D. Beguy, F. Odhiambo, C. Sacoor, H. D. Phuc, S. Punpuing and M. A. Collinson (2013), *Health and Demographic Surveillance Systems: Contributing to an Understanding of the Dynamics in Migration and Health*, Global Health Action 6.
Greif, M. J. and F. Nii-Amoo Dodoo (2011), Internal migration to Nairobi's slums: linking migrant streams to sexual risk behavior, *Health & Place*, **17**, 86–93.
Greif, M. J., F. Nii-Amoo Dodoo and A. Jayaraman (2010), Urbanisation, poverty and sexual behaviour: the tale of five African cities, *Urban Studies*, **48**(5), 947–957.
Hirsch, J. S. (2014), Labor migration, externalities and ethics: theorizing the meso-level determinants of HIV vulnerability, *Social Science & Medicine*, **100**, 38–45.
Kamndaya, M., L. Thomas, J. Vearey, B. Sartorius and L. Kazembe (2014), Material deprivation affects high sexual risk behavior among young people in urban slums, South Africa, *Journal of Urban Health*, **91**, 581–591.
Kamndaya, M., L. N. Kazembe, J. Vearey, C. W. Kabiru and L. Thomas (2015), Material deprivation and unemployment affect coercive sex among young people in the urban slums of Blantyre, Malawi: a multi-level approach, *Health & Place*, **33**, 90–100.
Kenyon, C., R. Colebunders, H. Voeten and M. Lurie (2014), Migration intensity has no effect on peak HIV prevalence: an ecological study, *BMC Infectious Diseases*, **14**, 350.
Kippax, S., N. Stephenson, R. G. Parker amd P. Aggleton (2013), Between individual agency and structure in HIV prevention: understanding the middle ground of social practice, *American Journal of Public Health*, **103**, 1367–1375.
Kurth, A. E., C. Celum, J. M. Baeten, S. H. Vermund and J. N. Wasserheit (2011), Combination HIV prevention: significance, challenges, and opportunities, *Current HIV/AIDS Reports*, **8**, 62–72.
Landau, L. B. and R. Amit (2014), Wither policy? Southern African perspectives on understanding law, 'refugee' policy and protection, *Journal of Refugee Studies*, **27**, 534–552.
Landau, L. B. and A. Wa Kabwe Segatti (2009), *Human Development Impacts of Migration: South Africa Case Study*, Human Development Research Paper 2009/5.
Landau, L. B., J. P. Misago and A. Wa Kabwe Segatti (2011a), *Responding to Human Mobility: Is Local Government Set up for Failure?* Johannesburg: African Centre for Migration & Society.
Landau, L. B, A. Segatti and J. P. Misago (2011b), *Mobility and Municipalities: Local Authorities, Local Impacts, and the Challenges of Movement, in: Contemporary Migration to South Africa: A Regional Development Issue*, Washington, DC: World Bank.
Lowicki-Zucca, M., P. B. Spiegel, S. Kelly, K-L. Dehne, N. Walker and P. D. Ghys (2008), Estimates of HIV burden in emergencies, *Sexually Transmitted Infections*, **84**, i42–i48.
Lurie, M. N. (2006), The epidemiology of migration and HIV/AIDS in South Africa, *Journal of Ethnic & Migration Studies*, **32**, 649–666.
Lurie, M. N. and B. G. Williams (2014), Migration and health in Southern Africa: 100 years and still circulating, *Health Psychology and Behavioral Medicine*, 2, 34–40.
McGrath, N., J. W. Eaton, M-L. Newell and V. Hosegood (2015), Migration, sexual behaviour, and HIV risk: a general population cohort in rural South Africa, *The Lancet*, **HIV 2**, e252–e259.
Mills, E. J., S. Singh, B. D. Nelson and J. B. Nachega (2006), The impact of conflict on HIV/AIDS in sub-Saharan Africa, *International Journal of STD and AIDS*, **17**, 713–717.
Misago, J. P., K. Takabvirwa, M. Kanyane and G. Siziba (2010), *Governing Migration*

and Urbanisation: Developing Approaches to Counter Poverty and Social Fragmentation (No. 25), Report ACMS, Wits, Johannesburg.

Mock, N. B., S. Duale, L. F. Brown, E. Mathys, H. C. O'Maonaigh, N. K. Abul-Husn and S. Elliott (2004), Conflict and HIV: a framework for risk assessment to prevent HIV in conflict-affected settings in Africa, *Emerging Themes in Epidemiology*, **1**, 6.

Mundandi, C., D. Vissers, H. Voeten, D. Habbema and S. Gregson (n.d.), No difference in HIV incidence and sexual behaviour between out-migrants and residents in rural Manicaland, Zimbabwe, *Tropical Medicine and International Health*, **11**, 705–711.

Nunez, L., J. Vearey and S. Drime (2010), *Who Cares? The Impact of HIV-Related Sickness on Migration Patterns in South Africa*, paper presented at the Urban Health Workshop, 13–16 January, Point Du Sud Bamako, Mali.

Núñez Carrasco, L., J. Vearey and S. Drimie (2011), Who cares? HIV-related sickness, urban–rural linkages, and the gendered role of care in return migration in South Africa, *Gender & Development*, **19**, 105–114.

Parker, R. G., D. Easton and C. H. Klein (2000), Structural barriers and facilitators in HIV prevention: a review of international research, *AIDS*, **14**, S22–S32.

Parkhurst, J. O. and M. Hunsmann (2015), Breaking out of silos – the need for critical paradigm reflection in HIV prevention, *Review of African Political Economy*, **42**, 477–487.

Richter, M., M. F. Chersich, J. Vearey, B. Sartorius, M. Temmerman and S. Luchters (2014), Migration status, work conditions and health utilization of female sex workers in three South African Cities, *Journal of Immigrant and Minority Health*, **16**, 7–17.

Roberts, B. and P. Patel (2010), Conflict, forced migration, sexual behavior, and HIV/AIDS, in F. Thomas, M. Haour-Knipe and P. Aggleton (eds.), *Mobility, Sexuality, and AIDS*, London: Routledge, pp. 55–66.

SADC Directorate for Social and Human Development and Special Programs (2009), *SADC Policy Framework for Population Mobility and Communicable Diseases in the SADC Region: Final Draft April 2009*, available online at www.arasa.info/files/pub_SADC%20 Policy_Framework_FINAL.pdf.

SADC Directorate for Social and Human Development and Special Programs (2012), *SADC Declaration on Tuberculosis in the Mining Sector*.

Seeley, J., C. H, Watts, S. Kippax, S. Russell, L. Heise and A. Whiteside (2012), Addressing the structural drivers of HIV: a luxury or necessity for programmes? *Journal of the International AIDS Society*, **15**.

Segatti, A. and L. Landau (eds.) (2011), *Contemporary Migration to South Africa: A Regional Development Issue*, Washington, DC: World Bank.

Spiegel, P. B., A. R. Bennedsen, J. Claass, L. Bruns, N. Patterson, D. Yiweza and M. Schilperoord (2007), Prevalence of HIV infection in conflict-affected and displaced people in seven sub-Saharan African countries: a systematic review, *The Lancet*, **369**, 2187–2195.

Todrys, K. and J. J. Amon (2009), Within but without: human rights and access to HIV prevention and treatment for internal migrants, *Globalization and Health*, **5**, 17.

UNAIDS (2014a), *Gap Report*, Geneva: UNAIDS.

UNAIDS (2014b), *Issues Brief: Local Epidemics*, Geneva: UNAIDS.

UNAIDS (2015), *AIDS by the Numbers 2015*, Geneva: UNAIDS.

Vearey, J. (2011a), *Challenging Urban Health: Towards an Improved Local Government Response to Migration, Informal Settlements, and HIV in Johannesburg, South Africa*, Global Health Action 4.

Vearey, J. (2011b), Migration and health in South Africa: implications for development, in A. Segatti and L. Landau (eds.), *Contemporary Migration to South Africa: A Regional Development Issue*, Washington, DC: World Bank.

Vearey, J. (2012), Learning from HIV: exploring migration and health in South Africa, *Global Public Health*, **7**, 58–70.

Vearey, J. (2013a), Migration, urban health and inequality in Johannesburg, in T. Bastia (ed.), *Migration and Inequality*, Routledge, London.

Vearey, J. (2013b), HIV, population mobility, and the post-conflict nexus: unpacking complexity, *International Peacekeeping*, **20**, 439–449.

Vearey, J. (2014), Healthy migration: a public health and development imperative for South(ern) Africa, *South African Medical Journal*, **104**, 663.

Vearey, J., I. Palmary, L. Núñez and S. Drime (2010), Urban health in Johannesburg: the importance of place in understanding intra-urban inequalities in a context of migration and HIV, *Health and Place*, **16**, 694–702.

Vearey, J., M. Richter, L. Núñez and K. Moyo (2011), South African HIV/AIDS programming overlooks migration, urban livelihoods, and informal workplaces, *African Journal of AIDS Research*, **10**, 381–391.

Weine, S. M. and A. B. Kashuba (2012), Labor migration and HIV risk: a systematic review of the literature, *AIDS and Behavior*, **16**, 1605–1621.

Welaga, P., V. Hosegood, R. Weiner, C. Hill, K. Herbst and M-L. Newell (2009), Coming home to die? The association between migration and mortality in rural South Africa, *BMC Public Health*, **9**, 193.

WHO (2008), *Closing the Gap in a Generation: Health Equity through Action on the Social Determinants of Health*, Geneva: Commission on Social Determinants of Health.

World Health Assembly (2008), World Health Assembly Resolution 61.17: Health of Migrants.

19 Infectious diseases in migrant populations in the European Union and the European Economic Area

Gemma A. Williams, Anna Odone, Taavi Tillmann, Anastasia Pharris, Dina Oksen, Bernd Rechel, Philipa Mladovsky, Sabrina Bacci, Rebecca Shadwick, Teymur Noori, Andreas Sandgren, Erika Duffell, Jonathan E. Suk, David Ingleby and Martin McKee

INTRODUCTION

In the past 30 years, morbidity and premature mortality from infectious diseases has declined substantially in Europe. However, progress has not been universal and some infectious diseases such as the human immunodeficiency virus (HIV), tuberculosis (TB) and hepatitis B still account for a considerable burden of disease in a number of countries (ECDC 2013b, 2013c; ECDC/WHO Europe, 2013a, 2013b). In recent years, inward migration from regions outside the European Union (EU) and the European Economic Area (EEA), where the prevalence of infectious diseases is high, has increasingly been viewed as a major barrier to reducing the spread of some infectious diseases in a number of member states.

Although migrants are often comparatively healthy overall due to healthier individuals being more likely to migrate (Rechel et al. 2013), evidence suggests that migrants in Europe, in particular those from countries with poor infectious disease prevention and control, are more vulnerable to specific infectious diseases than the native European population (Rechel et al. 2011). The pathways through which these migrant groups may be at higher risk of acquiring infectious diseases reflect a complex set of factors that occur throughout the migration process (Gushulak et al. 2010; Razum 2006; Rechel et al. 2013). Pre-migration, a migrant's health reflects patterns of disease in countries of origin and can be influenced by traumatic experiences during the migration journey. After arrival in the host country, poor living and working conditions increase the risk of exposure to a number of infectious diseases, while cultural factors such as language abilities, religion, gender roles and health beliefs will affect health and healthcare-seeking behaviours. Poor access to healthcare can be further exacerbated by legal restrictions in the host country, discrimination, lack of awareness of rights and entitlements, lack of familiarity with the health system and gaps in health literacy (Mladovsky et al. 2012, Rechel et al. 2013). Health risks to migrants may also continue for many years after arrival in Europe as a result of return travel to visit friends and relatives in countries of origin (Health Protection Services 2011).

In an era when migration to the EU/EEA is increasing, both in terms of size and diversity, it is inevitable that the epidemiology of infectious diseases in Europe is changing; this creates new challenges for the planning and delivery of health services, which need to adapt to accommodate diverse health needs (Rechel et al. 2013). Understanding and meeting the health needs of migrants affected by infectious diseases in Europe is crucial in order to protect both individual and public health (ECDC 2014). However, current understanding of the extent to which migrants in this region are actually affected by infectious diseases, and the patterns found in terms of subgroups affected and disease transmission, are limited due to a lack of data. Surveillance systems and surveys in most member states do not routinely collect or disaggregate data according to migrant status. In addition, comparisons of migrant health across Europe are challenging due to varied definitions of who constitutes a migrant, with definitions determined by national legislative, administrative and policy factors that vary between EU/EEA member states (Ingleby 2009; International Organization for Migration 2010). Further complications arise as there is a particular lack of data on certain types of migrants, such as asylum-seekers and irregular migrants.

With the goal of reducing these gaps in evidence and improving understanding on the burden of infectious diseases in migrant populations, the European Centre for Disease Prevention and Control (ECDC) recently published a report on key infectious diseases in migrant populations in the EU/EEA as part of their migrant health series (ECDC 2014). Using data from multiple sources including *The European Surveillance System* (TESSy) and a comprehensive literature review, this report assessed the burden of infectious diseases among migrant populations in the EU/EEA and evaluated the completeness, quality and usefulness of data reported to TESSy for disease-specific and migrant-specific variables. In this chapter, the findings of this report for HIV, TB, hepatitis B, measles, rubella and Chagas disease are explored. The chapter concludes with recommendations on how future policy and public health responses in the EU/EEA can be improved to reduce the infectious disease burden in vulnerable migrant groups.

HIV

Globally, an estimated 35.3 million people were living with HIV in 2012. The majority of people living with HIV reside in sub-Saharan Africa (25.0 million), with large numbers also found in South and South-East Asia (3.9 million), Latin American and the Caribbean (1.75 million) and Eastern Europe and Central Asia (1.3 million) (UNAIDS, 2013). HIV also remains a significant public health issue in the EU/EEA, with 151,890 HIV cases reported between 2007 and 2011 (ECDC 2014).

According to surveillance data, EU/EEA migrants from regions with high HIV prevalence rates are disproportionately affected by HIV in comparison to the native population and other migrant groups (Alvarez-Del Arco 2012). Of 123,883 HIV cases reported to TESSy during 2007–2011 with information on geographical origin, 39.9 per cent (48,613) were in migrants (ECDC 2014). Among HIV cases in migrants, the majority were from sub-Saharan Africa (54.3 per cent), with significant proportions from Latin America (12.2 per cent), Western Europe (9.5 per cent) and Central Europe (6.0 per cent). Data for 2011 shows that the proportion of cases among migrants varies considerably between countries, ranging from less than 1 per cent in Estonia, to more than 70 per cent in Sweden. Overall, during 2007–2011, 92 per cent of cases in migrants were reported by countries in Western Europe (ECDC 2014).

Between 2007 and 2011, the number of new HIV cases diagnosed in migrants rose slightly, with increased cases reported among migrants from Latin America and Central and Eastern Europe, but a decrease in cases among migrants from sub-Saharan Africa (ECDC 2014). These trends are likely to reflect changing patterns of migration within and to the EU/EEA, as well as differences in uptake of HIV testing. It may also reflect reduced incidence of HIV among migrants from some regions, in particular Sub-Saharan Africa, which saw a decline of 34 per cent in reported new HIV cases between 2001 and 2012 (UNAIDS 2013).

TESSy data shows that HIV cases in men outnumber those in women in native-born and migrant populations, with the exception of migrants from sub-Saharan Africa. Of all HIV cases reported during 2007–2011 with information available on geographic origin and gender, 73 per cent (90,762 cases) were among men; the overall male-to-female ratio was 2.7. Among migrant cases, the male-to-female ratio varied considerably, ranging from 24.3 in those originating from Australia and New Zealand, to 0.7 in cases from sub-Saharan Africa. The male–female ratio for migrants from sub-Saharan Africa diagnosed with HIV in Europe largely mirrors the male–female ratio in the region, where HIV prevalence is higher in women. For other regions, HIV infections among men predominate.

Predominant modes of transmission differ between subgroups of migrants depending on the region of origin. The majority of new HIV cases reported among migrants from Western Europe, Central Europe, East Asia and the Pacific, Australia and New Zealand were among MSM, while heterosexual transmission was the main transmission category for migrants from South and South-East Asia, North Africa and the Middle East, and the Caribbean. Overall, migrants accounted for a significant proportion of HIV cases with all modes of transmission. During 2007–2011, 58 per cent of all HIV cases where heterosexual transmission was the reported route of transmission, 57 per cent of cases of mother-to-child transmission, 23 per cent of cases with MSM as the route of transmission and 20 per cent of cases with injecting drug use as the route of transmission were among migrants (Figure 19.1).

A growing issue of concern in some EU/EEA countries is late diagnosis[1] of HIV among migrants from Latin America, Africa, the Middle East, Asia and the Pacific (ECDC 2014). Between 2007 and 2011, 37 per cent of native-born cases were diagnosed late, compared to 44 per cent of cases from Latin America, 46 per cent from North Africa and the Middle East, 46 per cent from the Caribbean, 51 per cent from East Asia and the

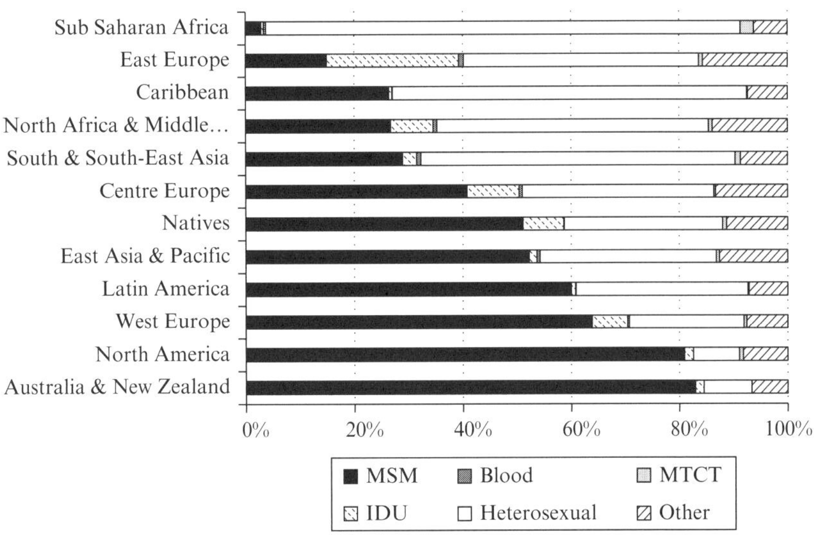

Source: ECDC 2014.

Figure 19.1 HIV transmission category by geographical origin, EU/EEA, 2007–2011 (n = 118 763 cases with information on geographical origin and transmission category)

Pacific, 51 per cent from sub-Saharan Africa and 55 per cent from South and South-East Asia (ECDC 2014). Only migrants from Western Europe, North America, Australia and New Zealand and Eastern and Central Europe had comparable or lower rates of late diagnosis than native-born cases.

There is also increasing evidence that migrant populations from countries with generalised HIV epidemics and migrant MSM are at higher risk of acquiring HIV infection after arrival in the EU/EEA. A recent ECDC report assessed the evidence for sexual transmission of HIV among migrant populations from countries with generalised HIV epidemics after arrival in the EU/EEA (ECDC 2013d). The report found evidence of ongoing HIV acquisition and transmission post-migration to Europe. Figures for the proportion of HIV infections acquired after migration ranged from 2 per cent among sub-Saharan Africans in Switzerland to 62 per cent among black Caribbean MSM in the United Kingdom.

Although many EU/EEA countries identify migrants as an important sub-population in their national response to HIV, few have adequate systems in place to monitor HIV among migrants (ECDC 2014). It is important that HIV surveillance among migrants is strengthened with improved completeness and reliable capture of variables such as country of birth, CD4 cell count at diagnosis, year of arrival, probable country of infection and route of transmission. This information will increase understanding of HIV infection by migrant status over time, of the probable country of infection and of key migrant sub-populations at greatest risk of HIV infection. Specific measures are also needed to ensure that HIV testing can be easily accessed by migrants at risk for HIV in order to reduce the proportion of this population that is undiagnosed or diagnosed late (ECDC 2014). It is crucial that any HIV testing is linked to appropriate treatment and care regardless of migrants' legal status to ensure the effectiveness of proactive testing strategies and the benefits of timely treatment.

TUBERCULOSIS

Tuberculosis (TB) is a major global public health concern. In 2013, there were an estimated 9 million cases of TB worldwide (WHO 2014). The majority of TB cases occur in low-income settings, predominantly in Asia (59 per cent) and Africa (26 per cent), but TB prevention and control remains a challenge in all countries (Abubakar et al. 2012; WHO 2014). In the EU/EEA, TB notification rates have declined over recent decades, but specific vulnerable subgroups of the population remain at high risk of acquiring TB infection and developing active disease (ECDC/WHO Europe 2013b). In particular, the share of foreign-born subjects in the total TB burden is increasing each year in many member states, representing a challenge for TB control programmes and a public health concern (Abubakar et al. 2012; Hollo et al. 2009).

Data from the ECDC and the WHO Global TB database show that 73,996 TB cases were reported in the EU/EEA in 2010, with 25.1 per cent classified as of 'foreign origin', 73.1 per cent as of 'native origin' and 1.7 per cent as of 'unknown origin' (ECDC 2014). The proportion of foreign-born cases among total notified TB cases varied considerably among countries, ranging from 0 per cent in Bulgaria and Romania to more than 80 per cent in Cyprus, Norway and Sweden. Migrant TB cases in 2010 mirrored the global burden of TB and occurred largely among those born in Asia (34 per cent), followed by those born in Africa (22 per cent) and Eastern Europe (13 per cent). Clearly, predominant countries or regions of origin will impact on TB prevalence among migrants in individual member states. For example, a study in the United Kingdom reported that 57 per cent of foreign-born TB cases in 2010 were from southern Asia and 27 per cent from sub-Saharan Africa (Health Protection Services 2011). However, in the Netherlands, the main countries of origin for TB cases were Somalia, Morocco and Turkey, which provide the largest migrant populations in the country (Borgdorff et al. 2010). In Italy, the largest share of TB cases in migrants were found to originate from the Middle East (36.6 per cent) and Africa (21.7 per cent), which are the most common regions of origin of migrants (Odone et al. 2011).

Published studies further show that TB incidence among migrants varies across Europe but is higher in foreign-born than native-born populations in most EU/EEA countries (Barniol et al. 2009; Borgdorff et al. 2010; Health Protection Services 2011). In Germany, TB incidence in 2005 in the foreign-born population was 27.4/100,000, which was 5.4 times higher than in native-born Germans (Barniol et al. 2009). In Italy, data from regional surveillance systems reported TB incidence in foreign-born subjects to be 100.7/100,000 (83.9/100,000 when the estimated 20 per cent of irregular migrants were added to the denominator), whereas incidence among native-born Italians was 6.5/100,000 (Odone et al. 2011). Although overall incidence has declined in the EU/EEA in the past ten years, the opposite trend is found among migrant populations (ECDC 2014).

Evidence from TESSy indicates that active TB disease occurs at significantly younger ages in migrants than in the native population (on average nine years younger, reflecting the different age distribution between foreign-born and native populations), with a slightly increased percentage of cases in female migrants when compared to natives (ECDC 2014).

Available data also suggests that migrants have a twofold increased risk of extra-pulmonary TB and may be at higher risk of TB-HIV co-infection (ECDC 2014). Foreign-born individuals represented more than 80 per cent of notified TB-HIV co-infected cases in England and Wales, and more than 60 per cent in Belgium, Denmark, France and the Netherlands (French et al. 2008). Lower percentages, of approximately 30 per cent, were reported in Italy and Spain. The fact that Northern European countries receive immigrants from countries with higher TB and HIV burdens compared with Italy and Spain may explain this difference.

TESSy data and epidemiological studies both show no significant differences in risk of multi-drug resistant (MDR) TB between foreign-born and native TB cases. Data reported to WHO and ECDC for 2010 shows that, at EU/EEA level, the proportion of TB cases that are resistant to isoniazid, rifampicin or both is lower in foreign-born cases than in native-born cases (ECDC 2014). Among TB cases for which origin is known, 3.1 per cent of foreign-born cases with drug susceptibility results had MDR-TB compared with 6.8 per cent of native-born cases (ECDC 2013a). More detailed analyses of country of origin for foreign-born MDR-TB cases suggest that the highest proportion of MDR-TB is found in people born in Eurasian countries (14.3 per cent), followed by those born in Northern Europe (13.9 per cent), Central Asia (12 per cent) and Eastern Europe (10.7 per cent).

Although TB represents a burden among migrants in the EU/EEA, there is no evidence to suggest that the presence of migrants with TB increases the burden of TB in the native population. In Germany, for example, the reported probability of TB transmission from foreign to native subjects in mixed clusters was low (Dahle et al. 2007). This may be due to low levels of social mixing between the two populations, as well as the efficacy of targeted prevention programmes (Barniol et al. 2009; Kamper-Jorgensen et al. 2012). A large nationally representative study in Denmark showed that TB transmission was actually 2.5 times more likely to occur from Danes to migrants than vice versa (Kamper-Jorgensen et al. 2012). In contrast, data from Spain estimated that in mixed clusters, 50 per cent of index cases were foreign-born, suggesting that transmission between communities might be a public health concern in some countries (Borrell et al. 2010).

According to TESSy data, migrants have twice as many unknown treatment outcomes at 12 months than non-migrants, and the proportion of TB cases achieving successful treatment outcomes at 12 months is lower among migrants (50 per cent) than among non-migrants (65 per cent) (ECDC 2014). This may reflect greater mobility than among the native-born population, deportation before treatment is completed, or barriers to follow-up care and adherence to treatment among migrants. In order to meet the goal of TB elimination in the EU/EEA, it is essential that a comprehensive approach to TB prevention and control that addresses both TB disease and individuals with latent TB infection is adopted (ECDC 2014). Priority must be given to ensuring that all individuals, irrespective of country of origin, have the right to prompt and continuous TB care of high quality.

HEPATITIS B

Worldwide, an estimated 2 billion people have been infected with the hepatitis B virus (HBV); of these, 240 million are estimated to have chronic infection[2] (WHO 2012). Hepatitis B prevalence is high in sub-Saharan Africa, Central and South-East Asia, the Pacific and South America. Southern areas of Eastern and Central Europe, the Middle East and India are classified as having intermediate prevalence and Western Europe and North America are classified as having low prevalence (WHO, 2012). In low-prevalence areas of Europe, migrants from countries with high and intermediate prevalence account for most reported cases of chronic hepatitis B (Haworth et al. 1999; Rossi et al. 2012; Vriend et al. 2012).

According to TESSy data, a total of 17,025 cases of hepatitis B were reported by 28 EU/EEA countries[3] in 2011 (ECDC 2013c). Only 18 of these countries provided data on whether cases were 'imported', 'indigenous' or of 'unknown' origin, covering 6,662 cases (39.1 per cent of all reported cases). Of these cases, more than half (52.6 per cent) were recorded as 'imported'. In all, 6.3 per cent of imported cases were acute infections and 81.5 per cent were chronic infections. Among acute hepatitis B cases, the proportion of imported cases ranged from 0 per cent in Austria, the Czech Republic, Germany, Greece, Hungary and Poland to 69.2 per cent in Finland. Among chronic cases, the proportion of imported cases ranged from 0 per cent in Estonia to 96.1 per cent in Sweden. During the period 2006–2011 there was an overall decline in notification rates for acute infection in the EU/EEA, but the opposite trend was observed for reported chronic infections (ECDC 2013c).

A higher prevalence of chronic infection among migrants than the native born population has also been found in a number of published studies from Denmark, Greece, Germany, Italy, Norway, Spain and the United Kingdom (Gjorup et al. 2003; Hahne et al. 2008; Chu et al. 2012; Lindh et al. 1993; Palumbo et al. 2008; Rimseliene et al. 2011). The prevalence of chronic infection in migrants in Europe and other countries with low endemicity was also assessed in a recent meta-analysis (Rossi et al. 2012). The authors estimated that almost 3.5 million migrants and refugees were chronically infected with HBV. The proportion of all migrants with chronic hepatitis B infection ranged from 3.7 per cent in Spain to 6.9 per cent in Ireland, with the largest absolute numbers in Germany (284,000 cases), Italy (201,000 cases), the United Kingdom (194,000 cases), Spain (128,000 cases) and France (114,000 cases) (Rossi et al. 2012). The meta-analysis also found that, as expected, the prevalence of HBV infection in migrants mirrored the prevalence in their country of origin (Rossi et al. 2012). In particular, prevalence of chronic infection was high in migrants from East Asia and the Pacific (11.3 per cent, 95%CI9.1–11.8) and sub-Saharan Africa (10.3 per cent, 95%CI10.3–12.4), intermediate in migrants from Eastern Europe (5.8 per cent, 95%CI4.3–7.9) and Central and South Asia (4.6 per cent, 95%CI2.6–7.8), and lower in migrants from Latin America (1.7 per cent, 95%CI1.1–2.7) and the Middle East and North Africa (1.7 per cent, 95%CI1.1–2.7) (Rossi et al. 2012).

Most individuals with hepatitis B from countries of high endemicity become infected at birth via vertical transmission from mother to child, or during early childhood, when the risk for chronic hepatitis B infection is greatest (Allaby 2010; Toy et al. 2008). Among 1,600 imported cases reported to TESSy in 2011 for which data on mode of transmission was available, 1,163 cases (72.7 per cent) were classified as mother-to-child transmission; 99.6 per cent of these cases were chronic. The findings of molecular epidemiology studies conducted in the Netherlands showed that genotypes of chronic HBV infection in migrants corresponded with HBV genotypes common in their countries of origin (Toy et al. 2008), suggesting that migrants from highly endemic countries are likely to have acquired their infection at birth or during childhood prior to migration. In contrast, the majority of hepatitis B cases in the native-born population occur in high-risk groups, such as injecting drug-users and MSM, and are acquired at an older age (Veldhuijzen et al. 2010).

The difficulties of drawing definitive conclusions or making meaningful cross-country comparisons on hepatitis B in migrants should be noted, in view of differences in national surveillance systems and the incompleteness of data in the EU/EEA (ECDC 2014). Using the importation status of a disease to assess the number of cases in migrants has significant limitations, as imported cases may also include infections acquired by native residents when travelling to an endemic country. Surveillance systems in the EU/EEA should be strengthened in order to capture more complete information on 'country of origin' of a case and to improve monitoring of trends over time. In addition, the majority of published studies have been conducted in a limited number of countries in Western Europe. More evidence is needed from a wider range of EU/EEA countries, as the relationship between risk of hepatitis B infection and country of origin means that host countries with different migration patterns will face different challenges in hepatitis B control. A better understanding of hepatitis B risk factors and distribution among migrants is essential to provide the basis for planning, implementation and evaluation of measures to reduce the burden of disease in this population.

Alongside strengthening the evidence base on hepatitis B in migrants, a consistent EU-wide approach to screening would be beneficial, as would be greater efforts to ensure that migrants have access to HBV diagnosis and appropriate follow up. Many migrants are likely to be unaware of their HBV status. Consideration should therefore be given to HBsAg testing of all persons born in countries with HBsAg prevalence of ≥2 per cent and referral of infected persons to care and of close contacts for testing and vaccination. This strategy is likely to be cost-effective and could capture a high proportion of foreign-born persons living with chronic hepatitis B in Europe (Veldhuijzen et al. 2010).

MEASLES AND RUBELLA

The availability of effective vaccines has led to a significant decline in reported measles and rubella cases in the EU/EEA in the past 30 years. However, despite these reductions, outbreaks and deaths continue in the region because vaccination coverage remains below the recommended level of 95 per cent of the population, leaving pockets of vulnerable groups unvaccinated (Lopalco 2010). Sub-optimal coverage rates often occur in at-risk groups, such as Roma, Irish travellers, vulnerable migrant populations and certain religious communities.

As is the case with hepatitis B, routine measles and rubella surveillance data captures the importation status of a disease, which indicates where an infection was acquired, rather than the country of birth of a case. This makes it difficult to establish whether cases are occurring in migrants specifically, although it makes it possible to trace the source of infection. Available TESSy data shows that in 2013, 10,271 measles cases were reported by 30 EU/EEA member states, with more than 95 per cent of total cases reported by France, Germany, Italy, Romania, Spain, Poland and the United Kingdom (ECDC 2014). Of these cases, 2.7 per cent (748 cases) were categorised as 'imported', 0.7 per cent (34 cases) 'import-related',[4] 88.9 per cent (9,132 cases) 'indigenous' and 8.1 per cent (827 cases) as of 'unknown' origin. During the period July 2011 to June 2012, a total of 22,835 rubella cases were reported to TESSy by 27 EU/EEA countries, with the majority of cases reported by Romania (17,517 cases) and Poland (5,106 cases) (ECDC 2012). Only 13 countries reported information on importation status for 201 rubella cases, with these data indicating that 8.5 per cent (17 cases) were categorised as 'imported', 47.3 per cent (95 cases) as 'indigenous' and 44.3 per cent (89 cases) as 'unknown' origin (ECDC 2014).

Few published studies are available on measles and rubella in migrant populations in the EU/EEA. In one study that has been conducted, national surveillance data from 32 European countries were analysed for 2006–2007 for a total of 12,132 reported measles cases (Muscat 2011). Of these, only 210 cases (1.7 per cent) were reported as 'imported'; 117 cases (56 per cent) were from another European country and 43 (20 per cent) were from Asia. The study further observed that measles outbreaks in Europe in 2005–2009 had been reported in vulnerable population groups, including Roma, Sinti, Traveller and specific religious communities as well as in migrants (Muscat 2011). A further report on a measles outbreak in Greece in 2010 noted that Roma communities from Greece and Bulgaria had a disproportionately high caseload (Pervanidou et al. 2010).

In one of the few studies assessing rubella in migrants, pregnant migrants in Spain were shown to be less likely to have antibodies against rubella than non-migrant pregnant women (92 per cent versus 97 per cent); migrant women from Latin America, Asia, sub-Saharan Africa and North Africa had the lowest levels of immunity (Ramos et al. 2012a). Another study in the region of Catalonia also found a statistically significant difference in the prevalence of rubella antibodies between migrant and native-born pregnant women (89 per cent versus 94.9 per cent) (Dominguez et al. 2007). Similar findings were also reported in a study of 13,136 pregnant women in the region of Aragon, which found that foreign-born women aged 15–19 years were most likely to lack rubella immunity, particularly if they were from Asia, although this finding was not statistically significant (Hernandez Diaz et al. 2011). A study in Sweden also found a correlation between migrant status and rubella immunity. The study analysed a dataset of 34,074 pregnant women in and around southern Stockholm for whom place of birth had been recorded, covering the period 2004–2006. Low levels of immunity were found in 2.8 per cent of Swedish-born women, 3.5 per cent of those born in other Nordic countries and 7.7 per cent of those born elsewhere (Kakoulidou et al. 2010).

Studies from a number of countries suggest that migrant children may be less likely to be vaccinated against measles and rubella than non-migrant children. Studies from Germany, using data from the representative German Health Interview and Examination Survey for Children and Adolescents, found that foreign-born children were three times as likely to be unvaccinated (Poethko-Müller and Mankertz 2012; Poethko-Müller et al. 2009). A Spanish study also found a statistically significant difference in immunisation rates between indigenous and immigrant children for both primary vaccination coverage (96.5 per cent and 85.0 per cent) and primary vaccination and booster dose coverage (88.6 per cent and 78.3 per cent) (Borras et al. 2007). Other studies in Spain have also reported lower vaccination rates among immigrant children (Cilleruelo et al. 2008).

Inadequate vaccination coverage, linked to poor access to health services for migrants and other populations, is identified as a major reason for measles and rubella outbreaks in Europe. Factors limiting access to health services include cultural and language barriers, socioeconomic exclusion and discrimination (Muscat 2011). Having parents who do not speak the language of the host country has also been identified as a risk factor for low vaccination coverage among children (Bouhamam et al. 2012; Riccardo et al. 2012). Studies highlight the need to improve vaccination coverage in migrants, including among adults who may not usually come into contact with the health system (Borras et al. 2007; Cilleruelo et al. 2008; Peña-Rey et al. 2009).

Limited information is available on measles and rubella among migrants in Europe. Routine national surveillance data reported to ECDC captures importation status of the disease but not country of birth of a case. In addition, few studies have been conducted to assess measles and rubella incidence and vaccination coverage in migrants. Those studies that have been conducted suggest that some migrant groups may be at elevated risk of measles, including socially and economically disadvantaged older children and young adults, mainly because of low vaccination coverage. Furthermore, there is evidence that levels of rubella immunity may be lower among pregnant women born abroad. To improve understanding of measles and rubella in migrants, it is important that surveillance data are strengthened to capture migrant relevant data, in particular country of birth. This information can help identify at-risk groups, which can inform efforts to improve vaccination coverage by improving the reach and uptake of immunisation services (ECDC 2014).

CHAGAS DISEASE

Chagas disease, also called American Trypanosomiasis, is a vector-borne disease caused by the *Trypanosoma cruzi* (*T. cruzi*) parasite. An estimated 10 million people are infected worldwide. Chagas disease is endemic only in the 21 Latin American countries where the vector is present; however, migration from Latin America means that there are also individuals with Chagas disease in Europe. Blood and organ donation as well as congenital transmission (from mother to child) are the main transmission risks in non-endemic countries (Schmunis and Yadon 2010).

Chagas disease is not systematically monitored by countries in the EU/EAA, but available data suggests that prevalence rates are high enough in some countries to warrant concern. Spain, Italy, the Netherlands, the United Kingdom, Germany and France have the highest number of estimated cases in Europe, with sporadic cases also reported in Austria, Croatia, Denmark, Germany, Luxembourg, the Netherlands, Norway, Portugal, Romania and Sweden (Schmunis and Yadon 2010).

Most studies on Chagas disease in Europe have been conducted in Spain, which has been the main destination for Latin American migration to Europe in the past decade. Several of these studies have assessed prevalence among pregnant women. One study found a prevalence rate of 3.96 per cent in 3,839 pregnant Latin American women in Madrid who were tested for *T. cruzi* infection from 2008 to 2010 (Flores-Chavez et al. 2011); the congenital transmission rate was 2.6 per cent. Another large hospital-based study, which tested 1,350 pregnant Latin American women between 2005 and 2007, found a prevalence rate of 3.4 per cent and a congenital transmission rate of 7.3 per cent (Munoz et al. 2009a). A further study, which tested 1,975 Latin American women and newborns during one year in Valencia, found a prevalence rate of 11.4 per cent and a congenital transmission rate of 3.5 per cent (Barona-Vilar et al. 2012). Other studies among Latin American migrant populations in general have found higher prevalence rates. For example, a study that tested 1,146 Latin Americans in Madrid attending hospitals found a prevalence rate of 31 per cent (Perez-Ayala et al., 2011); another study conducted in two centres for imported diseases in Barcelona found a prevalence rate of 41 per cent in a sample of 489 Latin American migrants (Munoz et al. 2009b). A cross-sectional study of a Paraguayan and Bolivian population living in Elche, Spain, found a prevalence rate of 6.5 per cent (Ramos et al. 2012b).

Prevalence data are also available from studies in other European countries. An Italian screening programme that included migrants, expatriates, travellers to endemic regions and children born to *T. cruzi* seropositive mothers attending a tropical disease centre had 876 participants of whom 4.2 per cent were *T. cruzi* positive (Angheben et al. 2011). In Switzerland, reported prevalence rates range from 2 per cent to 12.8 per cent and studies have generally found that participants were often awaiting regularisation (Chappuis et al. 2010; Jackson et al. 2009; Martinez de Tejada et al. 2009). A study in the Netherlands estimated that there were between 726 and 2,929 *T. cruzi* seropositive migrants, most of whom originated from Suriname (Bart et al. 2011). Irregular migrants appear to be especially at risk of Chagas disease in Europe. One study estimated that almost 45 per cent of cases in Europe are likely to be among irregular migrants (Basile et al. 2011), many of whom do not have access to healthcare.

There is currently low awareness of Chagas disease in Europe, and many cases may not be detected as most health professionals are not trained to diagnose and manage the disease (Basile et al. 2011; WHO 2009). There is a need to improve awareness and detection of Chagas disease in Europe and to improve access to healthcare for both legal and undocumented Latin American migrants, to ensure that the disease is diagnosed and treated. Key issues to be addressed in Europe are the prevention of transmission through blood, organ, tissue and cell donation by Latin American donors and prevention of congenital transmission in Latin American pregnant women who are infected with *T. cruzi.*

CONCLUSION

Drawing overall conclusions on infectious diseases in migrant populations in the EU/EEA is challenging as patterns and trends vary considerably depending on the disease in question and are confounded by the diversity of migrants and the changing patterns of migration both to and within Europe. Available evidence indicates that, overall, migrants in the EU/EEA have a higher burden of some infectious diseases, including HIV, TB and chronic hepatitis B, than the native-born population, but are less affected by others such as measles and rubella. The extent to which different migrant populations are affected by infectious diseases also depends on the disease in question, the country of destination and the region or country of origin. For example, Chagas disease disproportionately affects irregular migrants from Latin America, whereas the majority of migrant HIV cases in the EU/EEA are largely from sub-Saharan Africa and migrants with TB or chronic hepatitis B are mainly from Asia, Africa and other parts of the European region.

Although the findings presented in this chapter provide valuable insights into infectious diseases in migrant populations, it is important to note that they are to some extent limited by the incompleteness of surveillance data and limitations of published studies. In recent years, efforts have been made to harmonise data collected by national surveillance systems on migrant-specific variables such as 'country of birth', but the type and quality of data collected still varies between EU/EEA countries and reporting on migrant-specific variables is poor for the majority of diseases, with the exceptions of HIV and TB (ECDC 2014). Evidence from published studies is also incomplete, as research is often conducted in a narrow range of countries in Western Europe. Many studies also fail to explore how factors such as socioeconomic disadvantage and poor access to healthcare and prevention efforts may influence the progression of disease or acquisition of infection after arrival in Europe.

Understanding of infectious diseases in migrants can only be improved if all EU/EEA countries invest in further strengthening and harmonising surveillance systems to collect standardised case-based data on migrant-specific variables, in particular country of birth and probable country of infection. In addition, adding a variable on 'year of arrival' would help strengthen monitoring of post-arrival acquisition of infectious diseases. This is especially important for HIV and TB, as there is increasing evidence that migrants from some regions may be at risk of contracting HIV or reactivating latent TB after arrival in the EU/EEA. For measles and rubella it is equally important that more data are collected on vaccination coverage in the native and foreign-born population to ascertain if particular vulnerable migrant groups may be at risk of remaining unvaccinated. Alongside strengthening surveillance systems, it is important that more research is conducted in a wider range of European countries to help improve understanding of the epidemiology of infectious diseases among migrant populations.

Conducting more research and further strengthening surveillance systems in the EU/EEA is essential for planning, implementation and evaluation of appropriate and targeted infectious disease prevention and control interventions for at-risk migrant populations. In order to reduce the burden of infectious disease in migrant populations, it is essential that all migrants have equal access to preventive and curative health services. It is therefore vital that all member states ensure that all individuals, irrespective of country of origin and legal status, have the right to prompt testing and screening, linked to high-quality treatment and care.

ACKNOWLEDGEMENTS

The authors would like to extend their gratitude to Victoria Hernando, Débora Álvarez del Arco and Julia del Amo from the Instituto de Salud Carlos III, Madrid for helping to analyse the HIV TESSy data.

NOTES

1. Late diagnosis is defined as a CD4 cell count <350 cells/mm^3 or AIDS diagnosis.
2. Chronic infection is defined as the presence of the hepatitis B surface antigen (HBsAg) for more than six months.

3. Data were not reported by Belgium and Liechtenstein.
4. If the infection was acquired from a second person who acquired it following recent travel, then the secondary case is classified as 'import related'.

REFERENCES

Abubakar, I., H. R. Stagg, T. Cohen, P. Mangtani, L. C. Rodrigues, L. Pimpin, J. M. Watson, S. B. Squire and A. Zumla (2012), Controversies and unresolved issues in tuberculosis prevention and control: a low-burden-country perspective, *Journal of Infectious Diseases*, **205**(2), 293–300.

Allaby, M. (2010), *Screening for Hepatitis B and Hepatitis C Among Ethnic Minorities Born Outside the UK*, report for the National Screening Committee, National Health Service, available online at www.legacy.screening.nhs.uk/policydb_download.php?doc=127.

Alvarez-Del Arco, D., S. Monge, A. Azcoaga, I. Rio, V. Hernando, C. Gonzalez, B. Alejos, et al. (2012), HIV testing and counselling for migrant populations living in high-income countries: a systematic review, *European Journal of Public Health*, **23**(6), 1039–1045.

Angheben, A., M. Anselmi, F. Gobbi, S. Marocco, G. Monteiro, D. Buonfrate, et al. (2011), Chagas disease in Italy: breaking an epidemiological silence, *European Communicable Disease Bulletin*, **16**(37), 19969.

Barniol, J., S. Niemann, V. R. Louis, B. Brodhun, C. Dreweck, E. Richter, H. Becher, W. Haas and T. Junghanss (2009), Transmission dynamics of pulmonary tuberculosis between autochthonous and immigrant sub-populations, *BMC Infectious Diseases*, **9**(197).

Barona-Vilar, C., M. J. Gimenez-Marti, T. Fraile, C. Gonzalez-Steinbauer, C. Parada, A. Gil-Brusola et al. (2012), Prevalence of Trypanosoma cruzi infection in pregnant Latin American women and congenital transmission rate in a non-endemic area: the experience of the Valencian Health Programme (Spain), *Epidemiology and Infection*, **140**(10), 1896–1903.

Bart, A., C. J. Hodiamont, M. P. Grobusch, R. B. van den Brink, A. J. Smout and T. van Gool (2011), Chagas disease in the Netherlands: an estimate of the number of patients', *Ned Tijdschr Geneeskd*, **155**(A3170).

Basile, L., J. M. Jansa, Y. Carlier, D. D. Salamanca, A. Angheben and A. Bartoloni (2011), Chagas disease in European countries: the challenge of a surveillance system, *European Surveillance*, **16**(37), pii=19968.

Borgdorff, M. W., S. van den Hof, K. Kremer, L. Verhagen, N. Kalisvaart, C. Erkens and D. van Soolingen (2010), Progress towards tuberculosis elimination: secular trend, immigration and transmission, *European Respiratory Journal*, **36**(2), 339–347.

Borras, E., A. Dominguez, J. Batalla, N. Torner, N. Cardenosa, M. Nebot, A. Plasencia et al. (2007), Vaccination coverage in indigenous and immigrant children under 3 years of age in Catalonia (Spain), *Vaccine*, **25**(16), 3240–3243.

Borrell, S., M. Espanol, A. Orcau, G. Tudo, F. March, J. A. Cayla, J. M. Jansa, F. Alcaide, N. Martin-Casabona, M. Salvado, J. A. Martinez, R. Vidal, F. Sanchez, N. Altet, E. Rey, P. Coll and J. Gonzalez-Martin (2010), Tuberculosis transmission patterns among Spanish-born and foreign-born populations in the city of Barcelona, *Clinical Microbiology and Infection*, **16**(6), 568–74.

Bouhamam, N., R. Laporte, A. Boutin, M. Uters, V. Bremond, G. Noel, P. Rodier et al. (2012), Relationship between precariousness, social coverage, and vaccine coverage: survey among children consulting in pediatric emergency departments in France, *Archives De Pediatrie*, **19**(3), 242–247.

Chappuis, F., A. Mauris, M. Holst, P. Albajar-Vinas, A. O. Jannin J, Luquetti et al. (2010), Validation of a rapid immunochromatographic assay for diagnosis of Trypanosoma cruzi infection among Latin-American Migrants in Geneva, Switzerland, *Journal of Clinical Microbiology*, **48**(8), 2948–2952.

Cilleruelo, M. J., F. de Ory, J. Ruiz-Contreras, R. González-González, M. J. Mellado,

M. García-Hortelano, J. Villota et al. (2008), Internationally adopted children: what vaccines should they receive? *Vaccine*, **26**(46), 5784–5790.

Dahle, U. R., V. Eldholm, B. A. Winje, T. Mannsaker and E. Heldal, (2007), Impact of immigration on the molecular epidemiology of Mycobacterium tuberculosis in a low-incidence country, *American Journal of Respiratory and Critical Care Medicine*, **176**(9), 930–935.

Dominguez, A., P. Plans, J. Espuñes, J. Costa, N. Torner, N. Cardeñosa N et al. (2007), Rubella immune status of indigenous and immigrant pregnant women in Catalonia, Spain, *European Journal of Public Health*, **17**(6), 560–564.

ECDC (2012), Measles and rubella monitoring, August 2012, *Surveillance Report*, Stockholm: ECDC, available online at www.ecdc.europa.eu/en/publications/Publications/Forms/ECDC_DispForm.aspx?ID=940.

ECDC (2013a) *Annual Epidemiological Report 2012: Reporting on 2010 Surveillance Data and 2011 Epidemic Intelligence Data*, Surveillance Report, Stockholm: ECDC, available online at http://ecdc.europa.eu/en/publications/Publications/Annual-Epidemiological-Report-2012.pdf.

ECDC (2013b), *Annual Epidemiological Report 2013: Reporting on 2011 Surveillance Data and 2012 Epidemic Intelligence Data*, Surveillance Report, Stockholm: ECDC, available online at http://ecdc.europa.eu/en/publications/Publications/Annual-Epidemiological-Report-2013.pdf.

ECDC (2013c), *Hepatitis B and C Surveillance in Europe, 2006–2011*, Surveillance Report, Stockholm: ECDC, available online at http://ecdc.europa.eu/en/publications/Publications/Hepatitis-B-C-surveillance-report-2006-2011.pdf.

ECDC (2013d), *Migrant Health: Sexual Transmission of HIV Within Migrant Groups in the EU/EEA and Implications for Effective Interventions*, Technical Report, Stockholm: ECDC, available online at http://ecdc.europa.eu/en/publications/Publications/Migrant-health-sexual-transmission.pdf.

ECDC (2014), *Assessing the Burden of Key Infectious Diseases Among Migrant Populations*, Technical Report, Stockholm: ECDC, available online at http://ecdc.europa.eu/en/publications/Publications/assessing-burden-disease-migrant-populations.pdf.

ECDC/WHO Europe (2013a), *HIV/AIDS Surveillance in Europe 2012*, Surveillance Report, Stockholm: ECDC, available online at www.euro.who.int/__data/assets/pdf_file/0018/235440/e96953.pdf?ua=1.

ECDC/WHO Europe (2013b), *Tuberculosis Surveillance and Monitoring in Europe 2013*, Surveillance Report, Stockholm: ECDC, available online at http://ecdc.europa.eu/en/publications/Publications/Tuberculosis-surveillance-monitoring-2013.pdf.

Flores-Chavez, M. D., F. J. Merino, S. Garcia-Bujalance, P. Martin-Rabadan, P. Merino, I. Garcia-Bermejo et al. (2011), Surveillance of Chagas disease in pregnant women in Madrid, Spain, from 2008 to 2010, *European Communicable Disease Bulletin*, **16**(38).

French, C. E., J. R. Glynn, M. E. Kruijshaar, I. C. Ditah, V. Delpech and I. Abubakar (2008), The association between HIV and antituberculosis drug resistance, *European Respiratory Journal*, **32**(3), 718–725.

Gjorup, I. E., E. Smith, L. Borgwardt and P. Skinhoj (2003), Twenty-year survey of the epidemiology of hepatitis B in Denmark: effect of immigration, *Scandinavian Journal of Infectious Diseases*, **35** (4), 260–264.

Gushulak, B., P. Pace and J. Weekers (2010), Migration and health of migrants, in T. Koller (ed.), *Poverty and Social Exclusion in the WHO European Region: Health Systems Respond*, Copenhagen: WHO Regional Office for Europe, pp. 257–281.

Hahne, S. J., I. K. Veldhuijzen, L. J. Smits, N. Nagelkerke and M. J. van de Laar (2008), Hepatitis B virus transmission in the Netherlands: a population-based, hierarchical case-control study in a very low-incidence country, *Epidemiology and Infection*, **136**(2), 184–195.

Haworth, E. A., V. Soni Raleigh and R. Balarajan (1999), Cirrhosis and primary liver cancer amongst first generation migrants in England and Wales, *Ethnicity & Health*, **4**(1–2), 93–99.

Health Protection Services (2011), *Migrant Health: Infectious Diseases in Non-UK Born*

Populations in the United Kingdom, update to the baseline report, London: Health Protection Agency.
Hernandez Diaz, R., M. P. R. Val, A. M. Peral, M. L. R. Alfaro and M. B. A. Sancho (2011), Seroepidemiologic study of rubella in childbearing women in Aragon, Spain (2003–2007), *Gaceta Sanitaria*, **25**(1), 20–22.
Hollo, V., A. Amato-Gauci, C. Kodmon, and D. Manissero (2009), Tuberculosis in the EU and EEA/EFTA countries: what is the latest data telling us? *European Communicable Disease Bulletin*, **14**(11).
Ingleby, D. (2009), *Assisting Migrants and Communities (AMAC): Analysis of Social Determinants of Health and Health Inequalities: European Research on Migration and Health*. background paper developed within the framework of the IOM project, Geneva: International Organization for Migration, available online at www.migrant-health-europe.org/files/Research%20on%20Migrant%20Health_Background%20Paper.pdf.
International Organization for Migration (2010), *The Future of Migration: Building Capacities for Change*, World Migration Report 2010, Geneva: International Organization for Migration, available online at http://publications.iom.int/system/files/pdf/wmr_2010_english.pdf.
Jackson, Y., C. Myers, A. Diana, H. P. Marti, H. Wolff, F. Chappuis et al. (2009), Congenital transmission of Chagas disease in Latin American immigrants in Switzerland, *Emerging Infectious Diseases*, **15**(4), 601–603.
Chu, J. J., T. Wörmann, J. Popp, G. Pätzelt, M. K. Akmatov, A. Krämer and R. Reintjes (2012), Changing epidemiology of Hepatitis B and migration – a comparison of six Northern and North-Western European countries, *The European Journal of Public Health*, **23**(4), 642–647.
Kakoulidou, M., M. Forsgren, I. Lewensohn-Fuchs and K. Johansen (2010), Serum levels of rubella-specific antibodies in Swedish women following three decades of vaccination programmes, *Vaccine*, **4**, 1002–1007.
Kamper-Jorgensen, Z., A. B. Andersen, A. Kok-Jensen, M. Kamper-Jorgensen, I. C. Bygbjerg, P. H. Andersen, V. O. Thomsen and T. Lillebaek (2012), Migrant tuberculosis: the extent of transmission in a low burden country, *BMC Infectious Disease*, **12**(60).
Lindh, M., G. Norkrans, K. Stenqvist, K. Eriksson and J. Taranger (1993), Hepatitis B carriers in Sweden – effects of immigration, *Scandinavian Journal of Infectious Diseases*, **25**(4), 411–416.
Lopalco, P. L. and R. Martin (2010), Measles still spreads in Europe: who is responsible for the failure to vaccinate? *European Communicable Disease Bulletin*, **15**(17).
Martinez de Tejada, B., Y. Jackson, C. Paccolat and O. Irion (2009), Groupe Chagas Congenital G., *Revue Medicale Suisse*, **5**(222), 2091–2092.
Mladovsky, P., D. Ingleby, M. McKee and B. Rechel (2012), Good practices in migrant health: the European experience, *Clinical Medicine*, **12**(3), 248–252.
Munoz, J., O. Coll, T. Juncosa, M. Verges, M. del Pino, V. Fumado et al. (2009a), Prevalence and vertical transmission of Trypanosoma cruzi infection among pregnant Latin American women attending two maternity clinics in Barcelona, Spain, *Clinical Infectious Diseases*, **15**(12), 1736–1740.
Munoz, J., I. Gomez, J. Prat, M. Gallego, F. Gimeno, B. Trevino, P. Lopez-Chejade et al. (2009b), Clinical profile of Trypanosoma cruzi infection in a non-endemic setting: immigration and Chagas disease in Barcelona (Spain), *Acta Tropica*, **111**(1), 51–55.
Muscat, M, (2011), Who gets measles in Europe? *Journal of Infectious Diseases*, **204**, 353–365.
Odone, A., M. Ricco, M. Morandi, B. M. Borrini, C. Pasquarella and C. Signorelli, (2011), Epidemiology of tuberculosis in a low-incidence Italian region with high immigration rates: differences between not Italy-born and Italy-born TB cases, *BMC Public Health*, **11**, 376.
Palumbo, E., G. Scotto, D. C. Cibelli, G. Faleo, A. Saracin and G. Angarano (2008), Immigration and hepatitis B virus: epidemiological, clinical and therapeutic aspects, *Eastern Mediterranean Health Journal*, **14**(4), 784–790.
Peña-Rey, I., V. Martínez de Aragón, M. Mosquera, F. de Ory and J. E. Echevarría (2009),

Measles risk groups in Spain: implications for the European measles-elimination target, *Vaccine*, **27**(30), 3927–3934.

Perez-Ayala, A., J. A. Perez-Molina, F. Norman, M. Navarro, B. Monge-Maillo, M. Diaz-Menendez et al. (2011), Chagas disease in Latin American migrants: a Spanish challenge, *Clinical Microbiology and Infection*, **17**(7), 1108–1113.

Pervanidou, D., E. Horefti, S. Patrinos, T. Lytras, E. Triantafillou, A. Mentis, S. Bonovas et al. (2010), Spotlight on measles 2010: ongoing measles outbreak in Greece January–July 2010, *European Communicable Disease Bulletin*, **15**(30).

Poethko-Müller, C. and A. Mankertz (2012), Seroprevalence of measles-, mumps- and rubella-specific IgG antibodies in German children and adolescents and predictors for seronegativity, *PlOS One*, **7**(8).

Poethko-Müller, C., U. Ellert, R. Kuhnert, H. Neuhauser, M. Schlaud and L. Schenk (2009), Vaccination coverage against measles in German-born and foreign-born children and identification of unvaccinated subgroups in Germany, *Vaccine*, **27**(19), 2563–2569.

Ramos, J. M., A. Milla, J. C. Rodríguez and F. Gutiérrez (2012a), Rubella immune status among immigrant and non-immigrant women in Spain, *Journal of Medical Virology*, **84**(3), 548–550.

Ramos, J. M., Y. Ponce, I. Gallegos, M. Flores-Chavez, C. Canavate and F. Gutierrez (2012b), Trypanosoma cruzi infection in Elche (Spain): comparison of the seroprevalence in immigrants from Paraguay and Bolivia, *Pathogens and Global Health*, **106**(2), 102–106.

Razum, O. (2006), Commentary: of salmon and time travellers – musing on the mystery of migrant mortality, *International Journal of Epidemiology*, **35**(4), 919–921.

Rechel, B., P. Mladovsky, W. Devillé, B. Rijks, R. Petrova-Benedict and M. McKee (eds.) (2011), *Migration and Health in the European Union*, Maidenhead: Open University Press.

Rechel, B., P. Mladovsky, D. Ingleby, J. P. Mackenbach and M. McKee (2013), Migration and health in an increasingly diverse Europe, *Lancet*, **381**(9873), 1235–1245.

Riccardo, F., M. G. Dente, M. Kojouharova, M. Fabiani, V. Alfonsi, A. Kurchatova, N. Vladimirova et al. (2012), Migrant's access to immunization in Mediterranean countries, *Health Policy*, **105**(1), 17–24.

Rimseliene, G., O. Nilsen, H. Klovstad, H. Blystad and P. Aavitsland (2011), Epidemiology of acute and chronic hepatitis B virus infection in Norway, 1992–2009, *BMC Infectious Disease*, **11**(153).

Rossi, C., I. Shrier, L. Marshall, S. Cnossen, K. Schwartzman, M. B. Klein, G. Schwarzer and C. Greenaway (2012), Seroprevalence of chronic hepatitis B virus infection and prior immunity in immigrants and refugees: a systematic review and meta-analysis, *PLOS One*, **7**(9).

Schmunis G. A. and Z. E. Yadon (2010), Chagas disease: a Latin American health problem becoming a world health problem, *Acta Tropica*, **115**(1–2), 14–21.

Toy, M., I. K. Veldhuijzen, M. C. Mostert, R. A. de Man and J. H. Richardus (2008), Transmission routes of hepatitis B virus infection in chronic hepatitis B patients in the Netherlands, *Journal of Medical Virology*, **80**(3), 399–404.

UNAIDS (2013), *UNAIDS Report on the Global AIDS Epidemic*, Global Report, Joint United Nations Programme on HIV/AIDS (UNAIDS), available online at www.unaids.org/sites/default/files/en/media/unaids/contentassets/documents/epidemiology/2013/gr2013/UNAIDS_Global_Report_2013_en.pdf.

Veldhuijzen, I. K., M. Toy, S. J. Hahne, G. A. De Wit, S. W. Schalm, R. A. de Man and J. H. Richardus (2010), Screening and early treatment of migrants for chronic hepatitis B virus infection is cost-effective, *Gastroenterology*, **138**(2), 522–530.

Vriend, H. J., V. A. N. Veen, M. Prins, A. T. Urbanus, H. J. Boot, D. E. Coul and E. L. Op (2012), Hepatitis C virus prevalence in the Netherlands: migrants account for most infections, *Epidemiology and l Infection*, 1–8.

WHO (2009), *Control and Prevention of Chagas Disease in Europe*, Report of a WHO Informal Consultation (Jointly organised by WHO Headquarters and the WHO Regional Office for Europe), Geneva: WHO.

WHO (2012), *Hepatis B*, Fact sheet No. 204, available online at www.who.int/mediacentre/factsheets/fs204/en.
WHO (2014), *Global Tuberculosis Report 2014*, Geneva: WHO, available online at http://apps.who.int/iris/bitstream/10665/137094/1/9789241564809_eng.pdf.

PART VI

HEALTHCARE PROVISION

20 Health and wellbeing in refugee camps

Sarah Meyer, Cyril Bennouna and Lindsay Stark

INTRODUCTION

There are more people displaced by conflict and persecution today than at any other time in recorded history, and the numbers continue to grow rapidly. At the end of 2014, the United Nations High Commissioner for Refugees (UNHCR) estimated there were 59.5 million forced migrants[1] worldwide, up from 37.5 million just a decade earlier (UNHCR 2014). About a third (19.5 million) of individuals displaced by conflict and persecution cross a border and receive refugee status, a legal designation with special protections afforded under international law (UN General Assembly 1951). The remaining two-thirds (38.2 million) are internally displaced persons (IDPs) who remain within the borders and under legal regimes of their home countries, or asylum-seekers (1.8 million) whose refugee status has not been determined by the receiving government or the UNHCR.

There are three 'durable solutions' to resolve a refugee situation and thereby reduce the global total of refugees. First, refugees can be repatriated voluntarily to their home countries once the conflict or fear of persecution has subsided. This option, which is largely favored by host countries, is complicated given the increasing trend of conflicts to be prolonged and cyclical (Long 2014). The second solution, local integration, takes place when refugees become full legal, economic and cultural members of the host country. Local integration is rare, as many host countries do not want to take permanent responsibility for refugees, who may be considered threatening either to the country's security or economy (Hovel 2014). In 2014, for example, only 27 countries reported granting citizenship to refugees (*de jure* integration), covering a total of just 32,100 individuals (UNHCR 2014). *De facto* integration, whereby refugees settle in the host community informally, and outside of the law, is likely more common, especially in places where refugees and host communities share common ethnic, religious or linguistic identities; but altogether this phenomenon has not been well-documented (Hovel 2014).

The third durable solution is resettlement from the first country of asylum to a third country, with the United States, Canada and Australia together accounting for about 90 per cent of the world's resettlement capacity, and Northern Europe accounting for much of the rest (van Selm 2014). Resettlement countries enter into agreements with the UNHCR to accept a set number of refugees, and often set priorities within this number, such as refugees from particular regions, or with specific protection needs (for example, survivors of torture or women facing gender-based violence). The annual allotment of resettlement placements covers well under 1 per cent of all refugees, and between 2005 and 2014 it is estimated that only about 900,000 refugees were resettled around the world (UNHCR 2014; van Selm 2014).

Planned camps aim to shelter, protect and treat refugees temporarily as they wait to be repatriated, integrated or resettled. The frequent failure of these "durable solutions," however, means that, once they are granted asylum, individuals often remain refugees for years, even decades, and what were intended to be temporary camps have become sprawling, multigenerational settlements in many countries. The Dadaab camp complex in Kenya, for example, which was originally built in 1991 to accommodate 90,000 people, is now the most populous refugee camp in the world, with more than 250,000 refugees (UNHCR 2012a). The camps on the northern border of Thailand are of a similar nature, hosting multiple generations of refugees from Myanmar, the largest source country of refugees in Asia apart from Afghanistan. About 45 per cent of refugees worldwide now find themselves in protracted refugee situations such as these, and the average protracted situation lasts 25 years (UNHCR 2014), reflective of the failures to achieve durable solutions for refugees in these settings.

The considerable diversity of refugee situations makes it difficult to generalize about the "typical" refugee. Demographics and conditions in refugee camps vary widely, depending on the conflict that caused displacement, the preflight sociodemographics of the source country, the relationship between the source and host countries and other sociopolitical factors. The UNHCR has a non-discriminatory policy and so camps can often house people of many ethnicities, races and religions (UNHCR 2007). However, refugees with greater resources may have opportunities to avoid living in refugee camps in some cases, or to leave them more quickly, as in the case of Syrian refugees in Turkey (McClelland, 2014). Camps all over the world tend to have young populations, with 60 per cent of managed camp populations being children (UNHCR 2014). According to the available data, a little over half (54 per cent) of refugees in managed camps are female (UNHCR 2014). Depending on the policy of the host government, refugees living in camps may have permission to work and travel freely in the host country, or may face limitations on participation in the formal labor market or free travel outside of camp boundaries. Humanitarian services, including primary healthcare, food and nutrition programming, and education, are primarily delivered by international organizations and international and national non-governmental organizations, who are contracted by the UNHCR as "implementing partners" of programming in refugee camps.

The prolonged nature of these refugee situations and the paucity of "durable solutions" only exacerbate the fact that most refugees (86 per cent) are hosted in developing regions that are often themselves fragile, with a full 42 per cent entering countries whose gross domestic product per capita is below US$5,000 (purchasing power parity) (UNHCR 2014). Having little absorptive capacity, many host governments struggle to meet the basic needs of so many. Nevertheless, under the protection of the UNHCR, the agency mandated to protect refugees globally,[2] refugee populations sometimes receive services that are above the standards enjoyed by host communities (Orach and De Brouwere 2004). At times, host populations may consider refugees their competitors for scarce land, resources and economic opportunity, particularly when camps and urban dwellings are located close to, or interspersed with, their communities, or when there is already political or ethnic tension between refugee and local communities (Codjoe et al. 2013; Mabiso et al. 2014). In this way, the well-being of host communities is an important factor in planning for refugee population health (UNHCR 2007).

Less than a third (29.3 per cent) of today's refugees live in managed or planned camps (UNHCR 2014), and there is a growing trend towards refugees living in cities or with host communities in various arrangements. Despite this growing urbanization of refugee contexts globally (Spiegel et al. 2010), the health needs of refugees in managed or planned camps, often in settings with very limited resources, remains a major concern to the humanitarian community. This chapter focuses primarily on refugees in planned and managed camps, although it occasionally draws on research from internally displaced, urban, repatriated and resettled populations when there is a gap in the planned camp literature. While much of what follows will be applicable to IDPs, it should be noted that internal displacement can present unique challenges to population health (see, for example, Salama et al. 2001) that are outside the scope of this chapter. Most notable among these is that IDPs typically remain closer to the source of violence than refugees and that, without designated refugee protection, they continue to depend on their own government for protection, which in some cases has been deposed by hostile forces and in others is the primary perpetrator of violence. These factors not only place IDPs at risk but also make them difficult to reach for service-providers.

HEALTH AND WELLBEING IN REFUGEE CAMPS

The World Health Organization (WHO) defines health as "a complete state of physical, mental and social wellbeing, and not merely the absence of disease or infirmity" (WHO, 1948). The conditions of becoming a refugee—the harms experienced pre-flight, the conditions of the journey to a host country, and the subsequent conditions in refugee camps—may strike a blow at each of these elements of wellbeing.

The risks to individual- and population-level health in refugee camps are considerable. Challenges in meeting basic health standards in refugee settings, and lessons learned from humanitarian practice in major emergencies, have driven the field of humanitarian response to unprecedented growth and professionalization over the past two decades. The establishment of the Inter-Agency Standing Committee (IASC) in 1992 to coordinate humanitarian response globally and the 2005 Humanitarian Reform Agenda to improve collaboration, accountability, and standardization among humanitarian actors were important initiatives to institutionalize lessons learned from the field. The interagency Sphere Project introduced the *Humanitarian Charter and Minimum Standards in Disaster Response* in 1998, setting the bar for global humanitarian practice (McConnan 1998). Since then, the IASC and other interagency working groups have issued global standards on specific health issues, from HIV/AIDS (IASC 2010) and infant feeding (Emergency Nutrition Network 2007), to child protection (CPWG 2012), sexual and gender-based violence (IASC 2015b) and mental health and psychosocial support (IASC 2007). What is more, programs on humanitarian assistance, refugee health, and forced migration and health have found their homes in academic institutions across the world, training future generations of emergency response professionals and generating high-quality research on best methods and practices.

The following sections draw on this growing body of knowledge to further explore select topics in refugee health: communicable diseases, maternal and reproductive health, child health, food and nutrition, HIV/AIDS and protection from violence and abuse. The chapter ends with an exploration of advancements in the field of mental health and psychosocial support (MHPSS). The developments in MHPSS in emergencies in many ways echo the trajectory of change in the field of refugee health more broadly, and illustrate the ways in which research, programming, and policy interventions within the humanitarian sector can improve the health and wellbeing of individuals, families, and communities in refugee camps globally.

Communicable Diseases

Communicable diseases, such as diarrhea, respiratory infection, malaria, and measles are often the primary causes of mortality and morbidity in acute emergency settings (Connolly et al. 2004). A review of the impact of communicable diseases in complex emergencies notes that several risk factors for communicable diseases may operate "synergistically" in the acute phase of an emergency. These risk factors include "mass population movement and resettlement in temporary locations, overcrowding, economic and environmental degradation, impoverishment, scarcity of safe water, poor sanitation and waste management, absence of shelter, poor nutritional status as a result of food shortages, and poor access to health care," as well as "the collapse or overwhelming of public health infrastructure and absence of health services [which] hamper prevention and control programmes" (Connolly et al. 2004: 1974).

Many prevalent communicable diseases in refugee camp settings can be directly linked to living conditions and gaps in provision of basic needs and services to refugee populations. These proximate risk factors are often the cause of the vast majority of mortality and morbidity in the acute emergency phase (Checchi et al. 2008). For example, crowded living conditions and indoor fires for cooking and heating are associated with higher rates of acute respiratory infections, while malaria transmission can be facilitated and exacerbated by housing conditions in emergency settings. However, humanitarian agencies have also developed and implemented effective prevention and control interventions for communicable diseases, such that refugees in camp settings often have better access to interventions and reduced risk of communicable disease than individuals and communities in conflict-affected non-camp settings.

Key interventions—including shelter and site planning, water and sanitation, immunization and case management—have been found to be effective in reducing risk and preventing outbreaks of epidemics (Bigot et al. 1997). UNHCR's 2011 *Epidemic Preparedness and Response in Refugee Camp Settings* guidelines provide a basis for coordinated action to prepare and respond to a disease outbreak in a camp setting (UNHCR 2011). Several of the Sphere Standards relate to key actions in the control of, and response to, communicable diseases, including that "[p]eople have access to effective diagnosis and treatment for those infectious diseases that contribute most significantly to preventable excess morbidity and mortality" and "[o]utbreaks are prepared for, detected, investigated and controlled in a timely and effective manner" (Sphere Project 2011: 314, 316).

Despite these advances, as the UNHCR acknowledges in its guidelines, "[d]uring an acute emergency, the living conditions in camp settings present a favourable environment for epidemics of communicable disease. In more protracted refugee camp situations, even if the overall living condition of refugees has improved, many emergency standards (e.g. water availability, sanitation and living space) are often just met" (UNHCR 2011: 3). Communicable diseases therefore remain an important health challenge in refugee camps, particularly in the acute emergency phase.

Maternal and Reproductive Health

Policy and programming for maternal and reproductive health for refugees have developed considerably in the past two decades (Austin et al. 2008; Krause et al. 2000; Tanabe et al. 2015). The *Minimum Initial Service Package (MISP) for Reproductive Health in Crisis Situations*, published in 1996, is "a coordinated set of priority activities designed to prevent and manage the consequences of sexual violence; reduce HIV transmission; prevent excess maternal and newborn morbidity and mortality; and plan for comprehensive reproductive health services," and forms the basis of recommended priority interventions to improve maternal and reproductive health at the onset of an emergency (WRC, 2011: 3). The MISP includes coordination, prevention and clinical care for sexual and gender-based violence (SGBV), activities to reduce HIV transmission and prevention of excess maternal and neonatal morbidity and mortality. Since its development, the MISP has provided guidance for coordination and implementation of reproductive health interventions in a number of emergency settings, from Haiti to Chad to Syria (Krause et al. 2015).

While gaps in programming in emergency and post-emergency settings continue to exist, evidence shows that notable collaboration between humanitarian agencies, improved technical guidance and shifts in policies and programming to support maternal and reproductive health for refugees have improved safe motherhood, increased access to family planning and reduced reproductive health risks including unsafe abortion in camps globally (Austin et al. 2008; Hynes et al. 2002).

Prevalence and risk factors for maternal mortality and morbidity vary across refugee camps, with factors including stage of emergency, access to quality emergency obstetric care through district or national healthcare systems, and maternal health practices and cultural perspectives on pregnancy of refugees comprising some of the key influences (Hynes et al. 2002). Key interventions to reduce maternal mortality and morbidity include securing quality emergency obstetric care, skilled health workers, and the supplies needed to manage obstetric emergencies, and the establishment of referral systems, including transport, to ensure women with obstetric complications can be referred to a higher level of care from a health center in a refugee camp (Inter-Agency Working Group on Reproductive Health in Crises 2010).

Child Health

A review of epidemiological studies of child health in complex emergencies reveals a number of patterns that continue to hold true in refugee camps: first, in the vast majority of complex emergencies, the highest mortality rates are among children under the age of five; second, the most common causes of death among children in complex emergencies are the same major causes of death of children in countries with the highest child mortality rates (diarrheal diseases, acute respiratory infections, measles, malaria and severe malnutrition). The phase of emergency and access to quality health services significantly influence child health in refugee camps.

Some research, however, has shown significantly *lower* infant mortality rates in post-emergency refugee camps compared to host countries, and health services delivered by NGOs and UN agencies may allow refugees greater access to antenatal care, tetanus immunization, and attendance at births by a skilled birth attendant (Zimmerman et al. 2011). A retrospective study of refugees and IDPs in 52 post-emergency phase camps globally found similar patterns, whereby neonatal mortality rate and per centage of infants born with low birthweight was lower among refugees compared to country of origin or host country, concluding that "[b]etter access by camp residents to preventative and curative health care services, and to food and non-food items, as well as improvements in water supply and sanitation, may account for better reproductive health outcomes among post-emergency phase camp populations than in their respective host country and country-of-origin populations" (Hynes et al. 2002: 601).

Healthcare for children in refugee camps can be undermined, however, by fragmented, and poor quality and availability of health services, low levels of trained healthcare workers and exacerbation of "severity and magnitude of childhood diseases" (Moss et al. 2006: 58). WHO (2015) guidelines suggest that under-five child health in refugee camps be addressed through adapted integrated management of childhood illness (IMCI). The key principles and components of IMCI—training to improve case management skills of healthcare staff, improving overall healthcare systems, and improving family and community health practices—can be particularly challenging in refugee camp settings, given the unstable and irregular provision of healthcare staff, low quality of health systems, and lack of connections between refugee camp health systems and district health facilities (Moss et al. 2006). Therefore, while the WHO 2008 *Manual for the Health Care of Children in Humanitarian*

Emergencies utilizes the IMCI framework, the manual is adapted to account for differences in context in refugee camps, including adding sections on unintentional injuries and preventative measures, and combining IMCI with rapid triage procedures for emergency assessment and management (WHO 2008).

HIV and AIDS

While various aspects of refugee movement and displacement can increase vulnerability to HIV infection, the assumption that refugees are at higher risk than non-displaced populations, in country of origin or host countries, is not supported by existing data (Spiegel 2004). In particular, while displacement may certainly increase known risk-factors for HIV transmission—for example, breakdown of social structures, increased risk of sexual violence, and lack of access to health services—it may also be associated with *decreased* risks of HIV transmission, such as the improved health services and protection available in refugee camps (Spiegel 2004). Some data (relating to refugees from the DRC, Tanzania, and Zambia) indicate that refugees have higher odds of multiple partnership compared to host communities (Spiegel et al. 2014). However, data from 27 contexts in ten countries indicate, "no evidence that refugees reported consistently higher levels of risky sexual partnerships than host nationals living in the surrounding communities" (Spiegel et al. 2014: 767).

Levels of risk and vulnerability vary in the cycle of displacement (emergency, post-emergency, and durable solutions), all of which require different types of HIV interventions (UNAIDS and UNHCR 2005). One particular challenge in provision of HIV programs for refugees in camps is that funding and service-provision for HIV prevention and treatment for refugees are often provided separately to the healthcare system of the host country (UNAIDS and UNHCR 2005). Delivery of health services for refugees through parallel systems may limit the benefits of improved health services to local host communities, reduce sustainability of health services in protracted displacement settings, and cause conflict between refugees and host communities (Meyer et al. 2011).

The 2010 IASC *Guidelines for Addressing HIV in Humanitarian Settings* cover key humanitarian prevention, treatment, care, and support activities within the following fields: HIV awareness-raising and community support; health; protection; food security, nutrition, and livelihood support; education; shelter; camp coordination and camp management; water, sanitation, and hygiene; and HIV in the workplace (IASC 2010). The guidelines indicate key actions as part of emergency preparedness, minimum response and comprehensive response, including, for example, components of minimum response in the health sector—ensuring safe blood supply, provision of condoms, prevention and treatment of sexually transmitted diseases and prevention of mother-to-child transmission.

Food and Nutrition

Malnutrition caused by insufficient nutrient intake can increase vulnerability to, and mortality from, several communicable diseases (Moss et al. 2006). Insufficient nutrient intake in emergencies may be caused by lack of availability of food or lack of access to food due to distance of markets or price of food, but may also be due to patterns of distribution of food at the household level and incorrect infant feeding (Checchi et al. 2008). Provision of food rations in many refugee camps are designed to cover refugees' nutritional needs; however, food rations may be reduced due to donor funding, and refugees' food preferences and needs for non-food items may lead to them selling food rations in local markets. Severe acute malnutrition and moderate acute malnutrition prevalence—while varying considerably between and across countries and camps—continues in refugee camp settings, and therapeutic and supplementary feeding programs for under-fives are necessary (Doocy et al. 2011). Prevalence of acute malnutrition in refugee camps has varied widely; examples of prevalence estimates from refugee camps in Asia and Africa range from 12.1 per cent to 47 per cent (Young et al. 2004). In addition, micronutrient deficiencies may increase during emergencies, but have often received less attention in terms of programmatic response.

Decades of efforts towards increasing food security and reducing risk of malnutrition for refugees have resulted in widespread implementation of programs and guidelines to ensure adequate nutrition in refugee camps, including blanket food ration distribution and supplementary and therapeutic feeding programs (Doocy et al. 2011). The *Sphere Handbook* includes standards on food security and nutrition assessment, infant and young child feeding, management of acute malnutrition and micronutrient deficiencies, and food security, and has established minimum standards and indicators related to these topics (Sphere Project 2011). Suggested interventions to address micronutrient deficiencies include Vitamin A supplementation for children aged six to 15 months, fortification of food aid commodities and provision of food aid rations rich in micronutrients (Young et al. 2004). Nutrition interventions have evolved towards programs that "distinguish among different target groups, different nutrition concerns and timeframes, different commodities, and different modalities for distribution" (Webb et al. 2014: 36). There has been an overall paradigm shift to community-based management of malnutrition, compared to a previous paradigm focused on in-patient, facility-based treatment.

Data from UNHCR's Health Information System (from more than 90 refugee camps in 18 countries) indicate that supplementary feeding programs in refugee camps between 2007 and 2009 exceeded all UNHCR standards apart from length of enrollment, indicating high quality of feeding programs overall. However, there are some concerns related to coverage of growth monitoring and effective screening of children with severe acute malnutrition and moderate acute malnutrition (Doocy et al. 2011). Results of an evidence review of humanitarian health interventions found several studies of nutrition interventions to be of high quality; however, it noted a need for research to better understand the contextual factors leading to famine and malnutrition, alternatives to blanket supplementary feeding programs and the most effective way of delivering nutritional programs (Blanchet et al. 2013).

Protection

International protection is defined as actions the international community assumes in order to stand in for the protection governments should provide for their citizens. As the UNHCR states, "[s]ince, by definition, the basic rights of refugees are no longer protected by the governments of their home countries, the international community then assumes the responsibility of ensuring that those basic rights are respected. The phrase 'international protection' covers the gamut of activities through which refugees' rights are secured" (UNHCR 1999). Protection activities include ensuring physical security of refugees, often through provision of legal recognition of refugee status, to prevent *refoulement*,[3] prevention of recruitment into armed forces from refugee camps, and prevention of violence against refugees within refugee camps, either from other refugees or surrounding host communities (UNHCR 2006).

Protection and health concerns for refugees are linked in various areas, specifically, protection from sexual and gender-based violence (SGBV) and child protection. SGBV has emerged as a growing concern among humanitarian agencies, with UNHCR's 2003 *Conclusion on Protection from Sexual Abuse and Exploitation* noting:

> States, UNHCR and its implementing and operational partners [should] ensure that appropriate systems to prevent and respond to sexual and gender-based violence, including sexual abuse and exploitation, are in place, ensuring the needs of women and children, as well those of vulnerable persons, are addressed at all times.
>
> (UNHCR 2003)

SGBV may increase during displacement and risks may be exacerbated by conditions in refugee camps. For example, breakdown of social structures, discrimination against refugees in host countries, lay-out of refugee camps, modes of distribution of relief aid and lack of police protection may all be additional risks for SGBV in refugee camps (UNHCR 2003). A key concern is access to fuel and firewood, as women and girls may experience SGBV while gathering fuel and firewood in and around refugee camps (see, for example, Patrick 2011). Responses to this long-standing challenge have included provision of fuel-efficient stoves to households, to reduce the need for collection of firewood (Patrick, 2011).

Estimates of SGBV in refugee camps are often flawed, given reported data are often based on incident reports (for example, reporting to police), rather than population-based estimates of SGBV and that studies in this area are rarely conducted in refugee camps (Stark and Ager 2011). A meta-analysis of sexual violence against female refugees and IDPs in complex humanitarian emergencies (including but not limited to refugee camps) indicated a prevalence of more than 20 per cent of sexual violence across conflict-affected areas in 14 countries, which is expected to be an underestimate, given that underreporting of SGBV is common (Vu et al. 2014). Given the lack of baseline data, it is not possible to ascertain whether SGBV increases in refugee camp contexts. However, data from complex emergencies indicate that levels of intimate partner violence are higher than other types of SGBV, such as violence perpetrated by armed forces (Stark and Ager 2011).

Regardless of the methodological issues in assessing SGBV prevalence in refugee camps, it is clear that it is a prevalent and important concern, with serious health consequences for survivors. In recognition of this, humanitarian agencies have developed and consolidated recommended actions to prevent and mitigate SGBV in emergencies. The first iteration of consensus-based guidelines were the IASC *Guidelines for Gender-based Violence Interventions in Humanitarian Settings*, published in 2005, which aimed to establish standards for prevention and response to gender-based violence across all areas of humanitarian response (Ward 2014). The 2015 revision, *Guidelines for Integrating Gender-Based Violence Interventions in Humanitarian Action*, further promoted integration of SGBV prevention and mitigation within various sectors within humanitarian action, including food security and agriculture and housing, land and property, to ensure a holistic and comprehensive response to SGBV risks and impacts in humanitarian settings (IASC 2015b). There is some limited evidence for interventions to reduce risk and incidence of SGBV in humanitarian settings, although the quality of studies on interventions is low and studies have not been explicitly designed to assess reduction of risk or incidence in rigorous ways (Spangaro 2013).

Children may be particularly vulnerable to physical and sexual violence, neglect, abuse, and exploitation in refugee camps. The UNHCR's *Framework for the Protection of Children* includes key outcomes related to prevention of violence and abuse against children, including "[c]hildren are safe in homes and in the community and are protected by their family, community, teachers and humanitarian workers," and "children can report abuse and know where to get help" (UNHCR, 2012b). The *Minimum Standards for Child Protection in Humanitarian Settings* have established a framework of standards and indicators to establish principles and mechanisms for coordination, as well as integration of child protection principles within all sectors (CPWG 2012).

While data on prevalence of violence against children in low- and middle-income countries are improving (for example, Centers for Disease Control and UNICEF 2011), there are limited data concerning the prevalence of violence against children in refugee camps (Stark and Landis 2016). In a study of adolescent refugees from the DRC, aged 13–17, in Kiziba refugee camp in Rwanda, 72 per cent of adolescents reported having witnessed shouting and yelling at home, 18 per cent of adolescents reported having seen physical violence at home, and direct experience with violence at home was commonly reported, including being pushed, grabbed, or kicked (11 per cent); being hit, beaten, or spanked (19 per cent); and being beaten with a belt, paddle, stick, or other object (11 per cent). Twenty per cent of adolescents reported feeling unsafe in their home in the past week (Meyer et al. 2014). Other literature on consequences of violence and abuse experienced during conflict or in refugee settings often focuses on mental health and psychosocial impacts, and is addressed below.

FOCUS ON MENTAL HEALTH AND PSYCHOSOCIAL SUPPORT (MHPSS) IN REFUGEE CAMPS

Background to MHPSS in Refugee Camps

Despite the considerable mental health and psychosocial needs of refugees, the field of humanitarian response historically considered these needs subordinate to what were seen as more pressing "material" needs. As one expert has written: "A decade ago, mental health and psychosocial supports in international emergencies were relegated to the humanitarian ghetto and seen as things to be done after the 'real' humanitarian work of saving lives had been completed" (Wessells 2009: 842). This is not for a lack of contact between mental health professionals and refugees. For example, the mental health needs of resettled refugees after the Holocaust were widely recognized within a clinical framework (Ager 1993). American and European clinicians became increasingly preoccupied with the relationship between war trauma and anxiety, and when veterans returned from Vietnam exhibiting a patterned symptomology of flashbacks, intrusive memories, and restlessness, post-traumatic stress disorder (PTSD) was added to the Diagnostic and Statistics Manual and then the International Classification of Disease.

PTSD proved useful as a construct for describing the experiences of many refugees, and before too long, epidemiological researchers were assessing the frequency and distribution of PTSD in Cambodian, Hmong, Laotian and Vietnamese refugees (Ager 1993; Miller and Rasmussen 2010). This momentum helped to garner worldwide interest and funding in refugee mental health that continues to this day. This framework was primarily used in the field of humanitarian work in the health sector, and while a public health approach to the wider range of mental disorders and distress was sometimes employed in humanitarian work, the predominant approach in the health sector was vertical programming focused on PTSD (Wessells and van Ommeren 2008).

Many have found fault in the overly reductionist and inherently "Western," biomedical nature of the trauma model (Abramowitz and Kleinman 2008; Agger 2002; Summerfield 1999). Focusing narrowly on trauma and depression, it is argued, pathologizes natural responses to extreme circumstances, reducing refugees to victims or patients and overlooks their capacities for resilience (Miller and Rasmussen 2010). Moreover, applying a medical construct derived from European and American patients to other cultures is not always appropriate, and is often referred to as imperialistic (Pupavac 2002) or neo-colonial (Wessells 2009), as the fixation on standardized symptoms silences local idioms of distress and the prescription of Western therapies supplants endogenous mechanisms of healing. In some cases, this prescriptive approach risks prolonging or even intensifying symptoms rather than addressing them (Ager 1993).

The critics of the trauma model have advocated an alternative framework that attempts to reconcile the psychological and social experiences of refugees, to reflect the dynamic interplay between individuals and their environment (Meyer 2013). This "psychosocial approach," as it has come to be known, grew out of a human rights movement in Latin America and South Africa during the 1980s, and specifically the work of exiled psychologists and psychiatrists who developed community-based interventions to treat survivors of state terror, and in some cases, to document human rights abuses (Agger 2002; Miller and Rasmussen 2010). Advocates of the psychosocial approach started studying the indirect and somewhat hidden factors that affect mental health, both negatively and positively. In addition to trauma exposure, these more subtle "daily stressors," such as the disruption of social and family routines and the inability to meet other material needs, were thought to contribute significantly to psychological distress, and "protective factors," such as strong social networks, were thought to contribute to resilience. This approach was primarily embedded within the protection and social welfare sector of humanitarian action, and was rarely linked to health services or clinical mental health interventions (Wessells and van Ommeren 2008).

The conflict between these two general approaches to mental health in humanitarian contexts has often resulted in competition over funding, lack of collaboration between agencies and programs, and gaps in or overlap of provision of services. The humanitarian response in the Balkans became the subject of much criticism as the WHO identified more than 100 mental health projects operating without coordination in Bosnia alone, and organizations failed to monitor and evaluate their programs effectively (Abramowitz and Kleinman 2008; Mollica et al. 2004). Clinicians and researchers alike also struggled to define what exactly qualified as a psychosocial intervention, and what impacts such an intervention could be expected to have (PWG 2003; Strang and Ager 2003; van Ommeren et al., 2005). "Consequently," as one essay put it, "within a decade, the funding and legitimacy of emergency mental health care programmes became mired in paralyzing debates" (Abramowitz and Kleinman 2008: 220).

By the early 2000s, however, consensus began to emerge. The Sphere Project, which had been precipitated by the responses to the Balkans and to the 1994 genocide in Rwanda, initially excluded mental health in part due to expert disagreement in 2000 (Batniji et al. 2006), but added psychological and social interventions in the 2004 revision (Sphere Project, 2004). In the meantime, the Psychosocial Working Group (PWG), comprised of several academic and humanitarian partners, drafted a conceptual framework that attempted to reconcile the psychological, social and cultural conceptualizations of psychosocial wellbeing, and to form the basis for structuring cohesive programming and a unified research agenda (PWG 2003). A special interagency taskforce was established in 2005, and all these efforts culminated in the *IASC Guidelines on Mental Health and Psychosocial Support in Emergency Settings* (IASC 2007), which represent expert consensus based on the state of knowledge in the field. Since then, the guidelines have been widely adopted by humanitarian actors, researchers, and donors across the field, including the UNHCR (IASC

RG-MHPSS 2014; UNHCR 2013), and MHPSS, which describes "any type of local or outside support that aims to protect or promote psychosocial wellbeing and/or prevent or treat mental disorder" (IASC 2007: 16), has become a unifying principle.

Key Issues Affecting Mental Health and Psychosocial Wellbeing in Refugee Camps

The IASC Guidelines note that in emergencies, the percentage of people with a severe mental disorder is expected to increase 1 per cent above an estimated baseline of 2–3 per cent. The Intervention Pyramid—widely recognized as among the most influential contributions to the *MHPSS Guidelines*—reflects the expected breakdown of MHPSS needs, and appropriate interventions and responses to those needs (IASC RG-MHPSS 2014).

The bottom layer of the pyramid (Level 1), which applies to the broadest target populations and is focused on *prevention*, consists of interventions that are integrated within basic services, such as shelter or

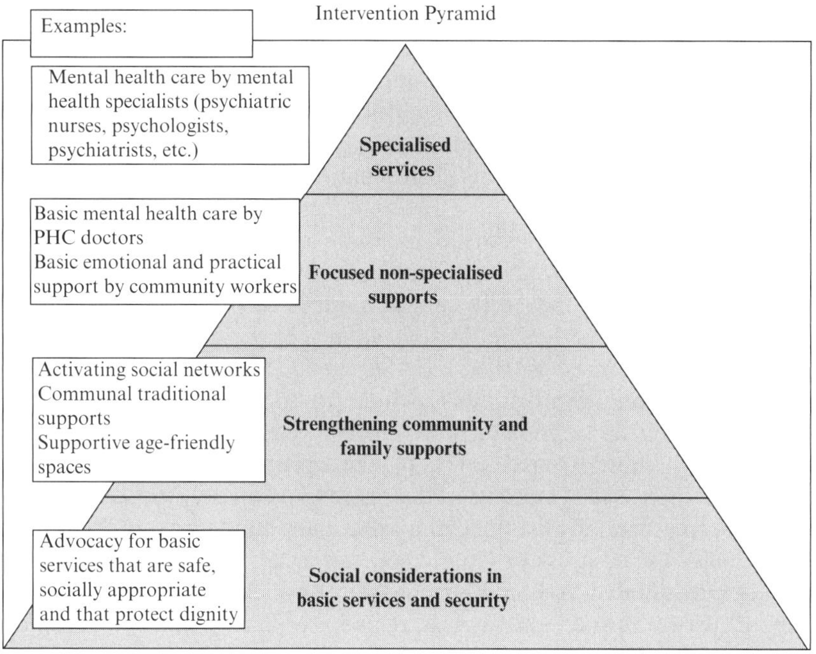

Figure 20.1 Intervention Pyramid for mental health and psychosocial support

water and sanitation. Level 2 interventions consist of strengthening community and family supports, such as family reintegration programs and child-friendly spaces. In line with this layer of the pyramid, research has indicated that social support, participation in community activities, and meaningful relationships can be important factors influencing refugee mental health and psychosocial wellbeing. For example, a systematic review concerning child soldiers examined multiple risk and protective factors, including social support, and concluded that "[f]indings indicate that social support and community acceptance may also promote successful reintegration and positive psychosocial adjustment" (Betancourt et al. 2013). In Adhikari and colleagues' study of risk and protective factors related to the reintegration of former child soldiers in Nepal, social support, especially at the community level, was found to be the most significant predictor of psychosocial wellbeing and mental health (Adhikari et al. 2014).

Another relevant outcome measure in line with Level 2 interventions is *functioning*, with instruments developed in various settings focusing on "activities that local people do to care for or contribute to the wellbeing of themselves, their families, and their communities" (AMHRG 2014). Reduced function is a central way in which mental health and psychosocial problems may affect individuals and those around them. Methodology designed to capture locally relevant aspects of functioning has been utilized in various studies of conflict-affected populations (Bolton and Tang 2002), ensuring that impacts of interventions are measured in ways relevant to affected populations (for example, Bass et al. 2013; Bolton et al. 2014).

Level 3 interventions provide focused—although non-specialized—supports, including mental health services provided by community health workers, targeted at the "still smaller number of people who additionally require more focused individual, family or group interventions by trained and supervised workers" (IASC 2007). Some relevant measures of need for Level 3 interventions include prevalence of common mental disorders, such as depression and anxiety. Research has identified a range of risk and protective factors for these problems. For example, risk factors for increased symptoms of depression and anxiety include torture, exposure to potentially traumatizing events, and time since conflict (Steel et al. 2009). Other stressors—described earlier as "daily hassles"—likely impact individuals who could benefit from Level 3 interventions. Strong support networks and family bonds, religious affiliation and active coping strategies are thought to be protective against PTSD, depression, and other anxiety disorders, although these likely vary by culture (Ager 1993; Betancourt and Khan 2008). Despite a commitment in the field to study protective and resilience factors, this topic still lacks a strong evidence base (Roberts and Brown 2011; Tol et al. 2012).

Level 4 interventions are specialized services provided by trained professionals, often targeting severe mental health *disorders*. There is limited epidemiological data on severe mental health disorders in refugee settings, including extreme forms of mood (e.g., bipolar I) and psychotic disorders (e.g., schizophrenia) (Jones et al. 2009); and even less is known about neurological disorders (e.g., epilepsy) and cognitive disabilities (e.g., dementia) (Kett and van Ommeren 2009). The relatively low global prevalence of these disorders and the clinical expertise needed for diagnosing and treating them have made severe mental health disorders a low priority for research and response (Jones et al. 2009). Analysis of health information systems data from 90 refugee camps across 15 countries found that visits for mental, neurological, and substance use problems are primarily for epilepsy and psychosis. This indicates the need to have services for severe mental disorders in refugee camps, but also that service utilization for emotional disorders such as depression and anxiety is low, and refugee healthcare services may not adequately address these needs through current approaches (Kane et al. 2014).

Effective Interventions in Refugee Camp Settings

A review of 160 reports of mental health and psychosocial support interventions in humanitarian contexts found that the most common interventions included basic counseling, promotion of community supports and child-friendly spaces, which were also the least frequently evaluated interventions (Tol et al. 2011). In turn, the specialized interventions at the top of the pyramid were the least frequently implemented but the most often evaluated. In recognition of the difficulties of implementing evidence-based mental health interventions in low-resource settings (including, but not limited to, refugee camps), the WHO and partners are developing and piloting low-intensity interventions for common mental health problems (for example, Dawson et al. 2015), ensuring that interventions can be delivered by para-professionals. A number of these interventions are currently being tested for feasibility, acceptability, and effectiveness. In addition, the recent release of mhGAP for humanitarian settings—an adaptation of the WHO's Mental Health Gap Action Plan—has added a practical tool for non-specialist healthcare providers, addressing acute stress, depression, PTSD, psychosis, and suicide risk, among other conditions, for humanitarian settings (Tol et al. 2013). There are growing efforts to evaluate commonly implemented Level 1 and 2 interventions, including community-based approaches such as child-friendly spaces, with assessments in refugee camps in Iraq, Uganda, Jordan, and Ethiopia indicating the feasibility of utilizing rigorous methods and the importance of employing these methods, including use of control groups, to more clearly understand the impacts of these interventions on protection and MHPSS outcomes (Metzler et al., 2013a, 2013b, 2014a, 2014b).

CONCLUSIONS

This chapter has outlined a number of the key issues affecting health in refugee camps: communicable disease, maternal and reproductive health, child health, HIV/AIDS, food and nutrition, protection, and, finally, mental health and psychosocial support. In each of these areas, there has been an evolution of programming and policy and development of consensus-based or evidence-based guidelines, often spurred by generation of data and evidence shedding light on the impact of specific interventions. Given the nature of protracted refugee situations globally, approaches to health in refugee camp settings should not be primarily or solely considered within a humanitarian relief framework (Spiegel et al. 2010). While the nature of displacement globally is changing, core challenges to health and wellbeing remain for individuals, households, and communities in refugee camps. Policy and practice is evolving, particularly in fields that have more recently consolidated evidence and guidelines, such as MHPSS, and careful and rigorous evaluation of the impact of interventions should be conducted, to improve interventions and refine best practice.

NOTES

1. This number does not include people forcibly displaced by natural disasters, climate change, economic crises, or development projects. It does, however, include 5.1 million Palestinian refugees not under the UNHCR's protection mandate.
2. Humanitarian response for IDPs and other non-refugee populations, on the other hand, are coordinated by the appointed Humanitarian Coordinator and the UN Office for the Coordination of Humanitarian Affairs (OCHA), (Joint UNHCR–OCHA Note on Mixed Situations: Coordination in Practice 2014; IASC 2015a).
3. *Refoulement* is addressed in Article 33 of the 1951 Convention, which prohibits states from expelling or returning (refouling) "a refugee in any manner whatsoever to the frontiers of territories where his (or her) life or freedom would be threatened on account of his race, religion, nationality, membership of a particular social group or political opinion" (UN General Assembly 1951).

REFERENCES

Abramowitz, S. and A. Kleinman (2008), Humanitarian intervention and cultural translation: a review of the IASC Guidelines on Mental Health and Psychosocial Support in Emergency Settings, *Intervention*, **6**(3), 219–227.

Adhikari, R. P., B. A. Kohrt, N. P. Luitel, N. Upadhaya, D. Gurung and M. J. Jordans (2014), Protective and risk factors of psychosocial wellbeing related to the reintegration of former child soldiers in Nepal, *Intervention*, **12**(3), 367–378.

Ager, A. (1993), *Mental Health Issues in Refugee Populations: A Review*, Cambridge, MA: Harvard Medical School, Department of Social Medicine.

Agger, I. (2002), *Therapeutic Approaches to the Treatment of Refugees: A Historical Perspective*, Working Paper.

AMHRG (2014), *Design, Implementation, Monitoring, and Evaluation of Mental Health and Psychosocial Assistance Programs for Trauma Survivors in Low Resource Countries: A User's Manual for Researchers and Program Implementers (Adult Version). Module 1: Qualitative Assessment*, available online at www.jhsph.edu/research/centers-and-institutes/center-for-refugee-and-disaster-response/response_service/AMHR/dime/VOT_DIME_MODULE1_FINAL.pdf.

Austin, J., S. Guy, L. Lee-Jones, T. McGinn and J. Schlecht (2008), Reproductive health: a right for refugees and internally displaced persons, *Reproductive Health Matters*, **16**(31), 10–21.

Bass, J. K., J. Annan, S. McIvor Murray, D. Kaysen, S. Griffiths, T. Cetinoglu, K. Wachter, L. K. Murray and P.A. Bolton (2013), Controlled trial of psychotherapy for Congolese survivors of sexual violence, *New England Journal of Medicine*, **368**(23), 2182–2191.

Batniji, R., M. van Ommeren and B. Saraceno (2006), Mental and social health in disasters: relating qualitative social science research and the Sphere standard, *Social Science and Medicine*, **62**(8), 1853–1864.

Betancourt, T. S. and K.T. Khan (2008), The mental health of children affected by armed conflict: protective processes and pathways to resilience, *International Review of Psychiatry*, **20**(3), 317–328.

Betancourt, T. S., I. Borisova, T. P. Williams, S. E. Meyers-Ohki, J. E. Rubin-Smith, J. Annan and B. A. Kohrt (2013), Psychosocial adjustment and mental health in former child soldiers – a systematic review of the literature and recommendations for future research, *Journal of Child Psychology and Psychiatry*, **54**(1), 17–36.

Bigot, A., L. Blok, M. Boelaert, Y. Chartier, P. Corijn, A. Davis, M. Deguerry, T. Dusauchoit, F. Fermon and A. Griekspoor (1997), *Refugee Health: An Approach to Emergency Situations*, London: Macmillan Education.

Blanchet, K., V. Sistenich, A. Ramesh, S. Frison, E. Warren, M. Hossain, A. Knight, C. Lewis, J. Smith, A. Woodward, M. Dahab, S. Pantuliano and B. Roberts (2013), *An Evidence Review of Research on Health Interventions in Humanitarian Crises*, Cardiff: Enhancing Learning and Research for Humanitarian Assistance (ELRHA).

Bolton, P. and A. M. Tang (2002), An alternative approach to cross-cultural function assessment, *Social Psychiatry and Psychiatric Epidemiology*, **37**(11), 537–543.

Bolton, P., J. K. Bass, G. A. Zangana, T. Kamal, S. M. Murray, D. Kaysen, C. W. Lejuez, K. Lindgren, S. Pagoto, L. K. Murray, S. S. van Wyk, A. M. A. Ahmed, N. M. M. Amin and M. Rosenblum (2014), A randomized controlled trial of mental health interventions for survivors of systematic violence in Kurdistan, Northern Iraq, *BMC Psychiatry*, **14**(1), 360.

Checchi, F., M. Gayer, R. F. Grais and E. J. Mills (2008), *HPN Network Paper 61: Public Health in Crisis-Affected Populations: A Practical Guide for Decision-Makers*, London: Overseas Development Institute.

Centers for Disease Control and UNICEF (2001), *Violence Against Children in Tanzania: Findings from a National Survey, 2009*, Dar es Salaam: UNICEF Tanzania.

CPWG (2012), *Minimum Standards for Protection of Children in Humanitarian Action*, Child Protection Area of Responsibility Working Group.

Codjoe, S. N. A., P. Quartey, C. A. Tagoe and H. E. Reed (2013), Perceptions of the impact of refugees on host communities: the case of Liberian refugees in Ghana, *Journal of International Migration and Integration*, **14**(3), 439–456.

Connolly, M. A., M. Gayer, M. J. Ryan, P. Salama, P. Spiegel and D. L. Heymann (2004), Communicable diseases in complex emergencies: impact and challenges, *The Lancet*, **364**(9449), 1974–1983.

Dawson, K. S., R. A. Bryant, M. Harper, A. Kuowei Tay, A. Rahman, A. Schafer and M. van Ommeren (2015), Problem Management Plus (PM+): a WHO transdiagnostic psychological intervention for common mental health problems, *World Psychiatry*, **14**(3), 354–357.

Doocy, S., H. Tappis, C. Haskew, C. Wilkinson and P. Spiegel (2011), Performance of UNHCR nutrition programs in post-emergency refugee camps, *Conflict and Health*, **5**(23).

Emergency Nutrition Network (2007), *Infant and Young Child Feeding in Emergencies: Infant and Young Child Feeding in Emergencies Core Group*, Oxford: IFE Core Group.

Hovel, L. (2014), Local integration, in E. Fiddian-Qasmiyeh, G. Loescher, K. Long and N. Sigona (eds.), *Oxford Handbook of Refugee and Forced Migration Studies*, Oxford: Oxford University Press.

Hynes, M., M. Sheik, H. G. Wilson and P. Spiegel (2002), Reproductive health indicators and outcomes among refugee and internally displaced persons in postemergency phase camps, *JAMA*, **288**(5), 595–603.

IASC (2005), *Guidelines for Gender-Based Violence Interventions in Humanitarian Settings: Focusing on Prevention of and Response to Sexual Violence in Emergencies*, Geneva: Inter-Agency Standing Committee.

IASC (2007), *IASC Guidelines on Mental Health and Psychosocial Support in Emergency Settings*, Geneva: Inter-Agency Standing Committee.

IASC (2010), *Guidelines for Addressing HIV in Humanitarian Settings*, Geneva: Inter-Agency Standing Committee.

IASC (2015a), *Reference Module for Cluster Coordination at Country Level*, Geneva: Inter-Agency Standing Committee.

IASC (2015b), *Guidelines for Integrating Gender-Based Violence Interventions in Humanitarian Action: Reducing Risk, Promoting Resilience and Aiding Recovery*, Geneva: Inter-Agency Standing Committee.

IASC RG-MHPSS (2014), *Review of the Implementation of the IASC Guidelines on Mental Health and Psychosocial Support in Emergency Settings*, Geneva: Inter-Agency Standing Committee Reference Group on Mental Health and Psychosocial Support.

Inter-Agency Working Group on Reproductive Health in Crises (2010), *Inter-agency Field Manual on Reproductive Health in Humanitarian Settings*.

Joint UNHCR-OCHA Note on Mixed Situations: Coordination in Practice (2014), available online at www.unhcr.org/53679e679.pdf.

Jones, L., J. B. Asare, M. El Masri, A. Mohanraj, H. Sherief and M. van Ommeren (2009), Severe mental disorders in complex emergencies, *The Lancet*, **374**(9690), 654–661.

Kane, J. C., P. Ventevogel, P. Spiegel, J. K. Bass, M. van Ommeren and W. A. Tol (2014), Mental, neurological, and substance use problems among refugees in primary health care: analysis of the Health Information System in 90 refugee camps, *BMC Medicine*, **12**, 228.

Kett, M. and M. van Ommeren (2009), Disability, conflict, and emergencies, *The Lancet*, **374**(9704), 1801–1803.

Krause, S., R. K. Jones and S. J. Purdin (2000), Programmatic responses to refugees' reproductive health needs, *International Family Planning Perspectives*, 181–187.

Krause, S., H. Williams, M. A. Onyango, S. Sami, W. Doedens, N. Giga, E. Stone and B. Tomczyk (2015), Reproductive health services for Syrian refugees in Zaatri Camp and Irbid City, Hashemite Kingdom of Jordan: an evaluation of the Minimum Initial Services Package, *Conflict and Health*, **9**(S1): S4.

Long, K. (2014), Rethinking 'durable' solutions, in E. Fiddian-Qasmiyeh, G. Loescher,

K. Long and N. Sigona (eds.), *Oxford Handbook of Refugee and Forced Migration Studies*, Oxford: Oxford University Press.

Mabiso, A., J. F. Maystadt, J. Vandercasteelen and K. Hirvonen (2014), Refugees, food security, and resilience in host communities, in *2020 Conference Paper*, pp. 1–41.

McClelland, M. (2014), How to build a perfect refugee camp, *The New York Times*, available online at www.nytimes.com/2014/02/16/magazine/how-to-build-a-perfect-refugee-camp.html.

McConnan, I. (1998), *Humanitarian Charter and Minimum Standards in Disaster Response*, Geneva: Sphere Project.

Metzler, J., R. Kaijuka, M. Vojta, K. Savage, M. Yamano, A. Schafer, G. Yu, G. Ebulu and A. Ager (2013a). *Evaluation of Child Friendly Spaces: Uganda Field Study Summary Report, July 2013*, Mailman School of Public Health, Columbia University, World Vision Uganda and World Vision International.

Metzler, J., K. Savage, M. Vojta, M. Yamano, A. Schafer and A. Ager (2013b), *Evaluation of Child Friendly Spaces: Ethiopia Field Study Summary Report February 2013*, Mailman School of Public Health, Columbia University, World Vision International, available online at http://washcluster.net/wp-content/uploads/sites/2/2013/03/WV-CU-CFS-Ethiopia-Field-Study-Summary-Report1.pdf.

Metzler, J., A. Atrooshi, E. Khudeda, D. Ali and A. Ager (2014a), *Evaluation of Child Friendly Spaces: Iraq Field Study Report: A MoLSA-Implemented CFS in Domiz Refugee Camp*, Save the Children and UNICEF.

Metzler, J., M. Ishaq, S. Hermosilla, E. Mumba and A. Ager (2014b), *Evaluation of Child Friendly Spaces: Jordan Field Study Report: A CFS Implemented by World Vision and partners in Zarqa, Jordan, February 2015*, Mailman School of Public Health, Columbia University and World Vision Jordan.

Meyer, S. (2013), *UNHCR's Mental Health and Psychosocial Support for Persons of Concern: Global Review – 2013*, Geneva: UNHCR.

Meyer, S., H. Tappis, W. Weiss, P. Spiegel and A. Vu (2011), Refugee site health service utilization: more needs to be done, *American Journal of Disaster Medicine*, **6**(4), 231–242.

Meyer, S., L. Muhorakeye and L. Stark (2014), *Measuring Impact through a Child Protection Index: Report of Pilot Study, Kiziba Camp, Rwanda*, CPC Learning Network, AVSI Rwanda and UNHCR.

Miller, K. E. and A. Rasmussen (2010), War exposure, daily stressors, and mental health in conflict and post-conflict settings: bridging the divide between trauma-focused and psychosocial frameworks, *Social Science and Medicine*, **70**(1), 7–16.

Mollica, R. F., B. L. Cardozo, H. J. Osofsky, B. Raphael, A. Ager and P. Salama (2004), Mental health in complex emergencies, *The Lancet*, **364**(9450), 2058–2067.

Moss, W. J., M. Ramakrishnan, D. Storms, A. Henderson Siegle, W. M. Weiss, I. Lejnev and L. Muhe (2006), Child health in complex emergencies, *Bulletin of the World Health Organization*, **84**(1), 58–64.

Orach, C. G. and V. De Brouwere (2004), Postemergency health services for refugee and host populations in Uganda, 1999–2002, *The Lancet*, **364**(9434), 611–612.

Patrick, E. (2011), *'We Have No Choice': Safe Access to Firewood and Alternative Energy in Eastern Democratic Republic of Congo Appraisal Report*, New York: Women's Refugee Commission.

PWG (2003), *Psychosocial Intervention in Complex Emergencies: A Conceptual Framework*, Psychosocial Working Group, available online at www.forcedmigration.org/psychosocial/papers/Conceptual%20Framework.pdf.

Pupavac, V. (2002), *Working Paper No. 59: Therapeutising Refugees, Pathologising Populations: International Psycho-Social Programmes in Kosovo*, Geneva: UNHCR.

Roberts, B. and J. Browne (2011), A Systematic Review of Factors Influencing the Psychological Health of Conflict-Affected Populations in Low- and Middle-Income Countries, *Global Public Health*, **6**(8), 814–829.

Salama, P., P. Spiegel and R. Brennan (2001), No less vulnerable: the internally displaced in humanitarian emergencies, *The Lancet*, **357**(9266), 1430–1431.

Spangaro, J., C. Adogu, G. Ranmuthugala, G. P. Davies, L. Steinacker and A. Zwi (2013), What evidence exists for initiatives to reduce risk and incidence of sexual violence in armed conflict and other humanitarian crises? A systematic review, *PLOS* One, **8**(5), e62600.

Sphere Project (2004), *Humanitarian Charter and Minimum Standards in Disaster Response*, Geneva: Sphere Project.

Sphere Project (2011), *Humanitarian Charter and Minimum Standards in Disaster Response*, Geneva: Sphere Project.

Spiegel, P. (2004), HIV/AIDS among conflict-affected and displaced populations: dispelling myths and taking action, *Disasters*, **28**(3), 322–339.

Spiegel, P. B., F. Checchi, S. Colombo and E. Paik (2010), Health-care needs of people affected by conflict: future trends and changing frameworks, *The Lancet*, **375**(9711), 341–345.

Spiegel, P. B., M. Schilperoord and M. Dahab (2014), High-risk sex and displacement among refugees and surrounding populations in 10 countries: the need for integrating interventions, *AIDS*, **28**(5), 761–771.

Stark, L. and A. Ager (2011), A systematic review of prevalence studies of gender-based violence in complex emergencies, *Trauma, Violence, and Abuse*, **12**(3), 127–134.

Stark, L. and D. Landis (2016) Violence against children in humanitarian settings: a literature review of population-based approaches, *Social Science and Medicine*, **152**, 125–137.

Steel, Z., T. Chey, D. Silove, C. Marnane, R. A. Bryant and M. van Ommeren (2009), Association of torture and other potentially traumatic events with mental health outcomes among populations exposed to mass conflict and displacement: a systematic review and meta-analysis, *JAMA*, **302**(5), 537–549.

Strang, A. B. and A. Ager (2003), Psychosocial interventions: some key issues facing practitioners, *Intervention*, **1**(3), 2–12.

Summerfield, D. (1999), A critique of seven assumptions behind psychological trauma programmes in war-affected areas, *Social Science and Medicine*, **48**(10), 1449–1462.

Tanabe, M., K. Schaus, S. Rastogi, S. K. Krause and P. Patel (2015), Tracking humanitarian funding for reproductive health: a systematic analysis of health and protection proposals from 2002–2013, *Conflict and Health*, **9**(S1), S2.

Tol, W. A., C. Barbui, A. Galappatti, D. Silove, T. S. Betancourt, R. Souza, A. Golaz and M. van Ommeren (2011), Mental health and psychosocial support in humanitarian settings: linking practice and research, *The Lancet*, **378**(9802), 1581–1591.

Tol, W. A., V. Patel, M. Tomlinson, F. Baingana, A. Galappatti, D. Silove, E. Sondorp, M. van Ommeren, M. G. Wessells and C. Panter-Brick (2012), Relevance or excellence? Setting research priorities for mental health and psychosocial support in humanitarian settings, *Harvard Review of Psychiatry*, **20**(1), 25–36.

Tol, W. A., C. Barbui and M. van Ommeren (2013), Management of acute stress, PTSD, and bereavement: WHO recommendations, *JAMA*, **310**(5), 477–478.

UNAIDS and UNHCR (2005), *Strategies to Support the HIV-Related Needs of Refugees and Host Populations*, Geneva: UNAIDS Best Practice Collection.

UN General Assembly (1951), *Convention Relating to the Status of Refugees*, United Nations, Treaty Series, 189, 137.

UNHCR (1999), *Protecting Refugees: A Fieldguide for NGOs*, Geneva: United Nations High Commissioner for Refugees.

UNHCR (2003), *Conclusion on Protection from Sexual Abuse and Exploitation*, Geneva: United Nations High Commissioner for Refugees, available online at www.unhcr.org/3f93b2c44.html.

UNHCR (2006), *Operational Protection in Camps and Settlements: A Reference Guide of Good Practices in the Protection of Refugees and Other Persons of Concern*, Geneva: United Nations High Commissioner for Refugees.

UNHCR (2007), *Handbook for Emergencies*, Geneva: United Nations High Commissioner for Refugees.

UNHCR (2011), *Epidemic Preparedness in Refugee Camp Settings: Guidance for Public Health Officers*, Geneva: United Nations High Commissioner for Refugees.
UNHCR (2012a), *Dadaab: World's Biggest Refugee Camp 20 Years Old*, available online at www.unhcr.org/4f439dbb9.html.
UNHCR (2012b), *Framework for the Protection of Children*, Geneva: United Nations High Commissioner for Refugees.
UNHCR (2013), *Operational Guidance Mental Health and Psychosocial Support: Programming for Refugee Operations*, Geneva: United Nations High Commissioner for Refugees.
UNHCR (2014), *World at War: UNHCR Global Trends – Forced Displacement in 2014*, Geneva: United Nations High Commissioner for Refugees.
van Ommeren, M., S. Saxena and B. Saraceno (2005), Mental and social health during and after acute emergencies: emerging consensus? *Bulletin of the World Health Organization*, **83**(1), 71–75.
van Selm, J. (2014), Refugee resettlement, in E. Fiddian-Qasmiyeh, G. Loescher, K. Long and N. Sigona (eds.), *Oxford Handbook of Refugee and Forced Migration Studies*, Oxford: Oxford University Press.
Vu, A., A. Adam, A. Wirtz, K. Pham, L. Rubenstein, N. Glass, C. Beyrer and S. Singh (2014), The prevalence of sexual violence among female refugees in complex humanitarian emergencies: a systematic review and meta-analysis, *PLOS Currents*, **6**.
Ward, J. (2014), *Revising the 2005 IASC Guidelines for Gender-Based Violence Interventions in Humanitarian Settings: Prioritising Accountability*, available online at www.odihpn.org/humanitarian-exchange-magazine/issue-60/revising-the-2005-iasc-guidelines-for-gender-based-violence-interventions-in-humanitarian-settings-prioritising-accountability.
Webb, P., E. Boyd, S. de Pee, L. Lenters, M. Bloem and W. Schultink (2014), Nutrition in emergencies: do we know what works? *Food Policy*, **49**, 33–40.
Wessells, M. (2009), Do no harm: toward contextually appropriate psychosocial support in international emergencies, *American Psychologist*, **64**(8), 842.
Wessells, M. and M. van Ommeren (2008), Developing inter-agency guidelines on mental health and psychosocial support in emergency settings, *Intervention*, **6**(3), 199–218.
WRC (2011), *Minimum Initial Service Package (MISP) for Reproductive Health in Crisis Situations: A Distance Learning Module*, Women's Refugee Commission, available online at www.unhcr.org/4e8d6b3b14.pdf.
WHO (1948), *WHO Definition of Health*, available online at www.who.int/about/definition/en/print.html.
WHO (2008), *Manual for the Health Care of Children in Humanitarian Emergencies*, Geneva: World Health Organization.
WHO (2015), *Integrated Management of Childhood Illness (IMCI)*, available online at www.who.int/maternal_child_adolescent/topics/child/imci/en.
Young, H., A. Borrel, D. Holland and P. Salama (2004), Public nutrition in complex emergencies, *The Lancet*, **364**(9448), 1899–1909.
Zimmerman, L., C. Packer and C. Robinson (2011), *Reproductive Health in Post-Emergency Refugee Camps*, available online at http://paa2011.princeton.edu/papers/110927.

21 Retirement migration and health: growing old in Spain

Kelly Hall

INTRODUCTION

The past few decades have seen a considerable increase in the number of older people retiring abroad. The migration of older people has generally been North to South; including from Northern to Southern Europe, and from Canada and the USA to Central and South America. Greater wealth and longevity in later life have led to longer periods of retirement, which enables older people to take on new challenges and pursue new opportunities including international travel or migration. For many individuals older age is seen as a 'third age' of life (Laslett 1991) during which new social and recreational activities can be pursued that are separate from the world of work. The movement of older people from one country to another has been conceptualised as 'international retirement migration' (King 2000), 'residential tourism' (O'Reilly 2000) and more recently, 'lifestyle migration' (Benson and O'Reilly 2009). 'Lifestyle migration' is a term that has been widely used by researchers across a range of disciplines to capture the movement of relatively affluent people across borders to improve their quality of life. Retirement for many older people can therefore provide the opportunity to move abroad, with Southern Europe remaining a key destination for British and other Northern European citizens.

This chapter considers the issue of retirement migration, with a particular focus on older British people in Spain. Spain has become a popular retirement destination for British citizens; its warm climate, lower living costs and relaxed pace of life has attracted those looking for a more fulfilling retirement. Most retirees are fit and healthy when they move to Spain, and subsequently most research on international retirement migration and lifestyle migration has focused on the reasons for moving, social networks and integration in the host country and the identities and lifestyles of healthy 'third age' retirees. However, old age can bring increased vulnerabilities, especially vulnerability to ill-health, disability and frailty, resulting in an abrupt end to the third age and the onset of the 'fourth age' of dependence and decline. This chapter therefore focuses on the health and care issues facing retired migrants who have entered the fourth age of life.

Drawing on research undertaken by the author and others, it concentrates on older British retirees in Spain who have experienced a decline in health and need access to health and social care. It considers how these migrants access health and social care services in Spain, including statutory and private services. It reviews the rights of retired migrants within the EU, in particular the exportability of healthcare rights from the UK to Spain. It also outlines the differences in statutory care and support services that are evident between Northern and Southern European countries that are often not recognised by older migrants. These differences result in a tension between expectations and reality underpinned by different cultural understandings of care. As such, older migrants often seek alternative routes to health and social care including through the voluntary sector in Spain and returning to the UK to access support in old age, which are also explored here.

RETIREMENT MIGRATION

While migration to rural and coastal areas within the UK remains a common choice for retirement (Lowe and Speakman 2006), growing numbers are choosing to retire abroad (Sriskandarajah and Drew 2006). This has been enabled through longer and healthier periods of retirement, combined with well-established tourist infrastructure, English media sources and cheaper travel making many destinations more accessible. Between 2008 and 2012, 24,000 British citizens of state pension age emigrated from the UK (Murray et al. 2012) and in 2009, 9.2 per cent of British pensioners lived abroad (Finch et al. 2010). While non-EU countries such as Australia and the USA remain popular migration choices for British citizens, especially those of working age, there is evidence of the continuing popularity of North–South retirement migration within Europe (e.g., King et al. 2000; Ackers and Dwyer 2002; O'Reilly 2007). The growing popularity of migration within the EU can be linked back to the 1992 Maastricht Treaty, which enabled the free movement of people within the EU and gave some EU migrants the ability to export their rights to healthcare and other social security schemes (discussed in more detail below). Popular Southern European destinations for older British people include Spain, France and Italy, which host a mix of permanent residents and second-home-owners.

International retirement migration has been noted as a particularly fluid and flexible form of migration, which can involve complex mobility patterns (Huber and O'Reilly 2004). As retired migrants are not constrained by paid work, many choose to split their time between different countries;

> **BOX 21.1 TYPOLOGY OF RETIRED MIGRANTS**
>
> ***Full/permanent residents***: these are migrants who have moved permanently, most of whom own property in the host country. They often have no intention of returning to their country of origin.
> ***Returning residents***: these are resident in the host country with regards to home, orientation and legal status but return to Britain each summer for between two and five months to escape the summer heat and crowds of tourists. Many own homes in both the host country and the UK and others stay with relatives or friends in the UK.
> ***Seasonal migrants/visitors***: these are resident in the UK with regards to home, orientation and legal status but spend up to six months in the host country. They usually have property in the UK and abroad. Generally, these elderly 'swallows' move south in the winter to escape the northern cold and move back north in the height of summer to avoid the heat.

for example, by spending six months in the host country and six months in the UK. A number of studies have attempted to devise typologies of international mobility based on movement characteristics and orientation towards home (e.g., O'Reilly 2000; King et al. 2000). Based on a review of these studies, Box 21.1 summarises three types of retired migrant. These categories are not always fixed, as some migrants move between them depending on their circumstances at the time. This therefore further indicates the flexibility of retired migrant lifestyles and for many, the country of residence is not always clear. There are subsequently large numbers of retired migrants that are undocumented in the host country.

SPAIN AS A POPULAR RETIREMENT DESTINATION

For many decades, Spain has been a popular retirement destination for older EU nationals, including Swedish (Gustafson 2001) and British nationals (O'Reilly 2000). Mass international tourism began in Spain upon the establishment of democracy following the death of the Spanish dictator General Franco in 1975. Traditionally a country of emigration, after 1975 immigration to Spain increased dramatically, and British people began to buy second or permanent homes (O'Reilly 2000). A familiarity with Spain through tourism has played a key role in the search for a retirement destination for retired migrants.

The migration of British people to Spain peaked in the early 2000s with around 60,000 British citizens moving there between 2003 and 2004, making it the second most common destination for British people of all ages (after Australia) and the most popular retirement destination (Finch et al. 2010). The number of British people moving to Spain, however, slowed after 2006, which coincided with the start of the recession and saw a decline in the value of the British pound against the euro, making living costs in Spain considerably higher than they were in the early 2000s.

The exact number of British people living in Spain remains unclear due to under-registration and fluid migration patterns, especially among older migrants as indicated above. Non-registration is a significant issue and the Consulate in Madrid have estimated that around 75 per cent of British people in Spain do not register with their local authority (Finch et al. 2010). Spanish registry data in 2015 indicates that there are 161,306 registered British citizens over the age of 55 living in Spain, of whom 104,368 are over the age of 65 (Instituto Nacional de Estadística, 2015). However, when non-registration is taken into account, it is estimated that there are nearly a million British people living in Spain permanently of whom around half are over 50 and 14 per cent are over 70 (Finch et al. 2010; Sriskandarajah and Drew 2006). Most older British people in Spain reside in coastal locations including the provinces of Alicante (Costa Blanca) and Malaga (Costa del Sol), as well as the Canary Islands and the Balearic Islands.

Spain has become a popular retirement destination for a number of reasons, which for most people include the warm and sunny climate. The Spanish climate is not only attractive in its own right but also enables a more outdoor and active lifestyle. In addition, the climate can reduce the negative effects of illnesses and disabilities, such as arthritis and rheumatism. Therefore, moving to Spain can enhance someone's quality of life or even elongate their life expectancy. Economic factors also feature highly in decisions over retiring to Spain. While living costs in Spain are converging with those in the UK (especially during the recent economic crisis) and vary depending on exchange rates, there are still some economic advantages to living in Spain over the UK. Cheaper living costs make it possible to acquire a good standard of living in Spain compared with the UK. This includes lower house prices, lower heating costs and the cheaper cost of eating out (Rodríguez et al. 2004; O'Reilly 2000).

GROWING OLD IN SPAIN: THE THIRD TO THE FOURTH AGE OF LIFE

Most retirees who move abroad are healthy, and are in what Laslett (1991) refers to as the 'third age' of life. The third age normally begins at the point of retirement and is the stage of life where personal goals, distinct from the world of work or childrearing, can be realised. It is therefore known as the age of personal achievement and fulfilment. Third agers often take up new interests and opportunities with international travel, second-home-ownership and migration being defining features of the third age for some people. Moving abroad in the third age can bring a multitude of opportunities for social engagement, including undertaking new social activities and making new friends. Spain has a wide variety of recreational activities and clubs that attract retired British people and, as such, older British migrants in Spain tend to have strong social networks (O'Reilly 2000). Despite their high level of social engagement, they are, however, largely segregated from the local Spanish people, living in purpose-built tourist and residential complexes, known as 'urbanisations'. Urbanisations generally lie outside of historic village centres and have their own shops, restaurants that cater to British tastes, as well as personal service outlets that sell British products (Huber and O'Reilly 2004). Such urbanisations are therefore host to large and segregated British communities in Spain, leading to little integration with the host community and a general lack of proficiency in Spanish. While older British migrants in Spain may not integrate or have Spanish friends, they have built a strong sense of community and have active social lives. Migrant social activities commonly include participation in British social clubs, from small activity groups to larger and more formal organisations such as the British Legion. Social clubs offer not only a source of enjoyment but present an opportunity to develop social networks, as they provide access to new friends and social contacts. They also allow people to share information and advice on living in Spain, including how to negotiate Spanish bureaucracy. For older migrants, social clubs are often an integral part of daily life.

Previous studies on retirement migration have tended to focus on those in the third age who are experiencing 'positive' or 'active' ageing (e.g., Oliver 2008; King et al. 2000; Casado-Diaz 2009), exploring the lives of those who are visible and active within British community life in Spain. However, healthy and active retired lifestyles in Spain can end abruptly with the onset of old age and a severe decline in health. This chapter therefore considers older retired migrants who have experienced a decline in health and as a result are frail, vulnerable and now require additional support and care. Laslett (1991) refers to the 'fourth age' of life, which begins when the third age ends; normally where a healthy and independent lifestyle is replaced with one of dependence and decline. The fourth age is normally associated with a decline in physical (or mental) health, with disability and frailty being common features. The fourth age has also been associated with 'deep old age' and while policymakers and academics have tried to link it with chronological age – for example, being over 75 or 85 years – in reality, the age at which someone reaches the fourth age varies from person to person. Nonetheless, what is evident is that as people become old, they become more vulnerable.

Vulnerability during old age has been widely associated with a decline in health (Grundy 2006; Bond and Corner 2004). When a health problem results in reduced mobility or an inability to look after oneself, the result can be physical and emotional dependence on other people, as well as on health and social care services including institutionalised care. Accessing sufficient medical support, social support and care in old age can therefore be vital. Family are often a crucial source of support for many older people, especially in Spain where a tradition of family care means that older Spanish people tend to be looked after by their younger extended family. However, for older British people living in Spain, family are normally located in the UK (or elsewhere) and therefore are not on hand to offer care and support following the onset of illness or a crisis. Subsequently, the availability of health and social care services in Spain is especially important.

HEALTHCARE IN SPAIN

In the post-Franco period, the quality and variation of healthcare available in Spain has increased dramatically. Following the creation of the Ministry of Health in 1977 and the General Health Care Act in 1986, a national health service was created. By the 1990s, universality of provision free at the point of delivery had been achieved. By 2002, although the Spanish social security system (Seguridad Sociale) has been retained at a national level, the compulsory health insurance system (El Instituto Nacional de Salud) was decentralised and healthcare is now provided by the 17 autonomous regions in Spain. Therefore, it is not possible to speak of a unified health system, but instead of 17 regional health services, with the national Ministry of Health assuming a coordinating role. Under this system, rights to healthcare are guaranteed for all Spaniards and foreign citizens resident in Spain (with some exceptions for retired migrants discussed below). The only costs for patients can be up to 40 per cent of the cost of prescriptions (which since 2012 includes pensioners) and there are charges for dental and psychiatric services. However, as each autonomous region has its own health network, health legislation and health plan, the level of care can differ between regions. Despite the recent economic recession and resulting cuts to the Spanish health system, the quality of Spanish healthcare is usually considered to be excellent (Hall 2011), often with shorter waiting times for non-emergency treatment and better-quality hospitals than in the UK.

In Spain, retired migrants must be covered by sickness insurance of some kind to have a right to residence. However, access to healthcare for retired migrants can vary according to age and status. British state pensioners are able to transfer their healthcare rights to Spain, giving them the same access to healthcare as a Spanish national. This is organised through reciprocal arrangements that exist between EU member states making any costs of healthcare recoverable against the country of origin. Older migrants who have worked in Spain prior to retiring there are also entitled to free healthcare through their status as a worker, giving them access to the same level of healthcare as a Spanish citizen. However, for migrants who have not yet reached state pension age and have never worked in Spain, automatic access to free and extended healthcare in Spain is not provided, meaning that once they become a resident in Spain, they cannot use Spanish healthcare services without paying the full cost of any services used.

By moving to Spain, British citizens also give up their rights to access healthcare in the UK. As a result, in order to retain access to the British National Health Service (NHS), some older migrants do not declare residency in Spain. Legido Quigley and La Parra (2007) refer to these unregistered migrants as a 'floating population' who have no clear healthcare provision in their chosen country of residence. This can become especially problematic for those with chronic conditions. Alternatively, Coldron and Ackers (2007) refer to these unregistered migrants as 'clandestine migrants' who manipulate the system to receive the best healthcare coverage to meet their needs. Despite living in Spain, many such people continue to use the British NHS and while in Spain may use the European Health Insurance Card (EHIC). The EHIC provides EU citizens with access to medical treatment when they travel to other EU countries; however, this should only be used by people who are visiting another country who need emergency medical treatment and not by migrants as an alternative source of healthcare. Coldron and Ackers (2007: 299) refer to migrants who use the EHIC as a source of healthcare as 'false tourists' and cite this as 'the darker side of active citizenship'. In addition to the implications for migrants with long-term conditions, it also has serious implications for the financing of state-funded healthcare systems. Funding for local services including social care is only provided for registered citizens in Spain and so non-registration can lead to a significant underfunding of services in areas with high numbers of older migrants.

Private healthcare is another option for migrants, especially early retirees who are resident in Spain. However, the high cost of private health insurance can be problematic for those on low incomes. Around 29 per cent of British people (of all ages) in Spain have private health insurance

(La Parra and Angel Mateo 2008) but this is likely to be lower among older British people, as premiums generally increase with age and medical needs, and can be of limited use when the need for long-term care arises as policies may exclude certain conditions or types of care.

SOCIAL CARE IN SPAIN

Social care, which includes support at home, day centres and nursing/residential homes, is normally provided by either Social Services or – for those with the financial means – private carers. Across Spain, the family and church were virtually the sole providers of Social Services until well into the 1970s, and to a great extent social care is still expected to be provided by the family today. In most of Southern Europe including Spain, the care of dependent elderly people is private and the responsibility of the nuclear and extended family and is not usually recognised as an activity to be covered by the public system. As a result, around 83 per cent of dependent older people in Spain receive informal care from family, which is 30 per cent more than in the UK (Costa-Font and Patxot 2005). There are, therefore, considerable differences in care practices between Spain and the UK and many British people appear to be moving to Spain expecting the same level of care as they would receive in the UK. This indicates the importance of cultural contexts when it comes to care and support and is especially important for frail older people.

Spanish Social Services do provide some care services including homecare, daycare centres, telecare and care homes. However, community care services are still in short supply, with district nursing services as well as palliative care being rare or non-existent (Age Concern 2005). Residential care has also expanded in Spain; however, state-funded long-term care places are very limited with places accommodating only around 2.8 per cent of the over 65 population in Spain (Royal British Legion 2009). Eligibility criteria for public nursing homes is based on income and need, although this varies from one region to another (Costa-Font and Patxot 2005) and Spanish citizens are usually prioritised.

Therefore, although Spain has ambitious social service and community development policies, there has not been widespread implementation (King et al. 2000). Private and voluntary organisations often fill these gaps in local health and care systems. There has been an expansion in the privatisation of care across Southern Europe, with private expenditure on institutional and community care in Spain being around 73 per cent of the total expenditure (Costa-Font and Patxot 2005). An extensive care market has developed in Spain and commercial solutions to elderly care needs have become established. From the end of the 1990s in many Southern European countries, a growing number of elderly people were being cared for by paid care workers. This includes a growth in private residential and nursing care for older people in Spain. However, this can be very expensive ranging from €1,500 to more than €5,000 a month. Even for those who can afford to pay for nursing homes, finding one where English is spoken may be difficult (Hardill et al. 2005). Therefore, British people living in Spain are entitled to access social care services to the same level as a Spanish citizen as long as they are registered with their local authority in Spain; however, as the level of social service provision in Spain is generally lower than in the UK, it can be very difficult to access. In addition, for those who can access care and support, language and cultural issues can create additional barriers.

LANGUAGE AND CULTURAL BARRIERS TO CARE IN SPAIN

When it comes to health and social care, there are therefore notable differences in services in Spain compared to the UK. Cultural differences that are underpinned by a model of family care in Spain are evident. This includes not only the differences in community care as explained above but also cultural differences within hospitals. For example, in a Spanish hospital, it is customary for the patient's family to provide basic nursing care, by undertaking duties such as feeding and washing the patient, while in the UK such duties would be performed by nursing staff (see Box 21.2).

Therefore, while hospital care is very good, hospital nursing practices

BOX 21.2 SPANISH HOSPITALS: CULTURAL DIFFERENCES IN CARE

In a Spanish hospital, care (e.g., washing, bathing and feeding) is expected to be performed by family members rather than nurses, as explained by an older British migrant in Spain:

> You have got to have someone in [hospital] with you. The nurses will not help you out at all . . . When [husband] was ill, the two girls [granddaughters] and [daughter] took turns to stay each night with him. You have to stay the night otherwise you don't get any help. When I wasn't there, the dinner, nobody gives them anything. And then they take it away. They don't feed you, they don't wash you . . . If you don't have anyone with you, you might as well die.

(adapted from Hall and Hardill 2014)

are very different to the UK. There is also little support following discharge from hospital, with very few community health services such as district nursing. The distribution of services can also vary by region; for example, hospital beds are also unevenly distributed, being scarcer in rural areas and in the South (Age Concern España 2006). Therefore, area of residence can greatly influence healthcare availability and in a similar fashion to the UK, many people have turned to the private sector.

An additional barrier for older British migrants looking to access health or social care services in Spain is the local language, which restricts access to doctors, social services and nursing homes. Integration with the Spanish community is low among older British people, especially those living in the Costa del Sol and Costa Blanca, and as indicated earlier, many older British people in Spain do not speak Spanish. Research conducted in the Costa del Sol shows that language is a significant problem for British people living there, with most only being able to interact on a superficial level (O'Reilly 2000). This is especially problematic when it comes to healthcare, as research by the Spanish Society of General Medicine (cited in Stevens 2006) found that fewer than 10 per cent of expatriates living in the Spanish Costas can communicate with medical staff and almost a third rely on hand gestures. Even those who have a reasonable understanding of the Spanish language are unlikely to understand complex medical terminology needed for a visit to the doctor or when receiving hospital treatment. It is especially important to fully understand what someone is being told when it comes to health and healthcare, and misunderstanding information from doctors can be potentially life-threatening, and can, for example, lead to someone taking the wrong medication or the wrong dose of a medication. Subsequently, the use of translators by older British people in Spain is high, especially for medical appointments; however, this can be very costly, especially for those who require long-term medical interventions. Translators are provided in some hospitals and also for those with private medical insurance. La Parra and Angel Mateo (2008) found that language problems in the public healthcare sector may also be the reason for a high use of private healthcare by British people in the Costa Blanca.

For those needing residential care, language and cultural barriers can be especially challenging. As noted above, acquiring a place in a state-funded residential or nursing home can be difficult due to their scarcity. If someone is able to find a place, most staff (and other residents) within care homes do not speak any English. This can leave older British people extremely vulnerable and isolated (Hall and Hardill 2014). While there are private care homes with English-speaking staff being established in Spain, as noted above, these can be very expensive and beyond the means of most older British migrants (see Box 21.3).

BOX 21.3 NURSING HOMES IN SPAIN

Accessing nursing homes is a common problem faced by older British people in Spain. Most find that due to limited state provision, the only homes available are private and subsequently very expensive costing between €1,500 and €5,000 per month. An interview with the daughter of an older disabled British person (both had migrated to Spain) highlighted the difficulties of accessing nursing homes in Spain:

> Interviewer: Is there any possibility of keeping [mother] in a nursing home in Spain?
> Daughter: It's over €2,000 a month.
> Interviewer: Have you looked into state-funded homes?
> Daughter: There aren't any. It's impossible. I have looked. I have looked. It was the first thing I tried. There are Spaniards queuing up for state homes so obviously they are going to give preference to a Spaniard anyway.

(adapted from Hall and Hardill 2014)

THE VOLUNTARY SECTOR IN SPAIN

A low level of statutory care in Spain has arguably led to an increased role of a British-run voluntary and community sector in Spain. The role of this sector in supporting older British people in Spain has been previously noted (Haas 2013), especially in supporting those with little kin support or financial means to pay for care (Oliver 2008). Charities and other non-governmental organisations are generally set up and run by the British community, with British (and some other English-speaking) volunteers supporting vulnerable British people with a range of activities, including accessing health and care services, translating at medical appointments and providing social or emotional support.

The voluntary and community sector is arguably able to bridge the gap between informal and formal care and support (Hall and Hardill 2014). While voluntary organisations do not tend to provide any personal or medical care, they are able to provide up-to-date information in English on health and care services, including supporting people to obtain care from Spanish social services, private carers and care homes.

There are a high proportion of ex-service personnel in Spain (Finch et al. 2010), and a range of British charities linked to HM Forces or occupations are active in Spain. For example, the Royal British Legion in the provinces of Malaga, Alicante and Valencia have well-developed voluntary welfare services. There are also a range of other British charities linked to HM Forces or occupations, such as the Royal Air Force

> **BOX 21.4 THE BRITISH VOLUNTARY SECTOR IN SPAIN**
>
> Age Concern España is a UK-based charity operating in Spain that provides specialist support and advice for British people over the age of 50 living there. It relies almost entirely on the unpaid work of members of the English-speaking community and on voluntary donations. They often play a key role in supporting older British people during times of crisis including ill-health, disability or following bereavement. This includes Elsa, who is disabled and speaks no Spanish so found it hard to cope when her husband died:
>
> > She has been so helpful this girl [Age Concern volunteer] she really has. I don't know what I would have done without her . . . every time I want something, and I have asked she has always come up with something, with a good answer.

or Royal Marines Benevolent Funds, which can provide subsidies and grants to British people living abroad. Hall (2011) found these funds were effectively utilised by many older British people in Spain, who often turn to these charities to access funding for care or alternatively funding and support when returning to the UK.

RETURNING TO THE UK FOR CARE

Following a decline in health or other crisis, some older British migrants return to the UK to access the support and care that they need (Hardill et al. 2005). Evidence suggests that care features prominently in the reason for a return move and the main reason older British people return from EU destinations is to use the national health and social care systems of their home country (Betty and Hall 2015; Hall and Hardill 2014). Some people make the positive decision to return as they feel it is the right option for them following a change in their circumstances and, as Ackers and Dwyer (2002) note, a return move for care may feature highly in the retirement 'plan' for older people living abroad. However, they also found that for others, returning was not a plan as such and presented itself as the result of a crisis. Some older British migrants may be forced to return to the UK when they can no longer live independently and there are no support systems (most frequently care) in the host country.

Another reason for returning is to be closer to family. While global communication and social networking can enable people to stay in regular contact with those in other countries, it is difficult to provide care at a distance. Bereavement can also trigger a return to the UK, as the death of a spouse or partner can result in isolation and loneliness (Betty and Hall 2015).

Alternatively, some moves are made to provide rather than to receive care. This may be either a return move to support children or care for grandchildren. Older migrants, especially women, may miss grandchildren and return to play a more active role in their lives. Return moves may also be made by adult children (who may themselves be retired) to support their elderly parents (Ackers and Dwyer 2002).

Returning to the UK following residency in another country is, however, not always straightforward. Residency restrictions, as well as the emotional, physical and financial impacts of returning, can result in significant challenges. There is some assistance for vulnerable or 'distressed' British nationals from organisations such as Age UK, the British Consulate and the Heathrow Travel Care Repatriation Project. These organisations have recognised the difficulties that older migrants can encounter when they return to the UK, especially vulnerable older people in need of immediate support upon return. Complex UK residency restrictions mean that if a British national decides to return to the UK permanently after taking up residency abroad, they may not be automatically eligible for any support. In order to claim support, anyone entering the UK, including returning British citizens, must have both a right to reside and be 'habitually resident'. While returning British citizens automatically have the right to reside, to be classed as 'habitually resident' they must pass the Habitual Residence Test (HRT). The HRT was introduced in August 1994 and only those who can demonstrate that they have a settled intention to stay can pass it. Depending on individual circumstances, passing the HRT can take from as little as a few days to three months. Upon passing the HRT, applications for any welfare benefits can take an additional two to three weeks (Age Concern 2007).

Returning to the UK can therefore be both lengthy and costly (financially and emotionally). However, this is something that people do not realise and instead expect to be able to gain instant access to UK support services (Age Concern 2007). Furthermore, people may not consider that if they have been living outside of the UK for a considerable period of time, there may have been changes to the health system and services they expect to receive, as well as the possible difficulties of reintegrating (Age Concern 2007).

CONCLUSION

Most British retirees are fit and healthy when they move to Spain, and are attracted by the warm and sunny climate that enables a more active outdoor lifestyle. While many older British people in Spain are not integrated into Spanish society, most enjoy active and fulfilling social lives as part of the British community, which is characterised by an abundance of social clubs and other activities. Research to date has generally focused on those in the 'third age' of life, by exploring the reasons for moving and the social lives and identities of migrants through the lens of 'active ageing' or 'lifestyle migration' (e.g., Benson and O'Reilly 2009; Oliver 2008; O'Reilly 2000; King et al. 2000). However, happy and fulfilling lives in Spain can end abruptly with the onset of illness or disability. A decline in health has been linked to increased vulnerability, resulting in dependence on other people. The need for health and social care services also becomes vital.

Older British people in Spain face a number of challenges with health and social care when compared to those living in the UK. British pensioners can exercise their rights as EU citizens enabling them access to free statutory healthcare in Spain; however, there are considerable cultural differences in services between the UK and Spain that many migrants do not anticipate. While Spanish healthcare is considered excellent, community and social care services are in short supply. A model of family care in Southern Europe means that nuclear and extended family normally care for their relatives in old age making the demand for statutory services much lower. For older British migrants who do not normally have family living close by, accessing support in old age can be difficult. A lack of preparation by older migrants in Spain has been highlighted in previous research (Hall 2011; Hall and Hardill 2014). This includes a poor understanding of the Spanish language, as well as Spanish culture, which can be a huge hindrance when trying to access support, especially at a time of crisis. The British community plays a key role in supporting older British people in Spain, especially British charities that are active in Spain. For example, Age Concern España provide support and advice to thousands of older British people in Spain each year (Hall 2008), including those who have experienced a severe decline in health or have been bereaved. Such services often supplement statutory services, and may fill the gap of family who live in the UK (or elsewhere), who can only provide support at a distance.

Older British people in Spain can therefore struggle to obtain the support that they need. While cultural differences in care are significant, an inability to speak Spanish and a lack of preparation by those moving to Spain form additional barriers. The British government is recognising the problems facing older British people in Spain and there is now a plethora of information for those who are moving abroad, including guidance on accessing healthcare in Spain. For example, the FCO's 'Know Before you Go' campaign is aimed at encouraging British travellers to be well-prepared before moving overseas. The British Consulate is also working alongside voluntary organisations in Spain, including Age Concern España, to provide information and support to older British people in Spain. However, it is up to migrants to access and utilise this information.

Research indicates that care is a key reason for returning to the UK, including to access statutory care that is not accessible in Spain, as well as informal care from family living in the UK. However, returning to the UK can present a number of challenges, especially when it is an unplanned return as a result of a crisis. This includes the physical, emotional and financial impacts of moving to another country. For those who have poor health or a disability, moving can be traumatic, especially for those who are unable to fly. Upon return to the UK, residency requirements and high demands on care services means that immediate access to support is not normally available. This indicates a need for older migrants to anticipate the challenges that they might face in old age, with a decline in health being likely, and to put support plans in place to navigate the challenges they may face.

This chapter has focused on the health and care issues faced by a subset of retired migrants, that of older British people in Spain. However, the issues and challenges around health and care identified here are not unique to this population. Indeed there are considerable numbers of British and other Northern European people (e.g., Norwegian, Danish, Dutch) living in Southern European countries including Spain, France and Italy who are also ageing, becoming frail and are in need of care. This population of Northern European retired migrants are also likely to be experiencing the same cultural differences in care that have been explored in this chapter. The ageing of retired migrants who have migrated from Northern to Southern European countries is therefore a significant issue. These 'well-off' lifestyle migrants are often ignored from research and policy and yet face some considerable challenges. It is therefore important for us to better understand their experiences so that appropriate care and support can be provided.

REFERENCES

Ackers, L. and P. Dwyer (2002), *Senior Citizenship? Retirement, Migration and Welfare in the European Union*, Bristol: Policy Press.

Age Concern (2005), *Retiring Abroad: What to Consider if You Are Planning to Leave the UK*, London: Age Concern England.

Age Concern (2007) *When the Sun Sets on Retirement Abroad*, Age Concern Conference, London, 17 May.

Age Concern España (2006), *Healthcare in the EEC*, Age Concern España.

Benson, M. and K. O'Reilly (eds.) (2009) *Lifestyle Migration: Expectations, Aspirations and Experiences*, Farnham: Ashgate.

Betty, C. and K. Hall (2015), The myth of no return? Why retired British migrants in Spain return to the UK, in K. Torkington, I. David and J. Sardinha (eds.), *Practising the Good Life Lifestyle Migration in Practices*, Cambridge: Scholars Publishing.

Bond, J. and L. Corner (2004), *Quality of Life and Older People*, Maidenhead: Open University Press.

Casado-Diaz, M. (2009) Social capital in the sun: bonding and bridging social capital among British retirees, in M. Benson and K. O'Reilly (eds.), *Lifestyle Migration: Expectations, Aspirations and Experiences*, Ashgate: Aldershot, pp. 87–102.

Coldron, K. and L. Ackers (2007), (Ab)using European citizenship? EU retired migrants and the exercise of healthcare rights, *Maastricht Journal of European and Comparative Law*, **3**, 287–302.

Costa-Font, J. and C. Patxot (2005), Design of the long-term care system in Spain: policy and financial constraints, *Social Policy & Society*, **4**(1), 11–20.

Finch, T., H. Andrew and M. Latorre (2010), *Global Brit: Making the Most of the British Diaspora*, Institute for Public Policy Research.

Grundy, E. (2006) Ageing and vulnerable elderly people: European perspectives, *Ageing and Society*, **26**, 5–34.

Gustafson, P. (2001) Retirement migration and transnational lifestyles, *Ageing and Society*, **21**(4), 371–394.

Haas, H. (2013), Volunteering in retirement migration: meanings and functions of charitable activities for older British residents in Spain, *Ageing and Society*, **33**, 1374–1400.

Hall, K. (2008), *Age Concern España: A Vital Resource for Older People in Spain*, Mallorca: Age Concern España.

Hall, K. (2011), *Retirement Migration, the Other Story: The Lived Experiences of Vulnerable, Older British Migrants in Spain*, PhD Thesis, Nottingham Trent University.

Hall, K. and I. Hardill (2014), Retirement migration, the 'other' story: caring for frail elderly British citizens in Spain, *Ageing and Society*, **36**(3), 562–585.

Hardill, I., J. Spradbery, J. Arnold-Boakes and M. L. Marrugat (2005), Severe health and social care issues among British migrants who retire to Spain, *Ageing and Society*, **25**, 769–783.

Huber, A. and K. O'Reilly (2004), The construction of *Heimat* under conditions of individualised modernity: Swiss and British elderly migrants in Spain, *Ageing and Society*, **24**(3), 327–352.

Instituto Nacional de Estadística (2015) *Explotación Estadística del Padrón*, available online at http://www.ine.es/jaxi/tabla.do?path=/t20/e245/p04/a2014/l1/&file=00000008.px&type=pcaxis&L=1.

King, R., T. Warnes and A. Williams (2000), *Sunset Lives: British Retirement Migration to the Mediterranean*, Oxford: Berg.

La Parra, D. and M. Angel Mateo (2008), Health status and access to healthcare of British nationals living on the Costa Blanca, Spain, *Ageing and Society*, **28**, 1–18.

Laslett, P. (1991), *A Fresh Map of Life: The Emergence of the Third Age*, Cambridge, MA: Harvard University Press.

Legido Quigley, H. and D. La Parra (2007), The health care needs of UK pensioners living in Spain: an agenda for research, *Euro Health*, **13**(4), 14–17.

Lowe P. and L. Speakman (eds.) (2006), *The Ageing Countryside: The Growing Older Population of Rural England*, London: Age Concern England.

Murray, R., D. Harding, T. Angus, R. Gillespie and H. Arora (2012), *Emigration from the UK*, 2nd edn, Research Report 68, November, London: Home Office.

Oliver, C. (2008), *Retirement Migration: Paradoxes of Ageing*, London: Routledge.

O'Reilly, K. (2000), *The British on the Costa del Sol: Transnational Identities and Local Communities*, London: Routledge.

O'Reilly, K. (2007), Intra-European migration and the mobility-enclosure dialectic, *Sociology*, **41**(2), 277–293.

Rodríguez, V., G. Fernández-Mayoralas and F. Rojo (2004), International retirement migration: retired Europeans living on the Costa del Sol, Spain, *Population Review*, **43**, 1–36
Royal British Legion (2009), *Caring in Spain Study into the Current and Future Care Needs of the British Ex-Service Community Permanently Resident in Spain*, Centre for Future Studies, February, available online at www.britishlegion.org.uk/media/138809/caringinspainreport.pdf.
Sriskandarajah, D. and C. Drew (2006), *Brits Abroad: Mapping the Scale and Nature of British Emigration*, London: Institute for Public Policy Research.
Stevens, J. (2006), Paradise turns to death trap for British expats in Spain, *The Observer*, 7 September.

22 Migrant children and young people's 'voice' in healthcare

Daniela Sime

INTRODUCTION

Across the UK and internationally there is a fast-growing commitment to listening to young people in decisions that affect their lives, including in public decision-making. The case for the importance of taking young people's views into account and facilitating their participation has been made on grounds of both principle and pragmatism. In the past, researchers have been criticised for considering them as 'objects of study' rather than seeking their experiences and their views on what is important to them and their lives. Prout (2001: 193) argued that children's voices should be listened to because they have their own consciousness as 'persons in their own right' and arguably experience the world in their own ways. Adopting adults' perspectives on matters that concern children and young people reflects historic approaches of power and regulation, and young people's generational positioning as less knowledgeable and in need of being controlled.

Children's distinct life experiences and competencies, including their ability to share their views if appropriate ways of involving them are identified, have been increasingly recognised by research and policymakers alike (Punch 2002). The 1989 United Nations Convention on the Rights of the Child (UNCRC) clearly affirms children and young people's rights to an adequate standard of living, the highest attainable standard of health and the right to be consulted and participate in decisions that have a direct impact on their lives. This means that including children and young people and taking into account their views is not only good practice, but also a matter of rights and entitlements, and public services have a duty to ensure that these rights are respected.

In a healthcare context, it is important to acknowledge that children and young people may experience health, illness and healthcare provision in significantly distinct ways to adults. The UNCRC states that rights should be ensured for all children and young people, irrespective of their various statuses, including nationality, ethnicity, language, social class or race. In today's globalised world, these statuses overlap and intersect for most, not always in positive ways, as children's health outcomes and wellbeing differ across diverse nations, ethnic and socioeconomic groups. The extent to which their rights to participation are ensured also depends on the ways in which they are thought of by others in the societies in which they live.

Children and young people's health and wellbeing is significant not only for their everyday lives, but also for the futures of the societies in which they live. In this context, listening to young people's views on provision of healthcare is key, to ensure that their needs are met and also to identify the challenges for services in meeting these needs. It is also important to ensure that all voices are heard, as certain groups are often more likely to be included in debates. Young people traditionally excluded are often on the periphery of society, for example, those living in extreme poverty, migrants, those affected by disabilities or mental health issues, or young people not in education. In many countries, certain groups also fall outside existing services, as rights to access public services might be restricted, as in the case of asylum-seekers, refugees or illegal migrants (Jayaweera 2010).

This chapter draws on research with Eastern European migrant children newly arrived in the UK in relation to experiences of healthcare provision post-migration. Although understanding users' views of healthcare provision is key to informing policy on health-related measures, the views of migrant groups, and in particular those of children and young people, are rarely explored. In order to address this gap, this chapter examines first the wider context of the physical and mental health status of migrant children and adults, the social determinants that influence migrant children's health outcomes and issues in their access to and use of healthcare services post-migration. The main focus is on children and young people's views of health service provision, the barriers they face in relation to health service use and the strategies migrant families adopt to overcome perceived shortcomings in provision, including adopting a transnational use of health services.

In the context of migration, young people's experiences of healthcare are significant because provision might need to adapt to meet their specific needs, as they may experience distinct barriers in terms of access and the quality of their experience. As already mentioned, children and young people are also entitled to healthcare rights, and effective policies need to be developed to ensure these rights are met. The chapter highlights the important role of migrants' active participation as users of health services, with a significant role for children and young people as cultural brokers for adults, and concludes that appropriate health policy and care delivery should take into account the needs and expectations of diverse populations.

SEEKING THE VIEWS OF CHILDREN AND YOUNG PEOPLE

In this chapter, I refer to migrant children and young people as those who were born in one country and then relocated to another country with their family, through planned rather than forced migration. I do not include refugee and asylum-seeking children, as their needs are acknowledged as more complex, due to the likely more traumatic nature of their migratory situations and legal status (Kohli 2006). Over the past two decades, research with children and young people has seen a significant shift in terms of how researchers perceive children and their ability to contribute to the research process, not only as research participants, but also as research partners and co-researchers (Kellett 2005). This has included an emphasis on the 'competent child' (or young person), and change in attitudes in relation to children and young people's ability to contribute as experts in their lives, often attributed to the rise of constructivist and interpretive theoretical perspectives in sociology (James and Prout 1997; James et al. 1998; 1998; Prout 2005). This 'new sociology of childhood' aims to reframe views of childhood as experienced, debated and defined in processes of social action that have children and young people as central actors.

While children's rights to participate have been enshrined in the United Nations Convention on the Rights of the Child (UNCRC) since 1989, it is only recently that children's and young people's views have been acknowledged as valid in their own right. There is now an expectation that research will consider children's rights to participate in investigating issues that affect them, including family legal procedures or initiatives to do with public places and the services they access. Prout (2001: 193) argued that taking notice of children's voices should be a matter of priority because 'it speaks to questions of flexibility and responsiveness in welfare and service provision and to debates about young people's engagement with key institutions such as schools'.

Articles 12 and 13 of the UNCRC explicitly address the right of children to be informed, involved and consulted in decisions that affect their lives, although the rights are expressed with several caveats, which have been criticised for the difficulties they pose for implementation (Bell 2008; Spyrou 2011). For example, Article 12 limits the right of participation to children who are 'capable of forming their own view', putting the responsibility on adults to decide on individual children's capability. This logically leads to questions around how capability should be established and by what measures and again puts adults in a position of power, as they make the judgement. Although Article 12 places the onus on adults to take responsibility for including children's views, it gives very little guidance on how this might be achieved. Similarly, Article 3, which discusses the best interests of the child as a key priority in any matters involving children, implies that adults need to prioritise children's protection and wellbeing. Nevertheless, these statements are not straightforward in their application, as adults need clear mechanisms to identify children who might be vulnerable and consider the ways in which ideas such as right to participation, protection and vulnerability are constructed across times, social groups and cultures (Rogoff 2003). Despite these caveats, the Convention provides a critical framework and a mechanism for empowering children in research and the shift in childhood studies has also been matched by a shift in wider policies on the inclusion of children's voice in governance at various levels. In the UK, for example, recent policies such as the Children and Families Bill 2013 in England (DfE 2013), and the Children and Young People (Scotland) Bill 2013 (Scottish Parliament 2013) emphasise the importance of giving children and young people an active role in decisions that concern their lives – for example, through contributing to improvement of local services – and place responsibility on services to create opportunities for consultation.

THE IMPACT OF MIGRATION ON THE HEALTH OF EASTERN EUROPEAN MIGRANTS

Migratory patterns to the UK have seen a significant change over the past two decades, in terms of migrants' country of origin, reasons for migration and settlement patterns (Castles and Miller 2013). Data from the last UK population census indicate that more than 7.5 million people, or 12 per cent of the UK population, were born abroad (ONS 2013), with the most common countries of birth being Poland, India and Pakistan. With the expansion of the European Union (EU) in the past decade, an increasing number of labour migrants to the UK now come from Central and Eastern Europe. Unlike in the past, when many adults migrated alone, a significant number of recently arrived European migrants have migrated together with their families, many of which include children and young people. Unlike people arriving from the non-EU countries, EU migrants have full entitlement to healthcare in the UK, as all 28 EU member states have either publicly sponsored or regulated universal healthcare. Since 2011, a directive on healthcare promotes cooperation between member states and access to safe and high-quality cross-border healthcare for European citizens (European Union 2011). However, despite free access to healthcare, comparatively little is known about EU migrants' health and wellbeing overall and their experiences of accessing healthcare provision post-migration.

The increase in the number of recently arrived migrants has led to debates about migrants' impact on the economy, the likely increase in demand for public services and, more broadly, the influence of migration on cultural values and national identity in receiving countries (Yuval-Davis 2011). Current debates on immigration often centre on the provision of public services (Spencer 2011). While some claim that increased migration has led to pressure on public services in the UK context (Institute of Community Cohesion 2007), others have raised concerns about migrants' low uptake of healthcare (Rolfe and Metcalf 2009; Collis et al. 2010), with some recent data suggesting that areas with increased rates of immigration have seen reduced waiting times for hospital outpatient referrals across England (Giuntella et al. 2015). It is generally perceived that European migrants are mostly young and healthy, which may explain their low service use. The 'healthy migrant effect' may also be due to self-selection, as migrants are likely to consider their health before deciding to move abroad. However, international research shows that in contrast with the 'healthy migrant effect' in the early stages of a migratory wave, migrants have a higher risk of deteriorating health over time through the so-called 'health acculturation' (Ronellenfitsch and Razum 2004), which occurs independently of improvements in their socioeconomic condition. Collis et al. (2010) also highlighted that many of the Eastern European countries that migrants leave from continue to focus on treatment rather than prevention in relation to key public health concerns, such as alcohol and tobacco use, obesity and low levels of physical activity, and mental health concerns. Increased stress and anxiety often triggered by the experience of migrating have also been linked to higher risks of developing somatic complaints and illnesses, such as heart disease, depression and anxiety (Robila 2010). Cultural differences might also affect health outcomes; for example, through perpetuating stigma around mental health issues, which can adversely impact on psychological and emotional health and attitudes to asking for professional help. One major factor in researching the effect of migration on individuals' health outcomes is the fact that data on migrants' health are scarce, mainly because migrants are not a homogenous group and country of birth and immigration status are not recorded consistently when health services are accessed.

While studies on the health of adult migrants are limited overall, studies on the health of migrant children in the UK are almost non-existent. Elsewhere, studies of migrant children have reported on the unique situations that contribute to their increased risk of poorer physical and mental health. The age at which they make the transition from one country to another has been highlighted as significant in how they adapt to the new country, with younger children faring better in terms of health and education outcomes (Chuang and Moreno 2013). Research with immigrant adolescents in Europe has reported on their difficulties concerning physical and mental health, and social isolation, with significantly higher scores on all scales of psychological distress and psychological problems (Sandhu and Mooza 2013). Like their parents, young Eastern European migrants may perceive mental health difficulties as taboo and worry about the stigma of accessing support, despite evidence that they present an increased risk of somatic complaints and illnesses such as depression, anxiety and suicide ideation in relation to non-migrant groups (Robila 2010). Beisser et al. (1998) have identified several unique situations that may contribute to the mental health issues of migrant youth. These include: adapting to family separation; disruption to education and language issues; and pressure to adapt to new customs while also conforming to their parents' expectations in relation to values from their homeland. Some migrant children also experience racism in schools and neighbourhoods (Devine 2009), which may result in poor self-esteem and self-worth and feelings of marginalisation.

Social determinants of health from individual characteristics (such as age, sex and constitutional factors), to social and community networks and socioeconomic and environmental conditions (such as education, housing, working conditions) play a key role in explaining the health practices and outcomes for migrant groups (Dahlgren and Whitehead 1991). Migrants' experiences are often polarised and aspects such as social class, types of jobs migrants engage in and the social capital available to them intersect in a multitude of ways in shaping their health outcomes (Ryan 2011). For migrants in low-skilled jobs, government measurements that restrict access to work and public services for certain groups and negative public perceptions of migrants can also significantly increase their disadvantage and contribute structurally and institutionally to poor health outcomes. Factors such as different expectations and cultural beliefs in relation to health have been shown to influence the health-related decision-making and behaviours of migrants from a wide range of socioeconomic backgrounds (Spencer et al. 2007; Son 2013; Thomas 2010). Migrants' health is thus influenced by a range of political, social and economic forces and one's status as recent migrant can be seen as an additional layer to those already identified by existing models of social determinants of health (Sime 2014).

CONDUCTING RESEARCH WITH YOUNG MIGRANTS

The impact of migration on children and young people's health and well-being, as well as their views on their access to healthcare provision and experiences of health services constitute a relatively new research area in a European context. Consideration of the most appropriate research approaches and techniques is therefore important in ensuring that participation is facilitated and does not become adult-led, restrictive or too burdensome for some young people. Thomson (2008) has outlined the advantages of doing participatory and visual research with children, as it allows them the means to take some control of the research process. By encouraging children's lead in the process of generating the data and in directing the discussion within interviews, children gain a voice and can influence the outcome of the research and its impact. Participatory and visual forms of research can also be effective methods for use with newly arrived young migrants, particularly where fluency in the language of the host population may be an issue. Researchers also need to consider their structural position, in terms of age, ethnicity and class, and how this can influence power relationships in the process and affect issues of access, consent, data collection, analysis and dissemination (Sime 2008).

Child-centred, qualitative research has clear advantages in giving migrant children a voice to inform current policy, practice and debates on global migration and social justice. However, researchers need to be mindful of migrant children's position within their families and society overall. Their participation is often hedged by constraints and controls (Sime 2015). In families, adults may want to ensure that children's participation is restricted to topics that families are comfortable with and non-intrusive in relation to family relationships, roles and rules, or adults may want to speak on behalf of their children.

In this chapter, I draw on data collected with 57 Eastern European children, aged seven to 16, who had lived in Scotland for less than three years at the time of the study. They were of both genders (31 girls and 26 boys) and from a range of socioeconomic backgrounds and the majority (48) were Polish, the main migratory group to the UK since 2004. Given children and young people's diverse competencies and preferences, a range of research methods and techniques were used to ensure that all involved were able to find the best tools to express their views. Fieldwork combined focus groups, individual interviews, diaries and photography. Focus groups have been shown to work well with children (Hennesy and Heary 2005), as they allow them to stimulate each other's ideas, and also allow the researcher to assess the extent to which the group shares beliefs and experiences. They were conducted in the children's own language (eight groups) and with interpreters present for multilingual groups (three groups), and covered children's access and views in relation to a range of services, including healthcare. Participants were encouraged to discuss first the experiences of a 'typical migrant family', a technique adopted in order to reduce the pressure of having to share personal stories, but still drawing on their knowledge and beliefs about migrants' lives in the UK. They could thus talk indirectly about what a migrant child 'would' experience, but also relate to their own experiences if they wished to. Child-centred activities were used, based on images of services children were likely to access – such as schools, medical centres, leisure centres, parks, etc. – and hands-on activities, to stimulate children's enthusiasm and engagement (Christensen and James 2000).

Following on from the focus groups, 23 in-depth family case studies were completed, including 29 children (six pairs of siblings were involved) and at least one parent in each family. The case studies included a majority of Polish children (n = 13), and five Lithuanian, four Slovak, two Bulgarian and two Romanian children, as well as one Hungarian, one Russian and one Czech family. In total, 15 girls and 14 boys were involved, with an average age of 11 (age range was 8–16 years old). All case studies consisted of visits to children's homes, as homes were seen as a more relaxed environment than public spaces. However, domestic spaces are not always under children and young people's control, as these are often shared spaces with other family members (Sime 2008). To increase children's sense of control over the process, we gave them the opportunity to take photographs of services they used and to complete a weekly diary. While some children and young people enjoyed these activities, others were more reluctant and preferred to just talk about their experiences. This highlights the importance of having a flexible set of tools and techniques that young people can choose from and the necessity of ensuring, on an ongoing basis, that young people are still in agreement to take part.

YOUNG MIGRANTS' HEALTH BEHAVIOURS AND ENGAGEMENT WITH HEALTH SERVICES POST-MIGRATION

Adult European migrants have been found to engage with health services less regularly than the majority population (Spencer et al. 2007; Collis et al. 2010). Despite public speculation that migrants add pressure on services (Delanti et al. 2011), there is very little systematic evidence in the UK on services accessed by migrants, patterns of use and views of services available. There is also limited evidence on how migrants' health behaviours alter as a result of family migration and changes to their family income and cultural influences in the new society. Children are strongly influenced by their families' ideas about health and healthy behaviours (Sime 2014). Shared values among individuals have a key role in the creation of social capital (Bassani 2007) and, in the case of migrant families, cultural values and knowledge shape their beliefs about health and health practices (Migge and Gillmartin, 2011).

Health behaviours and practices may appear to be private matters for individuals and families, but they are configured by a range of social contexts, which for children and young people consist of schools, family, peer group and neighbourhoods (Morrow 2010). While some authors claim that unchanged dietary habits, health beliefs and practices in migrant adults may be indicative of an emotional attachment to their home culture (Son 2013), others have emphasised the socioeconomic factors and inequalities that make positive health practices more affordable to the better-off (McKendrick et al. 2014; Nazroo 2014). Parents and children may also wish to adopt healthy behaviours and eating habits, but may be limited by the local availability and affordability of healthy foods or sports activities.

In our research, most of the children and young people gave largely positive accounts of their health overall and were confident in terms of accessing services available, such as GPs, pharmacies, hospitals and dentists. Most children were able to discuss particular aspects of the health system and health practices that they encountered in Scotland, often making comparisons with provision that they had encountered in their country of origin. Although sometimes they would differ in their assessment of quality of provision – for example, their perceptions of the competence of medical staff – they regularly commented on the better quality of the resources and equipment and the free prescriptions or services such as dental checks and eye tests available to all in Scotland:

> Zuzanna (12): Maybe the dentist and medication for kids is free here, so that's better. But maybe in Poland you get to see better doctors, not only GPs.
> Esther (13): I think that Polish doctors are better.
> Dzulieta (14): I think that it is the same here and there.
> Wioleta (14): I think that they have better equipment here.
>
> (Polish focus group)

While most children were registered with family doctors (or GPs), some were not, and were reliant on emergency services in case of illness. Some also said that they had kept registration with doctors and dentists in their country of origin. This reflected families' confidence in services they were familiar with, but also their precarious work conditions, which meant that return was also a possibility and families wanted to keep their registration with services in their own country:

> We haven't been here [in Scotland] long, so we didn't register yet with a doctor, but mum said we can go to the hospital in case of anything. But we are usually quite healthy.
>
> (Marta, Polish, 12)

> My mum says we might not stay here [in Scotland] long if she cannot find work, so we kept our doctor back in Poland, just in case.
>
> (Marek, Polish, 10)

Many children and young people commented on the child-centred approach to healthcare from the medical staff. This gave them a sense of empowerment and involvement in decisions on their care and was seen as good practice:

> I feel they talk to you more here [in the UK] and they ask you what you want, [they do] not just [ask] your mother.
>
> (Ana, 13, Bulgarian)

Children with chronic conditions commented on cross-cultural differences relating to the management of their conditions, and how they had to adapt to new views on suitable medication, practices and routines of engaging with medical staff. These included differences in medication that was prescribed for the same condition in different countries, the frequency of check-ups and the medical staff young people would interact with. One key aspect children and young people commented on was access to specialists, which seemed to be more routine in Eastern European countries even for minor conditions, while in the UK, their conditions were managed by GPs or local practice nurses. In addition to more immediate access, the issue of trust and reassurance that familiar doctors offered and the benefit of a shared language were other considerations when families decided to travel abroad to access healthcare. Ana, a Bulgarian teenager who had a chronic eye condition, explained how she perceived the long waiting times to see a specialist as frustrating and unhelpful, which in her case led to her mother's decision to travel to Bulgaria and see a specialist straight away:

> Well, here, you wait like months to get to a doctor . . . which is annoying . . . boring . . . you know you have an appointment, but it's so far away that you forget about it and just live your life and by the time your appointment comes, you are OK. So we went to see the Bulgarian doctor, the one that operated on

me. And she said it's OK if we wait and see how it goes, because it might get worse if they operate again. And I trust her more, I feel safer with her.

(Ana, 13, Bulgarian)

BARRIERS FOR YOUNG MIGRANTS' ACCESS TO HEALTH

It is clear from many studies that migrant families encounter a range of barriers that prevent them from accessing healthcare (Sime 2014; Robila 2010; Thomas 2010; Son 2013). In the UK context, with constant changes to rules around entitlements to access to healthcare, especially for non-EU migrants, young people and their families can face a constant struggle to understand the health system in their new country and the rules of engagement with service providers. In addition, the uncertainty over their families' entitlement to healthcare and treatment, especially immediately after their arrival, cultural differences in provision and approaches to treatment and language barriers can make the experiences of accessing health provision more difficult. In this section, we emphasise three types of barriers that research has identified as significant in relation to migrant groups, including lack of adequate information, cultural differences in the provision of care and the language barrier. I reflect on these from children and young people's perspective, as their experiences are often distinct from adults' own views and young people are often in the position of facilitating service access for their families, due to their access to information through schools and their competence in the majority language (Sime and Pietka-Nykaza 2015).

Lack of Adequate Information on Entitlements and Services Available

Children and young people's life experiences post-migration are configured by a range of factors, which include their parents' values, aspirations and employment opportunities. In our sample, most parents were in jobs below their level of qualification, often working in catering, food processing, agriculture or construction jobs. Many women were homemakers, due to their limited English language skills. This meant that many families relied on one income, often precarious and dependant on availability of work. Family income influences access to good-quality housing (Rolfe and Metcalf 2009) or the type of neighbourhoods in which migrants live (McGhee et al. 2013), meaning that migrant children and young people may become marginalised due to the complex interactions that result at the juncture of age, ethnicity, social class and place. Low income and poverty may lead to poor nutrition and substandard living conditions. By being forced to access low-cost accommodation in areas of high deprivation, migrants' access to services is affected by their status as new arrivals. Services are often of poorer quality in deprived areas and migrants may feel at risk in terms of personal safety when trying to access these (Spencer et al. 2007). In addition, the novelty of the new system and lack of direct experience of interacting with services in their new country may put them at a disadvantage in terms of access to information about services available.

In my research, I asked newly arrived migrant children if they accessed healthcare services available in the community, such as specialist or well-being clinics, pharmacies or spaces for leisure that could help promote better health. I report elsewhere the overall limited knowledge among new migrants of services available locally (Sime and Fox 2014; Sime 2015). Many families, newly arrived, were not certain of their entitlement to access health services, although all are free at point of use. They also relied on accident and emergency (A&E) care 'if something happened' and were not always registered with a doctor or dentist. Children from countries that had limited rights in terms of access to the employment market and welfare benefits at the time of the study (Romania and Bulgaria were not at the time EU members) were affected by their families' restricted access to healthcare. This meant that in some cases, families made deliberate decisions not to access care for fear of deportation and limited information on what health practitioners would and would not do in relation to their immigration status.

Information on access to health services is often mediated by schools, who send home information, bring interpreters into school to explain to parents what other services are available locally or actively mediate access for the families and, in some cases, help them register with doctors or dentists or fill in registration forms for families. In this process, children become important 'cultural brokers' for their families, translating information or exercising pressure on families to access provision, for example, to leisure facilities. As I show elsewhere (Sime and Pietka-Nykaza 2015), children's enhanced linguistic competence in English and regular contact with services through school positions them as 'experts' in the family and confers them a certain advantage over their parents, especially if the parents' linguistic competence is still developing. This reversal of social norms means that children can often have the main role in mediating their families' access to opportunities, which can also lead to increased ambivalence in children towards their parents' homeland language, culture and identity, as well as increasing pressure on children given the responsibility. Children and young people are also more likely to interact with other children through play and leisure time, and in so doing, enable the realisation of important social capital benefits (Putnam 2000). Participation in the community is also an opportunity for children to develop networks with other ethnic groups, and use these as sources of information and as a route to better access to community resources. However, networks of access to resources may be built in ways that privilege some 'insiders' (i.e., the established communities) over newcomers. For example, local children and young people may know of ongoing clubs, activities or have their own informal networks of getting together with friends to engage in leisure activities. In some cases, migrant children relied on information from their friends and their limited experience of services to assist with parents' decisions and actions. The roles young migrants have to take on to facilitate their families' engagement with local services therefore require complex skills and confidence and involve activities usually reserved for adults. These new roles may also pose increased pressure on them, including a risk to their mental health and wellbeing.

Cultural Differences in Provision and Rules of Engagement with Services

Previous experiences of the health system in the homeland will influence migrants' behaviours in relation to how the health system in the new country is accessed, expectations about how accessible services are and perceptions of the medical staff. I reported elsewhere (Sime 2014) on health practitioners' views that differences in provision led to disappointment among migrants, who often complained about waiting lists, restricted access to specialists and different approaches to treatment. A common complaint is on the perceived 'paracetamol culture', where practitioners prescribe mild painkillers for conditions commonly treated with antibiotics in other countries.

> I was very sick last year, and they give me only paracetamol, and I was ill for two months. It was something with my neck, I couldn't speak. I was in the hospital and they just give me that.
>
> (Agnieska, 15, Polish)

Perceived differences in approaches to treating conditions also led some families to adopt more informal approaches towards solving health problems, such as relying on family and friends for advice and treatment. These approaches included: emergency visits to the homeland to access doctors and dentists and to avoid 'waiting lists' in the UK or high charges for private care; or asking family members to post medicines or check a diagnosis with known medical staff in the homeland.

> Romek [son] got an allergy after the swimming pool, so I went to emergency. The woman looked at photos on the internet and then she gave me a prescription for some cream. But then I read the instructions and realised it was for scabies, so I called Agata, my friend, because her son had a similar problem, and I borrowed from her the cream that she got in Poland and it helped.
>
> (Dagmara, Polish mother)

> We couldn't get antibiotics here, and my mum was sure the doctor was wrong, so we called my auntie back home and she went to our local doctor [in Poland], told them what I have and then they posted me the medicine.
>
> (Marek, 14, Poland)

A key finding reported in the literature is that as migrants access better work and become more familiar with the system, they are able to build networks of support and become better-informed on existing services and how these operate. Research with Eastern European families (Sime and Fox 2014; McGhee et al. 2013), for example, has reported on families' narratives around temporary, transitional housing arrangements, such as residing in poorer areas, with a view of moving on to better opportunities once their work opportunities improve. As migrants strive to improve their work and living circumstances, their understanding and expectations of health services also change (Migge and Gilmartin 2011). In the case of children and young people, the influence of education, friendship groups and other members of the local community means that their health behaviours, attitudes to health and wellbeing and expectations of health services are also likely to change over time. In this context, practitioners need to be aware of the changing nature of migrants' expectations and health-related behaviours and values over time, to ensure provision is addressing their needs and takes into account their changing values and expectations.

The Language Barrier

Language is a key barrier to many migrants' access to health services. Migrants have different levels of competence in the language of their destination country and their developing competence in the majority language affects their ability to access information on services and entitlements, and their experience of interacting with medical practitioners and understanding treatment options. In our study, as children often developed their competence in English much more rapidly than their parents due to their school attendance, they were often asked by their parents to translate information materials or act as interpreters in medical appointments:

> When you don't understand, it's hard to know [what is available], like my mum when the nurses were visiting her, she said that she doesn't understand and they try to translate it, point it out until she will understand. Or if I am home, then I do it for her, tell her what they said, read the paperwork for her.
>
> (Klaudia, 13, Polish)

As discussed above, children and young people may feel under pressure to act as interpreters, and they may often give the impression of full competence in the new language, while lacking the full vocabulary to translate accurately. For practitioners, using children as interpreters is to be discouraged, for concerns over confidentiality and unreasonable pressure on children as well as their developing competence to interpret complex terminology and convey medical conversations accurately, and good practice would require professional interpreters to be booked for medical appointments. Working with families through an interpreter poses several challenges in terms of establishing rapport, collecting information, explaining treatment and time pressures, as appointments are usually time-limited. In addition, the cost of involving an interpreter or the limited availability of interpreters for less common minority languages may delay appointments and deter families from engaging with services. Research has also highlighted how migrants' feelings of unease about local care provision due to perceived social, cultural, religious and linguistic differences and lack of trust prompt people to seek care in more familiar contexts, such as from health providers in their country of origin (Glinos et al. 2010; Migge and Gilmartin 2011).

CONCLUSION

This chapter aimed to summarise the evidence on access to and experiences of formal health services from the perspective of migrant children, young people and their families. Many of the experiences that children and young people have post-migration are likely to have a direct impact on their wellbeing. As their quality of life is directly configured by their families' socioeconomic circumstances, the neighbourhoods in which they live and their friendship networks post-migration, there is an increasing need for local and central government policymakers to ensure a good quality of life and adequate access to health services for newly arrived migrant youth. There has been very little qualitative research or consultation to assess the extent to which newly arrived migrants engage successfully with health services and to elicit their views on experiences of health, access to healthcare and any barriers they encounter in accessing provision. Furthermore, data on migrants' health and use of health services is scarce and patchy, as country of origin, length of stay in the UK or immigration status are not recorded when individuals access healthcare. As mentioned at the beginning of this chapter, including children and young people and taking into account their views is not just good practice, it is a matter of social justice and public services have a duty to ensure that their rights are respected.

Working with young migrants in a health context poses specific challenges for practitioners and requires them to take a holistic approach. One significant challenge is to register young people with services such as GP practices and dentists, especially given the fact that they have little control at times over family decisions. Children and young people can, however, exert influence on their parents, mainly by translating information and finding out from their friends about services available, but the key issue seems to be around challenges to make adults understand services and trust available provision. Contrary to speculation in the media around practices such as 'health tourism' and pressure on health services due to increased migration to the UK, migrants seem to access a limited range of statutory provision and often find alternative routes to state provision, including private and transnational care. Acculturation plays another significant role in how migrant young people adopt or not healthy behaviours and practices – they may be more inclined to adopt new health practices, based on information they get from school, media and other sources in the new language, while still having less control over family decisions. Migrants' views of health services and expectations are often mapped on their prior experiences and this must be considered by healthcare professionals in the UK. It is clear that differences in provision and expectations about the rules of engagement with services need to be made more explicit to newly arrived migrants in order to better engage them in health-promoting behaviours and gain their trust. Practitioners need to review what prevents children and their families from making efficient use of the full range of health services. This suggests that health services need to be delivered in a culturally sensitive manner, with awareness of children and young people's position in families and communities.

It is evident that family migration poses significant challenges for children and young people and impacts on their health, health behaviours and wellbeing. For migrant children and young people, factors such as the migration experience (positive or negative), length of residence in the new country, socioeconomic position, age, gender and resilience may help explain different health behaviours and outcomes. Their varied attitudes to healthcare are likely to be influenced by their parents' social class before migration and socioeconomic situation post-migration, and their prior experiences of healthcare. To this extent, their views of healthcare need full consideration in order to inform policy and practitioners' behaviours. Healthcare providers must be sensitive and alert to the personal factors that affect migrant children and their families' decisions to engage with services and work with them to tailor provision whenever possible. Research shows that some families choose to use services transnationally or seek help from informal networks when they lack trust in health services in the new country. Accessing healthcare through multiple routes indicates the active role migrants adopt in making decisions about their use of healthcare provision and children and young people are often key actors within these decisions.

Migrant children are at a crossroads of influences in terms of the health behaviours they should adopt, attitudes about health service utilisation and levels of trust in health practitioners. While their parents might value more the healthcare system they are familiar with and they understand better, children will be expected to engage in sometimes different health behaviours by their schools and peer groups. Health practitioners working with newly arrived migrant children should be mindful of the multiple influences that impact on their expectations and beliefs and engage them in conversations to dispel any myths and address any concerns they might have. As young people develop their understanding of how healthcare operates in their new country, it is likely that their perceptions and beliefs will change over time. Also, as children's linguistic competence in English is sometimes more advanced than that of their parents due to their schooling, migrant children may in time become mediators of cultural knowledge about services available to their families (Sime and Fox 2014; Sime and Pietka-Nykaza 2015).

Transnational use of health services is a feature of family life for many European migrants, especially in the first few years after migration, and health practitioners need to be aware of children's exposure to possibly distinct cultures of practice. It is also important to highlight that not all children and young people coming from one country will have the same health experiences or outcomes. Existing research shows how different social and economic circumstances are the main contributing factors to children's unequal health outcomes (Morrow 2010; McKendrick et al. 2014). As a result, children and young people's health practices post-migration will take place in a range of new social arenas, while also influenced by their families' cultural values around health. There remains a need for substantial policy and practice development in relation to the health of migrant groups, with a specific focus on engagement of children and young people as an issue of rights and social justice, as well as good practice.

REFERENCES

Bassani, C. (2007), Five dimensions of social capital theory as they pertain to youth studies, *Journal of Youth Studies*, **10**(1), 17–34.
Bell, N. (2008), Ethics in child research: rights, reason and responsibilities, *Children's Geographies*, **6**(1), 7–20.
Beisser, M., M. Wood, C. Barwick, J. Berry, G. daCosta and W. Milne (1998), *After the Door has been Opened: Mental Health Issues Affecting Immigrants and Refugees in Canada*, Ottawa: Ministries of Multiculturalism and Citizenship and Health and Welfare.
Castles, S. and M. J. Miller (2013), *The Age of Migration: International Populations Movements in the Modern World*, 5th edn, London: Palgrave.
Christensen, P. and A. James (2000), *Research with Children: Perspectives and Practices*, London: Routledge.
Chuang, S. and R. P. Moreno (eds.) (2013), *Immigrant Children: Change, Adaptation and Cultural Transformation*, Maryland: Lexington Books.
Collis, A., N. Stott and D. Ross (2010), *Workers on the Move 3: European Migrant Workers and Health in the UK: The Evidence*, Norfolk: Keystone Development Trust.
Dahlgren, G. and M. Whitehead (1991), *Policies and Strategies to Promote Social Equity in Health*, Stockholm: Institute for Future Studies.
Delanti, G., R. Wodak and P. Jones (2011), *Identity, Belonging and Migration*, Liverpool: Liverpool University Press.
DfE (2013), *Children and Families Bill 2013*, London: Department of Education.
Devine, D. (2009), Mobilising capitals? Migrant children's negotiations of their everyday lives in the primary school, *British Journal of Sociology of Education*, **30**(5), 521–535.
European Union (2011), *Directive 2011/24/EU of the European Parliament and of the Council of 9th March 2011 on the Application of Patients' Rights in Cross-Border Healthcare*, Strasbourg.
Giuntella, O., C. Nicodemo and C. Vargas Silva (2015), *The Effects of Immigration on NHS Waiting Times*, available online at www.bsg.ox.ac.uk/research/working-paper-series/working-paper-005.
Glinos, I. A., R. Beaten, M. Herbe and G. Maarse (2010), A typology of cross-border patient mobility, *Health and Place*, **16**, 1145–1155.
Hennesy, E. and C. Heary (2005), Exploring children's views through focus groups, in S. Greene and D. Hogan (eds.), *Researching Children's Experience*, London: Sage, pp. 236–253.
Institute of Community Cohesion (2007), *Estimating the Scale and Impact of Migration at a Local Level*, London: Local Government Association.
James, A. and A. Prout (1997), *Constructing and Reconstructing Childhood*, London: Falmer.
James, A., C. Jenks and A. Prout (1998), *Theorising Childhood*, Cambridge: Polity Press.
Jayaweera, H. (2010), *Health and Access to Health Care of Migrants in the UK*, London: Race Equality Foundation.
Migge, B. and M. Gilmartin (2011), Migrants and healthcare: investigating patient mobility among migrants in Ireland, *Health & Place*, **17**, 1144–1149.
Kellett, M. (2005), *How to Develop Children as Researchers: A Step by Step Guide to Teaching the Research Process*, London: Paul Chapman.
Kohli, R. (2006), *Social Work with Unaccompanied Asylum Seeking Children*, New York: Palgrave Macmillan.
McGhee, D., S. Heath and P. Trevena (2013), Post-accession Polish migrants – their experiences of living in 'low-demand' social housing areas in Glasgow, *Environment and Planning*, **45**(2), 329–343.
McKendrick, J., G. Mooney, J. Dickie, G. Scott and P. Kelly (2014), *Poverty in Scotland: The Independence Referendum and Beyond*, London: Child Poverty Action Group.
Migge, B. and M. Gilmartin (2011), Migrants and healthcare: investigating patient mobility among migrants in Ireland, *Health & Place*, **17**, 1144–1149.
Morrow, V. (2010), Children's 'social capital': Implications for health and well-being, in

J. Rix, M. Nind, S. Kieron, K. Simmon and C. Walsh (eds.), *Equality, Participation and Inclusion*, 2nd edn, London: Routledge, pp. 271–285.
Nazroo, J. Y. (2014), *'If You Could Do One Thing. . .' Nine Local Actions to Reduce Health Inequalities*, London: British Academy, pp. 91–102.
ONS (2013), *Population by Country of Birth and Nationality Report*, Newport: Office for National Statistics.
Prout, A. (2001), Representing children: reflections on the Children 5–16 Programme, *Children & Society*, **15**, 193–201.
Prout, A. (2005), *The Future of Childhood*, London: Routledge.
Punch, S. (2002), Research with children: the same or different from research with adults? *Childhood*, **9**(3), 321–341.
Putnam, R. (2000), *Bowling Alone: The Collapse and Revival of American Community*, New York: Simon & Schuster.
Robila, M. (2010), *Eastern European Immigrant Families*, London: Routledge.
Rogoff, B. (2003), *The Cultural Nature of Human Development*, Maidenhead: Open University Press.
Rolfe, H. and H. Metcalf (2009), *Recent Migration into Scotland: The Evidence Base*, Edinburgh: National Institute of Economic and Social Research.
Ronellenfitsch, U. and O. Razum (2004), Deteriorating health satisfaction among immigrants from Eastern Europe to Germany, *International Journal of Equity in Health*, **3**(4), 1–10.
Ryan, L. (2011), Migrants' social networks and weak ties: accessing resources and constructing relationships post-migration, *The Sociological Review*, **59**(4), 707–724.
Sandhu, T. and F. Mooza (2013), Mental health of children of immigrants and ethnic minorities in Europe, *Adolescent Psychiatry*, **3**(1), 30–34.
Scottish Parliament (2013), *Children and Young People (Scotland) Bill*, Edinburgh: Scottish Parliament.
Sime, D. (2008), Ethical aspects of conducting research with children and young people in their homes, *Children's Geographies*, **6**(1), 63–78.
Sime, D. (2014), 'I think that Polish doctors are better': experiences with and views of health services in Scotland among newly arrived migrant children and their parents, *Health & Place*, **30**, 86–93.
Sime, D. (2015), Methodological aspects of conducting research with Eastern European children and young people, in T. Skelton, L. Holt and R. Evans (ed.), *Geographies of Children and Young People (Vol. 2), Methodological Approaches*, New York: Springer.
Sime, D. and R. Fox (2014), Migrant children, social capital and access to public services: transitions, negotiations and complex agencies, *Children & Society*, **29**(6), 524–534.
Sime, D. and E. Pietka-Nykaza (2015), Transnational intergenerationalities: cultural learning in Polish migrant families and its implications for pedagogy, *Language and Intercultural Communication*, **15**(2), 208–223.
Son, J. (2013), Assimilation and health service utilization of Korean immigrant women, *Qualitative Health Research*, **23**(11), 1528–1540.
Spencer, S. (2011), *The Migration Debate*, London: Polity Press.
Spencer, S., M. Ruhs, B. Anderson and B. Rogaly (2007), *Migrants' Lives Beyond the Workplace: The Experiences of Central and East Europeans in the UK*, York: Joseph Rowntree Foundation.
Spyrou, S. (2011), The limits of children's voices: from authenticity to critical, reflective representation, *Childhood*, **18**(2), 151–165.
Thomas, F. (2010), Transnational health and treatment networks: meaning, value and place in health seeking amongst southern African migrants in London, *Health and Place*, **16**, 606 612.
Thomson, P. (2008), *Doing Visual Research with Children and Young People*, London: Routledge.
Yuval-Davis, N. (2011), *The Politics of Belonging: Intersectional Contestations*, London: Sage.

23 Young migrants and sexual and reproductive healthcare

Jessica R. Botfield, Anthony B. Zwi and Christy E. Newman

INTRODUCTION

Young people from culturally diverse backgrounds, including migrants, refugees and international students, are at heightened risk of poor sexual and reproductive health. However while they have varied and sometimes complex health needs, these are often overlooked and sexual and reproductive health services underutilised (McMichael and Gifford 2009; Wray et al. 2014). This chapter reviews key issues relating to the sexual and reproductive health of young people from diverse migrant backgrounds, and emphasises the importance of appropriately engaging them through culturally sensitive approaches to sexual health promotion and service provision. Focusing on Australia as a case study in contemporary multiculturalism, it explores the complexities of designing effective healthcare systems that take into account their varied experiences and backgrounds, and reviews approaches to the promotion of sexual and reproductive health for these diverse communities. Reflecting on the mechanisms employed to engage culturally diverse young people with sexual and reproductive services, the chapter reinforces the importance of a youth-friendly setting and the promotion of cultural competence in sexual healthcare.

Given the complexity of the intersecting issues and experiences reviewed in this chapter, it is important to define the terminology used. The term 'migrant' in this chapter refers to people coming to Australia by choice, including for skilled migration and family reunion. International students and refugees are discussed separately, for the purposes of the chapter, due to their often unique experiences and needs. The term 'migrants' therefore refers to anyone who has chosen to leave their home country and move to Australia (primarily for work or family reunion purposes), and 'international students' as those coming to Australia to study on a temporary visa. A 'refugee' is someone who is outside the country of their nationality and is unable or unwilling to avail themselves of the protection of that country due to a well-founded fear of persecution. When referring to young people in the context of 'migrants' or 'refugees' in this chapter, they may personally fit under one of these terms, or their parents or grandparents do.

SEXUAL AND REPRODUCTIVE HEALTH IN YOUNG PEOPLE

'Sexual health' and 'reproductive health' overlap considerably. Sexual health pertains to pleasurable and safe sexual experiences, free of coercion, discrimination and violence, while reproductive health is focused on having a satisfying and safe sex life, with the freedom to decide if, when and how often to reproduce (Glasier et al. 2006). While offering a single definition of sexual and reproductive health is difficult due to the range and breadth of issues encompassed (Collumbien et al. 2012), the United Nations defines reproductive health, of which sexual health is a part, as 'a state of complete physical, mental and social well-being and not merely the absence of disease or infirmity, in all matters relating to the reproductive system and to its functions and processes' (United Nations 1995b). However, as with concepts of health generally, sexual and reproductive health relate not merely to the absence of disease (Temple-Smith and Gifford 2005; Hach 2012) but also include the promotion of wellbeing. It is centred around the availability of quality sexual and reproductive health services, eliminating preventable maternal and newborn mortality and morbidity, and addressing sexually transmitted infections, cervical cancer, sexual and gender-based violence, and the sexual and reproductive health needs of adolescents (Temmerman et al. 2014).

Health is a basic human right, and the right to sexual and reproductive health continues to gain recognition globally (Gruskin et al. 2014). The landmark International Conference on Population and Development held in 1994 placed rights at the heart of development, and affirmed sexual and reproductive health as a fundamental element within this agenda (DeJong 2000). The Conference endorsed a Programme of Action that recognised the importance of gender equality and equity, human rights and the empowerment of women (United Nations 1995b). This led to a shift from earlier policies targeting population control, to those that placed the individual at the centre and respected choice, rights and empowerment (World Health Organization 2014). The Fourth World Conference on Women was held the following year, and the Beijing Declaration and Platform for Action adopted, with the goal of advancing women's rights worldwide (United Nations 1995a). The UN Millennium Declaration was adopted in 2000 and eight Millennium Development Goals established for achievement by 2015; one of the eight goals focused on the promotion of gender equality and empowerment of women. The Sustainable Development Goals agreed in August 2015 reinforce these efforts towards promoting gender equality, as well as ensuring universal access to sexual and reproductive health and reproductive rights, and sexual and reproductive healthcare services (United Nations 2015).

There is also increasing awareness of the more specific sexual and reproductive health needs of young people (Williams and Davidson 2004). Worldwide there are 1.2 billion adolescents, young men and women aged 10–19 years (Cappa et al. 2012). As they make the transition from children to adults, they experience significant physical, psychological, emotional and economic changes (United Nations Children's Fund 2012), and are at heightened risk of sexual and reproductive ill-health (Bearinger et al. 2007; Glasier et al. 2006). Adolescents, however, may lack the cognitive capacity to make safe decisions, and may have limited understanding of their bodies or health. Many are disempowered and restricted by laws or customs, are vulnerable to sexual exploitation and high-risk behaviours (Badash 2006), and may have limited access to information, contraception and services (Kennedy et al. 2011). Furthermore, as young girls have immature reproductive and immune systems, they are more susceptible to sexually transmitted infections, and their lack of physical maturity and incomplete body growth makes them vulnerable during pregnancy and delivery (Bearinger et al. 2007). Adolescent girls in many countries are also at risk of harmful practices including female genital mutilation and early or forced marriage (United Nations Population Fund 2013; United Nations Children's Fund 2014), as well as exploitation by 'sugar daddies'; older men who provide material benefits or financial security in return for sexual relations (Silberschmidt and Rasch 2001). Economic pressures can also drive young men and women into sex work, with additional vulnerabilities due to their age and other forms of dependence, and reduced opportunities to protect themselves from harm. Variations in biological maturation, age of sexual debut, type and number of sexual partners, and use of contraceptive methods, along with educational and marital options and norms, create a myriad of factors that can both protect against sexually transmitted infections and early pregnancy, or increase a young person's risk of negative sexual and reproductive health outcomes (Bearinger et al. 2007). However, it is also important to appreciate that the research on young people and sexual health often emphasises these more negative aspects, particularly their vulnerabilities and risks. Young people's sexuality and sexual behaviour involve far more than this (Keys, Rosenthal, and Pitts 2013), and there is often little recognition of the considerable strengths, capabilities and assets that many young people draw on in navigating their complex social and sexual worlds (Persson and Newman 2012), particularly but not only in the context of migration.

RESPONDING TO CULTURE AND CONTEXT WITHIN SEXUAL HEALTH PROMOTION

Young people are not a homogeneous group, and it is widely recognised that diverse cultural, religious and social contexts and beliefs influence their health and the ways they access and use health information and services (Wray et al. 2014; Ussher et al. 2012; Khoei et al. 2008; Rawson and Liamputtong 2010; Rogers and Earnest 2014; Manderson et al. 2002). Ideas and values relating to sexual and reproductive health are likely to be shaped by the culture and society to which one belongs, or with which one identifies, and the factors that shape people's health will be strongly informed by their living conditions and social determinants of health (Keys et al. 2008).

Historically, much of the focus of sexual health research and policy centred on understanding and influencing community knowledge, attitudes and practices around sex. This was based on the belief that people are rational decision-makers when it comes to sex and health, and only needed information and skills in order to make health-promoting decisions (Aggleton 2004; Kippax et al. 2013). However, there has been a paradigm shift away from this focus on sexual behaviours and individual risk towards a greater recognition of the broader social and cultural settings within which these actions take place (Parker 2009; Aggleton 2004). Such thinking has reinforced wider recognition of social and cultural determinants of health and wellbeing, which is also important when examining the sexual health of diverse groups of young migrants.

While it is generally now acknowledged that society and culture shape our sexual experience and the ways in which we interpret and understand that experience (Parker 2009), the extent to which an individual's desires, practices and experiences are shaped by outside forces (social determinants) and how much they are a reflection of individual decisions to act (agency) are not so well understood or accepted. There is common understanding, however, that most human actions, thoughts and desires are influenced, if not determined, by key elements of social life including norms, values, networks, structures and institutions (Auerbach et al. 2011), and that these have a powerful influence on the regulation and governance of sexual behaviour and identity (Kippax 2008; Collumbien et al. 2012).

Studies that have focused on agency have examined the ways that individuals are able to pursue purposeful courses of action – they are able to imagine different paths of action and choose a particular path, either individually or collectively (Petesch et al. 2005). This has important implications when working with young people, and those from culturally diverse backgrounds, as an understanding of their sexual agency and its consequences can help enable the design of sexual health programmes that are informed by the realities of those they seek to support. Taking a more comprehensive and holistic approach to the promotion of sexual and reproductive health is essential in responding to the needs of young people from diverse migrant backgrounds, and requires that both individual needs and contextual factors be recognised and addressed (Aggleton 2004).

AUSTRALIA: A CASE STUDY IN CONTEMPORARY MULTICULTURALISM

When considering the sexual and reproductive health of young people from culturally and linguistically diverse backgrounds, Australia provides a useful case study due to the scale and diversity of its migration histories (Australian Bureau of Statistics 2015a). Australia today comprises an incredibly rich diversity of cultures, ethnicities and languages, with people from many different backgrounds coming into the country under a range of circumstances, including as migrants, refugees and international students. Although coming from a broad range of backgrounds and experiences, this provides a useful context within which to examine sexual and reproductive health issues in relation to diverse communities in a wealthy nation such as Australia.

Prior to 1788, Australia was populated by its Indigenous inhabitants, Aboriginal and Torres Strait Islander people. European colonisation and settlement in 1788 brought widespread violence and dispossession with consequent detrimental changes to indigenous society and culture (Australian Bureau of Statistics 2010; Aboriginal Heritage Office n.d.). Australia's cultural landscape began to further diversify from the mid-1940s following the end of World War II, when refugees from Eastern Europe began to resettle in the country. In more recent times (2013–2014) the primary countries of origin for offshore refugee and humanitarian entrants (those applying for humanitarian entry to Australia from outside of Australia) have been Afghanistan, Iraq, Burma and Syria (Refugee Council of Australia 2014b), and in 2015 Australia committed to resettling another 12,000 Syrian refugees from the widespread violence and displacement engulfing that country (Bourke 2015). International students also contribute to Australia's diversity, with just over 1,859,000 international students having undertaken study in Australia between 2002 and 2014. China and India were the top two contributing nationalities over this time (Department of Education and Training 2015). In 2013–2014, net overseas migration reflected an annual gain of 212,700 persons; of those migrating to Australia from non-Western countries, China and India were the top two countries of birth (Australian Bureau of Statistics 2015a, 2015b). Net overseas migration includes people entering Australia on temporary visas (such as student, visitor, working holiday) and permanent visas (such as family, skilled and humanitarian). Australia is now one of the most culturally diverse countries in the world, with nearly 30 per cent of its resident population, or 6.6 million people, born overseas (Australian Bureau of Statistics 2015b).

Migrants, refugees and international students will have had very different experiences prior to coming to Australia; most migrants and international students will have planned their move, while refugees will have fled to escape persecution. Despite these differences, each of these groups often still experience settlement challenges in Australia. These can include lack of adequate on-arrival information and support, difficulties with language acquisition and re-establishing themselves socially and professionally, loss of social and cultural networks, relationship conflict, discrimination and racism (Pittaway et al. 2009; Allotey et al. 2004; Iqbal et al. 2012; Poljski 2011). People living in a new country also often remain strongly anchored to traditional religious and cultural beliefs (Srikanthan and Reid 2008), while trying to navigate access to new ideas, information and services.

While marginalised young people from migrant or refugee backgrounds experience many of the same health concerns as the general youth population, their experiences are frequently more complex (Cummings and Kang 2012). They face the additional difficulties of displacement or migration and growing up between 'two cultures' (Chown et al. 2008; Lane 2008) – having to negotiate or accommodate the often conflicting expectations, priorities and values of their parents or family with those of their new society (Manderson et al. 2002). This can lead to stress, intergenerational disputes and a feeling of not completely belonging to either community (Iqbal et al. 2012). Humanitarian entrants to Australia also tend to be younger than the national Australian population and arrivals under other migration categories (Refugee Council of Australia 2014a; NSW Health 2011; Department of Immigration and Citizenship 2011), bringing an additional set of challenges. Family separation during the migration experience can mean an eldest child may have to take on responsibility as the head of a household, or children may assume these roles as they acculturate more quickly than their parents. Unaccompanied minors, young people under the age of 18 years who arrive in Australia without a parent or guardian, may similarly have to make decisions that would customarily fall to a parent (Refugee Council of Australia 2014a).

MIGRANT AND REFUGEE HEALTHCARE IN AUSTRALIA

Health services are acknowledged as vital elements to improving adolescent sexual and reproductive health (Bearinger et al. 2007; World Health Organization 2002; Tylee et al. 2007), and should therefore be accessible, acceptable and appropriate for young people, and include services for prevention, diagnosis, treatment and care (Bearinger et al. 2007).

Most healthcare for refugee and migrant communities in Australia is provided through mainstream health services (South Eastern Sydney Local Health District 2011; Finney Lamb and Smith 2002): any service 'that aims to cater for the broad population in the provision of its services and programs' (Department of Human Services 1998). Relevant mainstream services include general practitioners, youth health services and family planning and sexual health clinics, which vary by region, funding, structure, governance and service delivery (Kang and Sanci 2007). They have varying functions, such as education, health promotion and clinical services, and focus on one or more of a range of issues related to sexual and reproductive health. While mainstream health services have been developed with the needs of the majority population in mind, many refugees and migrants are routinely referred to them. It is vital, therefore, that such services ensure provision of accessible and culturally competent care that appreciates and responds effectively to the varying health needs people may present with (NSW Health 2011; Hach 2012).

General practice in particular is the cornerstone of primary healthcare for young people in Australia (Cummings and Kang 2012). General practitioners are viewed as the most accessible primary healthcare provider, and are usually a young person's first point of contact with the health system (Chown et al. 2008; Dadich et al. 2013). While a fee for services is levied by general practitioners, this may be covered in full or in part by the Medicare system, a federal government health scheme that enables access to healthcare for Australian citizens and some overseas visitors at little or no cost (Department of Human Services 2015). In Australia, general practitioners see approximately 2 million people under the age of 25 each year (Chown et al. 2008), including for issues related to sexual and reproductive health. However, they are facing increasing difficulties with more people coming from a growing range of culturally diverse backgrounds (Chown et al. 2008; Milosevic et al. 2012), especially when this encompasses those with more complex health needs (NSW Health 2011; Thomas et al. 2007).

Many health professionals also find working with young people challenging due to communication difficulties and uncertainty about medico-legal status for those under 18 years (Cummings and Kang 2012; Chown et al. 2008). This latter concern around medico-legal status is a common one, and is even more complex when working with culturally diverse communities. In 1986, the British case of *Gillick v West Norfolk and Wisbech Area Health Authority* established the legal precedent that the parental right to determine their child's treatment ends once a child under the age of 16 years is capable of fully understanding the medical treatment proposed. This common law principle is used in Australia (Bowles n.d.), and it is now generally accepted that most young people over the age of 16 are capable of giving their own informed consent. However there is still uncertainty in this area, particularly across different states and territories in Australia (Chown et al. 2008), and many young people have continued concerns about issues of confidentiality and potential disclosure to parents, which can be a barrier to them accessing health services (Booth et al. 2002, 2004; Sanci et al. 2005). This can be additionally complex for some culturally diverse young people, particularly those from migrant or refugee backgrounds, due to a range of additional factors including language barriers, lower health literacy and unfamiliarity with the health system.

CHALLENGES OF ENGAGING CULTURALLY DIVERSE YOUNG PEOPLE WITH SEXUAL AND REPRODUCTIVE HEALTH SERVICES

Young people can have complex health needs, and literature from Australian studies suggests that most do not seek healthcare as often as they could (Bernard et al. 2004; Kang et al. 2003; Skinner and Hickey 2003; Booth et al. 2008; Dadich et al. 2013). A study investigating the health concerns of adolescents in one state of Australia, for example, found that one-third of females and two-thirds of males would not seek help for any health concerns (Booth et al. 2002, 2004).

Sexual and reproductive health services are particularly underutilised, especially among culturally diverse communities in Australia (Ussher et al. 2012; Hach 2012; Wray et al. 2014; Martin et al. 2013; Manderson and Allotey 2003). This can be attributed to a number of sociocultural factors, including access to health-related information and services, the dynamics of the migration experience, and gender and cultural norms in different communities (Hach 2012).

Barriers to use of services for sexual and reproductive health needs can include the location and accessibility of services, level of dis/comfort in disclosing health concerns, attitudes of service providers (Booth et al. 2004), financial constraints (Hach 2012; Spike et al. 2011), and language barriers (Hach 2012; McMichael and Gifford 2009; McMichael 2008). Many young people, from any background, will not use a sexual and reproductive health clinic if they feel well or do not believe they are 'at risk' (Skinner and Hickey 2003), and for young migrants and refugees, unfamiliarity with the health system can further discourage service use (Hach 2012; McMichael 2008).

Challenges and barriers will also vary for different migrant and refugee groups and individuals for a myriad of reasons, including their length of time in Australia and visa status. For example, international students, including those from China and India (who represent the largest cohort of international students), experience raised rates of unplanned pregnancy and abortion and are at increased risk of intimate partner violence and sexually transmissible infections. However, their utilisation of health services is particularly low, largely due to limited understanding of the Australian health system and financial barriers, as well as generally lower health literacy, including that relating to sexual health, which is taboo within many countries (Poljski 2011; Reeders 2011). Unaccompanied minors also face challenges, often lacking the protection and support of a family (McMichael 2008) and requiring additional support and care (NSW Health 2011). Although Australia is often seen as a relatively safe and inclusive setting for lesbian, gay, bisexual, transgender and queer people, those from immigrant and refugee communities 'are a minority within a minority' in Australia (Victorian Department of Health 2013), and can experience added pressures and complexities, including tension between their religious beliefs and their sexuality, feeling unsafe at home, and having low levels of sexual health knowledge (Noto et al. 2014).

Young people from migrant or refugee backgrounds may not visit a general practitioner or local health clinic for sexual health concerns if the provider identifies with the same ethnicity or community, is of a different gender or if an interpreter is required (Rawson and Liamputtong 2009; McMichael and Gifford 2009; McMichael 2008). Sexual health services may also be perceived by some as culturally inappropriate for unmarried women, resulting in avoidance due to fear of others knowing they are interested in sexual health or engaging in premarital sexual activity (Ussher et al. 2012; Hach 2012).

WAYS FORWARD IN POLICY AND PRACTICE

While national and state policies on sexual and reproductive health issues in Australia focus on different priority groups (Botfield et al. 2015), several states are taking the lead in developing policies to address the needs of culturally diverse young people. In New South Wales (NSW), for example, the most populous state in Australia's Federation, the NSW Refugee Health Plan (2011–2016) identifies refugee youth as a priority population and sexual and reproductive health as a priority health issue. It seeks to implement strategies to ensure the delivery of safe, high-quality services to refugees through both refugee-specific health services and through accessible, culturally and linguistically competent mainstream health services. The Youth Health Policy (2011–2016) similarly aims to guide the NSW health system to support young people to achieve optimal health and wellbeing, and recognises the increasingly diverse community of young people that must be taken into consideration.

Within this policy context, innovative strategies are being developed to address the needs of young people and overcome barriers to access. Since 2006, the youth health service model has gained support through the national '*headspace*' initiative (Cummings and Kang 2012). This is a federally funded programme that allows young people to seek help early through new models of care provided in youth-friendly, integrated, multidisciplinary centres (Ministry of Health NSW 2010). Centres are built and designed with input from young people, and provide assistance with mental health, physical health (including sexual health), alcohol and drug, and work and study issues. There is a clear link between emotional distress, depression, substance abuse and sexual risk-taking behaviours in young people, and *headspace* is therefore an ideal setting for reaching those experiencing issues with relationships or sexuality, or at risk of sexually transmissible infections, who are unlikely to attend mainstream services and may therefore miss out on routine screening and advice. Sexual health assessments, advice, appropriate treatment and referral are available for *headspace* clients (Edwards et al. 2014). This service could be well-placed to more directly engage young people from migrant and refugee backgrounds.

Schools also play a critical role in shaping the health and wellbeing of young people, and are ideally placed to deliver sexuality education to educate young people about sexual and reproductive health (Smith et al. 2011; Goldman 2010). In Australia, sexuality and sexual health education is supported at a state level. In NSW, it is taught in all government schools, although to variable degrees, and is guided by the personal development, health and physical education syllabuses provided by the NSW Board of

Studies, Teaching and Educational Standards. This is a mandatory subject from Kindergarten to Year 10 (NSW Department of Education 2015a), and senior students then participate in *Crossroads*, a mandatory 25-hour programme (NSW Department of Education 2015b). Several family planning and sexual health services across Australia are also working with schools to support them in implementing sexuality and sexual health education (Family Planning NSW n.d.; Sexual Health and Family Planning ACT n.d.; SHine SA n.d.; Family Planning Victoria n.d.).

Despite widespread acceptance of the importance of sexual health education and a framework and support for its delivery, the amount of school-based education young people receive on sexual health in Australia is variable (Skinner and Hickey 2003), and inconsistencies in training, knowledge and confidence of teachers to adequately deliver sexual health education remain (Smith et al. 2011). A National Survey of Secondary Teachers of Sexuality Education, involving 300 secondary school teachers from every jurisdiction in Australia including government, Catholic and independent schools, found that 16 per cent of respondents reported having received no training in sexual health education (Smith et al. 2011). Furthermore, the majority of teachers teaching sexual health are female, which suggests there is a lack of male role models in the school setting to discuss these potentially sensitive and personal topics (Smith et al. 2011). In the Fifth National Survey of Secondary Students and Sexual Health, undertaken in 2013 with more than 2,000 Year 10, 11 and 12 students from a cross-section of schools across Australia, only 45 per cent found the sex education they received to be 'very' or 'extremely' relevant (Mitchell et al. 2014). A study exploring the acquisition of knowledge about sexual issues for Vietnamese young women in Australia similarly found that many felt sex education in school was inadequate and lacked the breadth of information they desired (Rawson and Liamputtong 2010). Young people's sexual pleasure is also largely unaddressed in sexuality education, as well as in society more generally (Keys, Rosenthal, and Pitts 2013).

However in contrast to these reports, a study with 142 young people from refugee backgrounds who had recently arrived in Australia reported that the sexuality education classes they had attended had increased their understanding of sexual health issues (McMichael and Gifford 2009). It is possible therefore, that despite its recognised shortcomings, for some young people from culturally diverse backgrounds, including young refugees and migrants, school-based sexuality education might be the best opportunity to increase their sexual health literacy, not only because it overcomes cultural mores and other barriers to discussing sexual health with parents, but also because it helps to overcome the difficulties they may face accessing information from other sources (McMichael 2008;

Rawson and Liamputtong 2010). However, it is also important to consider that not all young people arriving in Australia will have this opportunity to learn about sex and sexual health, as they may not attend secondary school upon their arrival, may not have the opportunity to 'catch up' on sexuality education programmes, or they may attend a school in which it is not offered (McMichael 2008, 2013). International students may also miss this opportunity if they have come from a country in which sexual health education is not provided or is not comprehensively covered (Reeders 2011; Poljski 2011), an issue that is particularly concerning given the often-new independence and subsequent risk-taking that can accompany student experience.

ACHIEVING YOUTH-FRIENDLINESS AND CULTURAL COMPETENCE IN SEXUAL HEALTH SERVICE SETTINGS

Youth-friendly Services

To improve the use of sexual and reproductive health services by young people, it is widely recognised that they should be tailored to their particular needs and preferences (Bender and Fulbright 2013; Braeken and Rondinelli 2012). Shaping the design and delivery of these services in this way is essential for increasing access and promoting health (Bender and Fulbright 2013). An approach advocated by many, both in the Australian and international contexts, is the establishment of 'youth-friendly' health services, particularly in the context of sexual and reproductive healthcare (Bearinger et al. 2007; Women's Health West 2010). While initially described as a framework for primary healthcare in low-income countries, there is growing recognition of the importance of this model in higher-income countries and specialist health services (Ambresin et al. 2013).

According to this framework, services should aim to be accessible, equitable, appropriate, comprehensive, efficient, effective and acceptable to young people (World Health Organization 2002), and cannot be considered youth-friendly if young people are not using them (Braeken and Rondinelli 2012). Examples of how a health service could be more youth-friendly include flexible opening hours, including outside school hours, close proximity to public transport, availability of male and female staff, option of bulk billing (no extra charges or out of pocket payment beyond government reimbursed amount), no Medicare card required, opportunity for 'dropping-in' and a welcoming and friendly atmosphere, including youth-specific visual 'branding' and information in the form of posters, images, reading material and brochures (Roberts and Crane 2012; Kang et al. 2005), that are available in a familiar language (World Health Organization 2012).

Ideally young people should also be involved in the development, implementation, review and evaluation of services in order to increase their sense of ownership and involvement in services (Kang et al. 2005; Ministry of Health NSW 2010). Youth participation can range from one-off consultations on specific issues, to surveys, focus groups and involvement on key committees (Kang et al. 2005), and may even extend to involving young people in designing their own sexual health education curriculum (University of South Australia n.d.).

Culturally Competent Services

Cultural competency has emerged as a potential strategy to contribute towards eliminating health disparities and improving quality of care. Culturally competent care aims to create a health system and workforce capable of delivering the highest quality care to all clients/patients, regardless of race, ethnicity, faith, culture or language proficiency (Betancourt et al. 2005). In multicultural societies such as Australia, sexual healthcare services must seek to be culturally sensitive at all times (Rawson and Liamputtong 2009), and this is typically well-recognised at national and state levels of government, as well as in professional frameworks that guide the practice of clinicians._ENREF_22

Cultural competence is an ongoing process whereby the provider works within a cultural context, which can involve the individual, their family and community, to provide care that is acceptable to the client/patient (Ngum Chi Watts et al. 2014). It entails understanding the importance of social and cultural influences on clients/patients' health beliefs and behaviours, consideration of how these interact at different levels of the healthcare system, and developing interventions that take these issues into account to ensure quality healthcare delivery to diverse populations. A framework for cultural competence should include organisational, structural and clinical interventions, as sociocultural barriers to care have been identified at these three levels (Betancourt et al. 2003). Providing culturally competent care is vital to successfully working with young refugees and migrants, and recognising methods such as sensitivity training, use of confidential and appropriate interpreter services, and hiring professionals who share clients/patients' ethnicity or language, if desirable, will help to enhance health outcomes (McKeary and Newbold 2010). Other strategies to address disparities in healthcare should include recruitment of minority community members into the health profession, development of interpreter services and language-appropriate health educational materials, and provider education on cross-cultural issues (Betancourt et al. 2003). Such initiatives could also involve the inclusion of young people in the design of strategies and delivery of services.

Diversity among young people represents a significant challenge for health services. The relationships between culture, development and health, and the expertise required by health professionals to provide culturally appropriate services, all play out in adolescent practice (Bennett et al. 2005). While highly visible communities are often labelled as belonging to a collective, homogenous group by appearance and/or experiences (Dean et al. 2012), a myriad of variations occur within and between cultures through factors such as cultural beliefs and practices, religion and level of acculturation. It is therefore important to acknowledge that culture is dynamic and relational, rather than static and fixed (Ussher et al. 2012). As refugees and migrants are not a homogeneous group, healthcare providers must recognise that the differential impact of factors including country of origin, language, culture, gender, age and migrant status leads to diverse health needs. Health is not a 'one size fits all', and providers should therefore respond to the unique needs of individuals (McKeary and Newbold 2010; Newman et al. 2013).

Providers must also be cautious not to stereotype those in their care, and recognise that differing value systems may influence decision-making in people of different cultures and backgrounds. This awareness must then be tempered by the understanding that each person and their situation is unique, and the values that an individual holds may not be the same as others, nor even of the official teachings of their religion or the cultural norms reported by others of the same religion or culture (Srikanthan and Reid 2008), including that of their parents. Sensitivity to the cultural, ethnic, religious, linguistic and social diversity among young people will help to avoid misunderstandings, improve patient/client satisfaction, and lead to better outcomes (Bennett et al. 2005).

Tervalon and Murray-Garcia (1998) suggest that healthcare providers should go beyond 'cultural competence' to being committed to, and actively engaging in, a lifelong process of self-reflection and self-critique, referred to as 'cultural humility'. Findings from a study exploring reproductive health providers' communication with Somali women in Finland, for example, highlighted the need for cultural competence in delivery of services to client/patients from different ethnic or cultural backgrounds, as well as a genuine passion to be flexible, to accept differences and a willingness to learn from each other (Tervalon and Murray-Garcia 1998; Degni et al. 2012). Campinha-Bacote (2002) similarly states that healthcare providers should go beyond saying they respect the values, beliefs and practices of their clients/patients, or providing a culturally specific intervention, to having a genuine motivation or passion to provide care that is culturally responsive. This includes having the desire to be open and flexible with others, to accept differences and build on similarities, and to be willing to learn from others as cultural informants, including young people from different cultural backgrounds.

CONCLUSION

While a number of populations experience barriers to accessing sexual and reproductive health promotion and care (Temple-Smith 2014), the factors influencing the experiences of young people from culturally diverse backgrounds in Australia reveal issues of significance to understanding the intersecting dynamics between migration and health. While migrants, refugees and international students come from a wide diversity of backgrounds and experiences, many face a range of often similar challenges in relation to their sexual and reproductive health. This chapter has reviewed this issue in the Australian context, and highlighted the importance of pursuing cultural competence in the provision of healthcare to an increasingly multicultural society. While the vulnerability of culturally diverse young people to poor sexual and reproductive health outcomes in Australia is widely recognised, knowledge gaps remain regarding their use of, and engagement with, appropriate healthcare (Botfield et al. 2015), including the strengths and assets they bring and the potential for this to be harnessed through lively policy and practice debates. An integrated and national approach is required, with a focus on the sexual and reproductive health of culturally diverse young people and all that this encompasses, in order to more effectively engage them with sexual and reproductive healthcare and improve health outcomes.

REFERENCES

Aboriginal Heritage Office (n.d.), *A Brief Aboriginal History*, Aboriginal Heritage Office, available online at, www.aboriginalheritage.org/history/history.

Aggleton, P. (2004), Sexuality, HIV prevention, vulnerability and risk, *Journal of Psychology and Human Sexuality*, **16**(1), 1–11.

Allotey, P., L. Manderson, S. Baho and L. Demian (2004), Reproductive health for resettling refugee and migrant women? *Health Issues*, **78**, 12–17.

Ambresin, A., K. Bennett, G. C. Patton, L. A. Sanci and S. M. Sawyer (2013), Assessment of youth-friendly health care: a systematic review of indicators drawn from young people's perspectives, *Journal of Adolescent Health*, **52**, 670e681.

Auerbach, J. D., J. O. Parkhurst and C. F. Caceres (2011), Addressing social drivers of HIV/

AIDS for the long-term response: conceptual and methodological considerations, *Global Public Health*, **6**(3), 293–309.
Australian Bureau of Statistics (2010), *Aboriginal and Torres Strait Islander Population*, Australian Bureau of Statistics, available online at www.abs.gov.au/ausstats/abs@.nsf/0/68AE74ED632E17A6CA2573D200110075?opendocument.
Australian Bureau of Statistics (2015a), *Migration, Australia, 2011–12 and 2012–13*, Australian Bureau of Statistics, available online at www.abs.gov.au/ausstats/abs@.nsf/Lookup/3412.0Chapter12011-12%20and%202012-13.
Australian Bureau of Statistics (2015b), *Migration, Australia: 2013–14*, Australian Bureau of Statistics, available online at www.abs.gov.au/ausstats/abs@.nsf/mf/3412.0.
Badash, M. (ed.) (2006), *Investing in the Next Generation: Reproductive Health for Youth*, Watertown, MA: Pathfinder International.
Bearinger, L. H., R. E. Sieving, J. Ferguson and V. Sharma (2007), Global perspectives on the sexual and reproductive health of adolescents: patterns, prevention, and potential, *The Lancet*, **369**(9568), 1220–1231.
Bender, S. S. and Y. K. Fulbright (2013), Content analysis: a review of perceived barriers to sexual and reproductive health services by young people, *The European Journal of Contraception and Reproductive Health Care*, **18**, 159–167.
Bennett, D. L., P. Chown and M. Kang (2005), Cultural diversity in adolescent health care, *Medical Journal of Australia*, **183**(8), 436–438.
Bernard, D., S. Quine, M. Kang, G. Alperstein, T. Usherwood, D. Bennett and M. Booth (2004), Access to primary health care for Australian adolescents: how congruent are the perspectives of health service providers and young people, and does it matter? *Australian and New Zealand Journal of Public Health*, **28**(5), 487–492.
Betancourt, J. R., A. R. Green, J. E. Carrillo and O. Ananeh-Firempong (2003), Defining cultural competence: a practical framework for addressing racial/ethnic disparities in health and health care, *Public Health Reports*, **118**(4), 293–302.
Betancourt, J. R., A. R. Green, J. E. Carrillo and E. R. Park (2005), Cultural competence and health care disparities: key perspectives and trends, *Health Affairs*, **24**(2), 499–505.
Booth, M. L., D. Bernard, S. Quine, M. Kang, T. Usherwood, G. Alperstein, L. Beasley and D. Bennett (2002), *Access to Health Care Among NSW Adolescents*, Westmead: NSW Centre for the Advancement of Adolescent Health.
Booth, M. L., D. Bernard, S. Quine, M. S. Kang, T. Usherwood, G. Alperstein and D. L. Bennett (2004), Access to health care among Australian adolescents young people's perspectives and their sociodemographic distribution, *Journal of Adolescent Health*, **34**, 97–103.
Booth, M. L., S. Knox and M. Kang (2008), Encounters between adolescents and general practice in Australia, *Journal of Paediatrics and Child Health*, **44**, 699–705.
Botfield, J. R., C. E. Newman and A. B. Zwi (2015), Young people from culturally diverse backgrounds and their use of services for sexual and reproductive health needs: A structured scoping review, *Sexual Health*, **13**(1), 1–9.
Bourke, L. (2015), Abbott government agrees to resettle 12,000 Syrian refugees in Australia, *The Sydney Morning Herald*, 9 September.
Bowles, K. (n.d.), *Age of Consent to Medical Treatment*, FindLaw Australia, available online at www.findlaw.com.au/articles/432/age-of-consent-to-medical-treatment.aspx.
Braeken, D. and I. Rondinelli (2012), Sexual and reproductive health needs of young people: Matching needs with systems, *International Journal of Gynecology and Obstetrics*, **119**, S60–S63.
Campinha-Bacote, J. (2002), The process of cultural competence in the delivery of healthcare services: a model of care, *Journal of Transcultural Nursing*, **13**(3), 181–184.
Cappa, C., T. Wardlaw, C. Langevin-Falcon and J. Diers (2012), Progress for children: a report card on adolescents, *The Lancet*, **379**(9834), 2323–2325.
Chown, P., M. Kang, L. Sanci, V. Newnham and D. L. Bennett (2008), *Adolescent Health: Enhancing the Skills of General Practitioners in Caring for Young People from Culturally Diverse Backgrounds*, GP Resource Kit, 2nd edn, Sydney: NSW Centre for the Advancement of Adolescent Health and Transcultural Mental Health Centre.

Collumbien, M., J. Busza, J. Cleland and O. Campbell (2012), *Social Science Methods for Research on Sexual and Reproductive Health*, Geneva: World Health Organization.

Cummings, M. and M. Kang (2012), Youth health services: improving access to primary care, *Australian Family Physician*, **41**(5), 339–341.

Dadich, A., C. Jarrett, L. Sanci, M. Kang and D. Bennett (2013), The promise of primary health reform for youth health, *Journal of Paediatrics and Child Health*, **49**, 887–890.

Dean, J., J. Wollin, D. Stewart, J. Debattista and M. Mitchell (2012), Hidden yet visible: methodological challenges researching sexual health in Sudanese refugee communities, *Culture, Health and Sexuality*, **14**(8), 911–924.

Degni, F., S. Suominen, N. Esse, W. El Ansari and K. Vehvila Inen-Julkunen (2012), Communication and cultural issues in providing reproductive health care to immigrant women: health care providers' experiences in meeting Somali women living in Finland, *Journal of Immigrant and Minority Health*, **14**, 330–343.

Dejong, J. (2000), The role and limitations of the Cairo International Conference on Population and Development, *Social Science & Medicine*, **51**, 941–953.

Department of Education and Training (2015), *International Students in Australia up to 2014*, Department of Education and Training, available online at https://internationaleducation.gov.au/research/Research-Snapshots/Documents/Total%20student%20counts%20to%202014.pdf.

Department of Human Services (1998), *Youth Assessment of Mainstream Health Services*, Victoria: Department of Human Services.

Department of Human Services (2015), *Medicare Services*, Victoria: Department of Human Services, available at www.humanservices.gov.au/customer/subjects/medicare-services.

Department of Immigration and Citizenship (2011), *A Significant Contribution: The Economic, Social and Civic Contributions of First and Second Generation Humanitarian Entrants. Summary of Findings* Victoria: Department of Immigration and Citizenship.

Edwards, C. A., M. L. Britton, L. Jenkins, D. J. Rickwood and K. E. Gillham (2014), Including a client sexual health pathway in a national youth mental health early intervention service – project rationale and implementation strategy, *Health Education Research*, **29**(2), 354–359.

Family Planning NSW (n.d.), *Teachers*, available online at https://www.fpnsw.org.au/health-information/teachers.

Family Planning Victoria (n.d.), *Schools & Teachers*, available online at www.fpv.org.au/schools.

Finney Lamb, C. and M. Smith (2002), Problems refugees face when accessing health services, *NSW Public Health Bulletin*, **13**(7), 161–163.

Glasier, A., A. M. Gulmezoglu, G. P. Schmid, C. G. Moreno and P. F. Van Look (2006), Sexual and reproductive health: a matter of life and death, *The Lancet*, **368**(9547), 1595–1607.

Goldman, J. D. G. (2010), The new sexuality education curriculum for Queensland primary schools, *Sex Education*, **10**(1), 47–66.

Gruskin, S., T. K. Sundari Ravindran and on behalf of the Rights-Oriented Research and Education Network for Sexual and Reproductive Health (2014), Realising the ICPD 20 years later: shifting the paradigms for research and education, *Global Public Health*, **9**(6), 647–652.

Hach, M. (2012), *Common Threads: The Sexual and Reproductive Health Experiences of Immigrant and Refugee Women in Australia*, Melbourne: Multicultural Centre for Women's Health.

Iqbal, N., A. Joyce, A. Russo and J. Earnest (2012), Resettlement experiences of Afghan Hazara female adolescents: a case study from Melbourne, Australia, *International Journal of Population Research*, **2012**.

Kang, M., D. Bernard, M. Booth, S. Quine, G. Alperstein, T. Usherwood and D. Bennett (2003), Access to primary health care for Australian young people: service provider perspectives, *British Journal of General Practice*, **53**, 947–952.

Kang, M., D. Bernard, T. Usherwood, S. Quine, G. Alperstein, H. Kerr-Roubicek, A. Elliott and D. Bennett (2005), *Final Report on Research Study: Access to Health Care Among Young People in New South Wales: Phase 2*, Sydney: NSW Centre for the Advancement of Adolescent Health.

Kang, M. and L. A. Sanci (2007), Primary health care for young people in Australia, *International Journal of Adolescent Medicine and Health*, **19**(3), 229–234.

Kennedy, E., N. Gray, P. Azzopardi and M. Creati (2011), Adolescent fertility and family planning in East Asia and the Pacific: a review of DHS reports, *Reproductive Health*, **8**, 11.

Keys, D., D. Rosenthal, H. Williams, S. Mallett, L. Jordan and D. Henning (2008), *Making it Real: Sexual Health Communication for Young People Living with Disadvantage*, Victoria: University of Melbourne, Family Planning Victoria.

Keys, D., D. Rosenthal, and M. Pitts (2013), Young people, sexual practice and meanings, in P. Aggleton, A. Ball, and Mane, P (eds), Sex, Drugs and Young People: International Perspectives. London: Routledge.

Khoei, E. M., A. Whelan and J. Cohen (2008), Sharing beliefs: what sexuality means to Muslim Iranian women living in Australia, *Culture, Health & Sexuality*, **10**(3), 237–248.

Kippax, S. (2008), Understanding and integrating the structural and biomedical determinants of HIV-infection: a way forward for prevention, *Current Opinion in HIV and AIDS*, **3**, 489–494.

Kippax, S., N. Stephenson, R. G. Parker and P. Aggleton (2013), Between individual agency and structure in HIV prevention: understanding the middle ground of social practice, *American Journal of Public Health*, **103**(8), 1367–1375.

Lane, C. (2008), *Adolescent Refugees and Migrants: A Reproductive Health Emergency*, Watertown, MA: Pathfinder International.

Manderson, L. and P. Allotey (2003), Storytelling, marginality, and community in Australia: how immigrants position their difference in health care settings, *Medical Anthropology: Cross-Cultural Studies in Health and Illness*, **22**(1), 1–21.

Manderson, L., M. Kelaher, N. Woelz-Stirling, J. Kaplan and K. Greene (2002), Sex, contraception and contradiction among young Filipinas in Australia, *Culture, Health & Sexuality: An International Journal for Research, Intervention and Care*, **4**(4), 381–391.

Martin, L., V. Knight, P. J. Read and A. Mcnulty, A. (2013), Fast-track services for all? The Preferences of Chinese-, Korean-, and Thai-speaking women attending a sexual health service, *Sexually Transmitted Diseases*, **40**(12), 929–932.

McKeary, M. and B. Newbold (2010), Barriers to care: the challenges for Canadian refugees and their health care providers, *Journal of Refugee Studies*, **23**(4), 523–545.

McMichael, C. (2008), *Promoting Sexual Health Amongst Resettled Youth with Refugee Backgrounds*, Melbourne: Refugee Health Research Centre.

McMichael, C. (2013), Unplanned but not unwanted? Teen pregnancy and parenthood among young people with refugee backgrounds, *Journal of Youth Studies*, **16**(5), 663–678.

McMichael, C. and S. Gifford (2009), 'It is good to know now. . . before it's too late': promoting sexual health literacy amongst resettled young people with refugee backgrounds, *Sexuality and Culture*, **13**(4), 218–236.

Milosevic, D., I. Cheng and M. M. Smith (2012), The NSW Refugee Health Service: improving refugee access to primary care, *Australian Family Physician*, **41**(3), 147–149.

Ministry of Health NSW (2010), *Youth Health Policy 2011–2016: Healthy Bodies, Healthy Minds, Vibrant Futures*, North Sydney: Ministry of Health, NSW.

Mitchell, A., K. Patrick, W. Heywood, P. Blackman and M. Pitts (2014), *5th National Survey of Australian Secondary Students and Sexual Health 2013*, Melbourne: Australian Research Centre in Sex, Health and Society, La Trobe University.

Newman, C. E., R. Gray, L. Brener, L. C. Jackson, P. Johnson, V. Saunders, M. Harris, P. Butow, and C. Treloar (2013), One size fits all? The discursive framing of cultural difference in health professional accounts of providing cancer care to Aboriginal people, *Ethnicity and Health*, **18**(4), 433–447.

Ngum Chi Watts, M. C., P. Liamputtong and M. Carolan (2014), Contraception knowledge and attitudes: truths and myths among African Australian teenage mothers in Greater Melbourne, Australia, *Journal of Clinical Nursing*, **23**(15–16), 2131–2141.

Noto, O., W. Leonard and A. Mitchell (2014), *'Nothing For Them': Understanding the Support Needs of LGBT Young People from Refugee and Newly Arrived Backgrounds*, Melbourne: Australian Research Centre in Sex, Health & Society, La Trobe University.
NSW Department of Education (2015a), *About Sexuality and Sexual Health Education in NSW Government Schools*, NSW Department of Education, available online at www.curriculumsupport.education.nsw.gov.au/sexual_health/assets/pdfs/sexualityedpolicyadvice.pdf.
NSW Department of Education (2015b), *Crossroads*, NSW Department of Education, available online at www.learning.schools.nsw.edu.au/crossroads/files/2015/03/Final_Crossroads_2March15-1caulki.pdf.
NSW Health (2011), *Refugee Health Plan 2011–2016*, North Sydney: Ministry of Health, NSW.
Parker, R. (2009), Sexuality, culture and society: shifting paradigms in sexuality research, *Culture, Health and Sexuality*, **11**(3), 251–266.
Persson, A.S., and C.E. Newman (2012), When HIV-positive children grow up: a critical analysis of the transition literature in developed countries, *Qualitative Health Research*, **22**(5), 656–667.
Petesch, P., C. Smulovitz and M. Walton (2005), Evaluating empowerment: a framework with cases from Latin America, in D. Narayan-Parker (ed.), *Measuring Empowerment: Cross-Disciplinary Perspectives*. Washington: World Bank.
Pittaway, E., C. Muli and S. Shteir (2009), 'I have a voice – hear me!' Findings of an Australian study examining the resettlement and integration experience of refugees and migrants from the Horn of Africa in Australia, *Refuge*, **26**(2), 133–146.
Poljski, C. (2011), *On Your Own: Sexual and Reproductive Health of Female International Students in Australia*, Melbourne: Multicultural Centre for Women's Health.
Rawson, H. and P. Liamputtong (2009), Influence of traditional Vietnamese culture on the utilisation of mainstream health services for sexual health issues by second-generation Vietnamese Australian young women, *Sex Health*, **6**(1), 75–81.
Rawson, H. and P. Liamputtong (2010), Culture and sex education: the acquisition of sexual knowledge for a group of Vietnamese Australian young women, *Ethnicity & Health*, **15**(4), 343–364.
Reeders, D. (2011), *Responding to Diversity: Meeting the Sexual and Reproductive Health Needs of International Students*, Melbourne: Centre for Culture, Ethnicity & Health.
Refugee Council of Australia (2014a), *Humanitarian Entrants in NSW*, Sydney: Refugee Council of Australia.
Refugee Council of Australia (2014b), *Refugee Council of Australia: Annual Report 2013/14*, Sydney: Refugee Council of Australia.
Roberts, S. and P. Crane (2012), *What Would it Take to Optimise Marginalised Young People's Sexual Health? A Conversational Journey with Youth Workers*, Queensland: Youth Affairs Network of Queensland.
Rogers, C. and J. Earnest (2014), A cross-generational study of contraception and reproductive health among Sudanese and Eritrean women in Brisbane, Australia, *Health Care for Women International*, **35**(3), 334–356.
Sanci, L. A., S. M. Sawyer, D. M. Haller, G. C. Patton and M. Kang (2005), Confidential health care for adolescents: reconciling clinical evidence with family values, *Medical Journal of Australia*, **183**(8), 410–414.
Sexual Health and Family Planning ACT (n.d.), *Schools Education Program*, Sexual Health and Family Planning ACT, available online at www.shfpact.org.au/community-health-promotion/school-s-educations-program.
SHine SA (n.d.), *Support for Schools*, SHine SA, available online at www.shinesa.org.au/support-for-schools.
Silberschmidt, M. and V. Rasch (2001), Adolescent girls, illegal abortions and 'sugar-daddies' in Dar es Salaam: vulnerable victims and active social agents, *Social Science & Medicine*, **52**, 1815–1826.
Skinner, S. R. and M. Hickey (2003), Current priorities for adolescent sexual and reproductive health in Australia, *Medical Journal of Australia*, **179**, 158–161.

Smith, A., M. Schlichthorst, A. Mitchell, J. Walsh, A. Lyons, P. Blackman and M. Pitts (2011), *Sexuality Education in Australian Secondary Schools 2010*, Melbourne: La Trobe University, the Australian Research Centre in Sex, Health & Society.
South Eastern Sydney Local Health District (2011), *Implementation Plan for the NSW Refugee Health Plan 2011 2016*, Sydney: South Eastern Sydney Local Health District.
Spike, E. A., M. M. Smith and M. F. Harris (2011), Access to primary health care services by community-based asylum seekers, *MJA*, **195**(4), 188–191.
Srikanthan, A. and R. L. Reid (2008), Religious and cultural influences on contraception, *Journal of Obstetrics and Gynaecology Canada*, **30**(2), 129–137.
Temmerman, M., R. Khosla and L. Say (2014), Sexual and reproductive health and rights: a global development, health, and human rights priority, *The Lancet*, **384**(9941), e30–e31.
Temple-Smith, M. (2014), *Sexual Health: A Multidisciplinary Approach*, Melbourne: IP Communications.
Temple-Smith, M. and S. Gifford (2005), *Sexual Health: An Australian Perspective*, Melbourne: IP Communications.
Tervalon, M. and J. Murray-Garcia (1998), Cultural humility versus cultural competence: a critical distinction in defining physician training outcomes in multicultural education, *Journal of Health Care for the Poor and Underserved*, **9**(2), 117–125.
Thomas, P., B. Milne, S. Raman and S. Shah (2007), Refugee youth: immunisation status and GP attendance, *Australian Family Physician*, **36**(7).
Tylee, A., D. M. Haller, T. Graham, R. Churchill and L. A. Sanci (2007), Youth-friendly primary-care services: how are we doing and what more needs to be done? *The Lancet*, **369**, 1565–1573.
United Nations (1995a), *Beijing Declaration and Platform for Action*, United Nations, available online at www.un.org/womenwatch/daw/beijing/pdf/BDPfA%20E.pdf.
United Nations (1995b), *Report of the International Conference on Population and Development*, Cairo, 5–13 September 1994, New York: United Nations.
United Nations (2015), *Transforming our World: The 2030 Agenda for Sustainable Development*, United Nations, available online at https://sustainabledevelopment.un.org/content/documents/7891Transforming%20Our%20World.pdf.
United Nations Children's Fund (2012), *Progress for Children: A Report Card on Adolescents*, New York: United Nations Children's Fund.
United Nations Children's Fund (2014), *A Statistical Snapshot of Violence against Adolescent Girls*, New York: UNICEF.
United Nations Population Fund (2013), *UNFPA Strategy on Adolescents and Youth: Towards Realizing the Full Potential of Adolescents and Youth*, New York: UNFPA.
University of South Australia (n.d.), *Engaging Young People in Sexuality Education Research Project*, University of South Australia, available online at www.youthsexuality.com.au.
Ussher, J. M., M. Rhyder-Obid, J. Perz, M. Rae, T. W. K. Wong and P. Newman (2012), Purity, privacy and procreation: constructions and experiences of sexual and reproductive health in Assyrian and Karen women living in Australia, *Sexuality & Culture*, **16**, 467–485.
Victorian Department of Health (2013), *Victorian Refugee Health and Wellbeing Action Plan: Consultation Summary*, Victoria: Department of Health.
Williams, H. and S. Davidson (2004), Improving adolescent sexual and reproductive health: a view from Australia: learning from world's best practice, *Sexual Health*, **1**, 95–105.
Women's Health West (2010), *Mapping and Needs Analysis: Sexual and Reproductive Health in the HealthWest Catchment*, Western Region Sexual and Reproductive Health Working Group.
World Health Organization (2002), *Adolescent Friendly Health Services: An Agenda for Change*, Geneva: World Health Organization.
World Health Organization (2012), *Making Health Services Adolescent Friendly: Developing National Quality Standards for Adolescent Friendly Health Services*, Geneva: World Health Organization, Department of Maternal, Newborn, Child and Adolescent Health.
World Health Organization (2014), *Sexual and Reproductive Health beyond 2014: Equality, Quality of Care and Accountability*, Geneva: World Health Organization.

Wray, A., J. M. Ussher and J. Perz (2014), Constructions and experiences of sexual health among young, heterosexual, unmarried Muslim women immigrants in Australia, *Culture, Health & Sexuality: An International Journal for Research, Intervention and Care*, **16**(1), 76–89.

24 Cultural competence in migrant healthcare

Felicity Thomas

INTRODUCTION

The increasing diversity of populations within countries across the globe creates new challenges for healthcare systems and providers. Although many migrants are young and healthy, they often face particular challenges and vulnerabilities that may undermine or threaten their health and wellbeing and impede access to appropriate healthcare services. Importantly, even when they are able to access healthcare, the specific needs they face may be poorly understood and inadequately responded to (Mladovsky et al. 2012), an issue known to have been exacerbated in countries that have experienced recent austerity measures (O'Donnell et al. 2013; Karanikolos et al. 2013). Responding effectively to these challenges therefore requires that health services adapt in order to provide for new populations and needs.

Studies undertaken in diverse contexts have found that barriers to effective healthcare for migrant populations can lead to adverse individual and public health outcomes, and can be economically harmful – both through the increased costs associated with delayed care, and through the loss of economic and social potential associated with better health (Bradby et al. 2015). In recognition of such issues, an initial set of recommendations was made in Europe through the Amsterdam Declaration 'Towards Migrant Friendly Hospitals in an Ethno-Culturally Diverse Europe' (see MFH 2004). This was followed in 2008, by a World Health Assembly resolution (WHA 61.17) on the health of migrants, which called on member states to develop migrant-sensitive health systems, to strengthen the collection of evidence and information to support policy formulation, and to promote equitable access to services, and was reiterated at the WHO High Level Meeting on Refugee and Migrant Health held in Rome in November 2015. Such strategies revolve around the concept of 'whole organisation approaches' in which the provision of culturally competent healthcare is viewed as much a task for organisations and systems as for individuals, and this thinking is central within the current European Health 2020 policy framework (WHO 2013). Yet although considerable progress has been made, there is still much to be done to ensure that such strategies are fully implemented.

In examining these issues, this chapter draws on literature and examples from Europe, an area that has experienced some of the largest growth rates of international migrants in recent years. It begins with an overview of the types of issues that influence migrant access to, and experience of health services. It then examines what is known about good practice in migrant healthcare, focusing in particular on the concepts of cultural competency and diversity sensitivity. The chapter ends by examining how cultural mediation can be effectively utilised by health providers and health users to provide more inclusive, relevant and effective healthcare.

ACCESSING HEALTHCARE

As has been demonstrated in a number of chapters in this volume, migrants often face a range of challenges accessing healthcare, despite international agreements in place to uphold the health-related rights of all. Refugees should, in theory, be able to access health services from their first country of registration for asylum. However, in practice, such rights may be delayed or denied during the initial asylum determination process. In Europe, governments tend to distinguish between 'asylum-seekers', whose claims for refuge are under consideration, and 'refugees', whose claims have been accepted. This in turn, can have major implications for accessing welfare and health services, and may reflect practical limitations on local service implementation rather than national policies of provision (Bradby et al. 2015). Rights to seek asylum also vary across Europe, with some nations refusing to recognise asylum claims for specific ethnic or national groups, or fast-tracking such applications to hasten the deportation process. The situation is particularly challenging for undocumented migrants who, being unable or unwilling to claim asylum, are often not deemed to be entitled to healthcare, despite evidence that they frequently experience considerable health issues (Schoevers et al. 2009, 2010; De Vito et al. 2015). There are also divergences in approach within countries. In Spain, for example, access to health services varies across regions, with some decentralised areas defying government policy to remove free primary healthcare to undocumented migrants (Rechel et al. 2013).

The role of healthcare providers also differs across the European region. In some countries, such as the UK and Ireland, for example, GPs have a key role as gatekeepers to secondary healthcare, unlike in Austria, where the healthcare system ensures free access to most specialist services, or in

Greece, where general practice is less common and less well acknowledged than other medical specialities (van den Muijsenbergh et al. 2014). While the European Union has a common framework around immigration policy, therefore, national legislation, interpretation of law and policy, varying migration histories and diverse approaches to 'integration' mean that considerable variation in healthcare rights and services continues to exist between and within countries.[1]

Even where healthcare entitlements are established, a range of other cross-cutting factors relating to the patient, the provider and/or the healthcare system may impede migrants' access to and effective use of formal healthcare services. In some areas of Europe, particularly in parts of the Commonwealth of Independent States (CIS) and within Southern Europe, for example, healthcare services remain relatively underdeveloped and, as a result, face major logistical difficulties responding to the significant flows of migrants witnessed in recent years. In other areas, policies of dispersal (such as used in the UK), and the use of accommodation centres (used in Germany and the Netherlands), can disrupt access to, and the effectiveness of, formal and sustained health services (Bradby et al. 2015). Many people are also faced with practical everyday constraints such as ensuring that basic needs – such as food and shelter – are met, as well as the logistical constraints of travelling to and from appointments (see for example, Hoyez, Chapter 9 in this volume; Parkinson and Behrouzan 2015), and the uncertainties and stresses of moving through, and location in, different countries, with varying health-care systems and rights.[2] Thus while many migrants entering Europe are often initially healthier than native-born residents, the combination of challenges and inequities they face can lead to a deterioration in health status over time (van den Muijsenbergh et al. 2014).

Research has found that a combination of structural, legal, institutional and cultural factors result in migrants making less use of public health facilities, screening and preventive programmes, as well as antenatal and homecare services, than the general population (Vermeer and van den Muijsenbergh 2010; Phillimore 2016). At the same time, research has found that when migrants cannot access primary healthcare, their use of emergency services is relatively high (Thomas et al. 2010). A further explanation for the relatively low uptake of healthcare services is that difficulties in communication can end up without mutual understanding being reached, leading to poorer compliance and decreased patient satisfaction (MacFarlane and de Brún 2010).

Other studies emphasise that this relates not only to language, but to ways of thinking about and understanding ill-health and effective responses to it. A number of studies within the social sciences, for example, have emphasised that the ways that people perceive healthcare services, as well as the informal networks they utilise to respond to health issues may also impact upon subjective understandings and responses relating to health service accessibility and use. Studies have also emphasised the importance of recognising how expectations around issues such as diet, hygiene, confidentiality, breaking of bad news, end-of-life decisions and human dignity can present very real dilemmas within daily healthcare practice (Ilkiliç 2015). As is demonstrated in case study 1, research has also shown that the individualistic approaches to healthcare adopted within Western biomedicine may at times be deemed inappropriate and even unhelpful for people drawing on different frameworks of understanding (ill-)health and wellbeing (see also Green et al. 2006; Thomas 2010, 2013; Gideon 2013). Such approaches recognise that experiences of health, and interactions between those who use and those who provide healthcare, are strongly influenced by cultural context, and that this in turn plays a key role in the provisioning of equitable healthcare (Napier et al. 2014; Chaturvedi et al. 2011; Abel et al. 2008).

CASE STUDY 1 SOMALI WOMEN'S EXPERIENCES OF HEALTHCARE

The largest diaspora of Somali refugees in the United States reside in Minnesota. Partnering with three community organisations in 2007–2008, Pavlish et al. (2010) implemented the Community Connections and Collaboration Project to address health disparities experienced by Somali women. The study found that the women's health beliefs contrasted sharply with the individualistic, biological models of understanding underpinning Western medicine. These diverging health beliefs resulted in differing expectations regarding treatment and healthcare interactions. When expectations remained unmet, the women and their healthcare providers reported multiple frustrations that often diminished perceived quality and productivity of healthcare. Such circumstances, as well as the cultural norms and stigma associated with particular issues within the Somali community, were found to exacerbate the difficulties the women faced in seeking support for sensitive issues such as those relating to depression, sexual health and reproductive decision-making.

(Pavlish et al. 2010)

It is vital therefore, to recognise that ensuring equity in healthcare is not just about increasing service provision, and that access to effective healthcare means more than just enabling people to get through the front door of the clinic or hospital. As Ingleby (2012) argued, when it comes to the responsiveness of services to the needs of diverse groups of patients (including migrants), equity involves offering '*different* care', rather than a 'one size fits all' approach to service provision that discriminates against those whose needs differ from the majority.

CULTURAL COMPETENCE

Ensuring the provision of healthcare that is sensitive to the needs of people from diverse backgrounds is commonly referred to as being 'culturally competent'. Yet, despite increasing attention being placed on the value of culturally competent healthcare, questions remain over its conceptualisation and how this can be best played out in practice. A large part of this challenge relates to often static and narrowly defined conceptualisations in which 'culture' is seen as synonymous with race and ethnicity, while the fluidity and constructed nature of culture and self-identity are overlooked (Owiti et al. 2014; Chiarenza 2012). Indeed, while concrete notions of culture and ethnicity may provide healthcare professionals with an important grounding in 'cultural awareness' and clearer guidance on working practice, it may also risk reducing the notion of cultural competence to a technical intervention, stereotyping and 'othering' patients, and wrongly labelling certain behaviours, responses and conditions as cultural traits (Owiti et al. 2014). Research has, for example, shown that assumptions made by healthcare providers on the basis of 'culture' can, whether consciously or unconsciously, shape behaviours during the clinical encounter and influence decisions made by professionals and patients. Differences in referral and treatment practices and patterns, for instance, have been found to be influenced by doctors' assumptions relating to the culture and socioeconomic background of patients. Joynt et al. (2013), for example, found that people from lower socioeconomic groups in the US were less likely to be given opioids for equivalent levels of pain than those from more affluent areas, and that black and Hispanic patients were also less likely to receive opioids, regardless of socioeconomic status. Such issues may be particularly problematic when culture is identified as an issue that is exclusive to migrants. Knipper, for example, argues that in Germany, assumptions around migration mean:

> It [migration] is a homogenising, morally charged category which fosters the false impression of a clear-cut boundary between non migrants and migrants, and obfuscates not only the huge heterogeneity of immigrants, but also the afflictions and desperate needs of some particular groups like undocumented migrants and refugees.
>
> (Knipper 2013: 376)

In response, it is increasingly recognised that more holistic definitions and understandings of culture are needed. The UNESCO definition for example,[3] has recently been adopted by the WHO Cultural Contexts of Health programme (see WHO 2015a) because it conceives of culture as a way of life, rather than simply as religious, social or ethnic characteristics that are delimited by geographical boundaries. Others have emphasised the value of incorporating 'cultural humility' into healthcare systems and responses. This concept not only recognises the wide array of often interconnected factors that impact on health experiences and outcomes, but also focuses on the need for healthcare workers to reflect on their own cultures and assumptions, and to actively seek to recognise the perspectives and experiences of patients (Chiarenza 2012).

CASE STUDY 2 FACTORS INFLUENCING MIGRANTS' USE OF HIV SERVICES

Late diagnosis of HIV and non-adherence to treatment regimens are known to limit treatment options and compromise effective health outcomes. A study undertaken with migrants from Southern Africa presenting for healthcare in London examined a range of factors that contributed to delayed diagnosis and non-adherence. The study found that many migrants faced logistical difficulties accessing basic healthcare, as well as fears relating to hospital charges and the potential for asylum applications to be compromised by an HIV-positive diagnosis.

At the same time, a number of migrants were found to rely on non-biomedical treatments that they sourced from wider transnational social networks. Such treatments were felt to provide important wellbeing benefits and enabled people to maintain supportive links with family and community members. Of those who had received an HIV-positive diagnosis, however, few discussed their use of such treatments with their HIV clinicians, potentially compromising the effectiveness of their antiretroviral treatment. When asked why, patients explained that they felt that their HIV clinician would judge them for using non-Western (and thus, in their eyes, non-'legitimate') medicine, and that they would be considered undeserving of further healthcare treatment and support.

(Thomas et al. 2010a, 2010b)

As is demonstrated in case study 2, ensuring people are able to access healthcare in a way that feels comfortable and non-judgemental is central to effective healthcare provision. Indeed, a recent shift towards the promotion of 'diversity sensitivity' in healthcare includes recognition of the role that background, experiences, language and culture play in fostering diversity between and within communities, and advocates that whatever its source – be it gender, ethnicity, age, socioeconomic status, religion, or sexual orientation – difference should be integrated into the delivery of effective and equitable health care for all patients (HPH Task Force MFH 2014).

While it is vital to ensure that the perspectives and experiences of patients are incorporated into healthcare practice, it is also vital that the perspectives of those who are *not* currently in, or using, the system are taken on-board. Understanding why people are not using healthcare is especially crucial since they may need to, and might be more willing to do so if it were better adapted to their needs (Ingleby 2012). Conventional methods of involving patient user groups to inform healthcare services (for example, through Patient and Public Involvement, see NIHR 2015) may therefore remain only partially effective in improving accessibility and experience for migrant groups. As Ingleby (2010) states, reaching out beyond existing patients to establish dialogue with migrant communities is also challenging, since it is often unclear who the 'community' encompasses and who can best represent it. Further work is therefore needed to develop effective ways of ensuring that the voices of migrants and other minority groups are heard so that they can play a key role in the co-production of their health and wellbeing.

GOOD PRACTICE IN HEALTHCARE

Although research on the provision of culturally competent healthcare remains limited, a number of important trends and findings have been observed. Diversity in the workforce, for example, has been found to strengthen provision of health services for migrants, with minority groups who are given a choice more likely to select health professionals from their own ethnic background and being generally more satisfied with the care they receive (Mladovsky et al 2012). While this trend points to the value of recruiting an ethnically diverse workforce, it is important to recognise that some migrants may choose to avoid healthcare workers from their own ethnic background, particularly in cases where health issues and experiences are stigmatised (Thomas et al. 2010a).

Other studies have emphasised the value of healthcare navigation in which people are guided through what may be complex and confusing processes and systems. Research across four European countries, for example, demonstrates that even migrants who have been settled in a host country for some time and know how to access health services can benefit greatly from guidance and support in system navigation (Green et al. 2014). Similarly, in the US, outreach attempts to provide navigational support for people with diabetes and/or hypertension have helped to re-engage people back into the healthcare system (see Wang et al. 2015).

Interpretation

Being understood and accepted is a key component of trust in the doctor–patient relationship, and is highly associated with patient satisfaction (van den Muijsenbergh et al. 2014; Anderson et al. 2003). Indeed, a systematic review found that good-quality, professional interpretation can improve perceptions of clinical care to a level almost equivalent to that received by patients with no language barriers (Karliner et al. 2007). The health professional's verbal behaviour – and especially the way in which the patient's experiences of illness are explored – affects to a large extent whether trust is built and maintained. This raises a number of questions regarding how trust and mutual understanding can be developed within consultations in which there is no shared language or culture between doctor and patient. Guidelines and training initiatives relating to the use of professional interpreters and intercultural competence are available across many European healthcare settings. However, evidence indicates that this varies enormously across the region, and that while language and cultural issues are commonly identified as a major problem for healthcare professionals, use is rarely made of professional, trained interpreters and cultural mediators in routine practice (see for example Martin and Phelan 2010), despite the known benefits of this approach and international requirements to ensure culturally appropriate healthcare (WHO 2010).

Reasons for this are unclear. However, research suggests that this is in part due to resource constraints – the Netherlands, for example, have recently withdrawn funding for formal interpreters (see van den Muijsenbergh et al. 2014) – and to poor organisational practice and prioritisation within healthcare systems. Indeed, research has shown that many healthcare providers 'get by' without training by drawing on informal strategies to support communication in consultations, such as using family/friends as interpreters (MacFarlane et al. 2014). Research undertaken for RESTORE, a cross-European project aimed at improving intercultural competence in healthcare, indicates that while such strategies can be effective, they also risk compromising migrants' access to, and experience of, healthcare, particularly when interpreting is of poor quality, when health issues are deemed sensitive or when sociocultural norms relating to issues such as gender and age negatively influence practices of care and support for particular households members (O'Donnell et al. 2008; van den Muijsenbergh et al. 2014).

In other cases, health services rely on telephone rather than more costly face-to-face interpretation. However, as discussed in the following section, communication relies on more than just verbal interaction, and important information may get lost when participants cannot see each other. This issue can be partially overcome through the use of videoconferencing. However, this may be difficult to implement in practice unless it can be arranged in advance, and even then, may prove difficult where consultations times are constrained.[4] Research has also shown that some healthcare professionals communicate differently with migrants compared to non-migrants, and that this then impacts on patient experience. In their study in the Netherlands for example, Meeuwesen et al. (2006) found that consultations with migrants were shorter than those with native-born populations, that GPs dominated discussions within consultations and that migrants were less demanding than non-migrant patients.

Intercultural Mediation

While ensuring good-quality interpretation is vital in supporting patient outcomes, being able to communicate verbally is not the only factor in establishing satisfactory interaction between patients and health providers. A small but growing body of research within the social sciences, for example, demonstrates how non-verbal gestures and body language can play an important role, not only in impacting on patient satisfaction, but in influencing health outcomes (see, for example, Lavelle et al. 2015; McCabe and Priebe 2008). At the same time, it is vital to recognise that even when language does not in itself present a barrier, migrants will not necessarily be familiar with the diverse health systems and norms of practice that determine health-seeking and health provision. Set alongside the challenging social, economic and political situation in which many migrants in Europe are living, and the ways that such circumstances can impact on health-seeking and health outcomes, it is important to look beyond the often fairly restricted role of interpretation to consider the role of cultural mediation.

The terms 'interpreter' and 'mediator' are often used interchangeably across Europe, yet while the roles are complementary, important differences exist. While interpreters are charged with facilitating verbal communication and understanding, the role of cultural mediators is more wide-ranging, and may be helpful even when language does not pose a barrier.[5] Cultural mediation can, for example, play an important role when tensions or anxieties exist between heath providers and healthcare users. This may be a result of a lack of cultural awareness or competence within the healthcare system and/or may result when a limited understanding of the healthcare system acts as a key barrier for migrant populations to benefit from health services (Martin and Phelan 2010). Cultural mediators can play an important role in informing patients of their entitlements to health and other support and welfare services, explaining how the health system works and encouraging them to voice their needs and concerns.

Cultural mediators may also take responsibility for facilitating effective and respectful dialogue between health providers and health users. Misunderstandings, inaccurate assumptions, stereotyping and judgemental attitudes on the part of both health providers and health users can result in tensions and even conflict, and engaging a cultural mediator has been found to prove useful in managing such situations, facilitating constructive relationships and fostering mutual understanding even in situations where tensions are already evident (Martin and Phelan 2010). Importantly, cultural mediators can help healthcare professionals to monitor the progress of their patients and ensure the provision of appropriate follow-up services and support within and beyond the health system. Cultural mediators in Spain, for example, are also used to help Roma children to access education, and help ensure school attendance (see VET4Roma 2015).

Because cultural mediators may be working with vulnerable people, it is important that strict codes of confidentiality, impartiality and professionalism are observed. While it is often helpful for mediators to come from the community requiring support, it is vital to recognise that fears of stigma and discrimination may result in some people preferring to use a mediator from a different community.

Training and Education of Health Workers

Despite increasing recognition of the potential of culturally competent healthcare provision, training to enable its implementation remains sparse and inconsistent across the European region. Where training in cultural mediation exists, for example, it varies in length from two-day to two-year programmes, and involves different content, focus and methods of delivery.

One of the main challenges recognised by those who run educational programmes on diversity and healthcare is being able to translate the notion of 'culture' into a helpful tool for medical training and practice (Knipper et al. 2010), and steer away from the inferior, 'exoticist' position that culture and diversity continue to hold within the field of (bio) medicine and health (Knipper 2013). Crucial within this, is that cultural competence training be integrated into day-to-day clinical practice, rather than seen as an occasional necessity reserved only for non-native 'others'. The following case study details an approach to training that has been praised within Germany.

CASE STUDY 3 TRAINING IN INTERCULTURAL CARE IN GERMANY

Until recently, issues of culture and ethnic diversity remained absent from medical education in Germany. In 2004, the Giessen University Medical School established a course dedicated to understanding ethnic diversity and the health-related needs of migrants. A key challenge facing the programme was how to deal with and 'fix' the ambiguous issue of 'culture' appropriately within medical education. Underpinning the course were two key themes: (1) recognition that perceiving 'ethnic groups' as culturally static, homogenous communities bound by common ancestry did not reflect the realities of people living hybrid identities in increasingly transnational social worlds; and (2) that social, economic and biographical factors often played a more direct role in influencing experiences of healthcare than cultural values and identities.

The course drew on ethnographic approaches that enabled trainee medical students to consider and understand patient's perspectives on (ill-)health and medical care, and the key issues that influenced this (e.g., legal status, social support networks, language skills, identity) and to reflect on and critique their own normative frameworks of (biomedical) understanding. An important principle of the course was to 'think global, teach local'. This meant that students were encouraged to learn about important issues affecting migration and health at global levels (e.g., epidemiology, legal frameworks and intercultural cooperation), at national levels (e.g., the history of migration and immigration policy in Germany) and at local levels. One particularly successful module enabled medical students to visit social workers supporting migrants in the local area. Through this, students were able to witness the living conditions of the migrants, and talk to them outside of the clinical setting.

Two further modules have also been designed to assist health workers to look beyond cultural assumptions. One provides knowledge about Islam in relation to medicine and helps students to reflect on their responses when they encounter what appears to be conflict between faith and medicine. The other focuses on the psychosomatic dimension of disease among migrants, and gets medical students to consider and communicate about the broader (non-medical) stresses facing their patients before inappropriately prescribing drugs such as antidepressants.

(Knipper et al. 2010)

Other studies have shown that training in cultural competence can result in a range of additional benefits. Case study 4 for example, stresses how the use of patient-centred narratives within assessment and treatment plans were felt by health professionals to improve doctor–patient engagement, increase medical compliance, hasten discharge from healthcare services and improve cost-effectiveness. While the perspectives of healthcare users were less clear-cut, some improvements were reported in levels of depression and anxiety as a result of engaging with the project.

CASE STUDY 4 CULTURAL CONSULTATION IN EAST LONDON

In the context of increasing challenges facing mental health services and in line with existing equalities guidance, the Cultural Consultation Service (CCS) was commissioned by Tower Hamlets NHS to provide cultural consultation in East London. Within this project, person-centred narratives were placed centrally in the patient assessment and treatment plans, as well as in therapeutic communications. Working across multiple levels of service delivery, the broad aims of the project were to: (1) improve clinical outcomes, service user outcomes and the experience of mental healthcare for patients from black and ethnic minorities; (2) improve the cultural competence of mental health professionals; and (3) work with commissioners to inform the development and improvement of services. In an evaluation of the project, clinicians reported that they found the CCS helpful because it allowed service users to share issues about life and illness experiences that were not previously known to staff. More specifically, clinicians felt the service had helped to provide: changes to treatment plan (71 per cent); improved engagement (50 per cent); increased medication compliance (21 per cent); and earlier discharge (7 per cent). Forty-five per cent of those clinicians who responded wanted to have a cultural consultant permanently based within their team and cited lack of resources as the main obstacle to implementing the recommendations of the CCS. No significant changes were found in service users' perceptions of their overall health. However, objective scoring methods reported some improvements in levels of depression and anxiety. The service was also cost-effective, with use of A&E services and psychiatrists reduced among those using the CCS.

(Palinski et al. 2012)

CONCLUSION

Migrants, like all other people, have a right to the highest attainable standards of health. Yet within the context of Europe, large-scale migration is taking place against a backdrop of austerity measures, and an increase in anti-immigration sentiment, greatly exacerbating what was already impeded access to health services. This chapter has argued that ensuring migrants have access to effective health services requires that such services take steps to adapt in order to better engage with, and respond to, migrants' subjectively experienced needs and priorities.

While the concept of culturally competent healthcare is gaining traction, challenges relating to its interpretation in practice remain. Indeed, as has been argued here, such notions may inadvertently fuel static conceptualisations in which culture is considered as synonymous with 'other' people, such as those from migrant backgrounds. Under such circumstances, assumptions made around 'culture' may result in inappropriate healthcare, and compromised health outcomes.

In order to help prevent such occurrences, a number of examples of good practice in healthcare provision and diversity sensitivity have been identified. This includes the importance of making available good-quality interpreting services, examining the potential role of cultural mediation and ensuring that training of health professionals involves a process of self-reflection in which embedded assumptions and ways of working can be challenged.

Efforts to ensure culturally competent healthcare that more effectively responds to patient's needs reflect a positive development in efforts to ensure health-related human rights. However, it is important to recognise that until the wider social, economic and structural disadvantages facing migrants are addressed, it remains only a partial solution to ongoing health inequalities.

NOTES

1. In response to the large-scale migration into Europe, the European Commission has recently developed a 'personal health record' – a template document that can help health-care providers reconstruct a past medical history for refugees who have no health documentation with them. This document has so far been developed in English and Arabic and measures have been taken to ensure the language used in the document is reassuring for refugees, who as a result of their experiences, may have an inherent suspicion of authority and be reluctant to carry a record of their transit route (WHO 2015b).
2. Recent research points to the difficulties that long-term migrants have navigating health-care, even when language is not an issue (see Green et al. 2014).
3. In its 2001 Universal Declaration on Cultural Diversity, UNESCO defined culture as 'the set of distinctive spiritual, material, intellectual and emotional features of society or a social group, and that it encompasses in addition to art and literature, lifestyles, ways of living together, value systems, traditions and beliefs' (see http://unesdoc.unesco.org/images/0012/001271/127162e.pdf).
4. In the UK, for example, GP consultations times last an average of 8–10 minutes per patient (NHS 2016).
5. In Spain, for example, cultural mediation has been in place for almost two decades to help people from the Roma population to access health services. Although the Roma in Spain speak Spanish, they face serious health inequities and discrimination, which hinder access and use of healthcare services.

REFERENCES

Abel, T. (2008), Cultural capital and social inequality in health, *Journal of Epidemiology and Community Health*, **62**(7), e13.

Anderson, L. M., S. C. Scrimshaw, M. T. Fullilove, J. E. Fielding and J. Normand (2003), Culturally competent healthcare systems: a systematic review, *American Journal of Preventive Medicine*, **24**(S3), 68–79.

Bradby, H., R. Humphris, D. Newall and J. Phillimore (2015), *Public Health Aspects of Migrant Health: A Review of the Evidence on Health Status for Refugees and Asylum Seekers in the European Region*, Copenhagen: HEN/WHO Regional Office for Europe.

Chaturvedi, S., N. K. Arora, R. Dasgupta and A. K. Patwari (2011), Are we reluctant to talk about cultural determinants? *The Indian Journal of Medical Research*, **133**(4), 361.
Chiarenza, A. (2012), Developments in the concept of 'cultural competence', in D. Ingleby, A. Chiarenza, W. Deville and I. Kotsioni (eds.), *Inequalities in Health Care for Migrants and Ethnic Minorities*, Cost Series on Health and Diversity, Antwerp: Garant.
De Vito, E., C. de Waure, M. L. Specchia and W. Ricciardi (2015), *Public Health Aspects of Migrant Health: A Review of the Evidence on Health Status for Undocumented Migrants in the European Region*, Copenhagen: HEN/WHO Regional Office for Europe.
Gideon, J. (2013), Access versus entitlements: health seeking for Latin American migrants in London', in F. Thomas and J. Gideon (eds.), *Migration, Health and Inequality*, London: Zed Books.
Green, G., H. Bradby, A. Chan and M. Lee (2006), 'We are not completely Westernised': dual medical systems and pathways to health care among Chinese migrant women in England, *Social Science and Medicine*, **62**,1498–1509.
Green, G., C. Davison, H. Bradby, K. Krause, F. Morente Mejias and G. Alex (2014), Pathways to care: how superdiversity shapes the need for navigational assistance, *Sociology of Health and Illness*, **36**(8), 1205–1219.
HPH Task Force Migrant Friendly Hospitals (2014), Standards for equity in health care for migrants and other vulnerable groups: self-assessment tool for pilot implementation, Task Force on Migrant-Friendly and Culturally Competent Health Care, Regional HPH Network of Emilia-Romagna, accessed online (6th July 2016) at http://steso.fi/data/documents/Equity_Standards_SAT_kasikirja.pdf.
Ilkiliç, I. (2015), Culture and ethical aspects of truth telling in a value pluralistic society, in W. Teays, J-S. Gordon and A. Dundes Renteln (eds.), *Global Bioethics and Human Rights*, Lanham: Rowman and Littlefield.
Ingleby, D. (2010), Adapting mental health services to the needs of migrants and ethnic minorities, in D. Bhugra and S. Gupta (eds.), *Migration and Mental Health*, London: Cambridge University Press, pp. 231–244.
Ingleby, D. (2012), Introduction, in D. Ingleby, A. Chiarenza, W. Deville and I. Kotsioni (eds.), *Inequalities in Health Care for Migrants and Ethnic Minorities*, Cost Series on Health and Diversity, Antwerp: Garant.
Joynt, M., M. K. Train, B. W. Robbins, J. S. Halterman, E. Caiola and R. J. Fortuna (2013), The impact of neighborhood socioeconomic status and race on the prescribing of opioids in emergency departments throughout the United States, *Journal of General Internal Medicine*, **28**(12), 1604–1610.
Karanikolos, M., P. Mladovsky, J. Cylus, S. Thomson, S. Basu, D. Stuckler, J. P. Mackenbach and M. McKee (2013), Financial crisis, austerity, and health in Europe, *The Lancet*, **381**(9874), 1323–1331.
Karliner, L. S., E. A. Jacobs, A. H. Chen and S. Mutha (2007), Do professional interpreters improve clinical care for patients with limited English proficiency? A systematic review of the literature, *Health Services Research*, **42**, 727–754.
Knipper, M. (2013), Joining ethnography and history in cultural competence training, *Culture, Medicine and Psychiatry*, **37**, 373–384.
Knipper, M., S. Akinci and N. Soydan (2010), Culture and healthcare in medical education: migrants' health and beyond, *GMS Zeitschrift fur Medizinische Ausbildung*, **27**(3), 1–6.
Lavelle M., S. Dimic, C. Wildgrube, R. McCabe and S. Priebe (2015), Non-verbal communication in meetings of psychiatrists and patients with schizophrenia, *Acta Psychiatrica Scandinavica*, **131**(3), 197–205.
MacFarlane, A. and T. de Brún (2010), Medical pluralism: biomedicines as ethnomedicines, in S. McClean and R. Moore (eds.), *Folk Healing and Healthcare Practices in Britain and Ireland: Stethoscopes, Wands and Crystals*, Oxford: Berghahn Books.
MacFarlane A, M. O'Reilly-de Brún, T. de Brún, C. Dowrick, C. O'Donnell, F. Mair, W. Spiegel, M. van den Muijsenbergh, E. van Weel Baumgarten, C. Lionis, C. Clissmann and on behalf of the RESTORE consortium (2014), Healthcare for migrants, participatory

health research and implementation science – better health policy and practice through inclusion: the RESTORE project, *European Journal of General Practice*, **20**, 148–152.

Martin, M. C. and M. Phelan (2010), Interpreters and cultural mediators – different but complementary roles, *Translocations: Migration and Social Change*, available online at http://doras.dcu.ie/16481/1/Martin_and_Phelan_Translocations.pdf.

McCabe, R. and S. Priebe (2008), Communication and psychosis: it's good to talk, but how? *British Journal of Psychiatry*, **192**(6), 404–405.

Meeuwesen, L., J. A. Harmsen, R. M. Bernsen and M. A. Bruijnzeels (2006), Do Dutch doctors communicate differently with immigrant patients than with Dutch patients? *Social Science and Medicine*, **63**, 2407–2417.

MFH (2004), *European Recommendations*, available online at www.mfh-eu.net/public/european_recommendations.htm.

Mladovsky, P., D. Ingleby, M. McKee and B. Rechel (2012), Good practices in migrant health: the European experience, *Clinical Medicine*, **12**(3), 248–252.

Napier, A.D., C. Ancarno, B. Butler, J. Calabrese, A. Chater, H. Chatterjee, F. Guesnet, R. Horne, S. Jacyna, S. Jadhav, A. Macdonald, U. Neuendorf, A. Parkhurst, R. Reynolds, G. Scambler, S. Shamdasani, S. Zafer Smith, J. Stougaard-Nielsen, L. Thomson, N. Tyler, A-M. Volkmann, T. Walker, J. Watson, A. Williams, C. Willott, J. Wilson and K. Woolf (2014), Culture and health, *The Lancet*, **384**, 1607–1639.

NHS (2016), *NHS General Practitioner (GP) Services*, available online at www.nhs.uk/NHSEngland/AboutNHSservices/doctors/Pages/gp-appointments.aspx.

NIHR (2015), *Patient and Public Involvement*, available online at www.nihr.ac.uk/funding/pgfar-patient-and-public-involvement.htm.

O'Donnell, C., N. Burns, C. Dowrick, C. Lionis and A. MacFarlane, on behalf of the RESTORE team (2013), Health-care access for migrants in Europe, *The Lancet*, **382**, 9890.

Owiti, J. A., A. Ajaz, B. De Jongh and K. S. Bhui (2014), Cultural consultation as a model for training multidisciplinary mental healthcare professionals in cultural competence skills: preliminary results, *Journal of Psychiatric and Mental Health Nursing*, **21**, 814–826.

Palinski, A., J. Owiti, M. Ascoli, B. De Jongh, J. Archer, P. Staples, N. Ahmed, A. Ajaz and K. Bhui (2012), *A Cultural Consultation Service in East London: Experiences and Outcomes from Implementation of an Innovative Service*, London: NHS Tower Hamlets and National Mental Health Development Unit.

Parkinson, S. and O. Behrouzan (2015), Negotiating health and life: Syrian refugees and the politics of access in Lebanon, *Social Science and Medicine*, **146**, 324–331.

Pavlish, C. L., S. Noor and J. Brandt (2010), Somali immigrant women and the American health care system: discordant beliefs, divergent expectations, and silent worries, *Social Science and Medicine*, **71**(2), 353–361.

Phillimore, J. (2016), Migrant maternity in an era of superdiversity: new migrants' access to, and experience of, antenatal care in the West Midlands, UK, *Social Science and Medicine*, **148**, 152–159.

Rechel, B., P. Mladovsky, D. Ingleby, J. P. Machenbach and M. McKee (2013), Migration and health in an increasingly diverse Europe, *The Lancet*, **381**, 1235–1245.

Schoevers, M. A., M. E. T. C. van den Muijsenbergh and A. L. Lagro-Janssen (2009), Self-reported health problems of female undocumented immigrants, tip of the iceberg self-rated health and health problems of undocumented migrant women in the Netherlands: a descriptive study, *Journal of Public Health Policy*, **55**, 409–422.

Schoevers, M. A., M. J. Loeffen, M. E. van den Muijsenbergh and A. L. Lagro-Janssen (2010), Health care utilization and problems in accessing health care of female undocumented immigrants in the Netherlands, *International Journal of Public Health*, **55**, 421–428.

Thomas, F. (2010), Transnational health and treatment networks: meaning, value and place in health seeking amongst southern African migrants in London, *Health and Place*, **16**(3), 606–612.

Thomas, F. (2013), Multiple medicaments: looking beyond structural inequalities in migrant healthcare, in F. Thomas, F. and J. Gideon (eds.), *Migration, Health and Inequality*, London: Zed Books.

Thomas, F., P. Aggleton and J. Anderson (2010a), 'If I cannot access services, then there is no reason for me to test': the impacts of health service charges on HIV testing and treatment amongst migrants in England, *Aids Care*, **22**(4), 526–531.
Thomas, F., P. Aggleton and J. Anderson (2010b), 'Experts', 'partners' and 'fools': exploring agency in HIV treatment seeking among African migrants in London, *Social Science and Medicine*, **70**(5), 736–743.
van den Muijsenbergh, M., E. van Weel-Baumgarten, E. Burns, C. O'Donnell, F. Mair, W. Spiegel, C. Lionis, C. Dowrick, M. O'Reilly-de Brún, T. de Brún and A. MacFarlane (2014), Communication in cross-cultural consultations in primary care in Europe: the case for improvement: the rationale for the RESTORE FP 7 project, *Primary Health Care Research and Development*, **15**(2), 122–133.
Vermeer, B. and van den M. E. T. C. Muijsenbergh (2010), The attendance of migrant women at the national breast cancer screening in the Netherlands, 1997–2008, *European Journal of Cancer Prevention*, **19**(3), 195–198.
VET4Roma (2015), *The Spanish Training Experience*, available online at http://mediation-4roma.eu/the-spanish-training-experience/#more-3406.
Wang, M. L., L. Gallivan, S. C. Lemon, A. Borg, J. Ramirez, B. Figueroa, A. McGuire and M. C. Rosal (2015), 'Navigating to health: evaluation of a community health center patient navigation program', *Preventive Medicine Reports*, **2**, 664–668.
WHO (2010), *Health of Migrants – The Way Forward: Report of a Global Consultation*, Geneva: World Health Organization.
WHO (2013), *Health 2020: A European Policy Framework and Strategy for the 21st Century*, Copenhagen: WHO Regional Office for Europe.
WHO (2015a), *Beyond Bias: Exploring the Cultural Contexts of Health and Well-being Measurement*, available online at www.euro.who.int/en/data-and-evidence/cultural-contexts-of-health/beyond-bias-exploring-the-cultural-contexts-of-health-and-well-being-measurement-2015.
WHO (2015b), *'Europe is Europe Because of Migration': Highlights from Day 2 of the High-Level Conference on Refugee and Migrant Health*, available online at www.euro.who.int/en/about-us/partners/news/news/2015/11/europe-is-europe-because-of-migration-highlights-from-day-2-of-the-high-level-conference-on-refugee-and-migrant-health.

PART VII

TRANSNATIONAL AND DIASPORIC NETWORKS

25 Transnational families, care and wellbeing

Loretta Baldassar, Majella Kilkey, Laura Merla and Raelene Wilding

TRANSNATIONAL FAMILIES AND CARE CIRCULATION[1]

Increasing numbers and types of migrants are separated from their family by distance and national borders. Even those family members who 'stay behind' become part of social relationships stretched across time and place, although they might never actually move at all. The notion of 'transnational families' emerged at the beginning of the twenty-first century to designate these new family forms, defined by Bryceson and Vuorela (2002: 18) as 'families that live some or most of the time separated from each other, yet hold together and create something that can be seen as a feeling of collective welfare and unity, namely "familyhood", even across national borders'.

The challenge of maintaining the feeling of collective welfare and unity in transnational families, friendships and support networks must be at the core of any discussion of migration and its impact on wellbeing. How do family members (broadly defined) support each other across distance? How do they perform their roles and duties as supportive friends, mothers and fathers, children, sisters and brothers, aunts and uncles, grandparents and so on? Our research leads us to argue that the exchange of care is one of the central processes (practices and performances) that maintains and sustains migrant family relationships – indeed all family relationships. For the purposes of this chapter, we focus on the ability of transnational family members to practise caregiving as a key feature of migrant wellbeing.

It must be noted that transnational families are not new. Throughout history there have been many and varied forms resulting from all types of mobility including emigration and immigration, colonial expansion and exploration and the separation of family members through entry into religious orders, the custom of apprenticeship and even the use of boarding schools (Yeates 2009). Rather, it is the scale and pattern of mobility that has been radically transformed (Castles et al. 2014). Contemporary forms of mobility include a diverse and overlapping set of population flows including:

- The large-scale flows of labour migrants, including the important phenomenon of migrant female domestic and care workers, which has radically feminised migration (see, for example, Parreñas 2001; Willis and Yeoh 2000).
- 'Forced' migrations, including of refugees and persons trafficked across international borders against their will (see, for example, Kneebone et al. 2014).
- The movement of skilled and professional migrants, often on temporary visas, including highly paid consular executives and expatriates as well as more middling professions such as nursing and trades (see, for example, Walsh 2008; Iredale 2002; Conradson and Latham 2005).
- The mostly rural–urban flows of internal migration are a feature of the so-called developing world. This form of migration in China today constitutes one of the largest movements of people in human history (see, for example, Cai et al. 2012).
- The movement of young people, both as working holiday visa holders and international students (see, for example, King and Raghuram 2013; Cairns 2010).
- The movement of people for lifestyle reasons, including so-called 'sunset' migrants, relocating in the retirement phase of the life-course (for example, Benson and O'Reilly 2009).
- The movement of people to form families via marriage migration (for example, Kim and Kilkey 2016).
- The category 'migrant' also blurs with other forms of mobile persons including commuter and fly-in/fly-out workforces that reflect the full spectrum of workers, from professionals to low-skilled (for example, Ralph 2014).

This complex range of migrant types has resulted in a tendency in the recent literature to refer to 'mobility' rather than 'migration' to better reflect this diversity (Urry 2007). What all these mobile types have in common, in terms of their wellbeing, is the desire and need to sustain their caregiving and receiving relationships across distance. The way people manage distance and its impact on family and friendship relationships has been revolutionised by the plethora of new communication technologies. Whereas in the past, transnational family members would stay in touch only by long-awaited letters that travelled by sea, today people can be 'virtually' constantly present in each other's lives. As Baldassar, Baldock and Wilding (2007: 13) write, 'the resulting idea of the "transnational family" is intended to capture the growing awareness that members of families retain their sense of collectivity and kinship in spite of being spread across multiple nations'.

Definitions and Key Concepts

Our definition of transnational families includes both nuclear and extended types whose members are actively engaged in family survival and maintenance, ranging from those whose involvement is extensive and constant to those whose roles are more marginal. We recognise too that these roles and the extent of engagement can change over time and across the lifecourse. For this reason, our definition of transnational caregiving includes a wide variety of care exchanges (Baldassar et al. 2007). Drawing on Finch and Mason's (1993) model of family support, five dimensions of care are distinguished: financial and material (including cash remittances or goods such as food and clothing, and paying household and other bills); practical (exchanging advice and assisting with tasks); emotional and moral aimed at improving psychological wellbeing; personal care (such as feeding and bathing); and accommodation (providing shelter and security). This multidimensional definition of care enables distinctions between caring practices that can be exchanged across borders through the use of communication technologies (typically financial and emotional), proximate caring practices that occur during visits, and proxy caring practices, involving the coordination of support provided by others (Kilkey and Merla 2014; Baldassar 2008; Wilding 2006). All these types of care can be exchanged in transnational settings, but to varying degrees and subject to a variety of factors, including gender, ethnic, class and power hierarchies, as well as national and international policy provisions in fields such as migration, care, communication and transport.

Transnational caregiving, just like caregiving in all families (whether separated by migration or not), binds members together in intergenerational networks of reciprocity and obligation, love and trust, that are simultaneously fraught with tension, contest and relations of unequal power. Baldassar and Merla (2014) point out how the exchange of care in families is inherently reciprocal and asymmetrical, governed by the 'norm of generalised reciprocity' – the expectation that the giving of care must ultimately be reciprocated, although it may not always be realised (Finch and Mason 1993). People may give care without measuring exactly the amount they receive, but with the expectation and obligation that care will be returned to them. This said, family members often carefully monitor these exchanges and they are governed by the multiple and constantly 'negotiated family commitments' and intimate and unequal power relations that characterise family life. For this reason, Baldassar et al. (2007) argue that all family caregiving (both proximate and distant) is mediated by a dialectic comprising the capacity (ability, opportunity), the culturally informed sense of obligation and the negotiated family commitments of individual members to provide care within family networks that are influenced by broader social and political contexts.

As care is given and returned at different times and to varying degrees across the life course, Baldassar and Merla (2014) argue that care could be described as circulating among family members over time as well as distance. This care circulation framework helps to capture all the actors involved in family life as well as the full extent of their care activity, including practical, emotional and symbolic, that defines their membership in a family. The care circulation framework helps to expand the more common focus on gendered dyads of care (e.g., mother–daughter) to consider multidirectional flows of care across more diverse kin, friendship and service networks. Relevant here are Kofman's (2012: 144) notions of social reproduction and global householding, which help to 'place care work within a wider landscape of activities . . . and to connect supposedly disparate circuits of mobility and migration, [labour, family and education], which are usually analysed separately'. Looking at migration and transnational family life through the lens of caregiving helps to sharpen our focus on wellbeing.

CARE CIRCULATION AND WELLBEING

The concept of care is strongly related to issues surrounding welfare and wellbeing, both at an individual and collective level. As Daly (2011) points out, care relates not only to the servicing of the needs of those who cannot take care of themselves as well as those who are able-bodied, it also emphasises in a broader sense the relational foundations of all social life. In other words, 'key elements of people's welfare inhere in their relations with others and the reciprocity around responses to need and the receipt of recognition and value for who people are' (Daly 2011: 47–48).

The capabilities approach offers a useful lens through which we can link care circulation in transnational families and wellbeing (Merla and Baldassar 2010). The capabilities approach proposes a multidimensional approach to wellbeing that attempts to account for both non-financial and non-material constituents (Robeyns 2007). Quality of life is defined as one's freedom to live the kind of life that, upon reflection, one finds valuable. Capabilities refer to 'what real opportunities you have regarding the life you may lead' (Sen 1987: 36). They represent people's potential functionings, or freedom to be and do what they want to be and do. These 'beings and doings' (or functionings) together constitute what makes a life valuable. Examples of capabilities include being well-fed, taking part in the community, being sheltered, relating to other people, working in the labour market, caring for others and being healthy (Robeyns 2003: 63). This approach takes diversity into consideration: it acknowledges that people differ in their capacity to transform the resources that are available to them into capabilities, depending on personal, social or environmental factors, such as physical and mental wellbeing, traditions, social norms, and public infrastructure. Sen's capabilities approach is a framework of thought rather than a fully specified theory, and does not provide a definite list of capabilities. It thus allows for the design of context-sensitive definitions of the criteria that influence people's wellbeing. In her attempt to apply the capabilities approach to gender equality, Robeyns (2003: 71–73) highlights the importance of care. Her list of capabilities includes elements such as unpaid domestic work and non-market (also called informal) care (that is, being able to raise children and to take care of others), and social relations (being able to be part of social networks and to give and receive social support). In our own work on transnational families, we have linked the capability to circulate care in transnational families with a series of interconnected capabilities that include mobility (being able to travel and send remittances), communication (being able to communicate across distance), social relations (having access to a supportive social network across distance), as well as time, money, education and knowledge, and appropriate housing (Merla and Baldassar 2010; Merla 2012; Kilkey and Merla 2014).

Thus, we define the circulation of care in transnational families as a capability that is strongly connected to wellbeing, as the following vignettes show. These four short case studies of transnational family care will help us underline that the ability to give and receive care to and from geographically distant relatives significantly impacts on the wellbeing of transnational family members – in terms of the provision of their care needs, of reciprocal care obligations and practices, and of identity recognition.

CASE STUDY 1 FLYING GRANDMOTHERS: THE CIRCULATION OF CARE ACROSS THE LIFE-COURSE

Eleonora, a 76-year-old woman born in the Dominican Republic, raised her seven children alone and also took care of the children of her daughters Eva and Elisa when they respectively migrated illegally to Belgium and the United States. When these grandchildren left to join their mothers abroad, Eleonora still continued to provide support to her distant relatives. During several years she acted as a 'flying grandmother' (Goulbourne and Chamberlain 2001) who regularly travelled to care for her relatives when necessary. In 1986, she spent three months in Belgium to take care of Eva during her final stage of pregnancy. Eva suffered from severe back problems, and the old lady travelled to Belgium every time she needed to undergo surgery. Eleonora also spent two to four months in Belgium caring for her grand-daughters; cooking, ironing, cleaning the house and walking the children to school. Over the years the two women have been able to get permanent citizenship, which has made it easier for Eleonora to travel back and forth. She also regularly travelled to the US to provide similar support to her American grandchildren.

Eleonora's children do their best to reciprocate the love and care they receive from their mother, and to support her financially. In 2003, they all received terrible news: Enrique, the youngest son living in the Dominican Republic, was diagnosed with stomach cancer. He died in hospital only a few weeks later. Elisa and Eva made an emergency trip to their homeland but sadly, they arrived the day after he passed away. The whole family rallied around Eleonora, who was terribly affected by her son's sudden death, and Eva decided to bring her mother to Belgium, where she cared for her for the next year. Eleonora moved back to her house and the frequency of her travel decreased as she became older. Two years ago she suffered from internal bleeding. Her local son and daughter took care of her. Once again, Eva rushed to her mother's side. She didn't trust the diagnosis of the local hospital and travelled to Belgium with her mother to undertake further medical examination. Eleonora soon recovered and moved back home a month later.

CASE STUDY 2 MIGRANT FILIAL OBLIGATION: CARE CIRCULATION ACROSS DISTANCE OVER TIME

Nacho left his native El Salvador in 1989 through a political refugee programme and migrated to Perth, Australia, with his wife and children. They had enjoyed a good socioeconomic situation in El Salvador. Nacho was an anaesthesiologist in a children's hospital, his wife managed a small coffee shop, and they had bought their own house in the capital, San Salvador. The decision to leave El Salvador was directly related to security: their lives were threatened because of their political activities. On arrival in Perth, Nacho was advised that, in order to have his qualifications recognised by the Australian education system, he had to pass English tests and repeat his university studies in medicine. Nacho did not have a good command of English and felt constrained instead to renounce his profession and take up a cleaning job, while his wife stayed at home to care for their four children. Later she took a cleaning job and he became the pastor of a Spanish-speaking evangelical church, while still working as a cleaner. The couple deeply suffered from their loss of social and economic status, and Nacho felt bad about leaving his ill mother behind.

When he lived in El Salvador, Nacho provided various degrees of financial, emotional, practical and personal care to his mother, and migration has not prevented him from continuing these contributions transnationally, in the form of regular and emergency remittances, as well as practical and emotional support. Nacho is very close to his mother, who suffers from diabetes and can hardly walk. His father died when he was a child, and his mother remarried and had another son. He had a difficult relationship with his mother when he was a teenager but they became very close when they both embraced Christianity – he was 17 at the time. He helped her financially and continued to help her after he got married, and shared all his worries with her. During the first year of his migration, Nacho called his mother three times a week from a public telephone. Later he bought a computer and mother and son chat every day on MSN, but Nacho still calls his mother on the phone, three times a month, because he likes to hear her voice. So far Nacho has not been able to visit his mother back home. When she had an accident in 2007, he wanted to visit her but she convinced him that it would be more useful to use that money to cover her medical expenses. Nacho deeply regrets not being able to hold his mother in his arms, but being a 'good' son who is 'there' for his mother, even from a distance, is particularly important for him, and partly helps him overcome the negative feelings arising from his social and economic downgrading in Australia.

CASE STUDY 3 REFUGEE TRANSNATIONAL CARE EXPERIENCE: THE LIMITS OF OBLIGATION

Mina migrated to Perth in the 1990s with her husband, Seyyad. Like him, she was born and lived in Kabul, where they owned a fruit and vegetable shop. Neither have any formal educational qualifications. They fled Afghanistan in the mid-1980s with their children and many of Seyyad's relatives to Pakistan. They eventually successfully applied to Australia's humanitarian programme. Mina had deeply mixed feelings about this opportunity for a better life because it meant leaving her elderly parents and six brothers behind in Iran. Mina is constantly trying to scrape together money to send to her family back home. However, with limited income, most of what they earn is taken up by their family's needs in Perth. Following the custom of traditional households, anything extra is given to Seyyad's family, who are also very needy. The distribution of meagre funds is a common dispute between Afghan couples. Men generally want to spend money on their families, as it is the duty of sons to care for their parents. Mina manages to phone her family once a month but is not able to send them any money, a situation that weighs heavily on her.

The dire economic circumstances of the Afghan refugees results in keen expressions of caregiving obligation as refugee families regularly restrict their own meagre subsistence in order to be able to support family abroad (one man mortgaged his house so that he could afford to help his parents in Iran). However, the limits of obligation and the pressures of economics are also evident. In cases where demands and obligations exceed capacity, a breakdown in networks can result as individuals attempt to shield themselves from obligations they cannot meet. Not surprisingly, a common complaint among Perth-based refugees was that their families (back home or in transit countries) did not understand the level of difficulty they faced in earning money. As Seyyad explained: 'They assume that we are wealthy because we live in a wealthy land.' Unsustainable obligation appears to result in a breakdown in social networks and obligation, although this may be temporary (Baldassar 2008).

CASE STUDY 4 TRANSNATIONAL FATHERS: THE SIGNIFICANCE OF BORDERS

We met David, a Polish national living in London, in 2010. He was one of the tens of thousands of Poles who had come to the UK after 1 May 2004, taking advantage of their newly found right, associated with membership of the European Union, to move and reside freely in the territory of any other EU member state (although, unlike the UK, most member states did not give this right in full until 2011). However, David had a long history of working irregularly in London prior to 2004, in order to support his wife and children back in Poland. David described migration in that period as 'sacrifice for the family', commenting 'I didn't really like England. In England I liked the pound.' Although he sent remittances home, he felt other aspects of his fathering and partnering role suffered because his irregular status and ensuing precarious labour market positioning meant that visits back to Poland were rare. This was compounded by poor communication technologies in that period – 'there was a time when from London to Poland you had to call for four hours just to get through' – as well as by poor transport networks.

David described 1 May 2004 as his day of 'freedom' to reunite his family. At first his wife came. The children were left in the care of their maternal grandmother in Poland while David's wife found employment and they saved enough to rent a family-sized accommodation. Because of improvements in the quality, availability and affordability in communication and transport networks, as well as their freedom to travel, David and his wife had daily contact with their children and managed the occasional quick visit. Their children arrived in September 2006, accompanied by their grandmother. While her intention had not been to remain in London, after observing the long working hours of her daughter and son-in-law, she stayed to help look after the children; David and his wife would find childcare prohibitively expensive, and in any case, their preference is to have their children cared for by family members (Kilkey et al. 2013).

These four vignettes provide a sense of the variety of migrant situations covered by the literature on transnational families, as well as highlighting some of the commonalities that cross these various family configurations. They all bring to the fore the important role that care exchanges play in the maintenance of family ties across distance and time. Care circulation can also put family ties under strain when care duties become too heavy, as in the case of the Afghan refugees mentioned here. Health issues in particular act as catalysts for the reactivation of sometimes dormant family connections, pushing kin to engage in more intense communications, emergency visits and sometimes prompting them to relocate for long periods of time in order to provide care for a dependent family member (Kilkey and Merla 2014; Wilding and Baldassar 2009; Baldassar 2014a). Being able to participate in routine care (such as the exchange of emotional support over the phone) and/or in crisis care is closely linked with definitions of the self as a 'good son', 'good daughter', 'good mother' or 'good grandparent' who fulfils his/her family obligations in accordance with culturally defined notions of filial/parental duty (Baldassar 2014b).

It is important to note that none of those case studies specifically deals with the important phenomenon of transnational mothering of young children, even if it is present in the stories of Eleonora and her daughters, and David and his wife. As the cases above suggest, our own research has focused on transnational elder care (Baldassar, Wilding, Merla) and transnational fathering (Kilkey). However, there is a vast literature on this issue that we wish to highlight here.

Transnational Mothering: De-demonising Distance

The transnational mothering literature in particular has highlighted the negative consequences of mother–child separation in the context of migration, including in terms of health, emotional distress and feelings of guilt, and stigmatisation (Parreñas 2005; Bonizzoni and Boccagni 2014). In the case of 'left-behind' children in particular, these negative consequences can be linked with cultural constructions of biological mothers as the only persons able to provide adequate care for children – thereby leading to the general assumption that substitute care 'would result in poor support being provided for children in terms of affection, nutrition, medical care, schooling, disciplining and control' (Bonizzoni and Boccagni 2014: 81). As Bonizzoni and Boccagni (2014) have shown, the quality of care provided by substitute carers depends on a variety of factors, including the sociodemographic profile of carers, the stage in the family life-cycle and the quality of interpersonal relationships. They further highlight that the impact of mothers' migration on children's wellbeing depends on two additional factors: the age of the child and the continuity and frequency of transnational practices.

The idea that only biological mothers can provide adequate care to children does not prevail in every society. The notion of 'family' indeed 'covers a multitude of senses of relatedness and connections' (Sørensen and Guarnizo 2007: 161), both within Western societies and across the globe. This richness is hidden from view in the dominant Western imaginary that identifies family with nuclear households bound up in notions of proximity and intimacy. As Sørensen and Guarnizo (2007) note, the tendency to identify the family with the domestic household has led researchers to assume that separation automatically leads to family disintegration, particularly when mothers leave husbands and children behind. The argument about the relative absence of anxiety related to physical separation in African as compared to Western cases is particularly instructive. For instance, Filho (2009: 525) argues that because of the set of imperatives that define migration in Cape Verdean society, families experience separation as less painful and disruptive than in the West, and this is due to 'the ethos that emphasizes a lack of anxiety in regard to physical separation between those who stay and those who leave, and the maintenance of a strong feeling of relatedness, acting as a bridge for the physical distance, by means of continuity of material obligations'. Similarly, Madianou and Miller (2012: 10) refer to 'anthropological accounts of many regions, such as the Caribbean, where the nuclear co-present family has never been the norm'. According to Segal, Caribbean migration 'should be understood as a form of extended kinship over space and time with frequent rather than one-time movements' (Segal 1996 in Nurse 2004: 4). The migration of women from the lower classes in Caribbean societies, for example, has been described as part of a system of circulation of care that is an integral and accepted aspect of family and kinship (Fog Olwig 2014).

Thus, the way transnational family members experience absence from loved ones is much more dependent on their interpretations of the quality of their relationships and on the socially constructed meanings of mobility and family than on the actual distance that separates them. This means that we need to revisit normative Western understandings of family, household, wellbeing, migration and the conceptualisation of human mobility more broadly.

Wall and Bolzman (2014) argue, for example, that the experience of physical separation and the feelings attached to having to deal with physical absence are not static, but change over time, depending not only on the objective situation of the migrant and his or her relatives, but also on subjective aspects including, among others, changes in migration and settlement projects, mutual expectations as well as the definition of self and of appropriate parenting at various stages. Drawing on extensive research data, they analyse the influence of life-stage on migration and transnational family life projects, including the impact on what they call 'care configurations'.

Different life-stages position migrants (both female and male) in a variety of caregiving configurations. Today it is not only young adults and couples who migrate and take on care responsibilities, in particular for spouses and young children left behind, but also middle-age migrants who care for close kin belonging to three or even four generations or elderly persons who migrate to be nearer their adult children. Contextualising transnational family life within the dynamics of the life-course is crucial to understanding the linkages between the migration project and the exchange of care across borders (Wall and Bolzman 2014: 74).

Wall and Bolzman argue that, in early adulthood, couples without children are focused on setting themselves up and often draw on support from their extended kin without needing to put much effort into caring for others. In contrast, couples with young children have intensive responsibilities to their children and often need to call on as much support as they can muster from their friendship and kin networks. They thus identify several patterns of transnational care within this category including caring migrant father, caring migrant parents and the caring young lone mother, who, within a short-stay and intensive-saving migration trajectory, leaves her young children with a close relative. In middle life, Wall and Bolzman identify the caring mother and caring grandmother, who migrates alone to support her older children and their families in the home country. As in proximate families, it is the absent long-distant father and the deprived lone mother who have the most precarious care networks. The latter are mothers who, in a situation of financial hardship in the host country, may develop weak care commitments in relation to the children left behind and they are therefore particularly at risk.

Clearly there are many factors that can facilitate and impede the ability of family members to exchange care across distance. In the final section of this chapter we consider the policy implications relevant to this issue. In the next section we go into some detail about how families actually manage to 'do' caring across distance.

NEW MEDIA AND TRANSNATIONAL CAREGIVING

Transnational families rely on similar practices and processes of caregiving as non-mobile families, and include a similarly broad range of caregiving relationships, including those between spouses (Mahler and Pessar 2001), those between mothers and fathers and their dependent children (Gardner 2012; Carling et al. 2012; Kilkey et al. 2013), and those between ageing parents and their adult children (Foner and Dreby 2011; Zontini 2012). Like families who live in close proximity, families dispersed across long distances make use of a range of new communication technologies to support their strategies of familyhood. In the process, they are arguably transforming the very nature of relationships and the foundations of human relatedness, intersubjectivity, autonomy and interdependence (Ling 2008).

The extraordinary uptake of new media means that social activities, social interactions and a sense of belonging need no longer be limited to local, proximate networks and communities. The emerging polymedia environment has transformed the ways in which caring relationships are experienced and practised, and not only by transnational families

(Madianou and Miller 2012). For example, the unprecedented recent adoption of mobile phones indicates a desire to maintain a sense of continuous co-presence with family and friends, providing an important foundation for ongoing practices of exchanging support, including visits, remittances, gifts and advice (Lee and Francis 2009). Social (and even intimate) life is no longer conducted wholly 'in place', within neat physical and territorial boundaries, but rather must now be conceived of as incorporating distant ties and connections. Indeed, there is a burgeoning field that examines the plethora of virtual communities that can provide support as well as sites of activism and solidarity (see, for example, Karatzogianni and Kuntsman 2012; Kwan 2007). This does not mean that place has become irrelevant, or that distant or virtual care can replace proximate care. It is clear that mobile lives are still lived by physical bodies that are 'in place', within specific regional, state and national borders (Kilkey and Merla 2014), with differential access to material, political and social resources both locally and at a distance (Wilding and Gifford 2013).

As a result of the transformations in new media, distance can no longer be presumed as a barrier to care and social interactions. Rather, it makes more sense to think of distance as a factor, to be considered alongside other factors that facilitate or inhibit social support and interaction (Litwak and Kulis 1987; Hjalm 2012). The perception and experience of distance has been transformed by the availability of diverse means of negotiating its effects (Wilding 2006). Similarly, the availability of diverse communication technologies must also be taken into account as a factor impacting upon who is called upon to care and what and how care is provided. While geographic distance might tend to prevent personal (hands-on) care and support, it may present no obstacle to the coordination of that support by others (Baldassar and Merla 2014). Similarly, distance is not necessarily a barrier to the exchange of emotional, practical (giving advice) or financial support on a daily basis (Baldassar and Wilding 2014). Furthermore, visits are often a feature of distant care relationships, providing the opportunity for intensive practical and personal care (Baldassar et al. 2007). Our past research questions assumptions that virtual forms of support tend to replace and therefore diminish proximate caregiving, instead demonstrating that virtual care practices may increase and expand proximate caregiving and vice versa. Indeed, new technologies can contribute to the possibility for geographic distance to actually bring people closer emotionally, by supporting the creation of the 'ideal distance for a relationship to flourish' (Madianou and Miller 2012: 146). Distance can encourage some people to put more effort into staying in touch than they would if they were living nearby (Baldassar et al. 2007).

This said, the ability to participate in distant care networks raises a number of equity issues surrounding capabilities (physical, economic, structural) and the uneven impact of the opportunities and costs of mobility and technologies on different sectors of the population (Cresswell 2010) in different parts of the world. Equally importantly, distant care is still profoundly gendered. It is mostly women who commit the time to do distant care, which is largely unpaid and often constrains women's choices to accept further employment (Wilding and Baldassar 2009).

Portability of Care

Madianou and Miller (2012) provide an important reminder that all forms of communication are mediated, not just those that occur across distance. The same point is warranted for caregiving, particularly as all forms of care rely on communication. Recent research indicates a plethora of new forms of caregiving that facilitate its portability. For example, in contrast to the letters that were relied on in the past, new media now facilitate forms of co-presence that come much closer to communicating the 'actual' person/relationship than the ideal form. A new lexicon is developing to define these new forms of sociality and to highlight their diverse features, including 'continuous' (Xu et al. 2011), 'streaming' (King-O'Riain 2014), and 'ambient' (Madianou 2015). In addition to these virtual forms of co-presence, which are delivered by social media and voice/video over internet platforms, Baldassar has proposed the notions of proxy and imagined co-presence. Proxy co-presence is provided by the 'special transnational objects' that are circulated, including photos and gifts, as well as the visits by family members who are a kind of proxy for the presence of other family members. Imagined co-presence refers to the sense of togetherness in all of the above and exemplified in 'praying' for family or 'keeping them in my thoughts' (Baldassar 2008; see also Davidson et al. 2012).

Contemporary transnational family members stay in touch through daily SMS and WhatsApp messages, regular email, Skype calls and Facebook posts. Visits home among the Italian post-war migrants Baldassar has researched have become annual or biennial events and these are practices that involve the second and third generations (Baldassar 2001). One of the most striking findings of our research has been the expansion of kinship networks that now often follows migration in families connected through new media. When in the past migration was characterised by the flow of information through key family members who formed a kind of hub, today it is a multiple and criss-crossing set of networks involving various and extended family members.

We now have conditions of polymedia (Madianou and Miller 2012) in which, for the first time in history, people have the choice of how and when to be in touch across distance such that the choices they make now become moral ones. A related finding is that the material means to be in touch across distance impacts on the cultural obligation to do so. The greater your level of access to the material world, the greater your moral obligation to reciprocate. In the past, it was perfectly acceptable to be in touch by occasional letters and very infrequent phone calls. Today, however, if you can afford to visit for a special anniversary or a funeral and you choose not to, how is that choice interpreted by family? Transnational families quickly establish new patterns and expectations of care exchange and communication that can be routine, ritualised and/or responsive to crises. The phatic function of communication exchange is especially relevant, with acts of communication acting as 'an emotional reminder of the distant significant other'. Caring through the acts of communication, writing SMS and email, maintaining the Facebook page, etc., become themselves constitutive of the actual relationships. For example, a distant grandparent relationship with grandchildren is constituted by their Skype calls. Sibling and other kin-like relationships are constituted by their Facebook activity. The SMS traffic between family members is constitutive of their sense of being a family.

Elsewhere (Baldassar and Wilding 2014), Madianou and Miller's point about ideal distance is extended to argue that the conditions of polymedia make it possible to achieve a sense of satisfactory care, which might be defined as an ideal of shared co-presence, where your ideal of being there for each other is met with the actual practice of being in touch. The sense that you are in touch enough suggests that polymedia environments can provide the conditions for adequate 'distant co-presence' and adequate 'distant care' (Baldassar and Wilding 2014). This idea resonates with Madianou and Miller's argument that 'as polymedia becomes more present and taken for granted, the range of encounters, including very direct webcam conversation, may approach the nuance of traditional co-presence in which the "actual person" is confronted more directly'. The idea that polymedia environments allow us to know the actual person despite distance and the passage of time, contrasts enormously with the historical limitations of communication technologies of the past.

Of course, achieving adequate forms of distant co-presence requires a number of resources that are not evenly distributed or equally available. Certainly, not all families enjoy the conditions of polymedia. The portability of care relies on access to mobility (to visit) and access to technology (to remain connected across distance); factors that social and other types of policies play an important role in mediating.

TRANSNATIONAL FAMILIES AND THE CIRCULATION OF CARE: POLICY CHALLENGES

Before examining more closely how policy mediates families' capabilities to care across distance, it is important to acknowledge the role they play in the formation of transnational families in the first place. Many migrants do not 'choose' to leave family members behind; rather they are forced to because migration policies create barriers for families to migrate together or to subsequently reunite. This is especially the case for labour migrants and refugees moving from poorer to richer parts of the globe. While migration policies vary significantly in rich countries, a common trend is to more tightly manage and control immigration flows. The motives for this vary too, but include a desire to restrict migration to only those persons seen as economically useful, a related desire to prevent 'welfare dependency' among immigrants and a desire to limit the long-term settlement of immigrants, especially among groups perceived to be difficult to 'integrate'/'assimilate' into the receiving country because of religious or 'cultural' differences. One result is that countries may permit the entry of a worker deemed instrumental to the economic needs of the country, but not allow (all) his or her dependants entry, or impose strict conditions on their entry that migrant workers find impossible to meet. In such cases, migrants and their families have little or no choice but to live apart.

For those families separated by borders, a significant issue is whether and how policies facilitate or impede their exchange of care and support. This remains a relatively recent and challenging question for policymakers who in the main continue to work within social policy environments that are nationally bounded and that assume that 'normal' family-life is too. Among the first to acknowledge that there was a policy dimension to the growth in transnational families were Baldassar, Baldock and Wilding (2007: 204) when they identified the capacity of family members to engage in caregiving as a key component of the dialectic mediating transnational caregiving practices (see above). Subsequent research has sought to unpack the 'capacity' component by identifying, first, the resources required for transnational caregiving, and second, the institutions through which those resources are in part derived.

Merla and Baldassar (2011) have identified six interconnected resources needed to underpin transnational caregiving. First, mobility, which refers to the ability to travel to receive or give care. Second, communication, which means being able to communicate at a distance and to send items across borders, and includes having the physical ability to communicate. Third, social relations, which refers to access to a social network of mutual support in the receiving and home country, which can represent a useful resource for the exchange of information about travel and accommodation, and can provide financial and practical support to carers and cared-for. Fourth, time-allocation, which involves having the capacity to take time for exchanging care. Fifth, education and knowledge, which refer to the possibility to learn how to use communication technologies and to learn the local language. It also includes having one's qualifications recognised, which can influence access to paid work and thus indirectly affect the ability to exchange care. Finally, paid work encompasses having access to a satisfying employment position and, if unemployed, to sufficient benefits in order to have the necessary funds to invest in caregiving. According to Merla (2012), these resources are positioned at three interconnected levels: it is through access to paid work, time-allocation, education and knowledge that family members are in turn able to communicate and be mobile. Social relations play a mediating role between these sets of resources, as they can help kin overcome obstacles to mobility and communication through money loans or the sharing of information on cheap flights and telephone cards. Kilkey and Merla (2014) subsequently added a seventh resource located at the same level as paid work, time allocation and education – appropriate housing, which is crucial for the settlement of migrant families, and can also be a prerequisite for eligibility to family reunification. Moreover, adequate housing is important for family members who travel to provide or receive proximate care, as issues such as lack of space and privacy can create tensions between visitors and their hosts. Appropriate housing, including appropriate institutional care, is also essential for care-receivers who remain in their home country.

The relevance of all seven of these resources to how families care transnationally is captured in the stories of Eleonora, Nacho, Mina and David set out earlier in the chapter. More or less explicit in those accounts was also the set of institutional arrangements, in both the home and the migrant-receiving societies that contribute to realising these resources. Here, the work of Kilkey and Merla (2014) is instructive. Starting with the premise articulated by the concept of 'care circulation' (Baldassar and Merla 2014) discussed above, that transnational families engage in proximate and transnational practices of care, that care flows are multidirectional, and that care relations are multigenerational, they develop the notion of a 'situated transnationalism' and draw on 'regime' theory, arguing that the capacity to care transnationally is influenced by migrants and their kin's respective positioning in the migration, welfare, gendered care and working-time regimes of their societies of origin and destination. By migration regime they refer to 'immigration policies – rules for entrance into a country (quotas and special arrangements), settlement and naturalisation rights, as well as employment, social, political and civil rights'

(Williams 2010: 390), and which also includes migration cultures in home and host societies. The welfare regime refers to the configuration of social protection for workers (Esping-Andersen 1990). The gendered care regime aims at capturing who is responsible for care, the nature of state support for non-familial care, and provisions for care leave (Williams 2010), as well as dominant national and local discourses – 'care cultures' – on what constitutes appropriate care (Williams and Gavanas 2008), and gender equality expectations and outcomes associated with care arrangements (Pfau-Effinger 2000). The working-time regime, finally, includes the set of legal, voluntary and customary regulations that influence working-time practice (Rubery et al. 1998: 72). Kilkey and Merla (2014) also highlight that policies around the regulation of cross-border transport, including its availability and affordability, and around the quality and accessibility of the communication infrastructure, especially telephone and internet, are also important. Moreover, they highlight that the institutional contexts within which transnational families' care arrangements are configured, are constituted in different levels and sites of governance. These include the global, the regional and the subnational, as well as the national. Moreover, those spaces are not separate and mutually exclusive entities, but are interconnected in a range of ways (Clarke 2005).

In addition to formal institutional structures, there are important areas of practice in the fields of health, social care and education that mediate the capacity for transnational care. Bacigalupe (2011), president of the American Family Therapy Academy, has drawn on some of our earlier research (for example, Baldassar et al. 2007; Baldassar 2008) to argue that new practice guidance is needed in medical settings to encourage and support medical staff to liaise with the distant kin of their patients (Bacigalupe and Lambe 2011). Currently, practice tends to privilege face-to-face communication, potentially discriminating against distant carers who may otherwise be integral to the support networks of patients. A similar argument could be made for social work and education practice, and in relation to transnational childcare, as well as transnational elder care.

CONCLUSIONS: THE MIXED IMPLICATIONS OF FAMILY CARE ON WELLBEING IN A TRANSNATIONAL CONTEXT

An analysis of transnational caregiving activity must be sensitive to the unevenness of reciprocal exchange, including the withholding and limiting of care. While the circulation of care involves reciprocal exchanges between family members, both the transnational and local care burdens fall most heavily on women, who generally receive less than they give (Ryan 2007). In this context, care and the ability to exchange it can be considered a form of social capital (or resource) that is unevenly distributed within families subject to cultural notions of gender and other roles, which intersect with and interrelate to the care regimes of the various nation-states and communities in which families reside. In addition, the care literature has rightfully highlighted how much care provision and heavy duties can be a burden and a source of high levels of stress. In the absence of other forms of support, and also often as a measure of the deep sense of obligation to care, some migrants make the decision to return to care for their ageing parents, despite the negative economic implications this might have (Baldassar 2014b).

What this growing field of research makes clear is that it is no longer possible to consider migration and health issues without paying attention to the dynamics of transnational family life. The wellbeing of migrants is no longer shaped only by the local care and policy regimes that are immediately visible to healthcare professionals and service providers. The everyday life of the migrant is also situated within non-local and transnational regimes that vary from family to family, depending on the country of origin, dispersal of kin, and life stages, resources and cultural contexts of family members. This represents a key challenge for social protection systems that have so far been largely conceived for citizens residing within the limits of a particular nation-state, and which need to be better adapted to the specific situations and needs of migrant workers who are engaged in the transnational circulation of care with relatives located in another country (Degavre and Merla, 2015).

NOTE

1. Some sections of this paper are drawn from Baldassar et al. (2014).

REFERENCES

Baldassar, L. (2001), *Visits Home: Migration Experiences between Italy and Australia*, Melbourne: Melbourne University Press.

Baldassar, L. (2008), Missing kin and longing to be together: emotions and the construction of co-presence in transnational relationships, *Journal of Intercultural Studies*, **29**(3), 247–266.

Baldassar, L. (2014a), Too sick to move: distant 'crisis' care in transnational families, *International Review of Sociology*, **24**(3), 391–405.

Baldassar, L. (2014b), Guilty feelings and the guilt trip: emotions and motivation in migration and transnational caregiving, *Journal of Emotions, Space and Society*, **16**, 81–89.

Baldassar, L. and L. Merla (eds.) (2014), *Transnational Families, Migration and the Circulation of Care: Understanding Mobility and Absence in Family Life*, New York and London: Routledge.

Baldassar, L. and R. Wilding (2014), Middle-class transnational caregiving: the circulation of care between family and extended kin networks in the Global North, in L. Baldassar and L. Merla (eds.), *Transnational Families, Migration and the Circulation of Care: Understanding Mobility and Absence in Family Life*, New York and London: Routledge.

Baldassar, L., C. Baldock and R. Wilding (2007), *Families Caring Across Borders: Migration, Aging and Transnational Caregiving*, Basingstoke: Palgrave Macmillan.

Baldassar, L., M. Kilkey, L. Merla and R. Wilding (2014), Transnational families, in J. Treas, J. Scott and M. Richards (eds.), *The Wiley-Blackwell Companion to the Sociology of Families*, Chichester: Wiley-Blackwell, pp. 155–175.

Bacigalupe, G. (2011), Is there a role for social technologies in collaborative healthcare? *Family, Systems, & Health*, **29**(1), 1–14.

Bacigalupe, G. and Lambe, S. (2011), Virtualizing intimacy: information communication technologies and transnational families in therapy, *Family Process*, **50**, 12–26.

Benson, M. and K. O'Reilly (eds.) (2009), *Lifestyle Migration. Expectations, Aspirations and Experiences*, Aldershot: Ashgate.

Bonizzoni, P. and P. Boccagni (2014), Care (and) circulation revisited: a conceptual map of diversity in transnational parenting, in L. Baldassar and L. Merla (eds.), *Transnational Families, Migration and the Circulation of Care: Understanding Mobility and Absence in Family Life*, New York and London: Routledge.

Bryceson, D. and U. Vuorela (2002), *The Transnational Family: New European Frontiers and Global Networks*, Oxford and New York: Berg.

Cai, F., Y. Du and M. Wang (2012), The largest migration in human history, *The Economist*, 24 February.

Cairns, D. (ed.) (2010), *Youth on the Move: European Youth and Geographical Mobility*, Wiesbaden: Springer.

Carling, J., C. Menjivar and L. Schmalzbauer (2012), Central themes in the study of transnational parenthood, *Journal of Ethnic and Migration Studies*, **38**, 191–217.

Castles, S., H. de Haas and M. Miller (2014), *The Age of Migration*, 5th edn, New York: Palgrave Macmillan.

Clarke, J. (2005), Welfare states as nation states: some conceptual reflections, *Social Policy and Society*, **4**(4), 407–415.

Conradson, D. and A. Latham (2005), Transnational urbanism: attending to everyday practices and mobilities, *Journal of Ethnic and Migration Studies*, **31**(2), 227–233.

Cresswell, T. (2010), Towards a politics of mobility, *Environment and Planning D: Society and Space*, **28**(1), 17–31.

Daly, M. (2011), *Welfare*, Cambridge and Malden: Polity Press.

Davidson, J., L. Bondi and M. M. Smith (eds.) (2012), *Emotional Geographies*, Aldershot: Ashgate.

Degavre, F. and L. Merla (2015), Defamilialisation of whom? Re-thinking defamilialisation in the light of global care chains and the transnational circulation of care, in M. Kilkey and E. Palenga-Möllenbeck (eds.), *Family Life in an Age of Migration and Mobility: Global Perspectives through the Life Course*, Basingstoke: Palgrave-Macmillan.

Esping-Andersen, G. (1990), *The Three Worlds of Welfare Capitalism*, Cambridge: Polity Press.

Filho, W. T. (2009), The conservative aspects of a centripetal diaspora: the case of the Cape Verdean Tabancas, *Africa*, **79**(4), 520–542.

Finch, J. and J. Mason (1993), *Negotiating Family Responsibilities*, London and New York: Tavistock, Routledge.

Fog Olwig, K. (2014), Migration and care – intimately related aspects of Caribbean family and kinship, in L. Baldassar and L. Merla (eds.), *Transnational Families, Migration and*

the Circulation of Care: Understanding Mobility and Absence in Family Life, London: Routledge.
Foner, N. and J. Dreby (2011), Relations between the generations in immigrant families, *Annual Review of Sociology*, **37**, 545–564.
Gardner, K. (2012), Transnational migration and the study of children, *Journal of Ethnic and Migration Studies*, **38**(6), 889–912.
Goulbourne, H. and M. Chamberlain (2001), *Caribbean Families in the Trans-Atlantic World*, London: Macmillan.
Hjalm, A. (2012), 'Because we know our limits': elderly parents' views on intergenerational proximity and intimacy, *Journal of Aging Studies*, **26**(3), 296–308.
Iredale, R. (2002), The migration of professionals: theories and typologies, *International Migration*, **39**(5), 7–26.
Karatzogianni, A. and A. Kuntsman (eds.) (2012), *Digital Cultures and the Politics of Emotion: Feelings, Affect and Technological Change*, Basingstoke: Palgrave.
Kwan, M. (2007), Affecting geospatial technologies, *The Professional Geographer*, **59**(1), 22–34.
King-O'Riain, R. C. (2014), Emotional streaming and transconnectivity: Skype and emotion practices in transnational families in Ireland, *Global Networks*, **15**(2), 256–273.
Kilkey, M. and L. Merla (2014), Situating transnational families' care-giving arrangements: the role of institutional contexts, *Global Networks*, **14**, 210–229.
Kilkey, M., A. Plomien and D. Perrons (2013), Migrant men's fathering practices and projects in national and transnational spaces: recent Polish male migrants to London, *International Migration*, **52**(1), 178–191.
Kim, G. and M. Kilkey (2016), Marriage migration policy as a social reproductive system: the South Korean experience, in M. Kilkey and E. Palenga-Möllenbeck (eds.), *Family Life in An Age of Migration and Mobility*, Basingstoke: Palgrave.
King, R. and P. Raghuram (2013), International student migration: mapping the field and new research agendas, *Population, Space and Place*, **19**(2), 127–137.
Kneebone, S., D. Stevens and L. Baldassar (eds.) (2014), *Conflicting Identities: Refugee Protection and the Role of Law*, London: Routledge.
Kofman, E. (2012), Rethinking care through social reproduction: articulating circuits of migration, *Social Politics: International Studies in Gender, State & Society*, **19**(1), 142–162.
Lee, H. and S. Francis (eds.) (2009), *Migration and Transnationalism: Pacific Perspectives*, Canberra: ANU E Press.
Ling, R. (2008), *New Tech, New Ties*, Cambridge, MA: MIT Press.
Litwak, E. and S. Kulis (1987), Technology, proximity and measures of kin support, *Journal of Marriage and the Family*, **49**(3), 649–661.
Madianou, M. (2015), Ambient co-presence: transnational family practices in polymedia environments, in L. Baldassar, M. Nedelcu, L. Merla and R. Wilding (eds.), Special issue on migration and ICTs: 'being together' and 'co-presence' in transnational family life, *Journal of Global Networks*.
Madianou, M. and D. Miller (2012), *Migration and New Media: Transnational Families and Polymedia*, London and New York: Routledge.
Mahler, S. J. and P. R. Pessar (2001), Gendered geographies of power: analyzing gender across transnational spaces, *Identities*, **7**(4), 441–459.
Merla, L. (2012), Salvadoran migrants in Australia: an analysis of transnational families' capability to care across borders, *International Migration*, published online.
Merla, L. and L. Baldassar (eds.) (2010), Les dynamiques de soin transnationales: entre émotions et considérations économiques, *Recherches sociologiques et anthropologiques*, **41**.
Merla, L. and L. Baldassar (2011), Transnational caregiving between Australia, Italy and El Salvador: the impact of institutions on the capability to care at a distance, in E. Addis, P. Villota, F. Degavre and J. Eriksen (eds.), *Gender and Well-Being: The Role of Institutions*, London: Ashgate, pp. 147–162.
Nurse, K. (2004), *Policy Paper: Diaspora, migration and development in the Caribbean*, New York: Focal.

Parreñas, R. (2001), *Servants of Globalisation*, Stanford: Stanford University Press.
Parreñas, R. (2005), *Children of Global Migration: Transnational Families and Gendered Woes*, Stanford: Stanford University Press.
Pfau-Effinger, B. (2000), Conclusion: Gender cultures, gender arrangements and social changes in the European context, in S. Duncan and B. Pfau-Effinger (eds.), *Gender, Economy and Culture in the European Union*, London and New York: Routledge.
Ralph, D. (2014), 'Always on the move, but going nowhere fast': motivations for 'Euro-commuting' between the Republic of Ireland and other EU states, *Journal of Ethnic and Migration Studies*, **41**(2), 176–195.
Robeyns I. (2003), Sen's capability approach and gender inequality: selecting relevant capabilities, *Feminist Economics*, **9**(2–3), 61–92.
Robeyns I. (2007), *Social Justice and the Gendered Division of Labour: Possibilities and Limits of the Capability Approach*, paper prepared for presentation at the Cost A34 Conference, Barcelona, 25–27 June.
Rubery, J., M. Smith and C. Fagan (1998), National working time regimes and equal opportunities, *Feminist Economics*, **4**(1), 71–101.
Ryan, L. (2007), Migrant women, social networks and motherhood: the experiences of Irish nurses in Britain, *Sociology*, **4**, 295–312.
Sen, A. (ed.) (1987), *The Standard of Living*, Cambridge: Cambridge University Press.
Sørensen, N. N. and L. Guarnizo (2007), *Transnational Family Life Across the Atlantic: The Experience of Colombian and Dominican Migrants in Europe Living Across Worlds: Diaspora, Development and Transnational Engagement*, Geneva: International Organization for Migration, pp. 151–176.
Urry, J. (2007), *Mobilities*, Cambridge: Polity Press.
Yeates, N. (2009), *Globalising Care Economies and Migrant Workers: Explorations in Global Care Chains*, Basingstoke: Palgrave.
Wall, K. and C. Bolzmann (2014), Mapping the new plurality of transnational families: a life-course perspective, in L. Baldassar and L. Merla (eds), *Transnational Families, Migration and the Circulation of Care: Understanding Mobility and Absence in Family Life*, New York and Abingdon: Routledge.
Walsh, K. (2008), Travelling together? Work, intimacy, and home amongst British expatriate couples in Dubai, in A. Coles and A. M. Fechter (eds.), *Gender and Family Among Transnational Professionals*, New York and London: Routledge, pp. 63–84.
Wilding, R. (2006), 'Virtual' intimacies? Families communicating across transnational contexts, *Global Networks*, **6**(2), 125–142.
Wilding, R. and L. Baldassar (2009), Transnational family–work balance: experiences of Australian migrants caring for ageing parents and young children across distance and borders, *Journal of Family Studies*, **15**(2), pp. 177–187.
Wilding, R. and S. Gifford (2013), Forced displacement, refugees and ICTs: transformations of place, power and social ties: introduction, *Journal of Refugee Studies*, **26**(4), 558–575.
Williams, F. (2010), Migration and care: themes, concepts and challenges, *Social Policy and Society*, **9**(3), 385–396.
Williams, F. and A. Gavanas (2008), The intersection of child care regimes and migration regimes: a three-country study, in H. Lutz (ed.), *Migration and Domestic Work: A European Perspective on a Global Theme*, Aldershot: Ashgate, pp. 13–28.
Willis, K. and B. Yeoh (eds.) (2000), *Gender and Migration*, Cheltenham: Edward Elgar Publishing.
Xu, B., W. Zhang and D. Li (2011), Copresence and its social-relational antecedents in computer-mediated communication: the case of instant messenger, *International Journal of Human-Computer Interaction*, **27**(10), 991–1009.
Zontini, E. (2012), Care arrangements of elderly transnational migrants: between family, community and the state, in C. Rogers and S. Weller (eds.), *Critical Approaches to Care: Understanding Caring Relations, Identities and Cultures*, New York: Routledge, pp. 171–182.

26 Knowledge transfer in the 'medical tourism' industry: the role of transnational migrant patients and health workers

Meghann Ormond

INTRODUCTION

'Medical tourism' denotes purposeful short-term travel from one's country of habitual residence to receive medical treatment paid for out-of-pocket in a country in which s/he does not habitually reside and within which s/he may not enjoy entitlements to healthcare beyond those availed to any other private consumer (Ormond 2014). Over the past 15 years, countries as diverse as India, Jamaica and the Philippines – keen to bank on rapidly increasing health and wellness consumption trends among the global middle classes – have been engaged in promoting 'medical tourism' and developing an industry around it in order to effectively attract healthcare consumers living outside of them. Proponents of 'medical tourism' have forcefully argued that potential benefits to lower- and middle-income destination countries include more foreign exchange earnings, diversified tourism offerings and a boost to the supply and quality of (private) medical care within these countries. In response, a growing number of stakeholders concentrated in Global South countries, like those mentioned above, have begun to develop their own 'medical tourism' plans and throw their hats into an already crowded, highly competitive global 'medical tourism' ring (Bookman and Bookman 2007; Connell 2011, 2013; see also Temenos and McCann 2013 on policy transfer).

Over the years, these destination countries' 'medical tourism' plans have also increasingly explicitly intersected with public and private sector policies and practices directed at attracting diverse forms of diasporic engagement and investment. Policy strategies abound at national, regional and local levels in migrants' places of origin to build and intensify transnational identity and solidarity in order to increase diasporic contributions, investments and spending. In recent years, this has involved a shift from focusing mainly on remittances and the transfer of material resources to harnessing, transferring and sharing migrants' acquired skills, knowledge and social capital back to their places of origin for the benefit of people living in them (e.g., return migration) (Faist 2008). This move towards developing both 'bonding' and 'bridging' social capital among diasporas reflects growing awareness of the range of power resources (e.g., economic, social, political, informational, moral and physical) that can be used to strategically embed places of origin in transnational networks that have the potential to avail them to new opportunity (Mitchell 1996; Opiniano and Castro 2006).

In spite of the significance of these shifts, Williams (2007a, 2007b) argues that insufficient scholarly attention has been given to the role of international migrants with different socioeconomic and politico-legal statuses in knowledge transfer. When attention is given to migrants' role in knowledge transfer and diffusion of innovation, it predominantly frames highly skilled migrants (e.g., those involved in information technology (IT), medicine, etc.) as the knowledgeable agents (see, e.g., Wang 2014). This racialised and gendered focus, however, overlooks the contributions of migrants engaged in unskilled, informal and heavily feminised care/emotional work – people who instead are often framed not as agents but rather as 'knowledge dupes' (Williams 2007b: 37). In response, Williams (2007a: 362) advances a more holistic approach to valorising human capital, 'whereby *all* international migrants are understood to be potential knowledge carriers or knowledgeable workers', regardless of their educational qualifications, income or occupation.

In this chapter, I build on earlier work on the nexus of migration and tourism (Williams and Hall 2000) – and more specifically migration and 'medical tourism' (Ormond 2012, 2013) – in order to explore the role of knowledge transfer by both migrant health workers and patients in these countries' developing 'medical tourism' industries. This focus allows me to take Williams' (2007a, 2007b) critical approach a step further by recognising migrants not only as knowledgeable (skilled or unskilled) workers but also as knowledgeable transnational citizens, family members and healthcare consumers. In the following sections, I review a wealth of recent literature in order to look in greater detail at the role of both migrant patients and migrant health workers in tacit knowledge transfer relative to the development of Global South destinations' 'medical tourism' industries. I then conclude the chapter by summarising and drawing lessons from the many examples of migrant knowledge transfer and barriers to it presented below.

MIGRANTS' ROLES IN HEALTH-RELATED TACIT KNOWLEDGE TRANSFER

In order to examine how knowledgeable migrant patients and health workers are engaged in the 'medical tourism' industry, let me first clarify what types of knowledge are held at a premium and what is being transferred. A distinction can be made between explicit knowledge, which is codified in documents and databases and is easily identified, stored and retrieved, and tacit knowledge, which encompasses intuitive understanding developed through experience and practice that 'cannot, or cannot easily, be expressed in explicit forms' (Williams 2007a: 30). In his work on the distinctive contribution that migrants can make in knowledge transfer and exchange, Williams (2007a, 2007b) predominantly draws on Blackler's (2002) four categories of tacit knowledge: embrained, embodied, encultured and embedded. *Embrained* knowledge involves mental models, conceptual skill and cognitive ability. *Embodied* knowledge comes from practical 'learning by doing' in specific contexts, which builds on physical presence and sensory information. *Encultured* knowledge involves shared understandings and values derived from socialisation and acculturation. Finally, *embedded* knowledge is not pre-given but rather emerges contextually through shared (organisational) rules and processes.

While these categories are transferable through international travel and migration, in practice they are not equally so. Embrained and embodied knowledge are more straightforwardly transferrable, with limited barriers to their implementation elsewhere (e.g., diagnostic and surgical procedures). Encultured and embedded knowledge (which do not merely serve as facilitators for the former two), however, derive from socially situated, localised experience. As a result, they are more difficult to enact outside of their generative contexts, leading to their partial transferability to other places and groups where shared meaning may be lacking or limited. Yet, their partial transferability can still be implemented productively. For example, migrants' translation of their experience – as patients and/or medical professionals – of how Country A's health system operates may be highly sought-after for comparison and emulation by those both using and working in the health system of Country B, even if most of those in Country B are not familiar with Country A.

Williams and Baláž (2008: 1925) found Blackler's typology particularly useful for examining skilled health worker (SHW) knowledge transfer because it acknowledges the range of knowledge necessary to the profession: academic knowledge (embrained), technical skill (embodied), cultural knowledge (encultured) and management skills (embedded). Yet, as noted earlier, in their physical boundary-spanning, migrants are 'distinctive knowledge bearers' (Williams 2007b: 366) with the potential to access, interpret and refine information gleaned from reflection on the intersections of their own unique range of transnational experiences, relationships, networks and resources that may be of use to other social actors. Blackler's typology, therefore, can also serve as a useful heuristic to reflect on the range of knowledge necessary for patients and their companions to pursue and receive medical care abroad. Scholars and practitioners alike have noted how both patients and their companions are increasingly savvy healthcare consumers. This is well-illustrated by Casey et al.'s (2013) study of how family and friends accompanying Canadian 'medical tourists' may assume different roles throughout their medical journeys: knowledge-broker, where information is transferred between patients and doctors; navigator, where information is gathered and care coordinated; and companion, where emotional and physical support are provided. The four types of tacit knowledge can be discerned in these roles: embrained (e.g., gathering, reflecting on and organising different medical perspectives on a medical concern or treatment), embodied (e.g., tailoring physical and emotional care to patients' specific constellations of ailments), encultured (e.g., sensitivity to and cross-cultural translation of cultural views and values related to illness and impairment and their treatment) and embedded (e.g., understanding and advocating for patients' rights, negotiating patient/doctor relations, etc.).

Patients

In delimiting 'medical tourism' as the purposeful short-term travel by people from their country of habitual residence for medical treatment in a country in which they do not habitually reside and within which they may not enjoy formal healthcare entitlements, we can distinguish 'medical tourists' from travellers whose temporary medical pursuits abroad are subsidised or reimbursed by the governments or insurers in their country of habitual residence usually as a result of bilateral or multilateral agreements (e.g., the European Union's 2011 Patients' Rights in Cross-Border Health Care Directive). The definition also differentiates 'medical tourists' from those engaging in not only short-term but also longer stays or settling permanently in receiving countries for reasons not primarily linked to medical treatment and who may or may not enjoy formal healthcare entitlements in the receiving country as a result of their political-legal status (e.g., economic migrants, students, return migrants, refugees and retirement migrants). Such discernment enables recognition of the great diversity of socioeconomic, political and legal statuses of people pursuing and receiving medical treatment abroad (Ormond 2014). Undermining attempts at introducing greater conceptual nuance, however, current recording practices in many countries promoted as 'medical tourism' destinations often do not effectively differentiate between these different statuses. Instead, published 'medical tourism' figures frequently lump *all* recipients of medical treatment with foreign passports together as 'medical tourists', effectively overestimating the volume of 'medical tourists' and paying limited regard to the diverse range of health issues and the urgency of care needs in the various places to which not only 'medical tourists' but also other (medical) travellers and migrants may be rooted.

The *de facto* diversity of statuses and origins of people receiving care abroad have been still further eclipsed by a widely pervasive imaginary of 'average medical tourists' as predominantly middle-class whites of non-migrant origin who, unhappy with medical care in their home countries in the Global North, combine short-term travel to world-class hospitals with leisure consumption (e.g., luxury hotel and resort stays, safari and city tours, etc.) in the Global South for treatment or care inaccessible to them back home. While some of those pursuing medical care abroad may in fact possess such origins and status, they are thought to be a minority. Recent work has shown that much 'medical tourism' – the purposeful short-term travel by people from their country of habitual residence for medical treatment in a country in which they do not habitually reside and within which they may not enjoy formal healthcare entitlements – is instead largely undertaken in the form of intra-regional and cross-border travel between lower- and middle-income countries within the Global South (Ormond and Sulianti 2014; Crush and Chikanda 2015). Yet the pervasive imaginary of 'average medical tourists' as middle-class whites from the Global North has profoundly shaped how policymakers, industry actors, journalists and everyday people have come to understand and legitimise the growing 'medical tourism' industry, including its key actors, its benefits and disadvantages, and how such transnational mobility links up healthcare issues and responsibilities at 'home' with those 'abroad'.

This chapter contributes to work that seeks to complicate the predominant 'average medical tourist' imaginary by paying attention to actually existing 'medical tourists', medical travellers and migrants, how they pursue and receive medical care, and their neither necessarily linear nor binary relationships to 'home' and 'abroad' (de Freitas 2005). Migrants of all types and their offspring are returning for longer or shorter periods to their places of origin or receiving care in countries with important diasporic centres that are meaningful to them. Short-term visitors are travelling with growing frequency from neighbouring countries with comparatively poorer healthcare offerings. Elite 'expat' executives and retirees are seeking out the best treatment options within the regions in the Global South in which they have settled. Such pursuits reveal a broader, richer transnational configuration of peoples and places around medical care – one that is far more socioeconomically polarised and ethnically, geographically and politico-legally diverse than the predominant 'medical tourist' imaginary.

In their study of UK residents' pursuit of treatment outside the UK and the EU, Hanefeld et al. (2015) looked not only at 'medical tourists' of British origin but also those of non-European migrant origin settled in the UK. In contrast with 'medical tourists' of British origin, respondents of Somali and Indian origin were found to be more familiar with both the UK's public and private health services and those in their countries of origin and third countries in which they or their family members had studied or lived previously. Having experienced a range of health systems in their lifetimes, they were thus better able to establish criteria for assessing and drawing comparisons between services as prospective healthcare consumers than those only familiar with the UK's socialised National Health Service (NHS). Studies by Bochaton (2015) and Ormond (2015), furthermore, point to how effective migrants' transnational social networks are, not only for amassing sufficient treatment funds for patients and providing them with accommodation and transport before and after treatment but also for word-of-mouth promotion of the best medical professionals and facilities.

In recognition of this, countries are seeking to develop 'medical tourism' by strategically targeting their diasporas, considered pioneering 'early adopters' capable of diffusing healthcare knowledge and innovative practices through their transnational networks. Indeed, several countries actively promoting themselves for years to the 'average medical tourist' described above have now begun to more explicitly acknowledge that their main markets from Global North countries are in fact predominantly diasporic in character (e.g., US-based people of Indian origin going to India (Connell 2011: 125); Germany-based people of Turkish origin going to Turkey (Turkish Directorate-General of Health 2012: 53–57); etc.) and to more aggressively target them.

The underlying logic of destinations like these is well illustrated by a 2012 plan designed by the Trinidad and Tobago Coalition of Services Industries:

> There are an estimated two million diaspora from the Southern Caribbean (mainly Trinidad and Barbados) living in the UK, USA and Canada. In most Caribbean countries, the estimate is there is the same number of diaspora as population nationally [. . .]. Therefore it is reasonable to assume that the diaspora of Trinidad and Tobago is around 1.3 million people plus their

> offspring (sometimes two generations). Given that the 1.3 million diaspora (first generation) are now aging, the need for medical care (and expenses it involves) is growing, medical facilities in Trinidad and Tobago could explicitly target this segment. Therefore, [. . . t]he specific target for 'Strategic Goal 3: Promotion of Medical Tourism to the Diaspora' will be to attract 4000 new diaspora patients per year – 2000 from the USA, 1500 from Canada and 500 from the UK after 3 years. This target would mean less than 0.3% of first generation diaspora travelling to Trinidad and Tobago for medical treatment and, if second/third generation were included, less than 0.1%. [However, t]he impact of 4000 diaspora patients, spending on average USD5000 per treatment, would generate USD20 million of revenue for private healthcare in Trinidad and Tobago.
>
> (Hellyer 2012: 12–13)

In this excerpt, we also see intentions by destination stakeholders to attract *diverse segments* of the diaspora. This not only includes first-generation migrants visiting friends and relatives (VFR) but also their second- and third-generation children and grandchildren who may have weaker links to these countries. The strategy of appealing to different age groups within the diaspora – both younger, economically active migrants and older, retired migrants considering whether they will remain in their countries of settlement, relocate to their countries of origin or circulate between these and other countries in their transnational networks (Warnes and Williams 2007; Sun 2014) – is supported by the development of medical and allied care services that anticipate diasporic consumers' diverse needs as they change and develop over the life-course.

Indeed, more and more stakeholders are tapping into the rapidly growing retirement migration market (and its return migration submarket) by developing property and lifestyle opportunities that complement their ongoing 'medical tourism' industry investments (see also Hall, Chapter 21 in this volume). Yet, developments must not only satisfy migrant retirees' nostalgic yearnings for the 'homeland' but also meet the standards of healthcare and security to which they have grown familiar in their lives abroad. Notes a representative of the Jamaican Diaspora Canada Foundation:

> I do not want to spend my twilight years in the cold. I would much prefer to spend it in Negril or Ocho Rios, but there are things you need to put in place. The fundamental right of every Jamaican is personal security, which is a problem in this country. Old people are afraid. When you reach 75 you want somewhere to come and retire that is sunny, where you can see a doctor and there is a clinic. We have the capacity to put those things in place. And there are also people in the diaspora who will come here and build those places, once the crime has been dealt with. Jamaicans will come any time, no matter what, but foreigners will not do that.
>
> (IMTJ 2013)

Effectively, although they are considered 'early adopters', the tacit knowledge that migrants – positioned in their countries of origin as medical care and lifestyle-focused consumers – bring with them of experience with comparatively better-organised health and public security systems in their countries of habitual residence may also at times render them more akin to 'mineshaft canaries' than pioneers. 'Medical tourism' destinations seeking not only to attract diasporic patients, therefore, have much to learn from these 'canaries' about how to best attract others in their habitual countries of residence.

At the same time, stakeholders in migrants' habitual countries of residence are increasingly aware of their transnational health pursuits. Authorities and doctors in European Union (EU) countries home to peoples of non-European descent have begun to raise concerns regarding the impacts of transnational healthcare pursuits not only on the health outcomes of 'medical tourists' and travellers but also on the health systems in their countries of residence more broadly. Similar to those outlined by Snyder et al. (2012) for Canada, their concerns include reduced continuity of care (e.g., a lack of records or communication between doctors in both countries) resulting in redundant or rival care (e.g., diagnostics, treatments and consultations), incomplete recovery or rehabilitation, the need to 'repair' health complications resulting from treatment abroad, the need to 'repair' trust between patients and providers in their country of residence and the need to undo 'mixed messages' (Nielsen et al. 2012; Şekercan et al. 2014).

At the same time, transnational care practices are also acknowledged to have the potential to supplement or even entirely replace care inaccessible or deficient in migrants' habitual countries of residence due to financial, legal, cultural and linguistic hurdles (Nielsen et al. 2012; Stan 2015). Studies in Denmark and the Netherlands have highlighted significant transnational medical pursuits by people of Turkish descent. Some 26.6 per cent of first-generation Turkish migrants living in Denmark for three or more years and an impressive 19.4 per cent of their descendants travelled abroad for at least some of their medical needs, compared with a mere 6.7 per cent of Danes of non-migrant origin (Nielsen et al. 2012).[1] Meanwhile, in the Netherlands, some 21.3 per cent of respondents of Turkish origin pursued healthcare abroad – more than double those of Moroccan origin (9.8 per cent) – and more than half of *all* respondents of non-European descent aged 55 and over reported healthcare consumption in their countries of origin within the last 15 years (Şekercan et al. 2014). Many of their healthcare pursuits in Turkey were considered to be motivated by disappointment with, and barriers to accessing, specific types of care in their habitual countries of residence.

Health Workers

The conventional range of international skilled health workers' (SHWs) mobilities can be discerned by length of stay (Wendland 2012). *Short-term stays* have traditionally comprised medical students and volunteers from the Global North engaging in what Wendland (2012) calls 'clinical tourism', brief stints of less than one year in understaffed and under-resourced destinations in the Global South in order to experience 'global health' issues first-hand. *Medium-term stays* have usually involved SHWs mainly from the Global South spending several years in Global North medical facilities for postgraduate specialty training or, alternatively, SHWs principally from the Global North being deployed by humanitarian or missionary organisations on two- to three-year tours in especially needy areas in the Global South (e.g., Médecins Sans Frontières). Finally, *long-term stays*, the most well-documented of all, have mostly included SHWs from the Global South who permanently migrate to the Global North. At first glance, these mobilities contrast with those described in the section above, where *patients* travel from one country to another in order to fulfil medical and other care needs. However, while studies of the globalisation of healthcare have largely attended separately to international *patient* and *SHW* mobilities, these can be quite intertwined and, together, have important and potentially novel repercussions on the people, places and health systems involved (Connell 2011).

When it comes to short-term SHW migration and travel, Wendland (2012) notes that the frequent rotation of 'clinical tourists' from the Global North means that the new treatment approaches they introduce can quickly circulate within Global South host hospitals, clinics and communities. However, 'clinical tourists' introduce medical perspectives and solutions that, although feasible in the Global North, may be out-of-reach in material and human resource-poor contexts. For this reason, among others, short-term SHW mobility has been the target of critique. Yet, the international 'medical tourism' industry has generated two novel forms of short-term, circular SHW migration that appear to bring even fewer concrete benefits to the local communities in their destinations. Linked to growth in offshoring 'medical tourism' practices meant to further minimise regulatory red tape and/or treatment costs, the first involves engagement in so-called 'time-share' medical practices, where doctors 'purchase the right to be the only individual offering a service for patients from a specific geographic region (typically where their main practice is based) and the right to practice for part of each year in an off-shore medical facility' (Snyder et al. 2015), and the second consists of doctors and nurses accompanying individual patients or groups of patients abroad in order to undertake their treatment. In making use of hospitals and clinical infrastructure that are independent and isolated from local healthcare staff and infrastructure in the destinations, neither of these forms offers potential for medical knowledge transfer or exchange.

Those involved in the organisation and delivery of healthcare in Global South countries frequently receive part of their formal education and training abroad. This is what Wendland (2012) refers to as 'medium-term' clinical mobility. During their sojourns, these SHWs have learned about, experienced and practised within health systems other than those of their countries of origin. This enables them to be able to bring home and potentially model good practices learned abroad, with many SHWs seeing themselves as 'secular missionaries' (Wendland 2012: 117). This type of brain circulation is especially prized in Global South countries' 'medical tourism' industries, since foreign patients are widely believed to prefer doctors and nurses who have trained and practiced in the Global North (e.g., the USA, UK, Canada, Australia and Japan) or in their own countries. Indeed, several 'medical tourism' destinations – such as India, Malaysia and the Philippines, which have large numbers of SHWs temporarily training and practising in Global North countries – explicitly showcase these medium-term SHW mobilities in promotional materials in order to highlight their destinations' world-class medical excellence and cultural competence (Ormond 2012, 2013; Walton-Roberts 2015). The Indian government, for example, places strategic value on Indian medical practitioners' training and experience abroad, specifically as regards their potential to contribute to 'private sector health provision in India, itself a generator of income for the country through the medical tourism that it has speeded up' (Raghuram 2008: 183). SHWs' medium-term sojourns, therefore, can constitute especially valuable sources of social, cultural and economic capital for their countries of origin. However, appreciation for SHWs' experience in foreign patients' habitual countries of residence cannot necessarily be taken for granted. Whittaker (2015), for example, notes that the 'medical tourists' and travellers from the Arabian Gulf countries she interviewed often expressed disdain for the Southeast Asians on temporary contracts who constitute the majority of SHWs in their home countries' medical facilities, yet they would highly praise the local SHWs in the Southeast Asian countries in which they pursue medical care.

Within a global context of severe SHW maldistribution and shortages, long-term international SHW migration has been described as a 'perverse subsidy' (Mackintosh et al. 2006) that disproportionately benefits recruiting countries in the Global North while depriving Global South source countries of valuable human capital in which they have heavily invested.

The effects of this on 'medical tourism' were explicit in my study of Indonesians travelling across the border to Malaysia for medical care (Ormond and Sulianti 2014; Ormond 2015). Living in a poor, peripheral part of Indonesia, my respondents were frustrated by the emigration of their best and brightest health workers to the capital city, Jakarta, and outside the country's borders. They decried the restrictions that the Indonesian government placed on recognising foreign medical education credentials for reducing the potential for Indonesian doctors trained abroad to return home and for foreign doctors to establish practices in their community. Thus, perceiving the local crop of Indonesian doctors to be inferior, they actively sought out alternatives in the form of distant regional missionary hospitals with a rotating staff of SHWs from the Global North or private hospitals in Malaysia and Singapore.

Yet long-term SHW migration can affect 'medical tourism' development in many other ways. Connell and Walton-Roberts (2015: 164) note that economically-motivated long-term SHW migration is far from a novel phenomenon: 'In south India, the Philippines and small island states, migration of SHWs has occurred over more than one generation, resulting in a "culture of migration" that becomes pervasive, normative, nurtured, and enhanced by the presence of overseas kin.' This has led to the development of multigenerational diasporic networks of SHWs. However, migrant knowledge transfer or 'brain gain' is not necessarily hindered by the permanent settlement of SHWs abroad. Indeed, Opiniano and Castro (2006) have highlighted the role of migrant associations and professional diasporic organisations in both knowledge networks (e.g., the Transfer of Knowledge Through Expatriate Nationals (TOKTEN) and *Balik* Scientist programmes in the Philippines). Diasporic investment in 'medical tourism' industry developments is also increasingly significant, enabled by social networks bringing together local and diasporic knowledge and investment. The mobilisation of charitable financial contributions and business investments by diasporic Jamaicans for the proposed Negril International Hospital in north-western Jamaica developed to serve the medical needs of diasporic Jamaican and non-Jamaican 'medical tourists' alongside those of resident Jamaicans is one example of this (IMTJ 2013). Walton-Roberts (2015) also shows how non-resident Indian (NRI) investment in Indian private healthcare and education as well as migrant Indian brain-circulation at the managerial level have worked together to internationalise Indian hospitals and medical education, effectively making a significant impact on the country's health system (see also Pandey et al. 2004). Her study indicates that not only migrant SHWs but also migrants with other forms of experience in the healthcare industry – such as management, sales and marketing – also bring new approaches and practices to the business of healthcare in their countries of origin as a result of their own migratory sojourns (e.g., 'medical tourism' facilitators such as IndUSHealth and MalaysiaHealthcare.com).

At the same time, the 'medical tourism' industry has been championed by international and national development organisations and government bodies for its potential to reduce the effects of long-term international SHW brain-drain. First, it is held to be able to help stem brain-drain by providing a greater number of more lucrative and better-resourced employment opportunities within SHWs' home countries (Connell 2011).[2] Second, it is used to legitimise investment in educating more SHWs in 'medical tourism' destinations. However, such logic rarely takes into account the length of time necessary to produce a sufficient number of competent nurses and medical professionals with the specialisations most in demand by 'medical tourists'. In light of this, destinations increasingly look to both diasporic and non-diasporic migrant health workers to either permanently or temporarily fill in the gaps. The 'medical tourism' industry has been used to justify governments' return migration campaigns targeting, among others, senior medical specialists practicing abroad in order to benefit from their knowledge, experience and prestigious foreign credentials. The Malaysian government's Returning Expert Programme (REP), for example, offers attractive fiscal incentives to senior Malaysian SHWs and permanent resident status to their non-Malaysian family members. In my 2012 study of Malaysian medical specialists who regularly work with 'medical tourists',[3] the significance of migrant SHWs' tacit knowledge transfer is explicit. Embrained, encultured and embedded knowledge are particularly well-illustrated in the following excerpt from an interview with a Malaysian specialist who returned to settle in his hometown:

> I have overseas qualifications, and a specialist qualification obtained overseas seems to be more sought-after than a specialist trained locally [. . .]. So, there seems to be confidence when you are trained in [. . .] a first-world country, trained in Australia. [. . .] People like us have an advantage. The other thing I realised is that the Australian system, which is the only system I can speak of, helped us a lot in terms of communication skills. [. . . It] really emphasises communication, and my seniors – Australian-Italians, Australian-Greeks and Australian-Maltese – were very smart people with a very high EQ [level of emotional intelligence]. They were my role models, showing me how to communicate with patients, showing me how to manage difficult situations. So, it was through them that I managed to develop my soft skills. When I got back, it wasn't a problem launching a private practice. I could take it on right away. I think that the Australian medical education taught us to have a holistic approach: you treat a disease, you treat a person – you don't treat a number. The patient is not a number – you call the patient by their name.

We also can see that Global South 'medical tourism' destinations are increasingly turning to migrant SHWs from both the Global North and South to fulfil their care labour needs. Snyder et al. (2015) point to growth in long-term international migration by SHWs *between* Global South countries. Low-wage Indian doctors, nurses and technicians, for example, are being hired to cover 75 per cent of the staffing needs in Health City Cayman Islands facilities. Matsuno (2009: 13), meanwhile, found that foreign nurses accounted for 40 per cent of all nurses in Malaysian private hospitals but only 2 per cent of all nurses country-wide. Furthermore, the growth of hospitals and care homes not only in the Global North but also the Global South has created new labour demands not only for SHWs but also for lower-wage, oftentimes less formally trained caregivers (e.g., orderlies, home care providers, etc.). Yet scant scholarly attention has been given to the locals and migrants employed in such jobs, although they are essential for 'medical tourism' industries. Finally, Snyder et al. (2015) also highlight the long-term settlement of so-called 'black sheep' or maverick SHWs from the Global North in Global South countries whose regulatory environments may facilitate medical practices unregulated elsewhere (e.g., experimental stem-cell therapies) or leave legal problems unresolved in their home countries unacknowledged. These recruitment and settlement strategies are opening 'medical tourism' destinations up to new directionalities of flows of tacit knowledge around health, illness, impairment and treatment with the potential to challenge standards and practices in local medical facilities and households.

CONCLUSIONS

Due to a dominant shared imaginary of who the 'average medical tourist' is and what he/she needs and desires, many 'medical tourism' industry stakeholders have been slow to – or perhaps still have yet to – acknowledge the actually existing diversity of people pursuing and receiving medical care outside of their usual countries of residence. For a long time, this conceptual blind spot has effectively precluded much of the potential of knowledge transfer by migrant patients to the developing 'medical tourism' industries in their countries of origin. Yet we are beginning to see greater awareness among stakeholders in both migrants' habitual countries of residence and other countries in which they choose to receive medical treatment of their practices, to the extent that migrants have become recognised by some as bellwethers for broader 'medical tourism' populations and trends. Migrants' diverse medical pursuits have underscored the need for policymakers and industry stakeholders to pay attention to the nuances of migration temporalities, employment statuses, integration trajectories, transnational social networks and stages of the life-course and how these in turn impact on engagements in (transnational) healthcare practices by economic migrants, refugees, international students, expatriates, retirement migrants, etc. (Ormond 2014; Stan 2015). Furthermore, the tacit knowledge that migrant patients, their families and communities have of different health systems, facilities and medical professionals puts them in a particularly unique position to assess the advantages and disadvantages of receiving treatment and care in different places.

Migrant health workers, meanwhile, bring another set of skills and knowledge to developing 'medical tourism' industries not only through return migration and brain circulation but also through diasporic professional knowledge transfer and investment. However, as with migrant patients, policymakers and industry stakeholders also have had – and continue – to work to eliminate another conceptual blind spot: namely, the existence of a much broader range of transnational health worker mobility existing both before the emergence of 'medical tourism' development plans and resulting from them. While destinations have banked on harnessing certain migrant SHWs' tacit knowledge to benefit the industry, a range of other entrepreneurial migrants with varied non-medical experience of healthcare operations have also recently come on to the scene, seeking to implement good practices and business models acquired elsewhere in their countries of origin. Still, other contributions by migrants – especially those engaging in care work considered 'unskilled' – have largely passed under the industry radar in spite of the growing relevance of caregiving in rapidly ageing societies around the world.

In sum, migrants are not only knowledgeable workers but they are also knowledgeable citizens, family members and consumers. Tapping into their diverse tacit healthcare knowledge can bring a range of stakeholders in countries of origin great insight, at both macro and micro levels, not only into how to improve on local healthcare delivery but also how to effectively respond to the needs and interests of 'medical tourists' as well as a range of travellers and migrants enfolded in developing 'medical tourism' industries.

NOTES

1. Danish national health insurance covered non-chronic medical and pharmaceutical expenses for all persons with permanent residence in Denmark until 2008. The impacts today of the 2008 legislation limiting non-EU coverage on Turkish migrants' healthcare pursuits outside of the EU remain unclear.
2. While there is little doubt that internal brain-drain is exacerbated by the privatisation of

healthcare, of which the 'medical tourism' industry is symbolic, further research needs to be done on the specific types of human resources required for medical tourism in order to substantiate such claims.
3. See Ormond and Sulianti (2014) and Ormond (2015) for study details.

REFERENCES

Blackler, F. (2002), 'Knowledge, knowledge work and organizations', in C. W. Choo and N. Bontis (eds.), *The Strategic Management of Intellectual Capital and Organizational Knowledge*, New York: Oxford University Press, pp. 47–62.

Bochaton, A. (2015), 'Cross-border mobility and social networks: Laotians seeking medical treatment along the Thai border', *Social Science & Medicine*, **124**, 364–373.

Bookman, M. Z. and K. R. Bookman (2007), *Medical Tourism in Developing Countries*, New York: Palgrave Macmillan.

Casey, V., V. A. Crooks, J. Snyder and L. Turner (2013), 'You're dealing with an emotionally charged individual. . .': an industry perspective on the challenges posed by medical tourists' informal caregiver-companions, *Global Health*, **9**(31).

Connell, J. (2011), *Medical Tourism*, London: CABI.

Connell, J. (2013), Medical tourism in the Caribbean Islands: a cure for economies in crisis? *Island Studies Journal*, **8**(1), 115–130.

Connell, J. and M. Walton-Roberts (2015), What about the workers? The missing geographies of health care, *Progress in Human Geography*, **40**, 158–176.

Crush, J. and A. Chikanda (2015), South–South medical tourism and the quest for health in Southern Africa, *Social Science & Medicine*, **124**, 313–320.

de Freitas, C. (2005), Health has no borders: Cape Verdean immigrants in the Netherlands and the transnational quest for health care across Europe, *International Journal of Migration, Health, and Social Care*, **1**(1), 19–36.

Faist, T. (2008), Migrants as transnational development agents: an inquiry into the newest round of the migration–development nexus, *Population, Space and Place*, **14**(1), 21–42.

Hanefeld, J., N. Lunt, R. Smith and D. Horsfall (2015), Why do medical tourists travel to where they do? The role of networks in determining medical travel, *Social Science & Medicine*, **124**, 356–363.

Hellyer, M. (2012), *Draft National Strategy for Medical Tourism*, Trinidad and Tobago Coalition of Services Industries, available online at http://c-nsc.org/download/trade_in_services/Trinidad%20and%20Tobago%20-%20Medical%20Tourism.pdf.

IMTJ (2013), Jamaica argues it is ready for medical tourism, *International Medical Travel Journal*, 4 October, available online at www.imtj.com/news/?entryid82=428628.

Mackintosh, M., K. Mensah, L. Henry and M. Rowson (2006), Aid, restitution and international fiscal redistribution in health care: Implications of health professionals' migration, *Journal of International Development*, **18**(6), 757–770.

Matsuno, A. (2009), Nurse migration: the Asian perspective, *ILO/EU Asian Programme on the Governance of Labour Migration Technical Note*, available online at http://www.ilo.org/wcmsp5/groups/public/---asia/---ro-bangkok/documents/publication/wcms_160629.pdf.

Mitchell, K. (1996), In whose interest? Transnational capital and the production of multiculturalism in Canada, in R. Wilson and W. Dissanayake (eds.), *Global/Local: Culture and the Production of the Transnational Imaginary*, Durham: Duke University Press, pp. 219–254.

Nielsen, S. S., S. Yazici, S. G. Petersen, A. L. Blaakilde and A. Krasnik (2012), Use of cross-border healthcare services among ethnic Danes, Turkish immigrants and Turkish descendants in Denmark: a combined survey and registry study, *BMC Health Services Research*, **12**(1).

Opiniano, J. M. and T. A. Castro (2006), Promoting knowledge transfer activities through

diaspora networks: a pilot study on the Philippines, in C. Wescott and J. M. Brinkerhoff (eds.), *Converting Migration Drains into Gains: Harnessing the Resources of Overseas Professionals*, Manila: Asian Development Bank, pp. 73–97.
Ormond, M. (2012), Claiming 'cultural competence': the promotion of multi-ethnic Malaysia as a medical tourism destination, in C. M. Hall (ed.), *Medical Tourism: The Ethics, Regulation, and Marketing of Health Mobility*, London: Routledge, pp. 187–200.
Ormond, M. (2013), Harnessing 'diasporic' medical mobilities, in F. Thomas and J. Gideon (eds.), *Migration, Health and Inequality*, London: Zed Books, pp. 150–162.
Ormond, M. (2014), Medical tourism, in A. A. Lew, C. M. Hall and A. Williams (eds.), *The Wiley-Blackwell Companion to Tourism*, Malden, MA: John Wiley & Sons, pp. 425–434.
Ormond, M. (2015), 'Solidarity by demand? Exit and voice in international medical travel – the case of Indonesia, *Social Science & Medicine*, **124**, 305–312.
Ormond, M. and D. Sulianti (2014), More than medical tourism: lessons from Indonesia and Malaysia on South–South intra-regional medical travel, *Current Issues in Tourism*, published online.
Pandey, A., A. Aggarwal, R. Devane and Y. Kuznetsov (2004), *India's Transformation To Knowledge-Based Economy: Evolving Role of the Indian Diaspora*, Washington, DC: World Bank, available online at http://info.worldbank.org/etools/docs/library/152386/abhishek.pdf.
Raghuram, P. (2008), Thinking UK's medical labour market transnationally, in J. Connell (ed.), *The International Migration of Health Workers*, London: Routledge, pp. 182–198.
Şekercan, A., M. Lamkaddem, M. B. Snijder, R. J. Peters and M. L. Essink-Bot (2014), Healthcare consumption by ethnic minority people in their country of origin, *The European Journal of Public Health*, **25**(S3).
Snyder, J., V. A. Crooks and R. Johnston (2012), Perceptions of the ethics of medical tourism: comparing patient and academic perspectives, *Public Health Ethics*, **5**(1), 38–46.
Snyder, J., V. A. Crooks, R. Johnston, K. Adams and R. Whitmore (2015), Medical tourism's impacts on health worker migration in the Caribbean: five examples and their implications for global justice, *Global Health Action*, **8**.
Stan, S. (2015), Transnational healthcare practices of Romanian migrants in Ireland: inequalities of access and the privatisation of healthcare services in Europe, *Social Science & Medicine*, **124**, 346–355.
Sun, K. C. Y. (2014), Transnational healthcare seeking: how ageing Taiwanese return migrants view homeland public benefits, *Global Networks*, **14**(4), 533–550.
Temenos, C. and E. McCann (2013), Geographies of policy mobilities, *Geography Compass*, **7**(5), 344–357.
Turkish Directorate-General of Health (2012), *Evaluation Report on Medical Tourism in Turkey, 2012*, Ankara: Department of Health Tourism, Republic of Turkey Ministry of Health, available online at www.saglikturizmi.gov.tr/admin/content_img/general/big_images/VY8HA0NDoT.pdf.
Walton-Roberts, M. (2015), International migration of health professionals and the marketization and privatization of health education in India: from push–pull to global political economy, *Social Science & Medicine*, **124**, 374–382.
Wang, D. (2014), Activating cross-border brokerage: interorganizational knowledge transfer through skilled return migration, *Administrative Science Quarterly*, **60**(1), 133–176.
Warnes, A. M. and A. Williams (2006), Older migrants in Europe: a new focus for migration studies, *Journal of Ethnic and Migration Studies*, **32**(8), 1257–1281.
Wendland, C. L. (2012), Moral maps and medical imaginaries: clinical tourism at Malawi's college of medicine, *American Anthropologist*, **114**(1), 108–122.
Whittaker, A. (2015), 'Outsourced' patients and their companions: stories from forced medical travellers, *Global Public Health*, **10**(4), 485–500.
Williams, A. M. (2007a), International labour migration and tacit knowledge transactions: a multi-level perspective, *Global Networks*, **7**(1), 29–50.
Williams, A. M. (2007b), Listen to me, learn with me: international migration and knowledge transfer, *British Journal of Industrial Relations*, **45**(2), 361–382.

Williams, A. M. and C. M. Hall (2000), Tourism and migration: new relationships between production and consumption, *Tourism Geographies*, **2**(1), 5–27.
Williams, A.M. and V. Baláž (2008), International return mobility, learning and knowledge transfer: a case study of Slovak doctors, *Social Science & Medicine*, **67**(11), 1924–1933.

27 End-of-life care and death of migrants

Lorena Núñez Carrasco

INTRODUCTION

The majority of contemporary literature on migration and health is concerned with examining the interaction between social determinants of health and conditions of migration at its various phases (pre-migration, migration and return), focusing on issues such as health inequalities and access to healthcare (Zimmerman et al. 2011). Literature on issues relating to end-of-life care for migrants has been relatively limited, and what exists has been produced mostly in the Global North, in countries with large, established and ageing immigrant populations, such as the USA and countries in Europe (WHO 2014: 218). Framed as part of palliative care provided by healthcare institutions, this work has mostly focused on how to more adequately respond in a culturally sensitive manner to the needs of dying immigrants and their families living in a host society (Searight and Gafford, 2005; Buiting et al. 2008). The interlocutors within these interventions are the family members of the sick, dying immigrant who are there to assist in the process and to facilitate a 'good death' (Andershed 2006).

In much of the Global South, the reality around end-of-life care is markedly different (WHO 2014). While family networks often play a crucial role in the provision of care and social support, formal systems of support are scarce (Gysels et al. 2011). In the case of migrants, not only is there a lack of formal and integrated responses to support end-of-life needs, but also a lack of literature that reflects on the particular needs that face this population group (Gysels et al. 2011). Understanding such issues is important, not only because the return movement of migrants in times of sickness adds significant complexity to the 'push and pull' factors that initially framed migration studies (Davies et al. 2011), but also because it can expose more clearly the social determinants of health and risk factors that migrants are exposed to throughout the migratory process (Davies et al. 2011).

The recent migrant crisis in Europe and the number of migrants and asylum-seekers that have very visibly encountered death in their journeys, has made the international community more aware of the dangers that threaten the lives of migrants while fleeing war and violence. These are children and adults whose bodies may never return to their families for burial and whose identities would not, in many cases, even be established. Less visible, however, are the predicaments of sick and dying migrants in contexts of more 'regular' forms of labour migration. While the term 'salmon bias' has been widely used to describe the movement back home of sick Hispanic migrants in the United States (Abraído-Lanza et al.1999), very little is documented on migrants' experiences and needs as they seek to undertake this journey, nor the predicaments that they face in the absence of more traditional networks of family support nearby.

The need for such understandings is particularly pressing when considered within the context of the generalised HIV/AIDS epidemic across much of sub-Saharan Africa. Out of the 36.9 million people living with HIV/AIDS in the world in 2015, 19 million were living in Eastern and Southern Africa and 6.5 million were living in Western and Central Africa (UNAIDS 2016). Within this population, the percentage of those who are migrants is not really known. Yet, the general growth of migration and high levels of chronic and infectious illness across the region means that there are reasons to believe that needs for end-of-life care for migrant populations are growing (IOM 2013). Furthermore, for migrants, refugees and asylum-seekers in the South, accessing formal healthcare is, in theory at least, often more difficult than for their counterparts in the North (Zimmerman et al. 2011).

This chapter examines the situation of sick and dying migrants in South Africa, a country that combines high prevalence of HIV and AIDS and a large number of migrants. It explores the symbolic, emotional and material resources migrants mobilise at a critical point in their lives and identifies the role played by various actors providing end-of-life care (families, NGOs, hospices, churches, social workers, bus drivers). A question of concern among all those involved is a death that occurs away from home. Central to these concerns is the notion of 'home' as the ultimate place of rest, so embedded in the ideal of a good death among many people from across Southern Africa (Núñez and Wheeler, 2012). This shared belief mobilises various actors in making return possible, before is too late. Yet, oftentimes, migrants do die away from home. The second part of this chapter therefore identifies the actors involved in managing a migrant's death in a foreign country (migrant communities, burial societies, and funeral parlours). It also examines their role in organising funerals and burials or an eventual repatriation following the death of a migrant. Overall, this work focuses on these agents' strategies to deal with the material, cultural, spiritual and practical needs that arise from sickness to avoid and to manage an eventual death *out of place*, in contexts often characterised by displacement, illegality, lack of social protection and poverty.

END-OF-LIFE CARE NEEDS AMONG MIGRANTS IN SOUTH AFRICA

Statistics from the Gauteng Department of Health (province including the cities of Johannesburg and Pretoria) shows that in the past 15 years (to June 2015), 35,226 permits were issued to export bodies of deceased migrants to their respective countries. Of these, 24,242 were issued to Zimbabwean nationals, 1,946 to Mozambican nationals and 1,762 to Malawian nationals – the remaining cases distributed among a large number of countries.[1] These figures are well representative of the broader migrant population in the country, as more than half of the total foreign migrants in South Africa concentrate in Gauteng. Figures from South Africa's 2011 Census indicate that 3.3 per cent (1.7 million, of the country's 51.7 million residents) were non-citizens, with almost 1 million (8 per cent) of Gauteng's population of 12.2 million comprised of non-citizens. While figures for repatriated bodies do not account for the total number of deaths of foreign migrants in the Gauteng Province – as there are an undetermined number of foreigners that are buried in the country – they are, however, indicative of the extent of the needs of care among terminally ill migrants. Indeed, the main causes of death among migrant populations are long-term and debilitating diseases such as heart-related conditions and TB, as well as conditions such as pneumonia and meningitis that are often associated with HIV/AIDS infection.[2] This shows that the majority of migrants die from diseases that are debilitating and often require care over relatively long periods of time. Furthermore, and as discussed within this chapter, there is room to assert that had they had access to healthcare and received proper treatment and care, many of these deaths could have been deferred or even avoided altogether.

RETURNING HOME TO DIE

In the Southern African region, available data uncover an important process of return migration, internally and across borders, in times of sickness (Clark et al. 2007). In most cases, sick migrants return home of their own volition.[3] Yet it has been argued that sick and dying circular migrants who return home to their rural families bring a burden of sickness and death for their communities (Collinson 2007). The return of sick migrants not only has an impact on the epidemiological profile of sending communities but also and importantly, it results in drainage of human and material resources that are channelled towards the provision of care. The burden of care from returning sick migrants is significant as often human and material resources, as well as healthcare infrastructure in sending areas (often rural) are scarcer and less developed than those of the receiving areas (often urban) (Welaga et al. 2009; Gysels et al. 2011).

In the context of the HIV/AIDS epidemic in sub-Saharan Africa, studies have focused on the impact of AIDS-related death in the affected households and have highlighted the role of women as prime carers for the sick (Upton 2003; Evans 2005; Thomas 2006). Studies that have examined care in the more specific context of migration have mostly focused on the needs of orphaned children (Monasch et al. 2004), yet relatively little has been written about the care provided to returning sick migrants in the region. We do not therefore know much about the dynamics that facilitate the return of sick migrants home, how that decision is made or the resulting impact of the burden of care in the receiving household (Núñez et al. 2010; Collinson et al. 2007). Indeed, the role played by the household of origin in the provision of care to sick returning migrants remains largely invisible and unaccounted for. In making this burden visible, structural factors need to be considered, such as the economic strain placed on the household when the sick migrant, unable to work, becomes dependent on the household they used to support. In addition, there is a symbolic burden that is brought about by migrants who return at a late stage of an AIDS-related illness to their rural families in circumstances in which HIV is perceived as a 'bad' and stigmatised disease, and a consequence of indecent behaviour of rural migrants in the city, such as found in rural Tanzania by Dilger's ethnographic study (Dilger 2008).

CARE BACK HOME

The provision of care available to sick migrants by their families and communities in the sending areas is influenced by structural factors at the household level. These relate to the availability of material resources and human care work as well as by less tangible and subjective factors such as mutual obligations within families that materialise in networks of reciprocity and support. The availability of care for migrants in times of sickness is a reflection of the logic through which social networks are mobilised across disparate places. The greater or lesser capacity of migrants to mobilise and receive care when sick is an outcome of this relation of reciprocity. These relationships and their associated obligations to provide care, however, may be weakened by conditions of poverty, by time and distance and, on occasion, by migrants' own intended disconnection (Worby 2010). While questions about who in the migrant's social network responds to their needs of care and support in times of sickness relate to relationships built in a lifetime, it is, as previously mentioned, generally the case that women become the prime carers for the sick. Indeed, a study conducted by Núñez et al. (2010) on migrant's intentions to return home should they become ill, showed that the availability of women's care work in sending communities was pivotal in migrants' decisions to return home when they found themselves sick and unable to work.

The next section explores the predicaments of sick migrants in the city of Johannesburg and identifies a range of formal and informal agents providing end-of-life care to this population. It highlights the place of home as a symbolic and material resource that mobilises these agents around making the return home possible. Yet, as shown, returning home is far from unproblematic, and is often even resisted by migrants reluctant to come back home sick and poor.

END-OF-LIFE CARE FOR SICK MIGRANTS

Under South African migration law, the issue of a temporary entry permit requires the payment of deposit as a guarantee that a visa applicant will return to their home country.[4] This money is meant to pay a return trip to the country of origin in case of disability, terminal illness or death of the foreign migrant. Such a deposit is paid by the employer in the case of work-related visas or by migrants themselves in the case of any other type of temporary visa. In the case of undocumented migrants, there is no such provision – a situation that relates to a significant number of migrants and asylum-seekers in South Africa (Mthembu-Salter et al. 2014). Lack of documentation contributes to a migrant's general lack of social protection, yet that is not the only factor. The difficulties migrants encounter in accessing healthcare in South Africa have been widely reported and barriers identified are economic, legal, linguistic and cultural (Vearey and Núñez, 2010). Furthermore, attitudes of the host society towards migrants are also reflected in the quality of care provided to them. A Human Rights Watch Report, for example, describes how refugee women in South Africa 'experience specific abuses – such as active discrimination and delayed or denied care' (HRW 2011: 1). Limitations on access to healthcare have been considered a determinant of health outcomes (IOM 2013). In this case, the lack of access to healthcare in cases of acute and chronic illness may worsen their conditions and hasten death.

The situation in South Africa is characteristic of many countries in the Global South in which migration takes place in the absence of social security. Consequently migrants – as well as locals – often have to deal with their needs of care and protection without recourse to state support.

Yet, unlike with locals, migrants' families and networks of support are often weak, fragmented or simply absent, unable to provide the care needed. For migrants, home is often elsewhere, yet when they find themselves sick, and especially when their illness is HIV/AIDS-related, many may choose not to return home to be cared for due to the stigma associated with the disease. In other circumstances, returning home without money to be cared for goes against something very fundamental to the ethos of migrants – the dream of returning home with money as a proof of the success of the migratory endeavour (Lundl 2008). In such situations, where there is a lack of institutional responses to ensure migrants' wellbeing, hospices, religious and civil charitable organisations are often the only entities responding to migrants' needs for care and support.

CARERS FOR POOR AND DESTITUTE SICK MIGRANTS

Catholic hospices such as Nazareth House and Mother Teresa are both located in Yeoville, an area in Johannesburg with the highest concentration of foreign nationals. They assist by offering palliative care to the destitute, poor and terminally ill migrants affected by TB and by AIDS-related illnesses. The NGO 'Ministry to Zimbabwean Immigrants' (MZI) was, until 2012, coordinating the repatriation of terminally ill migrants to Zimbabwe and worked closely with these hospices to facilitate their return. When migrants approached MZI for assistance, they were sent to either Nazareth House or Mother Theresa to receive palliative care until their health condition was stabilised. Both hospices continue to offer palliative care to terminally ill migrants affected by HIV/AIDS-related illnesses to help them recover to a level at which they are able to undertake the journey back home.

As explained by the social worker of Nazareth House, the possibility that a terminally ill and destitute migrant encounters death while on their premises is especially problematic. Repatriating a body is expensive and several potential difficulties arise if the body is buried locally as a pauper burial. The social worker expressed her reluctance to proceed to bury somebody in the absence of their family members in case the family came back to demand the body of their deceased relative. In order to avoid this complication, they currently only accept migrants in the hospice who come accompanied by a relative who takes responsibility for them in case of death.

Organisations such as these are driven by the conviction that it is best for terminally ill migrants to return home while they are still alive.

However, as mentioned, the stigma associated with HIV/AIDS is often explained as a key factor affecting a migrant's decision not to return home sick. The social worker at the Nazareth house explained the following:

> Some of them [the terminally ill migrants], they run away from their homes, some of them don't want families to know about their status [HIV/AIDS], admit it. They hide, they will tell you they have no one, so if something happens, we face a challenge. To bury this person, what about if the family comes – they can sue us? We don't have anything to cover ourselves. And at the same time if we take [them] to [the] mortuary the body is accumulating [may not be claimed for a long time with the associated costs of keeping it at the mortuary], we are between. It is not easy either way.
>
> (Núñez and Wheeler 2012: 218)

A variety of other circumstances may also influence a migrant's reluctance to go back home. For undocumented migrants, the homeless, for those wishing to avoid the stigma of HIV or those who do not have families in their home country, South Africa may be seen as the only option, and one that may slip out of reach forever if they leave. As the social worker at Nazareth House affirms:

> Those who don't want to go home, they came from the streets, so they don't mind going back to the streets – they are used to that kind of life. They say, at least, if they go home they can't come back. That's the reason that they don't want to go back, coming back [to Johannesburg] is the problem. You find that most of those that want to go back, they have family.
>
> (Núñez and Wheeler 2012: 218)

As a rule, these hospices host migrants for up to three months. However, more often than not this rule is broken and migrants stay longer, until their papers and accommodation are resolved. It is also common for migrants to return more than once to the hospices, each time they are particularly adversely affected by HIV/AIDS-related illness. Discontinuation of antiretroviral (ARV) treatment is often the reason why migrants keep returning to the hospices to be cared for, due to lack of awareness of the need to continue using ARVs also in times where health is good or because of the stigma around HIV/AIDS. Yet, the problem for migrants goes beyond individual barriers. While South Africa has protective policies that ensure universal access to ARVs, in reality, migrants face additional challenges to access and to remain in treatment. These relate to their own mobility and lack of papers, but more often to the fact that implementation of their rights to access treatment is deficient, and healthcare practitioners have different interpretations of the law and rights that may further limit treatment access (Vearey 2012).

The MZI assisted terminally ill Zimbabweans migrants to return home until 2012. Mr Khumalo who was in charge of the programme explained that it was in 2008, at the height of the economic and political crises in Zimbabwe, when many people – including the sick – migrated to South Africa. Driven by desperation, many ill migrants crossed the border hoping they would be able to access the healthcare they could not access in their own country, challenging the accepted notion common in the literature on migration that those who undertake the migratory journey are the fittest and healthiest (Zimmerman et al. 2011). Sick and frail, these migrants stayed with relatives or in shelters such as the Methodist Church in central Johannesburg. During this period there was an increase in xenophobic violence against migrants in South Africa (HRW 2009). Both survival as well as access to healthcare in South Africa proved to be difficult and many of those who came in desperation decided to return without having secured an income, in turn finding themselves in even more deteriorated health conditions. The same year, statistics show a peak in the number of migrants' bodies being repatriated,[5] which is demonstrative of the challenges sick migrants confronted at the time. Khumalo recalls the MZI was inundated with requests from terminally ill Zimbabweans to be assisted to return home. They assisted in the repatriation of approximately 100 terminally ill migrants that year, both adults and children. Numbers decreased as the situation in Zimbabwe became less critical. At the time, the MZI was working with a medical doctor who could provide ambulatory care to migrants and certify the medically critical condition of the ill migrant. Negotiations with the household back home were sometimes necessary to obtain agreement on them receiving the sick migrant to make sure they were taken in and cared for. Khumalo recalled how they also used to meet with communities of migrants to raise awareness on the need for them not to wait too long, not to stay in South Africa until they were too ill. As Khumalo describes, they used to explain to them that in all likelihood they would end up being buried as paupers. He was concerned with raising awareness on the cost of repatriation, something that would entail their relatives back home having to sell the livestock to pay for their return. Khumalo was driven by the conviction that:

> It was easier and more economic to send the person back home when they were still alive and it also gave them a chance to get closure at home, some needed to sort relationships, some needed to sort other things, some even had families.
> (interview, Danisa Khumalo, May 2015)

MZI organised and paid for the return of ill migrants, and counted on the assistance of sympathetic Zimbabwean bus drivers who understood the importance of returning home and were able to handle practical matters, such as how to return a dying migrant lacking proper documentation. While currently this is less frequent, cross-border drivers still play a vital role in transporting sick migrants in their buses to return them home to Zimbabwe. They do this on condition that the sick passenger comes accompanied by somebody that is able to take responsibility for the welfare of the patient. During my research, drivers shared anecdotes of cases where they had to drive with a sick passenger to a nearby hospital or to cross the border with a dead passenger pretending he or she was still alive, to avoid the administrative responsibility associated with repatriating a dead body in front of the authorities and the consequent interruption or delaying of the journey (interview, bus drivers, August 2015).

Such cases illustrate that while a death and burial at home is widely considered the ideal, in reality this is not always possible. As the following section examines, how a death in a foreign country is managed relates in part to the motivations and concerns of those involved in dealing with it. Involvement in facilitating the return of a dead migrant is mobilised by communities that share a national or ethnic identity or by a sentiment of solidarity that exists among some migrant communities.

A MIGRANT'S DEATH IN A FOREIGN COUNTRY

A good death is one that occurs at home and if that not possible, it needs to culminate with the deceased being buried at home. In the literature from across sub-Saharan Africa (see, for example, Geschiere 2005; Núñez and Wheeler 2012), the village is commonly accepted as being the rightful place to die and be buried, reaffirming urban connections to the village, and providing an opportunity for the celebration of family ties. The death of a migrant outside of their country or community of origin is generally referred to as a death *out of place* (Núñez & Wheeler 2012). Dying away from home concerns many Africans, as the culture and tradition around funerals and burials is often not adequately followed in host countries. This is in part due to the absence of knowledge among younger migrants relating to funerary rituals that would, in the home country, be undertaken by the older generation. It is also in part due to locally contextualised differences in the management and disposition of dead bodies. South Africa's sociocultural and legal environment and urban regulations, for example, prevent the Congolese community from performing particular elements of traditional cultural practices around death (Kwigomba 2013). As Kwigomba's study demonstrates, the lack of a culturally appropriate funeral has considerable impacts on wellbeing, creating feelings of isolation and loss among the Congolese migrant community.

The notion of 'good' and 'bad' death therefore not only refers to the time of the death and the cause of death but also, in this context, to the place of death and final resting place of the deceased. A death out of place brings about a prolonged sense of loss among family members. There are crucial absences that perpetuate this sense of loss and lack of closure, such as the absence of a body and the absence of a burial site. In some instances, when the dead body is not brought to the family for burial, they maintain the expectation that the person is still alive and will come back. A burial far from the homeland also represents for families the impossibility to observe practices such as visitation of the grave and talking to the deceased for advice (interview, funeral parlour, July 2015).

Migrants have long understood that dying and being buried out of place might remain an unfinished business, particularly if it meant that the required rituals for the spirit of the deceased to rest in peace were not observed. In view of this existential concern, many migrants have responded by creating and joining burial societies. In South Africa, these organisations became popular in the mining compounds of the Rand from the late nineteenth century onwards and remain popular to this day. As described by Lee (2011), the fear of dying and being buried away from home was a shared concern among miners in the mining compounds

> The prospect of being separated from one's ancestral home even in death – and buried without traditional burial rites administered through appropriate social and kin networks – was a fearful one, and motivated African migrants on the mines to construct South Africa's first burial societies to prevent such an eventuality. These informal funeral-finance associations tended to emphasize processes of ethnic identification already at work in mining compounds, and aided in the transport of the deceased body and mourners back to the society's 'home' area.
>
> (Lee 2011: 228)

The increase of membership to burial societies as a consequence of the HIV epidemic in South Africa has been observed in recent years, among both local and foreign populations (Collins and Leibbrandt 2007). Burial societies of cross-border migrants have incorporated new methods of ensuring that their associates are able to secure the return of the body back home (Vearey et al. 2011). As explained by Mr Sibaya, representative of a burial societies association, the affiliation of cross-border migrants to burial societies often takes place according to nationality or even, more specifically, according to the towns and villages migrants come from. Similar 'politics of place' are applied by the African diaspora in Britain where hometown associations of Cameroonians and Tanzanians are organised around specific regions of their countries of origin (Mercer and Page 2010). The logic of this affiliation is to maximise the resources invested in the returning of bodies back home. Yet among some migrant communities, there is no practice of joining burial societies. Among Congolese migrants in South Africa, for example, the discussion of death is not usually deemed culturally acceptable among young people, hence in a situation where elders are absent, provisions for death are not made (Kwigomba 2013).

REPATRIATION FOR BURIAL

> Burials also reflect the complicated relationship between humans, land and belonging.
>
> (Núñez and Wheeler 2012)

As indicated earlier, the Gauteng Department of Health has in recent years, issued more than 30,000 permits to export the bodies of deceased migrants, mostly across the borders to nearby countries (Zimbabwe, Mozambique and Malawi). This figure not only reveals the extent of the unmet needs of end-of-life care for migrants but also gives an indication of the relevance of home as a place of burial for African migrants. Importantly, they give an indication of the efforts and resources mobilised by migrants' families, burial societies and funeral parlours in the management of deaths among cross-border migrants.

Funeral parlours play a key role in interventions to provide a 'proper' funeral and burial that includes, where possible, the returning of the body to the deceased's home. While this is not necessarily different from the needs of internal migrants returning to their own villages, the management of a migrant's death in a foreign land often entails an active process undertaken by a community that shares these concerns, pools resources and works to make repatriation a possibility (Núñez and Wheeler 2012).

Funeral parlours are key agents in the process of repatriation as they facilitate organisation at a community level and assist families with the fulfilment of certain governmental, bureaucratic necessities for burial in or repatriation from the country through the processing of a myriad of documents. In their capacity to obtain this documentation, funeral parlours act as mediators between the foreign migrant and the state. Their role is particularly relevant in the case of undocumented migrants who in life would have most likely tried to avoid the gaze of the South African state (Núñez and Wheeler 2012).

Interestingly, these funeral parlours have resulted in a predominantly male-led funeral industry that has to some extent, displaced women's central role in the ritual care and treatment of the deceased (Lee 2011). The parlours' role in lengthening the time between death and burial has become especially significant in managing the funeral of foreigners. The refrigeration system of modern mortuaries and the embalming techniques of funeral parlours have been the key technological innovations that have extended the time between death and burial. An average of three weeks between death and burial now allows the body to be transported home and for family members to reunite for the occasion. Similarly, embalming and keeping the body in a mortuary for an undefined period of time is a key function of the repatriating parlours. This lengthening of time is crucial in that it enables the family of the deceased to be contacted, enables disputes to be resolved, and provides time for decisions to be made on how and where to proceed with the funeral and burial and for resources to be put together, while the funeral parlour assists in gathering the necessary documentation (Núñez and Wheeler 2012).

Funeral parlours may also assist in preserving the diverse cultural and traditional practices related to a death and burial. A recognised funeral parlour in the repatriation industry in South Africa for example, was the late Massasanya, a pioneer in the repatriation business. Employing Zimbabwean drivers that had both a cultural understanding of the need for repatriation and knowledge of how to transport bodily remains outside the country enabled them to perform important acts of cultural mediation between the two states. Over the 35 years Massasanya was active in the repatriation business, he gained familiarity with several burial traditions in the region, such as the traditional Ndebele practice of 'talking to the body' as it is transported home, by which the body is encouraged to continue on this cross-border journey and not to remain behind. A younger funeral parlour, 'NK', now follows Massasanya's principles and seeks to assist in bridging gaps in cultural knowledge between young migrants who are in South Africa and elders back home (Núñez and Wheeler 2012).

CLOSING REMARKS

The lack of institutional support offered to sick migrants in the Global South has been illustrated by the case of terminally ill migrants in South Africa. Due to their general lack of social protection, lack of access to healthcare and to networks of care in the city, sick migrants may opt to return home to be cared for by family members, or simply to die at home. In the absence of alternatives, a painful and difficult journey back home is undertaken by many poor, terminally ill migrants. This chapter has focused on the informal networks of care that emerge in contexts characterised by a lack of formal social support as they witness the plight of sick migrants in the city. It has presented the role of a number of charitable organisations and impromptu agents in Johannesburg motivated by religious principles and by culturally shared notions of home as the best place to be cared for and to die. The chapter has also shown the concerted efforts of several other agents that intervene when a migrant dies far from home in making the return of deceased migrants to be buried at home possible. Yet this work has also argued that many of these deaths are premature, resulting from the lack of access to care and support of terminally ill migrants.

The literature stresses the lack of an integrated perspective and response around migration and health from a policy perspective, indicating that these are often partial and disconnected (Davies et al. 2011). Clear questions are raised, for example, around migrants' rights to access supposedly 'universal' healthcare treatments such as antiretroviral drugs. By focusing on end-of-life care and death, this chapter also extends these critiques by making a further argument towards the need to attend to migration in the returning phase of the process. Finally, in advocating for the need to provide compassionate end-of-life care to migrants, it is vital that more attention is given to understanding how issues relating to responsibility – from the level of the individual to the state – can be effectively examined and addressed.

NOTES

1. Unpublished data, Gauteng Department of Health, provided to the author, June 2015.
2. As has been observed, HIV/AIDS as cause of death is often underreported, and opportunistic infections associated to AIDS are consigned instead. Unpublished data, Gauteng Department of Health, provided to the author, June 2015.
3. Countries such as South Korea and the Gulf States impose forced HIV testing to migrants. If migrants in such countries are found to be HIV-positive, they are deported, regardless of the limited capacity to treat and manage their conditions in their home countries (Davies et al. 2011).
4. Immigration Regulations, 2005, www.dha.gov.za/files/Government_Notice_on_Repatriation_Refunds.pdf.
5. This estimate is based on the data on exported dead bodies available for Gauteng (January 1995–June 2015).

REFERENCES

Abraído-Lanza, A. F., B. P. Dohrenwend, D. S. Ng-Mak and J. B. Turner (1999), The Latino mortality paradox: a test of the 'salmon bias' and healthy migrant hypotheses, *American Journal of Public Health*, **89**(10), 1543–1548.

Andershed, B. (2006), Relatives in end-of-life care – part 1: a systematic review of the literature the five last years, January 1999–February 2004, *Journal of Clinical Nursing*, **15**, 1158–1169.
Buiting, H. M., J. A.C. Rietjens, B. D. Onwuteaka-Philipsen, P. J. van der Maas, J. J. van Delden and A. van der Heide (2008), A comparison of physicians' end-of-life decision making for non-western migrants and Dutch natives in the Netherlands, *The European Journal of Public Health*, **18**(6), 681–687.
Clark, S. J, M. A. Collinson, K. Kahn, K. Drullinger and S. M. Tollman (2007), Returning home to die: circular labour migration and mortality in South Africa, *Scandinavian Journal of Public Health*, **35**, 35–44.
Collins, D. L. and M. Leibbrandt (2007), The financial impact of HIV/AIDS on poor households in South Africa, *AIDS*, **21**(S7), S75–S81.
Collinson M. A, S. M. Tollman and K. Kahn (2007), Migration, settlement change and health in post-apartheid South Africa: triangulating Agincourt demographic surveillance with National Census data, *Scandinavian Journal of Public Health*, **35**, 77–84.
Davies, A. A., R. M. Borland, C. Blake and H. E. West (2011), The dynamics of health and return migration, *PLOS Medicine*, **8**(6).
Dilger, H. (2008), 'We are all going to die': kinship, belonging, and the morality of HIV/AIDS-related illnesses and deaths in rural Tanzania, *Anthropological Quarterly*, **81**(1), 207–232.
Evans, R. (2005), Social networks, migration, and care inTanzania, *Journal of Children and Poverty*, **11**(2), 111–129.
Gerritsen, A., P. Bocquier, M. White, C. Mbacké, N. Alam, D. Beguy, F. Odhiambo and M. A. Collinson (2013), Health and demographic surveillance systems: contributing to an understanding of the dynamics in migration and health, *Global Health Action*, **6**(10).
Geschiere, P. J. (2005), Funerals and belonging: different patterns in South Cameroon, *African Studies*, **48**(2), 45–64.
Gysels, M., C. Pell, L. Straus and R. Pool (2011), End of life care in Sub-Saharan Africa: a systematic review of the qualitative literature, *BMC Palliative Care*, **10**(6).
HRW (2009), *No Healing Here: Violence, Discrimination and Barriers to Health for Migrants in South Africa*, New York: Human Rights Watch.
HRW (2011), *'Stop Making Excuses': Accountability for Maternal Health Care in South Africa*, New York: Human Rights Watch.
IOM (2013a), *World Migration Report 2013*, London: International Organization for Migration.
IOM (2013b), *A Rapid Assessment of Access to Health Care at Selected One Stop Borderposts (OSBP) in East Africa*, London: International Organization for Migration.
Kwigomba, D. (2013), *Managing the Final Journey Home: Exploring Perceptions, Experiences and Responses to Death among Congolese Migrants in Johannesburg*, Master's thesis, University of the Witwatersrand.
Lee, R. (2011), 'Death on the move': funerals, entrepreneurs and the rural urban nexus in South Africa, *Africa*, **81**(2), 226–247.
Lundl, C. (2008), 'To skip a step': new representation(s) of migration, success and politics in Senegalese rap and theatre, *Wiener Zeitschrift für kritische Afrikastudien*, **14**(8), 97–122.
Mazzucato, V., M. Kabki and Smith, L. (2006), Transnational migration and the economy of funeral: changing practices in Ghana, *Development and Change*, **37**(5), 1047–1072.
Mercer, C. and B. Page (2010), African home associations in Britain: between political belonging and moral conviviality, *African Diaspora*, **3**, 111–131.
Monasch, R. and J. T. Boerma (2004), Orphanhood and childcare patterns in sub-Saharan Africa: an analysis of national surveys from 40 countries, *AIDS*, **18**, S55–S65.
Mthembu-Salter, G., R. Amit, C. Gould and L. B. Landau (2014), Counting the cost of securitising South Africa's immigration regime, *Migrating Out of Poverty*, Arts B, University of Sussex.
Núñez, L. and B. Wheeler (2012), Chronicles of death out of place: management of migrant death in Johannesburg, *African Studies*, **71**(2), 212–233.

Núñez, L., J. Vearey and S. Drimie (2011), Who cares? HIV-related sickness, urban–rural linkages, and the gendered role of care in return migration in South Africa, *Gender & Development*, **19**(1), 105–114.

Robson, E., N. Ansell, U. S. Huber, W. T. S. Gould and L. van Blerk (2006), Young caregivers in the context of the HIV/AIDS pandemic in sub-Saharan Africa, *Population, Space and Place*, **12**(2), 93–111.

Searight, H. R. and J. Gafford (2005), Cultural diversity at the end of life: issues and guidelines for family physicians, *American Family Physician*, **71**(3), 515–522.

Thomas, F. (2006), Stigma, fatigue and social breakdown: exploring the impacts of HIV/AIDS on patient and carer well-being in the Caprivi Region, Namibia, Social Science & Medicine, **63**(12), 3174–3187.

UNAIDS (2016), *Fact Sheet Global Statistics 2015*, available online at www.unaids.org/sites/default/files/media_asset/UNAIDS_FactSheet_en.pdf.

Upton, R. L. (2003), 'Women have no tribe': connecting carework, gender, and migration in an era of HIV/AIDS in Botswana, *Gender & Society*, **17**(2), 314–322.

Vearey, J. (2012), Learning from HIV, *Global Public Health: An International Journal for Research, Policy and Practice*, **7**(1).

Vearey, J. and L. Núñez (2010), *Migration and Health in South Africa: A Review of the Current Situation and Recommendations for Achieving the World Health Assembly Resolution on the Health of Migrants*, Pretoria: IOM Regional Office for Southern Africa.

Vearey, J., M. Richter, L. Núñez and K. Moyo (2011), South African HIV/AIDS programming overlooks migration, urban livelihoods, and informal workplaces, *African Journal of AIDS Research*, **10**(S), 381–391.

Welaga, P., R. Hosegood, V. Weiner, C. Hill, K. Herbst and M. L. Newell (2009), Coming home to die? The association between migration and mortality in rural South Africa, *BMC Public Health 2009*, **9**(193).

WHO (2014), *Global Atlas of Palliative Care*, Geneva: World Health Organization.

Worby, E. (2010). Address unknown: the temporality of displacement and the ethics of disconnection among Zimbabwean migrants in Johannesburg, *Journal of Southern African Studies*, **36**(2), 417–431.

Zimmerman, C., L. Kiss and M. Hossain (2011), Migration and health: a framework for 21st century policy-making, *PLOS Medicine*, **8**(5).

Index